INTERNATIONAL INCIDENCE
OF CHILDHOOD CANCER

INTERNATIONAL AGENCY FOR RESEARCH ON CANCER

The International Agency for Research on Cancer (IARC) was established in 1965 by the World Health Assembly, as an independently financed organization within the framework of the World Health Organization. The headquarters of the Agency are at Lyon, France.

The Agency conducts a programme of research concentrating particularly on the epidemiology of cancer and the study of potential carcinogens in the human environment. Its field studies are supplemented by biological and chemical research carried out in the Agency's laboratories in Lyon and, through collaborative research agreements, in national research institutions in many countries. The Agency also conducts a programme for the education and training of personnel for cancer research.

The publications of the Agency are intended to contribute to the dissemination of authoritative information on different aspects of cancer research. A complete list is printed at the end of this book.

WORLD HEALTH ORGANIZATION

INTERNATIONAL AGENCY FOR RESEARCH ON CANCER

INTERNATIONAL INCIDENCE OF CHILDHOOD CANCER

EDITORS

D.M. PARKIN, C.A. STILLER, G.J. DRAPER, C.A. BIEBER,
B. TERRACINI AND J.L. YOUNG

IARC Scientific Publications No. 87

INTERNATIONAL AGENCY FOR RESEARCH ON CANCER

LYON   1988

Published by the International Agency for Research on Cancer,
150 cours Albert-Thomas, 69372 Lyon Cedex 08, France

Distributed by Oxford University Press, Walton Street, Oxford OX2 6DP, UK

Distributed in the USA by Oxford University Press, New York

ISBN 92 832 1187 1
ISSN 0300-5085

Printed in the United Kingdom

CONTENTS

CONTENTS

FOREWORD

The International Agency for Research on Cancer has for many years brought together data from cancer registries around the world in the series of volumes *Cancer Incidence in Five Continents*. These have served to point out the large geographic variations in the incidence of different cancers, variations linked, in the main, to the different environmental exposures of the inhabitants of the regions concerned. In the causation of many cancers of childhood, it is clear that exogenous factors play a relatively small part, and it may be that inheritance of a genetic predisposition to cancer, and spontaneous mutations of genes controlling cellular multiplication at a time of rapid cellular division have a more important role. The study of geographical and ethnic variation in the risk of childhood cancer is of great value in formulating hypotheses concerning the relative contribution of genetic susceptibility and environmental exposure to etiology.

This volume is the most extensive collection of data on the incidence of cancer in childhood that has ever been published. The comparisons of incidence presented in it are based on a classification reflecting the cells of origin of the neoplasms, rather than on the anatomical location of the resulting tumour. Since genetic alterations leading to cancerous proliferation are likely to affect these dividing cell lines, it is appropriate to base comparisons of risk on this classification, rather than on the anatomical location of the resulting tumour.

The editors of this volume are to be congratulated on the compilation and presentation of the data in this volume in a format such that appropriate comparisons can readily be made. The result is a considerable tribute to the collaborating research workers in over 50 countries of the world, who have agreed to make available for this international study results collected over many years. It is to be hoped that it will be possible to build on this collaboration in the future, to study the evolution of the geographical and ethnic variations in incidence which have been demonstrated.

Lorenzo Tomatis, M.D.

ACKNOWLEDGEMENTS

The editors would like to acknowledge the work of the following technical staff of IARC: Mr Patrick Maisonneuve, Mr Andrew Guljas and Mr Peter Ziegler. We are also greatly indebted to Mlle Odile Bouvy, who was responsible for co-ordinating the flow of data and correspondence and for managing the preparation of the manuscript, and to Miss Susan Medhurst of the Childhood Cancer Research Group for carrying out the administrative and secretarial work at Oxford.

We are grateful to Dr Elizabeth Lennox and Dr Bridget Caplan, who were responsible for coding the data from many of the centres.

The work of the Childhood Cancer Research Group was supported by the United Kingdom Department of Health and Social Security and Scottish Home and Health Department.

LIST OF CONTRIBUTORS
(PRINCIPAL INVESTIGATORS)

AFRICA

Madagascar
Dr P. Coulanges
Directeur de l'Institut Pasteur
Laboratoire d'Anatomie Pathologique
BP 1274
Tananarive

Malawi
Professor M.S.R. Hutt
Gwernvale Cottage
Brecon Road
Crickhowell
Powys NP8 1SE
United Kingdom

Morocco
Professor F. Msefer Alaoui
Service de Pédiatrie II
Hôpital d'Enfants
Rabat

Nigeria
Professor T.A. Junaid
Ibadan Cancer Registry
Department of Pathology
University College Hospital
Ibadan

Sudan
Dr A. Hidayatalla
Radiation and Isotope Centre
PO Box 677
Khartoum

Tanzania
Professor J. Shaba
Department of Pathology
Muhimbili Medical Centre
University of Dar es Salaam
Faculty of Medicine
Dar es Salaam

Tunisia
Dr N. Mourali
Director
Institut Salah Azaiz
Boulevard du 9 Avril
Bab Saadoun
Tunis

Uganda, Kampala
Professor R. Owor
Cancer Registry
Department of Pathology
Makerere University Medical School
PO Box 7072
Kampala

Uganda, West Nile
Dr E.H. Williams
45 Northcourt Avenue
Reading, Berks RG2 7HE
United Kingdom

Zimbabwe
Dr Molly E.G. Skinner
Radiotherapist
c/o Miss M. Hodges
21 Farm Close Road
Wheatley
Oxford OX9 1XD
United Kingdom

NORTH AMERICA

Canada (Atlantic Provinces)
Mrs Dorothy Robb
Department of Health
New Brunswick Provincial Tumour Registry
Saint John Regional Hospital
PO Box 2100
Saint John, New Brunswick
E2L 4L2

CONTRIBUTORS

Ms Thelma Croucher
Head, Health Records
Cancer Treatment and Research
Foundation of Nova Scotia
Halifax Clinic
5820 University Avenue
Halifax, Nova Scotia
B3H 1V7

Dr D.E. Dryer
Provincial Oncologist
Division of Cancer Control
Dept. of Health and Social Services
PO Box 2000
Charlottetown, PEI
C1A 7N8

Dr Sharon K. Buehler
Director
Provincial Tumour Registry
The Newfoundland Cancer Treatment
and Research Foundation
Prince Philip Drive
St John's, Newfoundland
A1B 3V6

Canada (Western Provinces)
Ms Mary McBride
British Columbia Cancer Registry
Cancer Control Agency of British Columbia
600 West 10th Avenue
Vancouver, British Columbia, V5Z 4E6

Dr G.B. Hill
Director
Alberta Cancer Board
Alberta Cancer Registry
Department of Epidemiology
& Preventive Medicine
11560 University Avenue
Edmonton, Alberta T6G 1Z2

Ms Diane Robson
Director of Data Services
Saskatchewan Cancer Foundation
2631 - 28th Avenue — Suite 400
Regina, Saskatchewan, S4S 6X3

Dr N.W. Choi
Director, Epidemiology and Biostatistics
Manitoba Cancer Treatment and Research
Foundation
100 Olivia Street
Winnipeg, Manitoba
R3E OV9

USA (Greater Delaware Valley)
Dr Greta R. Bunin
Children's Cancer Research Center
The Children's Hospital of Philadelphia
34th Street & Civic Center Boulevard
Philadelphia, PA 19104

USA (Los Angeles County)
Mr H.R. Menck
Los Angeles County
Cancer Surveillance Program
PMB-B105
USC School of Medicine
2025 Zonal Avenue
Los Angeles, CA 90033

USA (New York)
Dr W. S. Burnett
Director
Cancer Registry, State of New York
Department of Health,
Office of Public Health
The Governor Nelson A. Rockefeller
Empire State Plaza, Room 565
Albany, NY 12237

USA (SEER Program)
Dr D.F. Austin
Cancer Prevention Section
California Tumor Registry
Department of Health Services
5850 Shellmound Street, Suite 200
Emeryville, CA 94608

Dr J.T. Flannery
Cancer Registry
Chronic Disease Control Section
Connecticut State Department of Health
79 Elm Street
Hartford, CT 06115

Dr R.S. Greenberg
Atlanta Cancer Surveillance Center
Decatur
246 Sycamore Street, Suite 100
Atlanta, GA 30030

Dr P. Isaacson/Dr C. Platz
State Health Registry of Iowa
The University of Iowa
S.100 Westlawn
Iowa City, IA 52242

CONTRIBUTORS

Dr C.R. Key
New Mexico Tumor Registry
University of New Mexico
Medical Center
900 Camino de Salud NE
Albuquerque, NM 87131

Dr L.N. Kolonel
Hawaii Tumor Registry Cancer
Center of Hawaii
Epidemiology Research 1236
Lauhala Street, Room 402
Honolulu, HI 96813

Dr G. Marie Swanson
Metropolitan Detroit Cancer
Surveillance System
Division of Epidemiology
Michigan Cancer Foundation
110 East Warren Avenue
Detroit, MI 48201

Dr D.B. Thomas
Cancer Surveillance System
The Fred Hutchinson Cancer Research Center
1124 Columbia Street
Seattle, WA 98104

Dr D. West
Utah Cancer Registry
420 Chipeta Way, Suite 190
Salt Lake City, UT 84108

Dr J.L. Young
Chief, Demographic Analysis Section
Division of Cancer Prevention and Control
National Institutes of Health
National Cancer Institute
532B Blair Building
Bethesda, MD 20205

CENTRAL AND SOUTH AMERICA AND CARIBBEAN

Brazil (Fortaleza-Ceara)
Dr M. Gurgel Carlos da Silva
Registro de Cancer do Ceará
Rua Papi Junior, 1222
Bairro Rodolfo Teofilo
60000 Fortaleza-Ceará

Brazil (Recife-Pernambuco)
Dr M. Ricardo da Costa Carvalho
Registro de Cancer de Pernambuco
Faculdade de Medicina de Pernambuco
Departamento de Patologia
Cidade Universitaria
Recife-Pernambuco

Brazil (São Paulo)
Dr A. P. Mirra
Coordinator,
Registro de Cancer de São Paulo
Avenida Dr Arnaldo 715-1° Andar
01255 São Paulo

Colombia
Dr C. Cuello
Registro de Cancer de Cali
Department of Pathology
School of Medicine
University of Valle
Cali

Costa Rica
Dra Georgina Muñoz Leiva
Chief of Section
National Cancer Registry
Statistics Department
PO Box 745
Ministerio de Salud
San José

Dra Rafaela Sierra
Escuela de Biologia
Universidad de Costa Rica
Ciudad Universitaria
Rodrigo Facio
San José

Cuba
Dra Magali Caraballoso
Registro Nacional de Cancer
Instituto Nacional de Oncologia y Radiobiologia
29 y F Vedado
Habana

Jamaica
Dr B. Hanchard
Department of Pathology
University of the West Indies
Mona, Kingston 7

CONTRIBUTORS

Puerto Rico
Dr I. Martinez
Cancer Control Program
Department of Health
PO Box 9342
Santurce, PR 00908

ASIA

Bangladesh
Professor M.A. Rahim
Director, Cancer Epidemiology
   Research Project
Khan Mansion
21-Nawab Katra
Dhacca 2

China (Shanghai)
Dr Gao Yu Tang
Director
Shanghai Cancer Institute
2200 Xie Tu Road
Shanghai 200032

China (Taipei)
Dr Kuang Y. Chen
Cancer Registry
Cancer Therapy Center
Veterans General Hospital
Taipei
Taiwan, 11217

Hong Kong
Dr Y.F. Poon
Radiotherapy and Oncology Division
MHD Institute of Radiology and Oncology
Hong Kong Government
Queen Elizabeth Hospital
Wylie Road
Kowloon

India (Bangalore)
Dr M. Krishna Bhargava
Director
Kidwai Memorial Institute of Oncology
Hosur Road
Bangalore 560-029
Karnataka

India (Bombay)
Dr D.J. Jussawalla
Bombay Cancer Registry
Indian Cancer Society
74 Jerbai Wadia Road
Parel
Bombay- 400 012

India (Bombay, Tata Memorial Centre)
Dr P.B. Desai
Director and Chief of Surgery
Tata Memorial Centre
Dr Ernest Borges Marg
Parel, Bombay 400 012

Indonesia
Dr Soeripto
Department of Pathology
Medical Faculty, Gadjah Mada University
Yogyakarta

Iraq
Dr Asia Al-Fouadi
Central Public Health Laboratory
PO Box 862, Alwyia
Baghdad

Israel
Dr Leah Katz
Israel Cancer Registry
Israel Center for Registration
   of Cancer and Allied Diseases
20 King David Street
Jerusalem 91000

Japan (Kanagawa)
Dr R. Inoue
Department of Field Survey
Center for Adult Diseases of Kanagawa
54-2 Nakao, Asahi-ku
Yokohama

Japan (Miyagi)
Dr Yoshi Okuno
Miyagi Prefectural Cancer Registry
c/o Miyagi Cancer Society
Kamisugi 6-chome
Sendai 980

Japan (Osaka)
Ms Aya Hanai
Osaka Cancer Registry
Center for Adult Diseases
Higashinari-ku
Osaka 537

Kuwait
Dr Y.T. Omar
Director
Kuwait Cancer Control Centre
PO Box 42262
Shuwaikh
Kuwait

CONTRIBUTORS

Pakistan
Professor N.A. Jafarey
Department of Pathology
Jinnah Postgraduate Medical Centre
Karachi 35

Philippines
Dr T.P. Maramba
Central Tumor Registry
  of the Philippines
Philippine Cancer Society
PO Box 3066
310 San Rafael
Manila 2800

Dr A.V. Laudico
University of the Philippines
College of Medicine
Philippine General Hospital
Department of Surgery
Taft Avenue
Metro Manila D-2801

Singapore
Dr Lee Hin Peng
c/o Department of Pathology
National University Hospital
Lower Kent Ridge Road
Singapore 0511

Thailand
Ms Sineenat Sontipong
Chief, Planning and Statistics Division
National Cancer Institute
Rama VI Road
Bangkok 10400

Viet Nam
Dr Luong Tan Truong
Institut du Cancer
3 No Trang Long
Binh-Thanh
Ho Chi Minh City

EUROPE

Czechoslovakia
Dr I. Plesko
Cancer Research Institute
Slovak Academy of Sciences
Department of Pathology
Ul Csl. armady 21
812 32 Bratislava

Denmark
Dr Anne Prener
Danish Cancer Registry
Institute for Cancer Epidemiology
Landskronagade 66
2100 Copenhagen Ø

Finland
Dr L. Teppo
Finnish Cancer Registry
Liisankatu 21B
00170 Helsinki 17

France (Bas-Rhin)
Dr P. Schaffer
Registre Bas-Rhinois des Cancers
Faculté de Médecine
67085 Strasbourg Cédex

France (Lorraine)
Dr Marie-Chantal L'Huillier
Registre des Cancers de l'Enfant en Lorraine
Service de Pédiatrie II
Hôpital d'Enfants
Allée du Morvan
54511 Vandoeuvre Cedex

France (Provence-Alpes-Côte d'Azur and Corse)
Dr J.L. Bernard
Registre des Cancers de l'Enfant
Faculté de Médecine
27, Boulevard Jean Moulin
13385 Marseille Cedex 5

German Democratic Republic
Dr W. Staneczek
Nationales Krebsregister und Krebsstatistik
Academy of Sciences of the GDR
Sterndamm 13
1197 Berlin-Johannisthal

Germany, Federal Republic of
Professor J.H. Michaelis
Universität Mainz
Institut für Medizinische Statistik
  und Dokumentation
Postfach 3960
6500 Mainz

Germany, Federal Republic of (Saarland)
Mr H. Ziegler
Wirtschaftsdirektor
Statistisches Amt des Saarlandes
Postfach 409
6600 Saarbrücken 1

CONTRIBUTORS

Hungary
Dr T. Révész
Department of Paediatrics No II
Semmelweis University Medical School
Tüozoltó utca 7-9
1X Budapest

Italy
Dr G. Pastore
Registro dei Tumori Infantili
  della Provincia di Torino
Cattedra di Epidemiologia dei Tumori
Via Santena 7
10126 Torino

The Netherlands
Dr J.W.W. Coebergh
Dutch Childhood Leukaemia
  Study Group (DCLSG)
PO Box 60604
2506 LP The Hague

and

IKZ/SOOZ Cancer Registry
Europalaan 6a
5623 JL Eindhoven

Norway
Dr Froydis Langmark
Cancer Registry of Norway
Norwegian Radium Hospital
Montebello
Oslo 3

Poland
Professor Helena Gadomska
Professor of Oncology
Head of the Polish Cancer Registry
Cancer Centre of the Maria Sklodowska-Curie
  Institute
Wawelska 15, 02-034 Warsaw

Spain
Dr R. Peris-Bonet
Registro Nacional de Tumores Infantiles
Centro de Documentacion e Informatica
  Biomedica
Facultad de Medicina
Avenida de V. Bl. Ibáñez, no 17
46010 Valencia

Spain (Zaragoza)
Dr A. Zubiri
Registro del Cancer de Zaragoza
Calle Ramon y Cajal 68
Zaragoza 50004

Sweden
Dr T. Gunnarsson
Swedish Cancer Registry
The National Board of Health and Welfare
106 30 Stockholm

Switzerland
Dr F. Levi
Registre Vaudois de Tumeurs
CHUV BH 06
1011 Lausanne

Dr L. Raymond
Registre Genevois des Tumeurs
55 bld de la Cluse
1205 Genève

Dr Suzanne Pellaux
Registre Neuchâtelois des Tumeurs
Les Cadolles
2000 Neuchâtel

*United Kingdom (England and Wales,
and Scotland)*
Dr G.J. Draper
University of Oxford
Department of Paediatrics
Childhood Cancer Research Group
Radcliffe Infirmary
Oxford OX2 6HE

United Kingdom (Manchester)
Dr Jillian M. Birch
University of Manchester
Department of Epidemiology and Social
  Research
Christie Hospital and Holt Radium Institute
Manchester M20 9BX

Yugoslavia
Dr Vera Pompe-Kirn
Cancer Registry of Slovenia
Institute of Oncology
Zaloska 2, p.p. 17
61105 Ljubljana

OCEANIA

Australia (New South Wales)

Dr Joyce M. Ford
NSW Central Cancer Registry
Department of Health
PO Box 380
North Ryde, NSW 2113

CONTRIBUTORS

Australia (Queensland)
Dr W. McWhirter
University of Queensland
Department of Child Health
Royal Children's Hospital
Brisbane, Queensland 4029

Fiji
Dr L.M. Seruvatu
Consultant Government Pathologist
Ministry of Health
Government Buildings
Suva

New Zealand
Dr J. Fraser
Deputy Chief Health Statistician
Department of Health
National Health Statistics Centre
Private Bag 2
Upper Willis Street
Wellington

Papua New Guinea
Dr K. Jamrozik
The University of Western Australia
Department of Medicine
M. Block
Queen Elizabeth II
Medical Centre
Nedlands, Western Australia 6009
Australia

MAPS

Showing locations of areas covered by cancer registries from which data are presented in this volume.

Population-based registries are identified in red, non-population-based in blue.

1. AFRICA

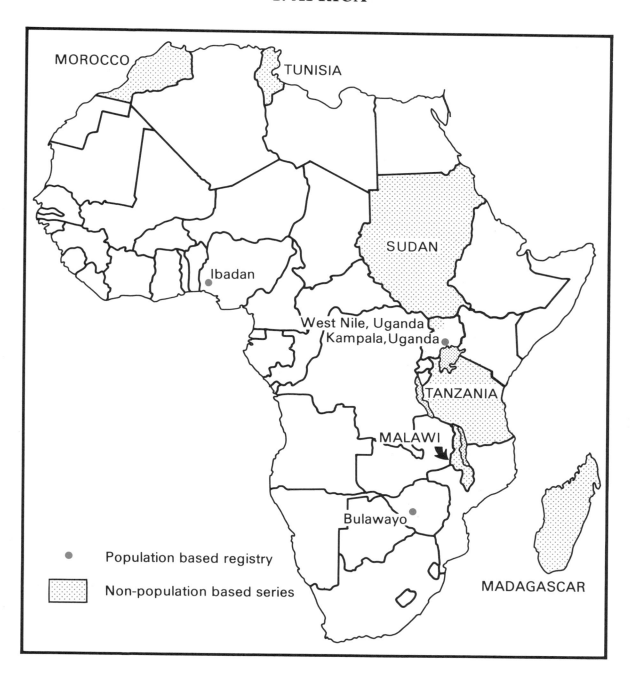

2. NORTH AMERICA

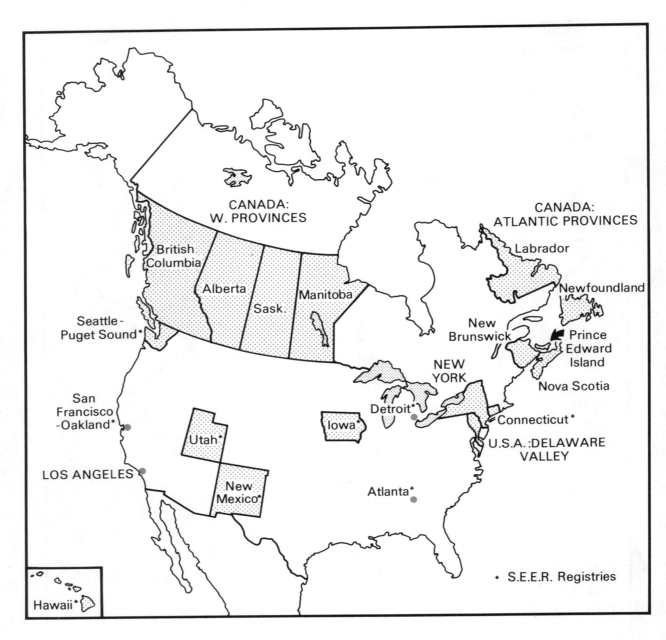

3. CENTRAL AND SOUTH AMERICA

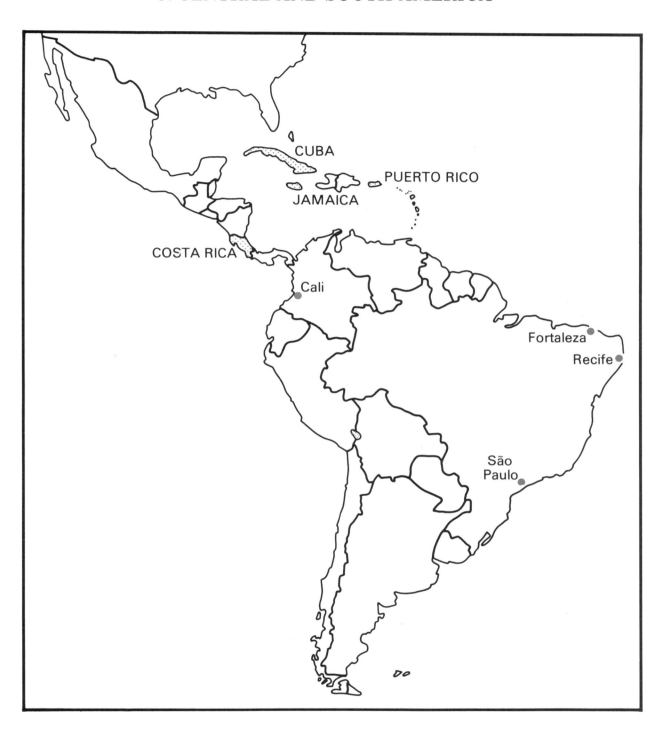

4. ASIA

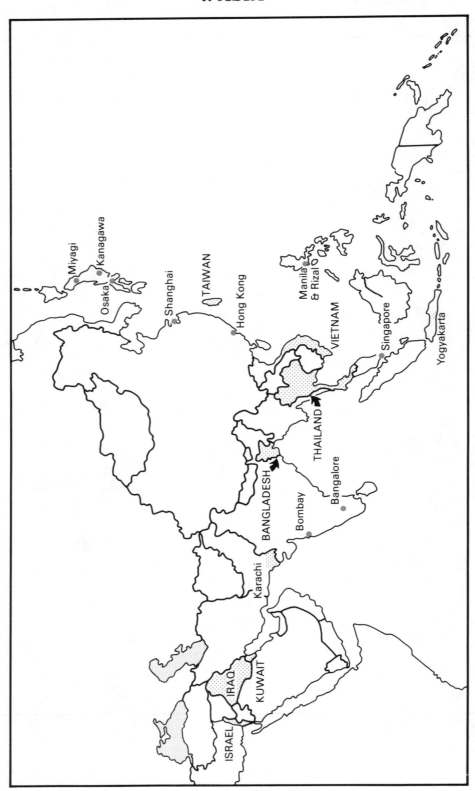

5. EUROPE

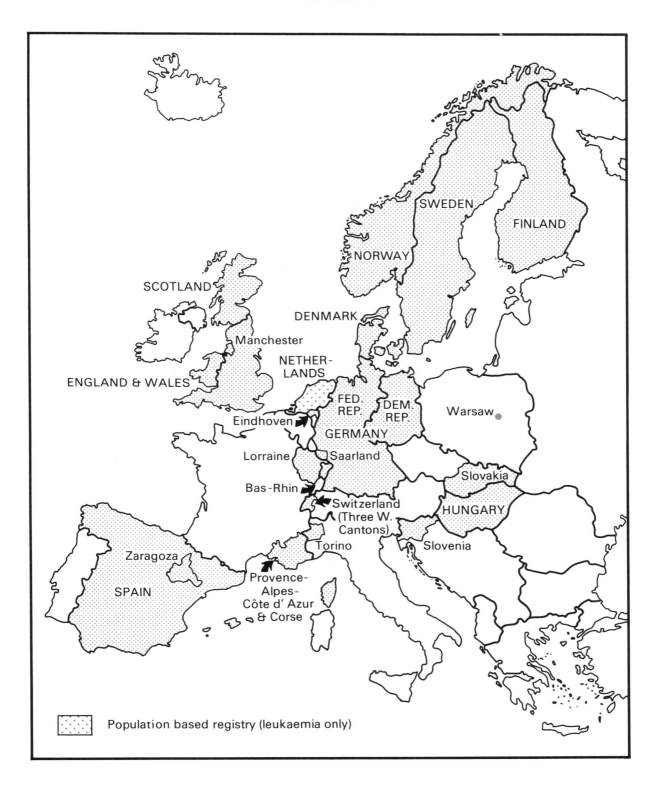

Population based registry (leukaemia only)

6. OCEANIA

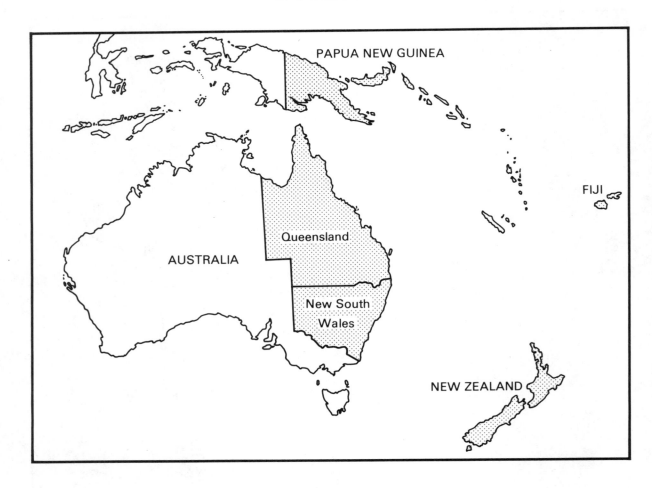

1. INTRODUCTION

The Editors

The term 'geographical epidemiology' is sometimes applied to studies of variations in disease frequency according to place of residence. In general terms, such variations may be ascribed to genetic factors (innate characteristics of the inhabitants of a particular place), or to factors in the environment, whether physical or social. Situations in which populations of (presumed) genetic similarity live in different geographical locations are thus particularly suitable for assessing the likely contributions of these two factors. This volume brings together data on the incidence of cancer in children from some 50 countries, grouped into six continents (Africa, North America, Central and South America and the Caribbean, Asia, Europe and Oceania). Where the populations concerned are of mixed racial composition, separate analyses have been carried out for the major ethnic groups concerned.

Many childhood cancers are more or less confined to this period of life, affecting cells which are actively dividing during early development. Several lines of evidence suggest a strong genetic component for these tumours. In addition, in areas of particularly high incidence, certain epithelial tumours of adults may appear in the childhood age-range (e.g., nasopharyngeal carcinoma, liver carcinoma), whereas others, including the major tumours of adults (stomach carcinoma, breast carcinoma), are exceedingly rare.

Within the last 15 years there have been several attempts to systematically review geographical and ethnic variations in the incidence of childhood tumours. The most comprehensive was that coordinated by the International Union Against Cancer (UICC) between 1971 and 1972, when data from some 60 centres around the world were collected (Miller, 1974). Although the results of this study have never been published in full, certain of the findings have been widely cited in Chapter 2 of this volume. Subsequently, Munoz (1976) analysed the data contained in *Cancer Incidence in Five Continents*, Vol. II, for the age-range 0–14 years, and Breslow and Langholz (1983) carried out a similar but more extensive analysis using the data from volumes I–IV, as well as that from the Surveillance, Epidemiology and End Results (SEER) Program in the USA. Finally, West (1984) attempted to use the WHO mortality data bank to study international variations in mortality rates. None of these studies is entirely satisfactory, for the following reasons:

1. Many centres, or cancer registries, have a population base too small to allow the recruitment of sufficient cases for the calculation of reliable incidence rates. Childhood cancers in general comprise only ½ to 3% of all neoplasms, depending on the age-structure of the population concerned.

2. The neoplasms chapter of the *International Classification of Diseases* (ICD), used in previous studies, is unsuited to the study of childhood cancer. In this age group, tumours are for the most part defined by their histology, rather than by their anatomical site, which forms the main axis of classification of the ICD.

3. Mortality rates suffer from all the defects of statistics based on death certificates. Furthermore, as a result of progress in treatment in recent years, the survival rate for several childhood cancers has greatly increased (see, e.g., Miller & McKay, 1984). Comparison of mortality rates is complicated by probable differences in survival between different geographical locations.

The decision to undertake an international study of the incidence of childhood cancer was the result of a meeting of investigators with a special interest in paediatric cancer, which took place during the International Union Against Cancer (UICC) conference in Seattle in 1982. The following year, a smaller working group met at the International Agency for Research on Cancer (IARC) in Lyon to consider the recommendations of the Seattle meeting, and to draft a study plan.

The methodology finally employed is described in Chapter 4. It involved requesting the collaboration of investigators throughout the world who were known to have data available on the incidence of childhood cancer, either via a specialized paediatric tumour registry, or through the medium of a general population-based cancer registry. In both cases, the participants were required to have a data base large enough to furnish an (arbitrary) minimum of 200 cases of cancer in the age group 0–14.

It is a tribute to the generosity and spirit of collaboration of researchers in this field that all but one of those approached agreed to participate in the study. The collaborating centres, with the name and address of the principal investigators, are listed on pages ix–xv, and their geographical location shown on the maps on pages xvi–xxii. A policy decision was taken at an early stage to include, mainly from developing countries, certain data sets which were not from population-based registries. For those case series, only the relative frequency of different tumour types can be calculated. However, it was considered preferable to provide data such as these rather than to confine the analysis to incidence rates, which would have greatly restricted geographical coverage of Africa and, to a lesser extent, Asia and Oceania.

Most of the data were collected in 1984-1985, and the variety of formats and classifications led to a lengthy period of analysis (Chapter 4). The adaptations of the coding system of the Manchester Children's Tumour Registry for international use (described by Marsden in Chapter 3), and the conversion of the data sets received into the categories finally chosen, were particularly time-consuming.

This volume is a tribute to the efforts of scientists and staff in cancer registries throughout the world, and to their generosity of spirit in providing the results of their labours, reviewing and revising the case listings and tables returned to them, and agreeing to the inclusion of an appraisal of their results in a Commentary accompanying the tables in this volume. The editors hope that the users of the data in this volume will feel able to cite the names of these contributors, whenever it is possible to do so.

References

Breslow, N.E. & Langholz, B. (1983) Childhood cancer incidence: geographic and temporal variations. *Int. J. Cancer*, *32*, 703-716

Miller, R.W. (1974) Childhood cancer epidemiology: two international activities. *Natl Cancer Inst. Monogr.*, *40*, 71-74

Miller, R.W. & McKay, F.W. (1984) Decline in US childhood cancer mortality. *J. Am. med. Assoc.*, *251*, 1567-1570

Muñoz, N. (1976) Geographical distribution of childhood tumours. *Tumori*, *62*, 145-156

West, R. (1984) Childhood cancer mortality: international comparisons 1955-74. *World Health Stat. Q.*, *37*, 98-127

2. GEOGRAPHICAL AND ETHNIC DIFFERENCES IN THE OCCURRENCE OF CHILDHOOD CANCER

Robert W. Miller

The first description of African lymphoma by Burkitt in 1958 is a classic of epidemiological research, which outshines all other findings concerning peculiarities in the occurrence of childhood cancer. Many interesting observations, however, have been made before and since, and a review of them will indicate the resources needed for detecting geographical and ethnic clustering in the future. Such studies can bring new understanding of cancer etiology and pathogenesis.

2.1 LEUKAEMIA

Mortality from leukaemia used to be a good measure of its incidence because survival was so short. Court Brown and Doll (1961) found that a peak in mortality from acute lymphocytic leukaemia (ALL) at 2-3 years of age emerged in England and Wales in 1920-1930, in the USA among Whites about 15 years later, and not at all in Blacks or Japanese. Later, in the 1960s, a peak began to emerge among Japanese. It is not known why these international differences occurred or why Blacks have not developed the peak. Presumably they are inherently resistant to whatever is the cause in other ethnic groups. (The peak, now at four years of age in the aforementioned groups, occurs at one year of age in Down's syndrome (Miller, 1970; Lashof & Stewart, 1965). Thus, these children develop leukaemia not only more often, but also earlier than usual.) Now that therapy has improved survival so dramatically, death-certificate data can no longer reveal changes in occurrence over time, and data from cancer registries must be used instead.

A peculiar cluster of acute monomyelogenous leukaemia (AMML) in Ankara, Turkey, was reported by Cavdar et al. in 1971. Chloroma of the eye was a common feature. The frequency of all forms of childhood leukaemia in Ankara was similar to that elsewhere in Europe and the USA, but the proportion due to AMML, 34%, was far above the usual 4%. The excess is at the expense of acute myelocytic leukaemia (AML), which accounted for only 4% of the cases. The reason for this shift in cell type was not revealed by cytogenetic, immunological or virological studies (Cavdar et al., 1978). AMML is also the only form of leukaemia for which patients with Fanconi's anaemia are at high risk (O'Gorman Hughes, 1974), and is the commonest form of leukaemia induced by alkylating agents used as treatment for cancer (Greene, 1985). Thus, clusters of AMML have been geographical, genetic, or drug-induced. Apparently, development of this form of leukaemia has something to do with alteration in host response.

2.2 LYMPHOMA

A surgeon's observation that a previously undescribed form of lymphoma occurred in clusters in tropical Africa provided a powerful stimulus to research in cancer epidemiology and virology. Other forms of lymphoma show peculiarities in geographical distribution. Hodgkin's disease had two age-peaks in all but one country studied by MacMahon in 1966. The exception was Japan, where cases early in life are rare, and the first age-peak is absent. This scarcity has also been observed among Japanese migrants to Hawaii (Nanba, personal communication), so that an inherent resistance appears to be responsible.

The distribution of Hodgkin's disease by subtype varies geographically; the more aggressive forms predominate in underdeveloped countries (Motawy & Omar, 1986). Subtypes of non-Hodgkin's lymphoma (NHL) have many geographical and ethnic dissimilarities (Magrath et al., 1984). For example, B-cell lymphomas are less frequent in Japan than in Western countries (Kadin et al., 1983). Japanese also have a seemingly reciprocal excess of certain autoimmune disorders; e.g., systemic lupus erythematosus, Hashimoto's thyroiditis and Takayasu's aortitis (Miller et al., 1981). As compared with Whites, Japanese appear to be protected against B-cell lymphomas, but predisposed to autoimmune disease.

Persons at high risk of lymphomas characteristically have immunosuppression, which may be inborn, as in Wiskott-Aldrich syndrome, ataxia-telangiectasia or the X-linked lymphoproliferative syndrome, or acquired, e.g., following the administration of drugs to organ-transplant patients, or infection with a virus, such as human immunodeficiency virus (HIV). Geographical clusters of lymphoma can be expected wherever severe immunosuppression occurs due to viruses, chemicals or inheritance.

2.3 THE UICC STUDY

With the discovery of Burkitt's lymphoma in mind, a simple survey was made to determine whether other forms of cancer had unusual frequencies elsewhere in the world. In the study, organized by Miller and Davies in 1971 under the auspices of the Union Internationale Contre le Cancer, information was sought on consecutive cases of cancer in patients under 15 years of age seen at medical centres in various parts of the world in recent years. The basic information consisted of age at diagnosis, sex, race and diagnosis by site and histological type. A few centres added information on co-existent congenital malformations and familial cancers. A total of 62 centres contributed information at their own expense. The number of children in individual series ranged from 32 to 3308 and the combined total was 37 374. At the National Cancer Institute in Bethesda, the data from each source were put into a standard format and compared with those from the population-based Manchester (England) registry. The contributors received tabulations of their own data, with an indication of the ways in which they differed from the Manchester series; they were encouraged to publish the results, and a few did so. When looked at in the aggregate, several peculiarities in occurrence stood out (Miller, 1977), and attention is drawn to these in subsequent subsections.

2.4 NEUROBLASTOMA

The biggest surprise from the UICC study was the finding of a near absence of neuroblastoma in Tanzania, 1959–1966, and the countries covered by the Kenya Regional Cancer Registry, 1968–1969. Rates could not be calculated, so a comparison was made with data from Manchester through the use of a ratio of neuroblastoma to Wilms' tumour. In Manchester the ratio was 1.35, whereas the lowest frequency in Africa gave a ratio of 0.09. In Uganda, Ibadan and the Dakar Regional Registry, the ratios were 0.25–0.45. In other parts of the world ratios below 0.5 were observed in Puerto Rico, Bombay and Cali (Colombia). The pathologists involved were all highly skilled, so that it is unlikely that neuroblastoma went unrecognized. A possible explanation is that, in these parts of the world, some inhibiting factor transmitted from the mother to the foetus or newborn infant enhances regression of neuroblastoma in situ, thus removing this potential precursor of clinical neuroblastoma.

2.5 RETINOBLASTOMA

In Manchester and in the USA, the frequency of neuroblastoma and of Wilms' tumour was coniderably higher than that of retinoblastoma, but in Israel, where diagnosis and reporting of cases are presumably similar, retinoblastoma was more frequent than the other two tumours. Similar high frequencies of retinoblastoma were reported in the Sudan, Uganda, Ibadan, Bombay and Karachi. Retinoblastoma was thus more frequent in certain parts of the Indian subcontinent and Africa than elsewhere. Other studies show no excess of bilateral (hereditary) cases, so the high frequency appears to be due to an environmental influence.

2.6 WILMS' TUMOUR

Wilms' tumour was thought to have a constant rate worldwide (Innis, 1972), but the All-Japan Children's Cancer Registry consistently shows the frequency there to be about half that elsewhere (Hirayama, 1980). The frequency of aniridia with Wilms' tumour in Japan is also said to be about half that in the USA and Europe (Kobayashi, personal communication). The possibility thus arises that the gene locus on the short arm of chromosome 11 may be less mutable in Japanese than in other ethnic groups.

2.7 BONE CANCER

In coding death certificates for bone cancer, the same numbers are used for all types. Hence, from coded data, Ewing's sarcoma cannot be distinguished from osteosarcoma. By recoding death-certificate diagnoses of bone cancer according to cell-type for all children in the USA who died of cancer during the 1960s, it was found that Blacks rarely develop Ewing's sarcoma (Fraumeni & Glass, 1970). The UICC study showed that Ewing's sarcoma is also rare among Blacks in Africa and among Chinese and Japanese. Data collected for the *Atlas of Cancer Mortality* in the People's Republic of China show this deficiency (Li *et al.*, 1980), as does the Bone Cancer Registry maintained by orthopaedic surgeons in Japan (Bone Tumor Committee of Japanese Orthopedic Association, 1982). Apparently Whites are much more susceptible than other races to this form of bone cancer. No such difference exists with regard to osteosarcoma.

2.8 TESTIS

The frequency of testicular cancer in Whites in the USA begins to rise at 15–19 years of age, reaching a tremendous peak at 25–29 years. There is no corresponding peak among Blacks (McKay *et al.*, 1982) or Japanese (Miller, 1987). These differences indicate that Whites are especially susceptible to various types of testicular cancer in adolescence and early adulthood. Small peaks in the frequency of embryonal cancer of the testis occur soon after birth among Whites in the USA and Japanese but not among Blacks in the USA (McKay *et al.*, 1982).

2.9 SKIN

The UICC study revealed that, at the Institut Salah Azaiz in Tunis, 14% of all cancer under 15 years of age was skin cancer in children with xeroderma pigmentosum (XP). This high frequency, equal to that for Wilms' tumour *plus* neuroblastoma in Europe and the USA, occurs throughout North Africa, but only the barest mention of it had been made in the medical literature (Marshall, 1964). The great excess of XP in North Africa was evident from the hundreds of cases which had been quickly assembled for laboratory research on the DNA repair defect in this disease. Ideally, protection from sunlight can prevent the skin cancers, so highly lethal among children in this part of the world.

2.10 BRAIN

Geographical or ethnic peculiarities in the occurrence of brain cancers are not easy to recognize because ascertainment and pathological classification are so variable from place to place. A noteworthy exception is pineal neoplasia of the teratomatous type, including germinomas, which are about 12 times more common in Japan than elsewhere (Koide *et al.*, 1980). In a small series of pineal tumours in Hawaii, a disproportionate number were in Japanese (Miller, 1971), a finding that suggests an inherent high risk that is not modified by the environment upon migration.

2.11 ADENOCARCINOMA OF THE VAGINA

One of the most notable adult-type cancers in childhood is clear-cell adenocarcinoma of the cervix or vagina due to maternal use of diethylstilboestrol (DES) during pregnancy. This neoplasm usually affects elderly women, but a cluster of four cases in Boston among young women in 1970 led to a case-control study that showed the relationship to the drug (Herbst *et al.*, 1979). The excess is detectable in the data of the Surveillance, Epidemiology and End Results (SEER) Program of the National Cancer Institute, 1973–1984, during which time 45 cases of clear-cell adenocarcinoma of the vagina or cervix in patients 15–29 years of age were reported (Kim & Miller, unpublished data). In 1984, new cases were still being diagnosed. The most recent year of birth was 1968.

2.12 NASOPHARYNGEAL CARCINOMA

In the UICC study, an excess of nasopharyngeal carcinoma (NPC) under 15 years of age was noted in data from the Institut Salah Azaiz, where 10% of childhood cancer was of this type. This was, of course, a reflection of the high rate of this neoplasm in Tunisia, related to infection with the Epstein-Barr virus (Old *et al.*, 1966), and is one of several such geographical clusters of NPC in various parts of the world.

2.13 HEPATOCELLULAR CARCINOMA

In Africa and Asia high rates of hepatocellular carcinoma occur, which are believed to result from chronic infection with hepatitis B virus (HBV). Immature liver cells are especially prone to develop chronic infection (Blumberg & London, 1985). Because the liver is less mature at birth in Africa than in China, the period of susceptibility to chronic HBV infection is longer.

2.14 CANCER CLUSTERS

Even rare events may cluster by chance. Childhood leukaemia is notorious in this respect. The Centers for Disease Control have investigated more than 100 cancer clusters, particularly of leukaemia, in the United States, but none could be traced to an environmental cause (Caldwell & Heath, 1976). To show how easy it is to find clusters, other investigators (Glass et al., 1968) made a scatter map of deaths due to leukaemia under 15 years of age in Los Angeles County, 1960–1964. By drawing boundaries as tightly as possible around groups of deaths, at least nine clusters could be created which were as large or larger than those described in the literature.

The other side of this story is that virtually all known human carcinogens were first recognized by alert clinicians who observed clusters of cancer and traced them to their causes. Examples include adenocarcinoma of the vagina caused by DES, already mentioned, mesothelioma from asbestos exposure, lung cancer from the manufacture of mustard gas, and liver neoplasia from oral contraceptives (Miller, 1978). Confirmation of clinical observations has come from special disease registries or cancer registries. In theory, cancer clusters due to environmental agents should be detectable from data in registries, but the unavoidable lag in registration and difficulties in sensing unusual aggregates from tables of numbers are handicaps. The new epidemic of Kaposi's sarcoma due to AIDS is detectable in the SEER data, but was noted much earlier by clinicians. The increase in the frequency of DES-induced clear-cell adenocarcinoma of the cervix or vagina among young women occurred before the SEER Program was initiated, so no change in rates can be detected in SEER data. The increase of 1–8 cases annually over two organ sites would not have attracted notice. Under the circumstances, the change in rates was more readily recognized by clinicians than by cancer registries.

2.15 ACTION REQUIRED IN THE FUTURE

First and foremost, clinicians need to be alert for peculiarities in cancer occurrence which may lead to a new understanding of their origins, be they inborn or environmentally induced. Epidemiological observations have been a tremendous stimulus to laboratory research, as human models for high risk of cancer have been found for which there are as yet no animal models. The same may be true eventually of observations concerning low risk of specific cancers, or differences in the subtypes or subsites involved among various ethnic groups. The SEER Program is a good source of data for use in ethnic comparisons of the more common cancers.

Childhood cancers, because of their low rates, accumulate slowly in this registry, so one must turn to international comparisons instead. Despite variations in ascertainment from one place to another, some peculiarities are so large that they show up in spite of differences in completeness of data collection — the low rates of neuroblastoma in central Africa, for example.

Special disease registries can be a great help in ethnic comparisons. Thus a variety of registries for specific cancers (e.g., for bone tumours, melanoma and thyroid cancer) or syndromes with high risk of cancer (e.g., xeroderma pigmentosum, immunodeficiency disorders and multiple endocrine neoplasia type I) exist in Japan. It may be appropriate to establish similar registries elsewhere in the world. In the absence of special disease registries, large case-series may suffice.

At the conclusion of the data collection phase of the UICC study of childhood cancer etiology, a one-day meeting was held in 1973 in Amsterdam at which a Study Group reviewed the findings and considered future activities. Among suggestions for the future were: (a) the development of check-lists to simplify hospital records concerning environmental and genetic influences and the association of specific cancers with other diseases; (b) the study of second primary cancers; (c) the establishment of an international registry for adult-type cancers in childhood, another for rare paediatric neoplasms, and still another for the children of long-term survivors of childhood cancer; (d) a study of the psychological effects among survivors of childhood cancer; (e) record-linkage of registries for cancer with registries for congenital malformations; and (f) the initiation of a childhood cancer etiology newsletter to be sent free of charge to interested people throughout the world. Most of these suggestions were put into effect under other auspices in the intervening years. The newsletter was published by the National Cancer Institute in Bethesda, 95 issues being produced at roughly monthly intervals.

References

Blumberg, B.S. & London, W.T. (1985) Hepatitis B virus and the prevention of primary cancer of the liver. *J. natl Cancer Inst.*, 74, 267-273

Bone Tumor Committee of Japanese Orthopedic Association (1982) *Bone Tumor Registry in Japan: The incidence of bone tumors in Japan*, Tokyo, National Cancer Center, pp. 122-123

Burkitt, D.P. (1958) A sarcoma involving the jaws of African children. *Br. J. Surg.*, 46, 218-223

Caldwell, G.G. & Heath, C.W. Jr (1976) Case clustering in cancer. *South. med. J.*, 69, 1598-1602

Cavdar, A.O., Arcasoy, A., Babacan, E., Gozdasoglu, S., Topuz, U. & Fraumeni, J.F. Jr (1978) Ocular granulocytic sarcoma (chloroma) with acute myelomonocytic leukaemia in Turkish children. *Cancer, 41*, 1606-1609

Cavdar, A.O., Arcasoy, A., Gozdasoglu, S. & Demirag, B. (1971) Chloroma-like ocular manifestations in Turkish children with acute myelomonocytic leukaemia. *Lancet, i*, 680-682

Court Brown, W.M. & Doll, R. (1961) Leukaemia in childhood and young adult life. Trends in relation to aetiology. *Br. Med. J., 1*, 981-988

Fraumeni, J.F. Jr & Glass, A.G. (1970) Rarity of Ewing's sarcoma among U.S. Negro children. *Lancet, i*, 366-367

Glass, A.G., Hill, J.A. & Miller, R.W. (1968) Significance of leukemia clusters. *J. Pediatr., 73*, 101-107

Greene, M.H. (1985) *Epidemiologic studies of therapy-related acute leukemia.* In: Castellani, A., ed., *Epidemiology and quantitation of environmental risks in humans from radiation and other agents — potential and limitations,* New York, Plenum Press, pp. 499-514

Herbst, A.L., Scully, R.E. & Robboy, S.J. (1979) Prenatal diethylstilbestrol exposure and human genital tract abnormalities. *Natl Cancer Inst. Monogr., 51*, 25-35

Hirayama, T. (1980) *Descriptive and analytical epidemiology of childhood malignancy in Japan.* In: Kobayashi, N., ed., *Recent advances in management of children with cancer,* Tokyo, The Children's Cancer Association of Japan, pp. 27-43

Innis, M.D. (1972) Nephroblastoma: possible index cancer of childhood. *Med. J. Aust., 1*, 18-20

Kadin, M.E., Berard, C.W., Nanba, K. & Wakasa, H. (1983) Lymphoproliferative diseases in Japan and western countries. *Hum. Pathol., 14*, 745-772

Koide, O., Watanabe, Y. & Sato, K. (1980) A pathological survey of intracranial germinoma and pinealoma in Japan. *Cancer, 45*, 2119-2130

Lashof, J.C. & Stewart, A. (1965) Oxford survey of childhood cancers. Progress report III: Leukaemia and Down's syndrome. *Mon. Bull. Minist. Health, 24*, 136-143

Li, F.P., Tu, J., Liu, F. & Shiang, E.L. (1980) Rarity of Ewing's sarcoma in China. *Lancet, i*, 1255

MacMahon, B. (1966) Epidemiology of Hodgkin's disease. *Cancer Res., 26*, 1189-1200

Magrath, I., O'Conor, G.T., & Ramot, B., ed., (1984) *Pathogenesis of leukemias and lymphomas: environmental influences,* New York, Raven Press, p. 399

Marshall, J. (1964) *Skin diseases in Africa,* Cape Town, Maske Miller, p. 91

McKay, F.W., Hanson, M.R. & Miller, R.W. (1982) Cancer mortality in the United States: 1950-1977. *Natl Cancer Inst. Monogr., 59*, 1-197

Miller, R.W. (1970) Neoplasia and Down's syndrome. *Ann. N.Y. Acad. Sci., 171*, 637-644

Miller, R.W. (1971) Relation between cancer and congenital malformations. The value of small series, with a note on pineal tumors in native and migrant Japanese. *Israel J. med. Sci., 7*, 1461-1464

Miller, R.W. (1977) *Ethnic differences in cancer occurrence: genetic and environmental influences with particular reference to neuroblastoma.* In: Mulvihill, J.J., Miller, R.W. & Fraumeni, J.F. Jr, eds, *Genetics of human cancer,* New York, Raven Press, pp. 1-14

Miller, R.W. (1978) *The discovery of human teratogens, carcinogens and mutagens. Lessons for the future.* In: Hollaender, A. & de Serres, F.J., eds, *Chemical mutagens: principles and methods for their detection,* Vol. 5, New York, Plenum, pp. 101-126

Miller, R.W. (1987) Report of a U.S.-Japan Cooperative Cancer Research Program. Workshop on adult-type cancer under age 30. *Jpn. J. Cancer Res.* (in press)

Miller, R.W., Gilman, P.A. & Sugano, H. (1981) Meeting highlights: differences in lymphocytic diseases in the United States and Japan. *J. natl Cancer Inst., 67*, 739

Motawy, M.S. & Omar, Y.T. (1986) Hodgkin's disease in children of Kuwait. *Cancer, 57*, 2255-2259

Old, L.J., Boyse, E.A., Oettgen, H.F., de Harven, E., Geering, G., Williamson, B. & Clifford, P. (1966) Precipitating antibody in human serum antigen in cultured Burkitt lymphoma cells. *Proc. natl. Acad. Sci., 56*, 1699-1704

O'Gorman Hughes, D.W. (1974) Aplastic anaemia in childhood. III. Constitutional aplastic anaemia and related cytopenias. *Med. J. Aust., 1*, 519-526

3. THE CLASSIFICATION OF CHILDHOOD TUMOURS

H.B. Marsden

Malignant tumours in children are relatively rare by comparison with those occurring in adult life but are nevertheless the most common cause of natural death in this age-range in England and Wales, being exceeded only by accidents. The improvement in therapeutic results during recent years has also led to the need for the assessment of morbidity and the provision of services accordingly.

Childhood neoplasms show differences from those seen in the adult both as regards sites of incidence and histological appearance. Primary epithelial involvement is relatively rare in the paediatric age group and many of the tumours have histological features which recall foetal development and are therefore designated 'embryonal'.

It is probable that the etiology of all neoplasms involves both genetic and extrinsic factors and that these may vary considerably in relation to particular tumours. Some, e.g., retinoblastoma, have a major genetic component while in others, e.g., carcinoma of the bronchus, extrinsic factors play a greater part. Considerable information is available on the factors leading to the development of some adult cancers but rather less with regard to tumours in childhood. The study of paediatric oncology is particularly important in helping to throw light on the genetic component in etiology and possibly also regarding the relationships between genetic and extrinsic factors. The young age of those involved, though tragic for those concerned, is helpful in undertaking family studies. The association of geographical and ethnic aspects together with family studies, as in Burkitt's lymphoma and nasopharyngeal carcinoma, may be most fruitful lines for further study.

The embryonal nature of many paediatric tumours, the resemblance to foetal tissue at varying stages of development and the association with malformations are aspects which need to be studied in order to understand the disorders of growth and tumour formation. In addition, studies in cyto-genetics and molecular biology may help to account for the presence of particular neoplasms of different histological type in the same pedigree.

In the past, a number of children's tumour registries have been set up, initially to assess the magnitude of the problem locally together with the requirements for the provision of a satisfactory service, and subsequently to assist in the study of etiological factors. It is important that centres interested in the field of paediatric oncology should be able to exchange information, and to this end a classification which may be widely used is required. Previous studies on paediatric oncology have been based on site rather than histology. Identification of the organ or anatomical site involved is of great importance in adults but less significant in paediatric oncology. It is highly probable that a neoplasm of the kidney in childhood is in fact a Wilms' tumour, although it is important that the other less frequent histological types of renal neoplasm are identified. As regards embryonal rhabdomyosarcoma, the primary tumour may be almost anywhere in the body, although the head, neck and pelvic regions are favoured sites for this neoplasm.

In order to fulfil the requirements for assessment based on histology, a new classification has been developed and is presented in this volume (see Annex). The *International Classification of Diseases for Oncology* (ICD-O) (World Health Organization, 1976) has been used as the basis for this classification, being regarded as more suitable than previous publications for such a study, particularly as regards the Morphology Section (M). Some reservations may be expressed concerning the Topography Section (T) in relation to paediatric oncology, as the emphasis is on regional anatomical identification. As an example, under T171, 'Connective tissue and other soft tissues', striated muscle, sympathetic and peripheral nervous system, blood vessels, synovia and adipose tissue, among others, are included under a common heading and there is considerable overlap between the subsections.

There are additional problems in topography relating to multiple neoplasms in paediatric oncology. Provision is made in ICD-O for the recording of multiple tumours, and it is recommended that they should be coded individually and given separate site codes. This is inappropriate for Wilms' tumour, retinoblastoma and neuroblastoma, where the site codes would be the same for additional neoplasms irrespective of whether there are multiple unilateral and/or bilateral tumours. In Wilms' tumour, there may be multiple unilateral and bilateral neoplasms, and to record four neoplasms with the same T-code would be inadequate to describe three tumours in one kidney and one in the other. From the point of view of genetic studies it is important that such details should be available.

The morphology (M) section of the ICD-O has been developed 'to include the terms for different types of neoplasm which have been defined and illustrated in widely accepted publications of tumour classification and which are in general usage throughout the world'. It is stressed that the ICD-O is a coded nomenclature rather than a classification scheme for tumours and the use of main and alternative terminology for particular neoplasms is an asset in the tables.

The classification scheme presented here was developed from that used by the Manchester Children's Tumour Registry (MCTR), with certain simplifications to adapt it for use in an international context. It has now been published elsewhere (Birch & Marsden, 1987). Leukaemias and other reticuloendothelial neoplasms comprise the largest numerical group. Intracranial tumours account for many of the solid neoplasms and, if the sympathetic nervous system is added, the total figure is over 40%. Embryonal tumours, including those of renal and mesenchymal origin, make up many of the remaining cases and there are important but numerically relatively small groups including those of epithelial origin.

Based on the above assessment, tumours have been divided into 12 diagnostic groups as follows:

I.   Leukaemias
II.   Lymphomas and other reticuloendothelial neoplasms
III.   Central nervous system and miscellaneous intracranial and intraspinal neoplasms
IV.   Sympathetic and allied nervous system tumours
V.   Retinoblastoma
VI.   Renal tumours
VII.   Hepatic tumours
VIII. Malignant bone tumours
IX.   Soft tissue sarcomas
X.   Germ-cell, trophoblastic and other gonadal neoplasms
XI.   Carcinomas and other malignant epithelial neoplasms
XII.   Other and unspecified malignant neoplasms

The tumours identified by an M-code in the classification are essentially malignant, although the inclusion of histiocytosis X in Group II and some benign intracranial and intraspinal neoplasms in Group III may not be in accordance with this statement. The borderline between benign and malignant tumours is difficult to establish in some cases; for example, regarding ependymomas, the ICD-O makes provision for benign tumours (5th digit 0) and uncertain whether benign or malignant, borderline malignancy (5th digit 1).

The distinction between benign and malignant tumours in childhood is blurred in other intracranial neoplasms apart from ependymomas. Astro-ocytomas in the MCTR are divided between juvenile and adult histological types. The juvenile cases are given the M-code 9421-9423. The 5th digit 3 (malignant, primary site) in ICD-O seems to be rather severe for such tumours, and there are examples where little change in the behaviour or extension of the lesion has taken place during many years without treatment apart from shunting of the cerebrospinal fluid. In adult astrocytomas (M-code 9400-9420) and glioblastic variants, the 5th digit 3, both as regards histological appearance and clinical behaviour, is more appropriate. For the purposes of the present study juvenile and adult astrocytoma are considered together, as many registries do not distinguish between these types. Optic nerve glioma is grouped with astrocytoma and identified by the T-code.

Renal tumours are thought to merit a separate diagnostic group. Wilms' tumour (M-code 8960) has received considerable attention in recent years in both genetic and molecular biological studies, and was at one time considered to be suitable for use as an index tumour in paediatric oncology. The widespread interest in clinical trials on paediatric renal neoplasms has led to the identification of other malignant tumours apart from the nephroblastoma. In the MCTR, an additional M-code has been inserted to identify the bone-metastasizing renal tumour, a term preferred to clear-celled sarcoma, as many of these neoplasms are not clear-celled and the histogenesis remains uncertain at this time. Similarly a code has also been introduced for the rhabdoid renal tumour. The second edition of ICD-O will include these codes, but in the present study these tumours will be included with Wilms' tumour. Mesoblastic nephroma has the same M-code as Wilms' tumour but receives the 5th digit of 1 (uncertain whether benign or malignant) as-opposed to 3 (malignant, primary site) for the nephroblastoma. This is thought to be appropriate, as the relationship between the two neoplasms is uncertain and, while the great majority of meso-blastic nephromas are benign or locally aggressive only, occasional examples of metastasis have been recorded. Many registries, however, do not register mesoblastic nephroma and this tumour is therefore not included in the present study. The subgroup 'other malignant renal tumours' allows for the inclusion of unspecified neoplasms, but such rare lesions as primary renal rhabdomyosarcoma or leiomyosarcoma would be placed in Group IX.

Hepatic tumours, although relatively infre-quent, constitute a clearly defined group (Group VII) and have been separately identified in view of the importance of genetic and familial studies relating to certain members of the group. Similarly retinoblastoma, being of exceptional interest, has been allocated a separate group (Group V).

Adrenocortical tumours might be considered to merit similar treatment, but the majority of adrenal neoplasms are of sympathetic nervous system ori-gin and the M-code 8370 allows for ready identi-fication.

Malignant bone tumours (Group VIII) com-prise a clearly defined diagnostic group and have received attention in view of the association be-tween osteosarcoma and retinoblastoma. In addi-tion, the osteosarcoma appears relatively un-common in Japan, while the same applies to Ewing's tumour in the black population of the United States.

Soft-tissue sarcomas (Group IX) constitute a difficult group. The embryonal rhabdomyo-sarcoma accounts for the great majority of such neoplasms but rare examples of a wide variety of specified tumours have been recorded. The M-code 8803, small-cell sarcoma, with the alternative title of round-cell sarcoma, in the 880 section (soft tissue tumours and sarcomas, NOS) in ICD-O might be considered suitable for Ewing's tumour of the soft parts. However, there are a number of soft-tissue round-cell neoplasms in children and it is felt that tumours having cytological features similar to those of the Ewing's tumour of bone should be

identified. For the purposes of the present study, therefore, we recommend the use of 9260/3 but with T-code appropriate to soft tissue. The M-code 9561/3 has been introduced for use in the MCTR for the Triton tumour (malignant Schwannoma with rhabdomyoblastic differentiation), and this will appear in the second edition of ICD-O. There are, however, other combined neoplasms, notably the gangliorhabdomyosarcoma, which overlaps two major diagnostic groups (IV and IX). The rarity of such neoplasms and the difficulty in deciding which major group to use has prevented the provision of a specific M-code in this case. The mesenchymal chondrosarcoma (M-code 9240) has been given a primary site in soft tissue. The soft-tissue osteosarcoma might receive similar treat-ment but on a histological basis is placed in Group VIII. There is, however, no M-code for the myxoid chondrosarcoma (parachordoma) of the soft tis-sues in ICD-O.

The germ-cell, trophoblastic and other gonadal neoplasms (Group X) do not require additional elaboration and, as stated above, provision is made for ready identification of important subgroups of Carcinoma and other malignant epithelial neo-plasms (Group XI), namely adrenocortical, thyroid and nasopharyngeal carcinoma, together with melano-matous neoplasms. At the same time, particular tumours, such as carcinoid and mucoepidermoid carcinoma, may be recorded.

It has been stressed earlier that ICD-O is 'a coded nomenclature and not a classification scheme for tumours', although there is some variation in the listing of tumours by cell type or tissue of origin. The M-codes listed in the present classification relating to carcinomas include many histological types which are presented in ICD-O and considered possible at a particular site. Car-cinomas which are thought to be inappropriate to such sites have not been so listed.

The final group (XII), Other malignant neo-plasms, contains rather a mixed bag of rare tumours, including mesothelioma and pneumo-blastoma, which are not thought to be appropriate for inclusion elsewhere. In the unspecified neo-plasms, important provision (M-code 9990) is made for the inclusion of cases lacking histological confirmation but with strong clinical probability. Unbiopsied CNS, renal, hepatic, bone and gonadal tumours are included with their respective groups. The M-codes 8002-8004 with the 5th digit 3 allow for cases of malignant tumours where small, giant or fusiform cells are not further identified.

In conclusion, the present classification is based on the incidence of childhood malignancy and is related to histological features. The ICD-O has been found to be suitable as a basis for such a classification and general groups, together with many specific tumour types, may be identified. There are spaces in the ICD-O for the insertion of additional M-codes and such insertions have been made at the MCTR. It is thought to be necessary that such additions should be made since, for example with renal tumours in childhood, it would be difficult to carry out an in-depth study without them at the present time. However, there should be general agreement regarding such insertions.

It is hoped that, by the use of the classification presented in this volume, information may be exchanged in order to assess problems locally, to provide an appropriate therapeutic service and to assist in the study of the etiological factors involved in paediatric oncology.

Acknowledgement

The Manchester Children's Tumour Registry is supported by the Cancer Research Campaign.

References

Birch, J.M. & Marsden, H.B. (1987) A classification scheme for childhood cancer. *Int. J. Cancer*, *40*, 620-624

World Health Organization (1976) *International Classification of Diseases for Oncology*, Geneva

ANNEX
INTERNATIONAL CLASSIFICATION SCHEME
FOR CHILDHOOD CANCER

It should be noted that, in this Annex, the ICD-O T-code refers to the site of the **primary** tumour. The presence of a behaviour code /6 implies that the histological diagnosis (M-code) is based on the biopsy of a metastasis; nevertheless, the associated T-code refers to the known (or suspected) primary site from which the metastasis derived.

Diagnostic group	ICD-O M-code First 4 digits	ICD-O M-code 5th digits	ICD-O T-code
I. Leukaemias			
(a) Acute lymphocytic leukaemia	9821,9824	3	
(b) Other lymphoid leukaemia	9820,9822,9823, 9825,9850	3	
(c) Acute non-lymphocytic leukaemia	9840,9841,9861, 9864,9866,9891, 9894	3	
(d) Chronic myeloid leukaemia	9863	3	
(e) Other and unspecified leukaemia	9800-9804, 9810,9830,9842, 9860,9862,9865, 9870-9890,9892, 9893,9900-9940	3	
II. Lymphomas and other reticuloendothelial neoplasms			
(a) Hodgkin's disease	9650-9662	3,6,9	
(b) Non-Hodgkin lymphoma	9591,9602-9642, 9690-9701	3,6,9	
(c) Burkitt's lymphoma	9750	3,6,9	
(d) Unspecified lymphomas	9590,9600,9601	3,6,9	
(e) Histiocytosis X	9722 (also SNOMED morphology codes 77860,77910,77920)	3,6,9	
(f) Other reticuloendothelial neoplasms	9710-9721, 9730-9741	3,6,9	
III. Central nervous system and miscellaneous intracranial and intraspinal neoplasms			
(a) Ependymoma	9383,9390-9394	0,1,3,6,9	
(b) Astrocytoma	9380	3,6,9	192.0
	9381,9400-9441	3,6,9	
(c) Medulloblastoma	9470-9480	3,6,9	
(d) Other glioma	9380	3,6,9	191.0-191.9, 192.1-192.9
	9382,9384, 9442-9460, 9481	1,3,6,9	

—13—

Diagnostic group	ICD-O M-code First 4 digits	ICD-O M-code 5th digits	ICD-O T-code
(e) Miscellaneous intracranial and intraspinal neoplasms	8270-8281,8300, 9350-9362,9505, 9530-9539	0,1,3,6,9	
	9060-9102	0,1	191.0-192.9, 194.3,194.4
	8000-8004	3,6,9	191.0-192.9, 194.3,194.4
	9990	0,1,3,6,9	191.0-192.9, 194.3,194.4
IV. Sympathetic nervous system tumours			
(a) Neuroblastoma and ganglioneuroblastoma	9490,9500	3,6,9	
(b) Other	8680,8693-8710, 9501-9504, 9520-9523	3,6,9	
V. Retinoblastoma	9510-9512	3,6,9	
VI. Renal tumours			
(a) Wilms' tumour	8960	3,6,9	
(b) Renal carcinoma	8010-8041,8043, 8050,8120,8122, 8130,8140,8230, 8231,8260,8310	3,6,9	189.0
	8312	3,6,9	
(c) Other and unspecified malignant renal tumours	8961,8962	3,6,9	
	8000-8004,9990	3,6,9	189.0
VII. Hepatic tumours			
(a) Hepatoblastoma	8970	3,6,9	
(b) Hepatic carcinoma	8010-8041,8043, 8140,8230,8231, 8260	3,6,9	155.0, 155.1
	8160-8180	3,6,9	
(c) Other and unspecified malignant hepatic tumours	8000-8004,9990	3,6,9	155.0, 155.1
VIII. Malignant bone tumours			
(a) Osteosarcoma	9180-9190	3,6,9	
(b) Chondrosarcoma	9220-9230	3,6,9	
	9240	3,6,9	170.0-170.9, 199.9
(c) Ewing's sarcoma	9260	3,6,9	170.0-170.9, 199.9
(d) Other and unspecified malignant bone tumours	8812,9250, 9261-9330,9370	3,6,9	
	8000-8004, 8800,8801, 8803,9990	3,6,9	170.0-170.9

Diagnostic group	ICD-O M-code First 4 digits	ICD-O M-code 5th digits	ICD-O T-code
IX. Soft-tissue sarcomas			
(a) Rhabdomyosarcoma, embryonal sarcoma and soft-tissue Ewing's tumour	8900-8920,8991	3,6,9	
	9260	3,6,9	140.0-169.9 171.0-195.8
(b) Fibrosarcoma, neurofibro- sarcoma, and other fibromatous neoplasms	8810,8811, 8813-8832,9540, 9560	3,6,9	
(c) Other soft-tissue sarcoma	8840-8895,8990, 9040-9044, 9120-9170,9251, 9581	3,6,9	
	9240	3,6,9	140.0-169.9, 171.0-195.8
	8800-8804	3,6,9	140.0-169.9, 171.0-199.9
X. Germ-cell, trophoblastic and other gonadal neoplasms			
(a) Non-gonadal germ-cell and trophoblastic neoplasms	9060-9102	3,6,9	140.0-182.8, 183.2-185.9, 187.1-199.9
(b) Gonadal germ-cell and trophoblastic neoplasms	9060-9102	3,6,9	183.0,186.0, 186.9
(c) Gonadal carcinoma	8010-8041,8043, 8140,8230,8231, 8260,8310,8440, 8480,8481	3,6,9	183.0,186.0, 186.9
	8381,8441-8471	3,6,9	
(d) Other and unspecified malignant gonadal tumours	8600-8650,9000	3,6,9	
	8000-8004,9990	3,6,9	183.0, 186.0, 186.9
XI. Carcinoma and other malignant epithelial neoplasms			
(a) Adrenocortical carcinoma	8370	3,6,9	194.0
(b) Thyroid carcinoma	8010-8041,8043, 8050,8070,8140, 8230,8231,8260, 8290,8480,8510	3,6,9	193.9
	8330-8350,8511	3,6,9	
(c) Nasopharyngeal carcinoma	8010-8041,8043, 8070-8082,8120, 8140,8480,8560	3,6,9	147.0-147.9
(d) Melanomatous neoplasms	8720-8780	3,6,9	
(e) Other carcinoma	8010-8154, 8190-8310, 8320-8323,8380 8390-8440, 8480-8510, 8512-8580, 8940	3,6,9	140.0-146.9, 148.0-154.8, 156.0-165.9, 173.0-182.8, 183.2-185.9, 187.1-188.9, 189.1-192.9, 194.1-195.8 199.9

Diagnostic group	ICD-O M-code First 4 digits	ICD-O M-code 5th digits	ICD-O T-code
XII. Other and unspecified malignant neoplasms			
	8930,8950,8951, 8980,8981,9020, 9050-9053,9110, 9580	3,6,9	
	8000-8004,9990	3,6,9	140.0-154.8, 156.0-169.9, 171.0-182.8, 183.2-185.9, 187.1-188.9, 189.1-190.9, 193.9-194.1, 194.5-199.9

[a]Systematized Nomenclature of Medicine, Chicago, IL, College of American Pathologists (1976)

We believe that, in the above classification, we have included virtually all possible types of carcinoma (M codes 8010-8580) occurring in the kidney, liver, ovary, testis, adrenal cortex, thyroid and nasopharynx. However, if verified carcinomas of other morphological types should be found in any of these sites, we recommend that, for statistical purposes, they be included with the other carcinomas of the same site.

4. MATERIALS AND METHODS OF THE STUDY

D.M. Parkin

4.1 CONTRIBUTORS

This volume contains contributions from some 50 different countries. The objective of the editors was to include data from as many general population-based or childhood tumour registries as possible, provided that the number of cases available for analysis was 200 or more, in order to permit an extensive analysis of geographical variations in the incidence of childhood cancer. The time period to which the incidence rates were to refer was chosen so as to correspond as closely as possible to the decade 1970–1979. Furthermore, since the classification system to be used for childhood cancers (see Chapter 3) requires data on both site and histological type, contributors were asked to supply such information.

In practice, there have been several deviations from this study plan. Firstly, in some regions of the world, notably Africa and parts of Asia, there are no population-based cancer registries which could provide information on incidence rates of childhood cancer. It was therefore decided to accept, from such regions, large case series deriving from hospital-based or histopathology-based registries. Although these do not relate to a defined population, they can provide useful information on the relative frequency of different cancers in children which would otherwise be unavailable.

Secondly, in some countries many cancer registries are in operation, and it would have been possible to reproduce rates from several of these —for example, in the USA and Great Britain. Whilst this might be of value in illustrating regional differences in the incidence of certain tumours of the adult, the variation in incidence of childhood cancers in subnational populations (of similar ethnic background) is likely to be of much less importance. Thus, in general, we chose to present information from the larger or longer established registries in a country (as in the case of Australia), or to present the pooled results from national collaborative projects, such as the SEER Program in the USA or the National Registry of Childhood Tumours of Great Britain, which rely on an input from regional registries, rather than to present the data of the original registries themselves. However, the results from certain large regional registries which do not participate in national projects have been included in addition (e.g., Los Angeles, New York), as well as those from specialized childhood tumour registries providing high quality information over long time periods (e.g., Greater Delaware Valley Pediatric Tumor Registry, Manchester Children's Tumour Registry).

It proved impossible to restrict the time period to 1970–1979. Although several contributors provided information strictly in accordance with this request, many preferred that the analysis of their data should incorporate later and/or earlier years in addition. Several registries which were established after 1970 preferred that their results subsequent to 1979 should be included, so that incidence rates would be based on the maximum number of cases possible. For other registries with a small population base, the period analysed had to be extended to cover years before 1970 in order to include sufficient cases to meet the requirement of a minimum number of 200. In general, however, the small differences in time periods between the data sets in this volume are unlikely to account for much of the variation in incidence rates observed.

4.2 INFORMATION SUPPLIED

The contributing centres were each asked to supply three sets of information:
(1) A listing of cases registered
(2) The population at risk
(3) Information concerning the registry (area, methods, etc.)

4.2.1 Cases registered

The data provided comprised one record for each case of childhood cancer registered, with the following 10 variables:

(1) Registration number (to identify the case in the registry's files).

(2) Date of birth (or age in years).

(3) Date of incidence.

(4) Sex.

(5) Ethnic group.

(6) Site of primary tumour, with laterality for eye and kidney.

(7) Site code.

(8) Histopathological diagnosis (if available).

(9) Morphology code.

(10) Basis of diagnosis.

Item (5) was optional for those registries having populations comprising one or more distinct ethnic or tribal groups; religious group was occasionally substituted.

A specific request was made to provide information on the site of the *primary* tumour, rather than of any metastatic deposits which might have been subjected to biopsy. The topography code (item 7) corresponded to this site; where the localization of the primary was unknown, the appropriate code for 'unknown primary site' was used.

For those centres which had recorded it, the laterality of tumours of the eye and kidney was requested. However, for many centres, it was clear that laterality had not been systematically recorded, so that the results reported relate only to those cases for which laterality is mentioned.

For registries which keep their data on a computer, the file of cases was supplied either on magnetic tape or diskette. In this case, the site item (6) and histology item (8) in *words* were usually unavailable, because they were stored only in coded form.

Some smaller registries, principally in Africa, Asia and Oceania, provided their data as case listings on special forms, with the diagnosis given in words. For some of these, site and histology had also been coded, and this was checked before the stage of data entry. For 12 centres, coding of site and histology according to ICD-O was carried out by experienced coding staff employed specifically for this study.

A wide variety of coding schemes for site and histology had been used. Several registries provided data sets corresponding to more than one scheme (because of changes in practice during the period considered).

Site of tumour was invariably coded according to one of the revisions of the *International Classification of Diseases* — 7th, 8th or 9th — or the topography section of ICD-O. It was necessary, however, to ensure that the site code referred to the site of the primary tumour, so that the subsequent conversions to the childhood classification scheme were possible.

There were numerous coding schemes for histology. The most frequently used, especially in recent years, is the morphology section of ICD-O. However, in addition, data sets were received coded according to the *Systematized Nomenclature of Pathology* (College of American Pathologists, 1965) and to the *Manual of Tumour Nomenclature and Coding* (American Cancer Society, 1968), and also to other schemes specially developed by the registries concerned.

4.2.2 Population at risk

Population-based registries were asked to supply information on the composition of the population of the area from which the cases were drawn. The population by sex and age, in the maximum detail possible, was requested. Thus age was to be given in one of three formats preferably by single year of age, or as five-year age-groups (0—4, 5—9, 10—14), separating, if possible, the population aged less than one year from that aged 1—4.

Figures for as many years as possible relating to the period from which the cases were drawn were requested. In addition, the contributors were requested to indicate the source(s) of the population data.

4.2.3 Registry profile

The contributors were asked to complete a questionnaire providing information about the registry itself.

Population-based registries were asked to specify the geographical region covered by the registry; non-population-based registries were asked to list their sources of data (hospitals, laboratories) and to indicate sources of childhood cancer cases in their region which did *not* report to the registry. Details of registration procedures, including methods of data collection, and information on the types of tumour registered (especially whether benign or borderline neoplasms were included) were requested. Finally, the contributors were asked for a brief description of the geography and demography of the region covered by the registry.

4.3 CLASSIFICATION

The classification scheme used in this study is an adaptation for international use of that of the Manchester Children's Tumour Registry, described in the preceding chapter. It depends on the allocation of tumours coded by site and histology according to ICD-O, to 12 major diagnostic groups, and to 40 subgroups within those groups.

The first stage in the analysis therefore required all cases from the different data sets received to be coded according to ICD-O. For data sets using alternative coding schemes, the nearest ICD-O equivalent codes were allocated by means of a set of computer programs. For certain registries with individualistic coding schemes, it was sometimes necessary to request information on the histological type of groups of tumours identified by a single code, since allocation of an ICD-O equivalent unique to the categories in the childhood classification was not feasible.

The data were then subjected to various checks, firstly to ensure that the codes used (either the original codes or ICD-O equivalents) were valid, and then to identify various combinations of codes (sex-site, sex-histology, age-site, age-histology, site-histology) which were impossible or unlikely. Listings of impossible or unlikely combinations were returned to contributors for verification, and appropriate corrections made.

Finally, each case was allocated to one of the diagnostic groups described in Chapter 3, according to the conversion scheme shown in the Annex (pages 13—16). As noted in this Annex, the types of carcinoma normally found in kidney, liver, testis, ovary, adrenal cortex, thyroid and nasopharynx are incorporated into the conversions shown. However, some histologically verified carcinomas of other cell types were occasionally reported, and, if confirmed, were included with other carcinomas of the same site for statistical purposes.

It should be noted that, under the classification scheme, the following tumours are excluded from subsequent analyses:

(1) Carcinoid tumours, unless specified as malignant.
(2) Plasmacytomas, unless specified as malignant.

(3) Mixed salivary tumours (ICD-O code 8940/0).
(4) Teratoma NOS. (ICD-O code 9080/1) *unless* intracranial or intraspinal
(5) Various melanomatous lesions, e.g., juvenile melanoma (8770/0), precancerous melanosis (8741/2).

Unless specifically stated to the contrary in the corresponding text, the following tumours are included:

(1) Histiocytosis X, Hand-Schuller-Christian disease, and eosinophilic granuloma of bone (Group IIe).
(2) Pituitary adenomas and craniopharyngiomas.
(3) Meningiomas.
(4) Benign or unspecified tumours if intracranial/intraspinal, and no histological diagnosis is available (ICD-O codes 9990/0 and 9990/1).

4.4 ANALYSIS AND PRESENTATION

4.4.1 Main tables

For each contributing centre, the distribution of registered cases amongst the 12 diagnostic groups and their subgroups is given separately for males and females, and where appropriate for different racial groups.

Numbers. For all registries, the number of cases by age-group is given. The age-groups are 0 (less than one year of age), 1—4, 5—9 and 10—14. (Two registries in Africa — the Radiation and Isotope Centre, Khartoum, and the Bulawayo Cancer Registry, Zimbabwe — made no distinction between children aged less than one, and those aged one year; a single category (0—4) has been used for these centres.)

The figures for 'All ages' are occasionally greater than the sum of those for the component age-groups. This occurs when cases are registered as 'Child, age not known'; in this case the figure in the column 'All' is marked with a special symbol ($\boxtimes$).

Relative frequency. Three indices are included:

(i) *Crude* percentage: the percentage contribution of the particular group or subgroup to the total case series;

(ii) *Adjusted* percentage: the age-standardized cancer ratio (ASCAR) (see below);

(iii) *Group* percentage: the percentage contribution of each subgroup category to the total of the individual diagnostic group.

The crude and adjusted frequencies are calculated from the total number of cases in the series. When these are used for purposes of comparison between centres, it should be noted that some case series exclude certain tumour types; in particular, leukaemias are omitted from certain histopathology-based data sets.

Age-standardized cancer ratio. The relative frequency of different cancers differs considerably by age-group. In childhood, for example, some cancers are almost entirely confined to the under-fives (e.g., retinoblastoma) while others, such as bone sarcomas, are most common in the oldest age group (10–14) Thus, the proportion of different cancers in a case series will be strongly dependent on the age-composition of the population.

To permit comparison of summary percentages between case series which may have differing age compositions, the age-standardized cancer ratio (ASCAR) devised by Tuyns (1968) has been used. This is analogous to the direct standardization of rates, in that a standard population (or case series) is used, to which the observed age-specific proportions are applied.

The standard population for the study of childhood cancer was derived as the mean of the percentage of cases in each age-group (0–4, 5–9, 10–14) in 15 large registries (three in each continent) from *Cancer Incidence in Five Continents*, Volumes III and IV (Waterhouse *et al.*, 1976, 1982). The averages were rounded to give the following standard:

Age group	Age (years)	Percent
1	0–4	40
2	5–9	30
3	10–14	30
	0-14	100

The ASCAR is thus calculated as

$$40 \times (n_1/N_1) + 30 \times (n_2/N_2) + 30 \times (n_3/N_3)$$

where

n_i = number of cases in the given diagnostic group, or subgroup, in age-group i

N_i = total cases (all causes) in age-group i.

Incidence rates. Incidence rates are presented only for population-based registries, where it is believed that registration of new cancers arising in a defined population is reasonably complete, and there is good knowledge of the population at risk.

There are a few exceptions to these rules: rates for a few centres which are of particular interest have been presented even though they are only estimates of the true incidence, because of known under-enumeration of cases (e.g., Fiji), or inaccuracies in the denominator populations, as in the three African registries — Ibadan, Kampala and Bulawayo. In such cases, a cautionary note has been inserted in the text, and the summary tables include the incidence rates only for the 12 main diagnostic groups.

All rates are annual and expressed *per million* population at risk.

Age-specific rates are presented separately for age 0 (less than 1) when appropriate population denominators were available, otherwise the youngest age-group is 0–4. These are calculated by dividing the observed number of cases in the age category concerned, by the number of years of observation and the average population for the period concerned (see Section 4.4.2, below). Thus,

$$r_i = \frac{n_i}{Y \times P_i} \times 10^6$$

where

r_i = age-specific rate for age-group,

n_i = number of cases in age-group i,

Y = number of years of observation,

P_i = average population at risk, in age group i.

The crude rate is the total number of cases (all ages 0–14), divided by the number of years and the average population (aged 0–14) for the period in question.

The adjusted rate (age-adjusted rate) has been calculated by the direct method, using the world standard population for the age-groups under 15 (Waterhouse *et al.*, 1982). The standard population is:

Age group	Age (years)	Population
0	0	2400
1	1–4	9600
2	5–9	10000
3	10–14	9000
	0–14	31000

Where the population at risk in age-group 0 (age less than 1) is known, and using the same notation as above, the age-standardized rate (ASR) can be calculated as follows:

$$ASR = [(r_0 \times 2.4) + (r_1 \times 9.6) + (r_2 \times 10) + (r_3 \times 9)] / 31$$

The cumulative rate (Day, 1982) is the sum over each year of age of the age-specific incidence rates from birth to age 14. It is thus equivalent to an age-standardized rate, where each age-specific rate is given the same weight. Because only a minority of registries provided populations at risk by individual years of age, the actual calculation for each centre uses the age-specific rates shown in the corresponding table. Thus, where the incidence rate for age 0 is present, and using the same notation, the cumulative rate is:

$$\text{Cumulative rate} = r_0 + (4 \times r_1) + (5 \times r_2) + (5 \times r_3)$$

The cumulative rate is an approximation to the cumulative risk; the latter is the risk of an individual developing the cancer in question before the age of 15, if no other causes of death were in operation. It is here expressed per million, like all the other rates.

Histologically verified. The figures for 'histologically verified' indicate the percentage of those cases for which the basis of diagnosis was known, that had been diagnosed on histological grounds. 'Histology' includes the examination of tissue sections from biopsy of the primary tumour or of a metastasis, or of cytological or haematological specimens.

4.4.2 Population at risk

As mentioned in section 4.2.2, contributors were asked to supply information on the population at risk in as much detail, and for as many years within (or close to) the period of registration as possible.

A great variety of data were received, ranging from annual estimates by single year of age, to a single point estimate within a relatively long period.

For each registry, linear interpolation was used to provide estimates of the populations for those years for which actual data had not been provided. The total person-years at risk within each age-group and sex was then calculated, and divided by the number of years of observation, to yield the average population, by age-group and sex, for the period concerned.

These average populations appear with the entry for each registry, either for three age-groups (0—4, 5—9, 10—14) or, whenever possible, for age 0 (less than one) separately from ages 1—4.

The sources of the data from which these averages have been calculated are specified.

4.4.3 Text and commentary

Each table of data is accompanied by a textual description of the registry, its methodology and the area and population covered. This is based on the written descriptions and questionnaire responses provided by each contributor. An attempt has been made to draw the reader's attention to any features which may lead to unusual results — for example, the exclusion of certain tumour types from the registration process. For the non-population-based registries, the nature and sources of the case series are given, together with an indication of the ways in which these may not be representative of all incident cancers in the country of origin concerned.

The commentary for each centre has been written by the editors. We have avoided any discussion of the interpretation of the data since it is our hope and assumption that this will be done separately both by contributors to this volume and by others. In these commentaries, the rates for the major diagnostic groups are compared with those for other similar populations and attention is drawn to any particularly unusual features. Comparisons with general features of the rates for, e.g., Europe or Africa can most easily be made by reference to the summary tables in Chapter 6.

Sex ratios have been computed using age-standardized rates where these are available, but otherwise from total numbers.

In making the comparisons between registries and ethnic groups we have not used statistical significance tests. In most cases this would, in fact, not be appropriate, since any uncertainties about the true values of the rates are likely to arise from problems such as incompleteness of ascertainment or the validity of the population data rather than from chance fluctuations leading to statistical imprecision in the estimated rates. In assessing the validity of our comments we have relied mainly on the occurrence of consistent patterns in different registries.

Most of the comments about special features of the findings for a particular registry are discussed in a more general context in Chapter 2.

Finally, a brief bibliography of previous publications by the registry or from the region/country concerned on the descriptive epidemiology of childhood cancers in that region/country, is also included.

4.4.4 Summary tables

Age-standardized and cumulative rates. These rates for males, females and both sexes combined are shown for each diagnostic group, and for certain subgroups for 65 populations. Rates based on fewer than 10 cases are shown in light type. Where no cases were present, a '−' is shown. As already mentioned, incidence rates for four registries (Bulawayo, Fiji, Ibadan, Kampala) should be considered as approximations. They are given only for the 12 major diagnostic groups.

Ratio tables. These express the simple ratios of *numbers* of cases in different diagnostic categories within the same registry. Since this calculation requires only that numbers of cases are known (the population at risk is not required), the ratio tables include entries for *all* registries, not just for those which are population-based. Only those data sets for which a main table (section 4.4.1) has been produced are used as entries in the ratio tables.

Where one of the categories used to calculate the ratio contains no cases, a '−' is entered in the table.

Three tables have been prepared, as follows:

1. *Lymphoma distribution.* This summarizes the percentage contributions to the category Lymphomas and other reticuloendothelial neoplasms (Group II) of Hodgkin's disease, Burkitt's lymphoma and Other lymphomas.

2. *Lymphoma:leukaemia ratio.* This shows the ratio of the number of cases of lymphoma (Group II) to leukaemia (Group I).

3. *Embryonal and bone tumour ratios.* The cases for males and females have been combined. The following three figures are shown for each centre:
   — the ratio of neuroblastoma to Wilms' tumour,
   — the ratio of retinoblastoma to Wilms' tumour,
   — the ratio of Ewing's sarcoma to osteosarcoma.

4.4.5 Appendix tables

Five sets of appendix tables are included, to provide further details on certain of the diagnostic subgroups, and particularly the precise breakdown of the total number of cases by histological type (or site).

Miscellaneous intracranial and intraspinal neoplasms (Group IIIe). This category contains certain well-defined histological and clinical entities (e.g., craniopharyngioma, pinealoma), as well as malignant neoplasms of undetermined nature, and intranant neoplasms of undetermined nature, and intracranial neoplasms of benign or uncertain nature with no histological diagnosis (ICD-O codes 9990/0 and 9990/1). The table shows the breakdown of registered cases into eight histologically defined categories.

Soft tissue sarcomas (Group IX). The table shows the breakdown of registered cases into 11 histologically defined categories, nine of which are subsumed in the subgroup 'Other soft-tissue sarcomas' (Group IXc) in the main tables.

Melanoma (Group XId). The site of registered melanomatous neoplasms (ICD-O codes 8720-8780) is given, including the numbers of ocular melanomas.

Miscellaneous carcinomas. This table shows the location of the miscellaneous carcinomas and malignant epithelial neoplasms which fall into Group XI, with the exclusion of the melanomas.

It should be noted that carcinomas of certain organs appear in other diagnostic groups, e.g., Renal carcinoma (VIb), Hepatic carcinoma (VIIb), Gonadal carcinoma (Xc), and so do not feature in this table.

Other and unspecified tumours. The sites of these tumours are shown. The category includes a few rare tumours of specified cell type (e.g., mesothelial neoplasms), but the great majority are unspecified (ICD-O codes 8000 and 9990).

References

American Cancer Society (1968) *Manual of tumour nomenclature and coding*, New York, NY

College of American Pathologists (1965) *Systematized nomenclature of pathology*, Chicago, IL

Day, N.E. (1982) *Cumulative rate and cumulative risk*. In: Waterhouse, J., Muir, C., Shanmugaratnam, K. & Powell, J., eds, *Cancer Incidence in Five Continents*, Vol. IV (*IARC Scientific Publications* No.42), Lyon, International Agency for Research on Cancer, pp. 668-670

Tuyns, A.J. (1968) Studies on cancer relative frequencies (ratio studies): A method for computing an age-standardized cancer ratio. *Int. J. Cancer*, *3*, 397-403

Waterhouse, J., Muir, C.S., Correa, P. & Powell, J., eds (1976) *Cancer Incidence in Five Continents*, Vol. III (*IARC Scientific Publications* No.15), Lyon, International Agency for Research on Cancer

Waterhouse, J., Muir, C.S., Shanmugaratnam, K. & Powell, J., eds (1982) *Cancer Incidence in Five Continents*, Vol. IV (*IARC Scientific Publications* No.42), Lyon, International Agency for Research on Cancer

5. LIST OF TABLES

AFRICA

Madagascar	Institut Pasteur, 1959-1983[1]
Malawi	Histopathology Registry, 1976-1980[1]
Morocco	Children's Hospital, Rabat, 1983-1985[1]
Nigeria	Ibadan, 1960-1984[1]
	1960-1969[2]
Sudan	Radiation and Isotope Centre, Khartoum
	Arab, 1967-1984[1,4]
	Sudanic, 1967-1984[1,4]
Tanzania	1980-1981[1]
Tunisia	Institut Salah-Azaiz, 1969-1982[1]
Uganda	Kampala, 1968-1982[1]
	1968-1982[2]
	West Nile, 1961-1978[1]
Zimbabwe	Bulawayo, 1963-1977[1,4]
	Bulawayo, residents only, 1963-1977[2,4]

NORTH AMERICA

Canada	Atlantic Provinces, 1970-1979
	Western Provinces, 1970-1979
USA	Greater Delaware Valley,
	White, 1970-1979
	Non-White, 1970-1979
	Los Angeles,
	Black, 1972-1983
	Hispanic, 1972-1983
	Other White, 1972-1983
	New York (City and State),
	White, 1976-1982
	Black, 1976-1982
	SEER Program,
	White, 1973-1982
	Black, 1973-1982

CENTRAL AND SOUTH AMERICA AND CARIBBEAN

Brazil	Fortaleza, 1978-1980
	Recife, 1967-1979
	São Paulo, 1969-1978
Colombia	Cali, 1977-1981
Costa Rica	1980-1983
Cuba	1970-1981
Jamaica	1968-1981
Puerto Rico	1973-1982

ASIA

Bangladesh	Cancer Epidemiology Research Program,
	1970-1981[1]
China	Shanghai, 1972-1979
	Taipei, 1983-1984
Hong Kong	1974-1979
India	Bangalore, 1982-1984
	Bombay Cancer Registry, 1970-1979
	Tata Memorial Hospital,
	Bombay, 1970-1979[1]
Indonesia	Yogyakarta Pathology Registry,
	1973-1983[1]
Iraq	Baghdad, 1976-1984[1]
Israel	Jews, 1970-1979
	Non-Jews, 1970-1979
Japan	Kanagawa, 1975-1979
	Miyagi, 1971-1979
	Osaka, 1971-1980
Kuwait	Kuwaiti, 1974-1982
	Non-Kuwaiti, 1974-1982
Pakistan	Jinnah Post Graduate Medical Centre,
	1979-1983[1]
Philippines	Metro Manila and Rizal Province,
	1980-1982
Singapore	Chinese, 1968-1982
	Malay, 1968-1982
Thailand	1971-1980[1]
Viet Nam	Ho Chi Minh City, 1976-1980[1,4]

EUROPE

Czechoslovakia	Slovakia, 1970-1979
Denmark	1978-1982
Finland	1970-1979
France	Bas Rhin, 1975-1984
	Paediatric Registries, 1983-1985
	Lorraine, 1983-1985[2]
	Provence-Alpes-Côte-d'Azur and
	Corsica, 1984-1985[2]
German D.R.	1976-1980
Germany F.R.	Children's Tumour Registry, 1982-1984
	Saarland, 1967-1982
Hungary	1975-1984
Italy	Torino, 1967-1981

—23—

---

[1]Table without rates
[2]Short table with rates
[3]Leukaemia only
[4]Age-group '0-4' for numbers of cases (special format)

AFRICA

MADAGASCAR

Anatomo-Pathology Laboratory, Institut Pasteur, 1959–1983

P. Coulanges

The series comprises all the cases of childhood cancer diagnosed on the basis of histopathology in the laboratories of the Institut Pasteur for a 25-year period, 1959-1983. A description of the service provided by the anatomo-pathology service of the Institut Pasteur of Madagascar has been published (Coulanges et al., 1979). The laboratory has provided a pathology service (primarily histopathology) for the island continuously since 1954. Between 1954 and 1968, it was the only such facility in the island, and provided a free service to all hospitals and clinics. In 1968 a pathology department was opened in the Befelatanana General Hospital in the capital, Tananarive, and another soon afterwards in the military hospital (Girard et Robic), also in the capital. After 1976, when a University chair in anatomo-pathology was created, the Institut officially provided a service for three of the six provinces only (Tuléar, Fianarantsoa and Diégo Suarez). In fact, it continued to receive specimens from the whole island, and since 1981, the Institut Pasteur has again taken over the work arising from the General Hospital and now provides a histopathology service for the whole island. Until 1968, specimens were also received from Reunion and the Comoros.

Almost all the histopathology work of the laboratory concerns biopsy material derived from surgical procedures; cytological and bone marrow specimens are rare (only three cases of leukaemia appear in the series), and necropsy examinations are very infrequent. Furthermore, major surgical procedures such as thoracic surgery and neurosurgery are carried out only in the capital; the level of experience and competence in provincial hospitals is very variable.

Madagascar is a large island (587 000 square kilometres) in the Indian Ocean. The majority of the country is a high plateau at an altitude of 1000–2000 m. On the east coast, in the north, the climate is moist and tropical; in the west, the climate is dry and tropical, with a semi-desert region in the south. The country is predominantly agricultural, with a few industries in the major towns.

The inhabitants (Malagaches) are a homogeneous group, speaking a single language, and are ethnically of Indonesian origin. There are 19 family or tribal groupings of various sizes. Approximately 80% of the population are Christian, the remainder predominantly animist with very few Moslems (mainly from the Comoros).

The population at the census of 1975 was estimated at 7.53 million, of whom 44.5% were aged less than 15. Approximately 98.6% of the population are Malagaches. The series reported here comprises 555 cases, of whom approximately 89% are Malagaches and 7% Comorians; there were 11 cases in Europeans and other races.

Several previous reports of results relating to cancers diagnosed in the laboratory have been published (Brygoo & Dodin, 1967; Mayoux et al., 1970; Coulanges et al., 1979).

Commentary

The data are presented as numbers of cases and relative frequencies only since, although the Institut Pasteur provides a histopathology service for the whole of Madagascar, it is not a population-based registry. There were only three cases of leukaemia in the series, and only 10 brain and spinal tumours. These very low numbers are almost certainly not a true reflection of the incidence rates for these two diagnostic groups. The largest diagnostic group was the lymphomas, accounting for 38% of all cases; for almost half of these, the sections have been recently reviewed and reclassified. Over half were non-Hodgkin lymphomas and a quarter were Hodgkin's disease; only 9% of lymphomas were of the Burkitt's type. The second largest diagnostic group was retinoblastoma (19% of the total); of the 107 cases, 92 (86%) were stated to be unilateral and

Contd p. 28

—25—

Madagascar, Institut Pasteur   1959 – 1983   MALE

DIAGNOSTIC GROUP	NUMBER OF CASES					REL. FREQUENCY (%)			HV (%)
	0	1-4	5-9	10-14	All	Crude	Adj.	Group	
TOTAL	8	117	104	84	313	100.0	100.0	100.0	
I. LEUKAEMIAS	0	1	1	1	3	1.0	1.0	100.0	100.0
Acute lymphocytic	0	0	0	1	1	0.3	0.4	33.3	100.0
Other lymphocytic	0	0	0	0	0	-	-	-	-
Acute non-lymphocytic	0	0	0	0	0	-	-	-	-
Chronic myeloid	0	0	0	0	0	-	-	-	-
Other and unspecified	0	1	1	0	2	0.6	0.6	66.7	100.0
II. LYMPHOMAS	2	30	62	47	141	45.0	44.9	100.0	100.0
Hodgkin's disease	0	6	19	18	43	13.7	13.8	30.5	100.0
Non-Hodgkin lymphoma	1	18	34	26	79	25.2	25.2	56.0	100.0
Burkitt's lymphoma	0	3	7	1	11	3.5	3.3	7.8	100.0
Unspecified lymphoma	0	3	1	2	6	1.9	2.0	4.3	100.0
Histiocytosis X	1	0	0	0	1	0.3	0.3	0.7	100.0
Other reticuloendothelial	0	0	1	0	1	0.3	0.3	0.7	100.0
III. BRAIN AND SPINAL	1	0	3	0	4	1.3	1.2	100.0	100.0
Ependymoma	0	0	0	0	0	-	-	-	
Astrocytoma	0	0	2	0	2	0.6	0.6	50.0	100.0
Medulloblastoma	0	0	0	0	0	-	-	-	
Other glioma	1	0	1	0	2	0.6	0.6	50.0	100.0
Other and unspecified *	0	0	0	0	0	-	-	-	
IV. SYMPATHETIC N.S.	0	0	3	0	3	1.0	0.9	100.0	100.0
Neuroblastoma	0	0	3	0	3	1.0	0.9	100.0	100.0
Other	0	0	0	0	0	-	-	-	
V. RETINOBLASTOMA	1	42	6	1	50	16.0	15.8	100.0	100.0
VI. KIDNEY	1	15	8	2	26	8.3	8.1	100.0	100.0
Wilms' tumour	1	15	7	2	25	8.0	7.9	96.2	100.0
Renal carcinoma	0	0	1	0	1	0.3	0.3	3.8	100.0
Other and unspecified	0	0	0	0	0	-	-	-	
VII. LIVER	0	1	0	1	2	0.6	0.7	100.0	100.0
Hepatoblastoma	0	0	0	0	0	-	-	-	
Hepatic carcinoma	0	1	0	1	2	0.6	0.7	100.0	100.0
Other and unspecified	0	0	0	0	0	-	-	-	
VIII. BONE	0	3	5	10	18	5.8	6.0	100.0	100.0
Osteosarcoma	0	0	1	7	8	2.6	2.8	44.4	100.0
Chondrosarcoma	0	0	0	0	0	-	-	-	
Ewing's sarcoma	0	1	3	2	6	1.9	1.9	33.3	100.0
Other and unspecified	0	2	1	1	4	1.3	1.3	22.2	100.0
IX. SOFT TISSUE SARCOMAS	1	14	14	10	39	12.5	12.4	100.0	100.0
Rhabdomyosarcoma	0	6	3	0	9	2.9	2.8	23.1	100.0
Fibrosarcoma	0	1	5	4	10	3.2	3.2	25.6	100.0
Other and unspecified	1	7	6	6	20	6.4	6.4	51.3	100.0
X. GONADAL & GERM CELL	1	5	1	2	9	2.9	2.9	100.0	100.0
Non-gonadal germ cell	0	0	1	0	1	0.3	0.3	11.1	100.0
Gonadal germ cell	1	4	0	1	6	1.9	2.0	66.7	100.0
Gonadal carcinoma	0	1	0	0	1	0.3	0.3	11.1	100.0
Other and unspecified	0	0	0	1	1	0.3	0.4	11.1	100.0
XI. EPITHELIAL NEOPLASMS	1	1	0	9	11	3.5	3.9	100.0	100.0
Adrenocortical carcinoma	0	0	0	0	0	-	-	-	
Thyroid carcinoma	0	0	0	1	1	0.3	0.4	9.1	100.0
Nasopharyngeal carcinoma	0	0	0	1	1				
Melanoma	0	1	0	3	4	1.3	1.4	36.4	100.0
Other carcinoma	1	0	0	5	6	1.9	2.1	54.5	100.0
XII. OTHER	0	5	1	1	7	2.2	2.2	100.0	100.0

* Specified as malignant

FEMALE

Madagascar, Institut Pasteur   1959 – 1983

DIAGNOSTIC GROUP	NUMBER OF CASES					REL. FREQUENCY(%)			HV(%)
	0	1-4	5-9	10-14	All	Crude	Adj.	Group	
TOTAL	14	103	62	63	242	100.0	100.0	100.0	100.0
I. LEUKAEMIAS	0	0	0	0	0	–	–	–	–
Acute lymphocytic	0	0	0	0	0	–	–	–	–
Other lymphocytic	0	0	0	0	0	–	–	–	–
Acute non-lymphocytic	0	0	0	0	0	–	–	–	–
Chronic myeloid	0	0	0	0	0	–	–	–	–
Other and unspecified	0	0	0	0	0	–	–	–	–
II. LYMPHOMAS	4	20	24	25	73	30.2	31.7	100.0	100.0
Hodgkin's disease	0	1	6	3	10	4.1	4.7	13.7	100.0
Non-Hodgkin lymphoma	2	13	11	17	43	17.8	18.5	58.9	100.0
Burkitt's lymphoma	0	1	4	3	8	3.3	3.7	11.0	100.0
Unspecified lymphoma	1	2	2	1	6	2.5	2.5	8.2	100.0
Histiocytosis X	1	1	0	0	2	0.8	0.7	2.7	100.0
Other reticuloendothelial	0	2	1	1	4	1.7	1.6	5.5	100.0
III. BRAIN AND SPINAL	0	0	3	2	5	2.1	2.4	100.0	100.0
Ependymoma	0	0	0	0	0	–	–	–	–
Astrocytoma	0	0	1	1	2	0.8	1.0	40.0	100.0
Medulloblastoma	0	0	1	0	1	0.4	0.5	20.0	100.0
Other glioma	0	0	0	1	1	0.4	0.5	20.0	100.0
Other and unspecified *	0	0	1	0	1	0.4	0.5	20.0	100.0
IV. SYMPATHETIC N.S.	0	0	4	1	5	2.1	2.4	100.0	100.0
Neuroblastoma	0	0	4	1	5	2.1	2.4	100.0	100.0
Other	0	0	0	0	0	–	–	–	–
V. RETINOBLASTOMA	0	45	8	3	56	23.1	20.7	100.0	100.0
VI. KIDNEY	1	14	6	1	22	9.1	8.5	100.0	100.0
Wilms' tumour	1	14	6	1	22	9.1	8.5	100.0	100.0
Renal carcinoma	0	0	0	0	0	–	–	–	–
Other and unspecified	0	0	0	0	0	–	–	–	–
VII. LIVER	0	1	1	1	3	1.2	1.3	100.0	100.0
Hepatoblastoma	0	0	0	0	0	–	–	–	–
Hepatic carcinoma	0	1	0	1	2	0.8	0.8	66.7	100.0
Other and unspecified	0	0	1	0	1	0.4	0.5	33.3	100.0
VIII. BONE	1	3	3	3	10	4.1	4.2	100.0	100.0
Osteosarcoma	1	3	2	0	6	2.5	2.6	60.0	100.0
Chondrosarcoma	0	0	0	0	0	–	–	–	–
Ewing's sarcoma	0	0	1	2	3	1.2	1.3	30.0	100.0
Other and unspecified	0	0	0	1	1	0.4	0.3	10.0	100.0
IX. SOFT TISSUE SARCOMAS	5	11	5	12	33	13.6	13.6	100.0	100.0
Rhabdomyosarcoma	1	5	3	0	9	3.7	3.5	27.3	100.0
Fibrosarcoma	2	5	0	4	11	4.5	4.3	33.3	100.0
Other and unspecified	2	1	2	8	13	5.4	5.8	39.4	100.0
X. GONADAL & GERM CELL	2	1	5	8	16	6.6	7.3	100.0	100.0
Non-gonadal germ cell	1	0	0	1	2	0.8	0.8	12.5	100.0
Gonadal germ cell	1	1	1	4	7	2.9	3.1	43.8	100.0
Gonadal carcinoma	0	0	2	3	5	2.1	2.4	31.3	100.0
Other and unspecified	0	0	2	0	2	0.8	1.0	12.5	100.0
XI. EPITHELIAL NEOPLASMS	0	1	0	4	5	2.1	2.2	100.0	100.0
Adrenocortical carcinoma	0	0	0	0	0	–	–	–	–
Thyroid carcinoma	0	0	0	0	0	–	–	–	–
Nasopharyngeal carcinoma	0	0	0	0	0	–	–	–	–
Melanoma	0	0	0	2	2	0.8	1.0	40.0	100.0
Other carcinoma	0	1	0	2	3	1.2	1.3	60.0	100.0
XII. OTHER	1	7	3	3	14	5.8	5.6	100.0	100.0
* Specified as malignant	0	0	1	0	1	0.4	0.5	100.0	100.0

only one (1%) bilateral; laterality was not given for
the remaining 14 (13%). Kidney tumours, nearly all
of which were Wilms' tumour, were slightly less
than half as frequent as retinoblastoma. Neuroblastoma and liver tumours were both very rare.

References

Brygoo, E.R. & Dodin, A. (1967) Le cancer à Madagascar. A
    propos de cinq mille sept cent quatre vingt cas diag-
    nostiqués à l'Institut Pasteur de Madagascar de 1954 à
    1966 inclus. *Méd. trop.*, *27*, 139-149

Coulanges, P., Rakotonirina-Randriambeloma, P.J., Gueguen,
    A. & Randriamalala, J.C. (1979) Le cancer à Madagascar.
    Arch. Inst. Pasteur, Madagascar, *48*, 171-212

Mayoux, A.M., Coulanges, P. & Brygoo E.R. (1970) Les
    tumeurs solides de l'enfant et du jeune adulte à Mada-
    gascar. *Arch. Inst. Pasteur, Madagascar*, *39*, 141-172

MALAWI

Register of Tumour Pathology, 1976–1980

M.S.R. Hutt

In 1968 the only resident histopathologist in Malawi left the country, and arrangements were therefore made whereby all the diagnostic pathology for the country was done in St Thomas's Hospital, London. A description of this unusual service has been published recently (Hutt & Spencer, 1982). The data presented here represent information derived from tissue specimens diagnosed as malignant during the five-year period 1976-1980, from governmental and mission hospitals throughout the country. Haematological specimens and bone-marrow biopsies are not included. An attempt has been made to eliminate duplicate specimens derived from the same case.

The data reproduced here are for the 238 cases of malignant disease where the age of the patient was recorded as 0–14 (or specified as 'child').

The population of Malawi at the 1977 census was given as 5.5 million, of whom 44.6% were children (1.23 million boys and 1.25 million girls). The crude rate of incidence (all sites combined) can be estimated from these figures as 19.1 per million (both sexes); this is clearly a considerable under-estimate of the true rate, and indicates the restricted and probably selective nature of hospital attendance and biopsy of cancer cases.

Commentary

For the reasons explained above, only one case of leukaemia is included in the data from this registry; no brain tumours were registered. Of the 238 registered cases, 85 (36%) were lymphomas, 53 being Burkitt's lymphoma, while 12 cases of Kaposi's sarcoma were registered, all in boys. Retinoblastoma, which accounts for 25 (11%) of the registered tumours, appears to have a high frequency but the degree of incompleteness of registration makes it difficult to be sure of this; no information on the laterality of these tumours is available. Three of the miscellaneous carcinomas were in the bladder.

Reference

Hutt, M.S.R. & Spencer, H. (1982) Histopathology services for developing countries. *Br. med. J.*, *283*, 1327-1329

Malawi, Histopathology Registry   1976 - 1980   MALE

DIAGNOSTIC GROUP	NUMBER OF CASES					REL. FREQUENCY(%)			HV(%)
	0	1-4	5-9	10-14	All	Crude	Adj.	Group	
TOTAL	1	38	58	41	138	100.0	100.0	100.0	100.0
I. LEUKAEMIAS	0	0	0	0	0	—	—	—	—
Acute lymphocytic	0	0	0	0	0	—	—	—	—
Other lymphocytic	0	0	0	0	0	—	—	—	—
Acute non-lymphocytic	0	0	0	0	0	—	—	—	—
Chronic myeloid	0	0	0	0	0	—	—	—	—
Other and unspecified	0	0	0	0	0	—	—	—	—
II. LYMPHOMAS	0	6	28	23	57	41.3	37.5	100.0	100.0
Hodgkin's disease	0	0	1	2	3	2.2	2.0	5.3	100.0
Non-Hodgkin lymphoma	0	3	1	0	4	2.9	2.3	7.0	100.0
Burkitt's lymphoma	0	5	18	13	36	26.1	24.0	63.2	100.0
Unspecified lymphoma	0	1	6	7	14	10.1	9.3	24.6	100.0
Histiocytosis X	0	0	0	0	0	.	—	—	—
Other reticuloendothelial	0	0	0	0	0	—	—	—	—
III. BRAIN AND SPINAL	0	0	0	0	0	—	—	—	—
Ependymoma	0	0	0	0	0	—	—	—	—
Astrocytoma	0	0	0	0	0	—	—	—	—
Medulloblastoma	0	0	0	0	0	—	—	—	—
Other glioma	0	0	0	0	0	—	—	—	—
Other and unspecified *	0	0	0	0	0	—	—	—	—
IV. SYMPATHETIC N.S.	0	2	0	0	2	1.4	2.1	100.0	100.0
Neuroblastoma	0	2	0	0	2	1.4	2.1	100.0	100.0
Other	0	0	0	0	0	—	—	—	—
V. RETINOBLASTOMA	0	10	4	0	14	10.1	12.3	100.0	100.0
VI. KIDNEY	0	9	6	1	16	11.6	13.1	100.0	100.0
Wilms' tumour	0	9	6	1	16	11.6	13.1	100.0	100.0
Renal carcinoma	0	0	0	0	0	—	—	—	—
Other and unspecified	0	0	0	0	0	—	—	—	—
VII. LIVER	0	0	0	0	0	—	—	—	—
Hepatoblastoma	0	0	0	0	0	—	—	—	—
Hepatic carcinoma	0	0	0	0	0	—	—	—	—
Other and unspecified	0	0	0	0	0	—	—	—	—
VIII.BONE	0	0	3	6	9	6.5	5.9	100.0	100.0
Osteosarcoma	0	0	3	2	5	3.6	3.0	55.6	100.0
Chondrosarcoma	0	0	0	0	0	—	—	—	—
Ewing's sarcoma	0	0	0	0	0	—	—	—	—
Other and unspecified	0	0	0	4	4	2.9	2.9	44.4	100.0
IX. SOFT TISSUE SARCOMAS	1	9	9	7	26	18.8	20.0	100.0	100.0
Rhabdomyosarcoma	1	3	4	2	10	7.2	7.6	38.5	100.0
Fibrosarcoma	0	1	0	1	2	1.4	1.8	7.7	100.0
Other and unspecified	0	5	5	4	14	10.1	10.6	53.8	100.0
X. GONADAL & GERM CELL	0	1	0	0	1	0.7	1.0	100.0	100.0
Non-gonadal germ cell	0	0	0	0	0	—	—	—	—
Gonadal germ cell	0	1	0	0	1	0.7	1.0	100.0	100.0
Gonadal carcinoma	0	0	0	0	0	—	—	—	—
Other and unspecified	0	0	0	0	0	—	—	—	—
XI. EPITHELIAL NEOPLASMS	0	1	6	3	10	7.2	6.3	100.0	100.0
Adrenocortical carcinoma	0	0	1	0	1	0.7	0.5	10.0	100.0
Thyroid carcinoma	0	0	0	0	0	—	—	—	—
Nasopharyngeal carcinoma	0	0	0	2	2	1.4	1.5	20.0	100.0
Melanoma	0	0	1	0	1	0.7	0.5	10.0	100.0
Other carcinoma	0	1	4	1	6	4.3	3.8	60.0	100.0
XII. OTHER	0	0	2	1	3	2.2	1.8	100.0	100.0
	0	0	0	0	0	—	—	—	—

* Specified as malignant
¤ Includes age unknown

FEMALE

Malawi, Histopathology Registry   1976 – 1980

DIAGNOSTIC GROUP	NUMBER OF CASES					REL. FREQUENCY(%)			HV(%)
	0	1-4	5-9	10-14	All	Crude	Adj.	Group	
TOTAL	4	29	29	37	100¤	100.0	100.0	100.0	100.0
I. LEUKAEMIAS	0	0	1	0	1	1.0	1.0	100.0	100.0
Acute lymphocytic	0	0	0	0	0	-	-	-	-
Other lymphocytic	0	0	0	0	0	-	-	-	-
Acute non-lymphocytic	0	0	0	0	0	-	-	-	-
Chronic myeloid	0	0	0	0	0	-	-	-	-
Other and unspecified	0	0	1	0	1	1.0	1.0	100.0	100.0
II. LYMPHOMAS	0	3	13	12	28	28.0	26.8	100.0	100.0
Hodgkin's disease	0	1	1	1	3	3.0	3.1	10.7	100.0
Non-Hodgkin lymphoma	0	1	10	6	17	17.0	16.4	60.7	100.0
Burkitt's lymphoma	0	1	2	5	8	8.0	7.3	28.6	100.0
Unspecified lymphoma	0	0	0	0	0	-	-	-	-
Histiocytosis X	0	0	0	0	0	-	-	-	-
Other reticuloendothelial	0	0	0	0	0	-	-	-	-
III. BRAIN AND SPINAL	0	0	0	0	0	-	-	-	-
Ependymoma	0	0	0	0	0	-	-	-	-
Astrocytoma	0	0	0	0	0	-	-	-	-
Medulloblastoma	0	0	0	0	0	-	-	-	-
Other glioma	0	0	0	0	0	-	-	-	-
Other and unspecified *	0	0	0	0	0	-	-	-	-
IV. SYMPATHETIC N.S.	1	1	0	1	3	3.0	3.2	100.0	100.0
Neuroblastoma	1	1	0	1	3	3.0	3.2	100.0	100.0
Other	0	0	0	0	0	-	-	-	-
V. RETINOBLASTOMA	1	7	3	0	11	11.0	12.8	100.0	100.0
VI. KIDNEY	0	8	2	2	12	12.0	13.4	100.0	100.0
Wilms' tumour	0	8	2	1	11	11.0	12.6	91.7	100.0
Renal carcinoma	0	0	0	0	0	-	-	-	-
Other and unspecified	0	0	0	1	1	1.0	0.8	8.3	100.0
VII. LIVER	1	0	0	2	3	3.0	2.8	100.0	100.0
Hepatoblastoma	1	0	0	0	1	1.0	1.2	33.3	100.0
Hepatic carcinoma	0	0	0	2	2	2.0	1.6	66.7	100.0
Other and unspecified	0	0	0	0	0	-	-	-	-
VIII. BONE	0	0	0	2	3¤	3.0	1.6	100.0	100.0
Osteosarcoma	0	0	0	2	3¤	3.0	1.6	100.0	100.0
Chondrosarcoma	0	0	0	0	0	-	-	-	-
Ewing's sarcoma	0	0	0	0	0	-	-	-	-
Other and unspecified	0	0	0	0	0	-	-	-	-
IX. SOFT TISSUE SARCOMAS	1	6	5	2	14	14.0	15.3	100.0	100.0
Rhabdomyosarcoma	1	5	3	0	9	9.0	10.4	64.3	100.0
Fibrosarcoma	0	1	2	0	3	3.0	2.7	21.4	100.0
Other and unspecified	0	0	0	2	2	2.0	2.2	14.3	100.0
X. GONADAL & GERM CELL	0	0	1	0	1	1.0	1.0	100.0	100.0
Non-gonadal germ cell	0	0	1	0	1	1.0	1.0	100.0	100.0
Gonadal germ cell	0	0	0	0	0	-	-	-	-
Gonadal carcinoma	0	0	0	0	0	-	-	-	-
Other and unspecified	0	0	0	0	0	-	-	-	-
XI. EPITHELIAL NEOPLASMS	0	4	3	13	20	20.0	18.5	100.0	100.0
Adrenocortical carcinoma	0	0	0	0	0	-	-	-	-
Thyroid carcinoma	0	0	0	0	0	-	-	-	-
Nasopharyngeal carcinoma	0	0	2	0	2	2.0	2.1	10.0	100.0
Melanoma	0	4	1	13	18	18.0	16.4	90.0	100.0
Other carcinoma	0	0	0	0	0	-	-	-	-
XII. OTHER	0	0	1	3	4	4.0	3.5	100.0	-

* Specified as malignant
¤ Includes age unknown

MOROCCO

Rabat: Hospital for Children, 1983–1985

F. Msefer Alaoui

The Hospital for Children in Rabat provides specialized services for the northern part of the country, where over 94% of the patients live. The hospital has 500 beds and, in addition to general paediatrics, has specialized units for gastro-enterology, nephrology, oncohaematology and children's surgery. In 1985, there were almost 14 000 new admissions. The hospital is part of a university hospital complex in which, in addition, there are two maternity hospitals, a general hospital (medicine and surgery), a specialist hospital (ENT, ophthalmology, neurology, neurosurgery), a psychiatric hospital, a tuberculosis hospital, a hospital for rheumatology and rehabilitation, and the National Institute for Oncology. The Institute does not admit children, but is responsible for the radiotherapy of children in the other hospitals (including the Hospital for Children).

The cases included in the series here represent those treated for cancer at the Hospital for Children over a three-year period, and also cases of childhood cancer diagnosed and treated in the ophthalmology and otorhinolaryngology services of the neighbouring specialist hospital. However, cases treated in the neurosurgical departments of this latter hospital and of the main general hospital of the city are not included. With the exception of many brain tumours, it is likely that most children receiving in-patient treatment for cancer in the region of Rabat and the northern part of Morocco are included in this series. However, many children with cancer never receive hospital treatment. This is due to the large distances that patients may have to travel and the difficulties of doing so, and the continued use of traditional medicine. Many cases arrive at hospital at an advanced stage of the disease, and have very short survival times; it is probable that a large number die without ever reaching hospital.

The cases are all Moroccan, of the Moslem religion, and predominantly of middle to low socioeconomic status.

The size of the population from which the cases are drawn is unknown. In 1985, the total population of the country was approximately 22 million, about 46% of whom were children; the distribution of this childhood population by age-group was 38% aged 0–4, 32% aged 5–9 and 30% aged 10–14.

Commentary

As the data are drawn mainly from the Hospital for Children, it seems likely that under-ascertainment would be more pronounced in the 10–14 age-group. The largest diagnostic group was the lymphomas. Of these, 34% were Hodgkin disease, 46% non-Hodgkin lymphoma and 21% Burkitt's lymphoma. The ratio of males to females for both Hodgkin's disease and non-Hodgkin's lymphoma was over 4, but Burkitt's lymphoma had a sex ratio of only 1.3. Wilms' tumour was the most frequent embryonal tumour, and there was a somewhat smaller number of neuroblastomas. Retinoblastoma may be somewhat under-enumerated since most of the cases included in this series were those admitted to hospital for enucleation, and many parents refuse such treatment. There were 12 cases (3% of the series) of nasopharyngeal carcinoma; as this tumour occurs mainly in the 10–14 age-group, this may be an underestimate of the true relative frequency.

Morocco, Children's Hospital, Rabat   1983 – 1985   MALE

DIAGNOSTIC GROUP	NUMBER OF CASES					REL. FREQUENCY(%)			HV(%)
	0	1-4	5-9	10-14	All	Crude	Adj.	Group	
TOTAL	14	105	105	67	296¤	100.0	100.0	100.0	90.8
I. LEUKAEMIAS	5	19	28	18	70	23.6	24.1	100.0	100.0
Acute lymphocytic	1	14	23	13	51	17.2	17.4	72.9	100.0
Other lymphocytic	0	0	0	0	0	-	-	-	-
Acute non-lymphocytic	3	3	3	3	14	4.7	4.8	20.0	100.0
Chronic myeloid	0	0	0	2	2	0.7	0.9	2.9	100.0
Other and unspecified	1	2	0	0	3	1.0	1.0	4.3	100.0
II. LYMPHOMAS	0	30	51	29	112¤	37.8	37.6	100.0	91.1
Hodgkin's disease	0	4	22	14	41¤	13.9	13.9	36.6	100.0
Non-Hodgkin lymphoma	0	21	22	10	54¤	18.2	17.8	48.2	81.5
Burkitt's lymphoma	0	5	7	5	17	5.7	5.9	15.2	100.0
Unspecified lymphoma	0	0	0	0	0	-	-	-	-
Histiocytosis X	0	0	0	0	0	-	-	-	-
Other reticuloendothelial	0	0	0	0	0	-	-	-	-
III. BRAIN AND SPINAL	0	5	1	1	7	2.4	2.4	100.0	42.9
Ependymoma	0	0	0	0	0	-	-	-	-
Astrocytoma	0	2	0	1	3	1.0	1.1	42.9	66.7
Medulloblastoma	0	3	1	0	4	1.4	1.3	57.1	25.0
Other glioma	0	0	0	0	0	-	-	-	-
Other and unspecified *	0	0	0	0	0	-	-	-	-
IV. SYMPATHETIC N.S.	3	15	8	1	27	9.1	8.8	100.0	74.1
Neuroblastoma	3	15	7	1	26	8.8	8.5	96.3	73.1
Other	0	0	1	0	1	0.3	0.3	3.7	100.0
V. RETINOBLASTOMA	0	4	4	0	11¤	3.7	2.5	100.0	87.5
VI. KIDNEY	5	22	6	1	34	11.5	11.2	100.0	85.3
Wilms' tumour	5	22	6	0	33	11.1	10.8	97.1	84.8
Renal carcinoma	0	0	0	1	1	0.3	0.4	2.9	100.0
Other and unspecified	0	0	0	0	0	-	-	-	-
VII. LIVER	0	0	0	0	0	-	-	-	-
Hepatoblastoma	0	0	0	0	0	-	-	-	-
Hepatic carcinoma	0	0	0	0	0	-	-	-	-
Other and unspecified	0	0	0	0	0	-	-	-	-
VIII. BONE	0	0	3	5	8	2.7	3.1	100.0	100.0
Osteosarcoma	0	0	2	3	5	1.7	1.9	62.5	100.0
Chondrosarcoma	0	0	0	0	0	-	-	-	-
Ewing's sarcoma	0	0	1	1	2	0.7	0.7	25.0	100.0
Other and unspecified	0	0	0	1	1	0.3	0.4	12.5	100.0
IX. SOFT TISSUE SARCOMAS	0	6	1	1	8	2.7	2.8	100.0	100.0
Rhabdomyosarcoma	0	5	1	1	7	2.4	2.4	87.5	100.0
Fibrosarcoma	0	0	0	0	0	-	-	-	-
Other and unspecified	0	1	0	0	1	0.3	0.3	12.5	100.0
X. GONADAL & GERM CELL	1	3	0	0	4	1.4	1.3	100.0	100.0
Non-gonadal germ cell	0	0	0	0	0	-	-	-	-
Gonadal germ cell	1	3	0	0	4	1.4	1.3	100.0	100.0
Gonadal carcinoma	0	0	0	0	0	-	-	-	-
Other and unspecified	0	0	0	0	0	-	-	-	-
XI. EPITHELIAL NEOPLASMS	0	1	3	11	15	5.1	6.1	100.0	100.0
Adrenocortical carcinoma	0	0	0	0	0	-	-	-	-
Thyroid carcinoma	0	0	0	0	0	-	-	-	-
Nasopharyngeal carcinoma	0	0	2	7	9	3.0	3.7	60.0	100.0
Melanoma	0	0	0	0	0	-	-	-	-
Other carcinoma	0	1	1	4	6	2.0	2.4	40.0	100.0
XII. OTHER	0	0	0	0	0	-	-	-	-

* Specified as malignant
¤ Includes age unknown

Morocco, Children's Hospital, Rabat   1983 - 1985   FEMALE

DIAGNOSTIC GROUP	NUMBER OF CASES					REL. FREQUENCY(%)			HV(%)
	0	1-4	5-9	10-14	All	Crude	Adj.	Group	
TOTAL	8	66	38	32	148¤	100.0	100.0	100.0	88.2
I. LEUKAEMIAS	0	12	11	8	31	20.9	22.7	100.0	100.0
Acute lymphocytic	0	8	10	6	24	16.2	17.8	77.4	100.0
Other lymphocytic	0	0	0	0	0	-	-	-	-
Acute non-lymphocytic	0	2	0	1	3	2.0	2.0	9.7	100.0
Chronic myeloid	0	0	1	1	2	1.4	1.7	6.5	100.0
Other and unspecified	0	2	0	0	2	1.4	1.1	6.5	100.0
II. LYMPHOMAS	0	12	13	8	33	22.3	24.2	100.0	97.0
Hodgkin's disease	0	0	5	3	8	5.4	6.8	24.2	100.0
Non-Hodgkin lymphoma	0	8	2	2	12	8.1	7.8	36.4	91.7
Burkitt's lymphoma	0	4	6	3	13	8.8	9.7	39.4	100.0
Unspecified lymphoma	0	0	0	0	0	-	-	-	-
Histiocytosis X	0	0	0	0	0	-	-	-	-
Other reticuloendothelial	0	0	0	0	0	-	-	-	-
III. BRAIN AND SPINAL	0	4	1	3	8	5.4	5.8	100.0	25.0
Ependymoma	0	0	0	0	0	-	-	-	-
Astrocytoma	0	2	0	3	5	3.4	3.9	62.5	-
Medulloblastoma	0	1	1	0	2	1.4	1.3	25.0	50.0
Other glioma	0	1	0	0	1	0.7	0.5	12.5	100.0
Other and unspecified *	0	0	0	0	0	-	-	-	-
IV. SYMPATHETIC N.S.	1	9	3	0	13	8.8	7.8	100.0	84.6
Neuroblastoma	1	9	3	0	13	8.8	7.8	100.0	84.6
Other	0	0	0	0	0	-	-	-	-
V. RETINOBLASTOMA	1	3	2	0	10¤	6.8	3.7	100.0	50.0
VI. KIDNEY	5	13	2	1	21	14.2	12.2	100.0	81.0
Wilms' tumour	5	13	2	1	21	14.2	12.2	100.0	81.0
Renal carcinoma	0	0	0	0	0	-	-	-	-
Other and unspecified	0	0	0	0	0	-	-	-	-
VII. LIVER	0	3	0	0	3	2.0	1.6	100.0	66.7
Hepatoblastoma	0	3	0	0	3	2.0	1.6	100.0	66.7
Hepatic carcinoma	0	0	0	0	0	-	-	-	-
Other and unspecified	0	0	0	0	0	-	-	-	-
VIII. BONE	0	2	3	3	8	5.4	6.3	100.0	100.0
Osteosarcoma	0	0	2	0	2	1.4	1.6	25.0	100.0
Chondrosarcoma	0	0	0	1	1	0.7	0.9	12.5	100.0
Ewing's sarcoma	0	1	1	1	3	2.0	2.3	37.5	100.0
Other and unspecified	0	1	0	1	2	1.4	1.5	25.0	100.0
IX. SOFT TISSUE SARCOMAS	1	7	2	2	12	8.1	7.8	100.0	100.0
Rhabdomyosarcoma	0	7	2	2	11	7.4	7.2	91.7	100.0
Fibrosarcoma	1	0	0	0	1	0.7	0.5	8.3	100.0
Other and unspecified	0	0	0	0	0	-	-	-	-
X. GONADAL & GERM CELL	0	1	1	3	5	3.4	4.1	100.0	100.0
Non-gonadal germ cell	0	1	1	0	2	1.4	1.3	40.0	100.0
Gonadal germ cell	0	0	0	3	3	2.0	2.8	60.0	100.0
Gonadal carcinoma	0	0	0	0	0	-	-	-	-
Other and unspecified	0	0	0	0	0	-	-	-	-
XI. EPITHELIAL NEOPLASMS	0	0	0	4	4	2.7	3.8	100.0	100.0
Adrenocortical carcinoma	0	0	0	0	0	-	-	-	-
Thyroid carcinoma	0	0	0	0	0	-	-	-	-
Nasopharyngeal carcinoma	0	0	0	3	3	2.0	2.8	75.0	100.0
Melanoma	0	0	0	0	0	-	-	-	-
Other carcinoma	0	0	0	1	1	0.7	0.9	25.0	100.0
XII. OTHER	0	0	0	0	0	-	-	-	-

* Specified as malignant
¤ Includes age unknown

NIGERIA

Ibadan Cancer Registry, 1960–1984

T.A. Junaid & B.O. Babalola

The Cancer Registry of Ibadan was initiated in April 1960 by the late Professor G.M. Edington, the then head of the Pathology Department, University College Hospital (UCH), Ibadan, where the registry is located. The objective was to record cancer incidence in Ibadan and its environs for health planners, physicians in the teaching hospital and research workers. It was also hoped that the collected data would provide a basis for geographical comparisons of cancer incidence.

Case finding is effected through regular visits by Registry staff to clinics and wards of all hospitals in Ibadan, and by consultation of surgical pathology records, surgical operation lists and autopsy reports in UCH. Notification is voluntary.

All activities in the Registry are carried out manually and this causes considerable delay in data retrieval. In addition, financial support is limited to the payment of staff salaries by the University of Ibadan.

The Registry separates registrations of patients into Ibadan and non-Ibadan residents for the purpose of calculating rates. Ibadan residents are defined as persons who have been living in the city, which covers an area of about 70 square kilometres, for at least one year prior to diagnosis of cancer.

Although a national census was held in 1973, the figures are not available. The 1963 census figures give a population at risk of 627 379. Using an annual rate of growth of 2.5%, the present population of Ibadan has been estimated at about one million. Ibadan residents include Moslems, Christians and traditionalists; most, however, are Moslems. They are predominantly Yoruba, who engage in subsistence farming and small-scale trading. There is a growing number of small-scale and medium-sized industrial projects within and around the city. These include a motor assembly plant, breweries, soft-drink factories, a flour mill and food-processing plants. Air pollution is minimal but water pollution by human and animal wastes is widespread.

The Registry is aware that registration of cancer cases is incomplete, as the hospital and other health facilities in Ibadan are inadequate for complete coverage of the population. Consequently, a sizeable proportion of the population of this rural-cum-urban city relies on practitioners of traditional medicine; cancer data from this source are unobtainable.

An analysis of the relative frequencies of the principal types of childhood cancer during 1960–1972 was published by Williams (1975). These relative frequencies were compared by Olisa et al. (1975) with those observed in a series of black children in the United States and with registry data from the United Kingdom and Uganda. Estimates of childhood leukaemia incidence rates from a clinical survey carried out in 1978–1982 have also been published (Williams & Bangboye, 1983).

Because of the unavailability of population figures from the 1973 census, the data from the Registry are presented in two sets of tables. These are: (i) numbers of cases with rates (based on the 1963 census) for broad diagnostic groups, 1960–1969 only; (ii) numbers of cases and relative frequencies only, for the detailed diagnostic classification, covering the whole period 1960–1984.

Population

Population data are based on the 1963 census.

AVERAGE ANNUAL POPULATION: 1960–1969

Age	Male	Female
0–4	35897	35340
5–9	29437	30073
10–14	27036	23801
0–14	92370	89214

Contd p. 41

Nigeria, Ibadan   1960 - 1984   MALE

DIAGNOSTIC GROUP	NUMBER OF CASES					REL. FREQUENCY(%)			HV(%)
	0	1-4	5-9	10-14	All	Crude	Adj.	Group	
TOTAL	25	125	249	186	585	100.0	100.0	100.0	77.3
I. LEUKAEMIAS	0	10	20	30	60	10.3	9.9	100.0	60.0
Acute lymphocytic	0	6	7	9	22	3.8	3.9	36.7	81.8
Other lymphocytic	0	0	0	0	0	-	-	-	-
Acute non-lymphocytic	0	0	5	10	15	2.6	2.2	25.0	66.7
Chronic myeloid	0	1	1	1	3	0.5	0.5	5.0	100.0
Other and unspecified	0	3	7	10	20	3.4	3.3	33.3	25.0
II. LYMPHOMAS	3	37	178	131	349	59.7	53.2	100.0	75.6
Hodgkin's disease	0	3	10	15	28	4.8	4.4	8.0	89.3
Non-Hodgkin lymphoma	1	2	8	11	22	3.8	3.5	6.3	95.5
Burkitt's lymphoma	1	30	154	90	275	47.0	41.3	78.8	72.7
Unspecified lymphoma	1	2	6	15	24	4.1	3.9	6.9	75.0
Histiocytosis X	0	0	0	0	0	-	-	-	-
Other reticuloendothelial	0	0	0	0	0	-	-	-	-
III. BRAIN AND SPINAL	1	7	13	6	27	4.6	4.7	100.0	59.3
Ependymoma	0	0	0	0	0	-	-	-	-
Astrocytoma	0	2	4	0	6	1.0	1.0	22.2	100.0
Medulloblastoma	0	0	0	2	2	0.3	0.3	7.4	100.0
Other glioma	0	0	0	0	0	-	-	-	-
Other and unspecified *	1	5	9	4	19	3.2	3.3	70.4	42.1
IV. SYMPATHETIC N.S.	9	8	6	1	24	4.1	5.4	100.0	95.8
Neuroblastoma	9	8	6	1	24	4.1	5.4	100.0	95.8
Other	0	0	0	0	0	-	-	-	-
V. RETINOBLASTOMA	1	23	7	2	33	5.6	7.6	100.0	100.0
VI. KIDNEY	8	26	11	0	45	7.7	10.4	100.0	91.1
Wilms' tumour	7	24	10	0	41	7.0	9.5	91.1	95.1
Renal carcinoma	0	1	0	0	1	0.2	0.3	2.2	100.0
Other and unspecified	1	1	1	0	3	0.5	0.7	6.7	33.3
VII. LIVER	1	1	1	4	7	1.2	1.3	100.0	100.0
Hepatoblastoma	1	0	0	1	2	0.3	0.4	28.6	100.0
Hepatic carcinoma	0	1	1	3	5	0.9	0.9	71.4	100.0
Other and unspecified	0	0	0	0	0	-	-	-	-
VIII. BONE	0	0	0	4	4	0.7	0.6	100.0	75.0
Osteosarcoma	0	0	0	3	3	0.5	0.5	75.0	66.7
Chondrosarcoma	0	0	0	1	1	0.2	0.2	25.0	100.0
Ewing's sarcoma	0	0	0	0	0	-	-	-	-
Other and unspecified	0	0	0	0	0	-	-	-	-
IX. SOFT TISSUE SARCOMAS	1	10	8	5	24	4.1	4.7	100.0	95.8
Rhabdomyosarcoma	0	8	3	3	14	2.4	3.0	58.3	100.0
Fibrosarcoma	0	2	3	1	6	1.0	1.1	25.0	100.0
Other and unspecified	1	0	2	1	4	0.7	0.7	16.7	75.0
X. GONADAL & GERM CELL	0	0	0	0	0	-	-	-	-
Non-gonadal germ cell	0	0	0	0	0	-	-	-	-
Gonadal germ cell	0	0	0	0	0	-	-	-	-
Gonadal carcinoma	0	0	0	0	0	-	-	-	-
Other and unspecified	0	0	0	0	0	-	-	-	-
XI. EPITHELIAL NEOPLASMS	0	0	2	2	4	0.7	0.6	100.0	100.0
Adrenocortical carcinoma	0	0	0	0	0	-	-	-	-
Thyroid carcinoma	0	0	1	1	2	0.3	0.3	50.0	100.0
Nasopharyngeal carcinoma	0	0	0	0	0	-	-	-	-
Melanoma	0	0	1	0	1	0.2	0.1	25.0	100.0
Other carcinoma	0	0	0	1	1	0.2	0.2	25.0	100.0
XII. OTHER	1	3	3	1	8	1.4	1.6	100.0	25.0

* Specified as malignant | 0 | 3 | 6 | 3 | 12 | 2.1 | 2.0 | 100.0 | 16.7

Nigeria, Ibadan   1960 – 1984   FEMALE

DIAGNOSTIC GROUP	NUMBER OF CASES					REL. FREQUENCY(%)			HV(%)
	0	1-4	5-9	10-14	All	Crude	Adj.	Group	
TOTAL	10	97	146	119	372	100.0	100.0	100.0	77.2
I. LEUKAEMIAS	0	6	6	14	26	7.0	7.0	100.0	73.1
Acute lymphocytic	0	2	2	7	11	3.0	2.9	42.3	72.7
Other lymphocytic	0	0	1	0	1	0.3	0.2	3.8	100.0
Acute non-lymphocytic	0	2	3	3	8	2.2	2.1	30.8	87.5
Chronic myeloid	0	0	0	0	0	-	-	-	-
Other and unspecified	0	2	0	4	6	1.6	1.8	23.1	50.0
II. LYMPHOMAS	0	20	96	74	190	51.1	45.9	100.0	70.0
Hodgkin's disease	0	0	2	5	7	1.9	1.7	3.7	85.7
Non-Hodgkin lymphoma	0	1	2	3	6	1.6	1.5	3.2	100.0
Burkitt's lymphoma	0	19	90	62	171	46.0	41.2	90.0	67.8
Unspecified lymphoma	0	0	2	4	6	1.6	1.4	3.2	83.3
Histiocytosis X	0	0	0	0	0	-	-	-	-
Other reticuloendothelial	0	0	0	0	0	-	-	-	-
III. BRAIN AND SPINAL	0	3	10	7	20	5.4	4.9	100.0	65.0
Ependymoma	0	0	0	1	1	0.3	0.3	5.0	100.0
Astrocytoma	0	0	3	1	4	1.1	0.9	20.0	100.0
Medulloblastoma	0	0	1	0	1	0.3	0.2	5.0	100.0
Other glioma	0	1	2	0	3	0.8	0.8	15.0	100.0
Other and unspecified *	0	2	4	5	11	3.0	2.8	55.0	36.4
IV. SYMPATHETIC N.S.	2	7	5	4	18	4.8	5.4	100.0	100.0
Neuroblastoma	2	7	4	4	17	4.6	5.2	94.4	100.0
Other	0	0	1	0	1	0.3	0.2	5.6	100.0
V. RETINOBLASTOMA	1	28	5	0	34	9.1	11.9	100.0	97.1
VI. KIDNEY	0	22	8	1	31	8.3	10.1	100.0	93.5
Wilms' tumour	0	19	7	0	26	7.0	8.5	83.9	100.0
Renal carcinoma	0	1	0	1	2	0.5	0.6	6.5	100.0
Other and unspecified	0	2	1	0	3	0.8	1.0	9.7	33.3
VII. LIVER	0	0	1	2	3	0.8	0.7	100.0	100.0
Hepatoblastoma	0	0	1	1	2	0.5	0.5	66.7	100.0
Hepatic carcinoma	0	0	0	1	1	0.3	0.3	33.3	100.0
Other and unspecified	0	0	0	0	0	-	-	-	-
VIII. BONE	0	1	1	1	3	0.8	0.8	100.0	100.0
Osteosarcoma	0	0	1	1	2	0.5	0.5	66.7	100.0
Chondrosarcoma	0	0	0	0	0	-	-	-	-
Ewing's sarcoma	0	0	0	0	0	-	-	-	-
Other and unspecified	0	1	0	0	1	0.3	0.4	33.3	100.0
IX. SOFT TISSUE SARCOMAS	5	5	7	5	22	5.9	6.4	100.0	95.5
Rhabdomyosarcoma	1	4	5	3	13	3.5	3.7	59.1	100.0
Fibrosarcoma	1	1	0	1	3	0.8	1.0	13.6	100.0
Other and unspecified	3	0	2	1	6	1.6	1.8	27.3	83.3
X. GONADAL & GERM CELL	1	0	1	2	4	1.1	1.1	100.0	100.0
Non-gonadal germ cell	1	0	0	0	1	0.3	0.4	25.0	100.0
Gonadal germ cell	0	0	0	1	1	0.3	0.3	25.0	100.0
Gonadal carcinoma	0	0	1	0	1	0.3	0.2	25.0	100.0
Other and unspecified	0	0	0	1	1	0.3	0.3	25.0	100.0
XI. EPITHELIAL NEOPLASMS	0	0	1	5	6	1.6	1.5	100.0	100.0
Adrenocortical carcinoma	0	0	0	0	0	-	-	-	-
Thyroid carcinoma	0	0	1	2	3	0.8	0.7	50.0	100.0
Nasopharyngeal carcinoma	0	0	0	1	1	0.3	0.3	16.7	100.0
Melanoma	0	0	0	0	0	-	-	-	-
Other carcinoma	0	0	0	2	2	0.5	0.5	33.3	100.0
XII. OTHER	1	5	5	4	15	4.0	4.3	100.0	33.3
* Specified as malignant	0	1	4	4	9	2.4	2.2	100.0	22.2

Nigeria, Ibadan

1960 – 1969

MALE

DIAGNOSTIC GROUP	NUMBER OF CASES					REL. FREQUENCY(%)			RATES PER MILLION					Cum	HV(%)
	0	1-4	5-9	10-14	All	Crude	Adj.	Group	0-4	5-9	10-14	Crude	Adj.		
TOTAL	8	38	79	58	183	100.0	100.0	100.0	128.1	268.4	214.5	198.1	198.5	3055	92.9
I. LEUKAEMIAS	0	2	3	12	17	9.3	9.1	100.0	5.6	10.2	44.4	18.4	18.3	301	100.0
II. LYMPHOMAS	0	13	59	41	113	61.7	54.9	100.0	36.2	200.4	151.6	122.3	122.7	1941	91.2
III. BRAIN AND SPINAL	1	0	4	0	5	2.7	2.4	100.0	2.8	13.6	-	5.4	5.5	82	80.0
IV. SYMPATHETIC N.S.	3	3	3	0	9	4.9	6.4	100.0	16.7	10.2	-	9.7	9.8	135	88.9
V. RETINOBLASTOMA	0	5	1	0	6	3.3	4.7	100.0	13.9	3.4	-	6.5	6.5	87	100.0
VI. KIDNEY	2	9	3	0	14	7.7	10.7	100.0	30.6	10.2	-	15.2	15.1	204	100.0
VII. LIVER	1	1	0	2	4	2.2	2.8	100.0	5.6	-	7.4	4.3	4.3	65	100.0
VIII. BONE	0	0	0	2	2	1.1	1.0	100.0	-	-	7.4	2.2	2.1	37	50.0
IX. SOFT TISSUE SARCOMAS	1	5	5	1	12	6.6	7.6	100.0	16.7	17.0	3.7	13.0	13.0	187	100.0
X. GONADAL & GERM CELL	0	0	0	0	0	-	-	-	-	-	-	-	-	-	-
XI. EPITHELIAL NEOPLASMS	0	0	0	0	0	-	-	-	-	-	-	-	-	-	-
XIII. OTHER	0	0	1	0	1	0.5	0.4	100.0	-	3.4	-	1.1	1.1	17	100.0

Nigeria, Ibadan

1960 – 1969

FEMALE

DIAGNOSTIC GROUP	NUMBER OF CASES					REL. FREQUENCY(%)			RATES PER MILLION					Cum	HV(%)
	0	1-4	5-9	10-14	All	Crude	Adj.	Group	0-4	5-9	10-14	Crude	Adj.		
TOTAL	1	22	42	34	99	100.0	100.0	100.0	65.1	139.7	142.9	111.0	111.7	1738	90.9
I. LEUKAEMIAS	0	0	2	2	4	4.0	3.2	100.0	-	6.7	8.4	4.5	4.6	75	100.0
II. LYMPHOMAS	0	6	31	25	62	62.6	54.6	100.0	17.0	103.1	105.0	69.5	70.3	1125	90.3
III. BRAIN AND SPINAL	0	0	2	2	4	4.0	3.2	100.0	-	6.7	8.4	4.5	4.6	75	100.0
IV. SYMPATHETIC N.S.	0	1	1	0	2	2.0	2.5	100.0	2.8	3.3	-	2.2	2.2	31	100.0
V. RETINOBLASTOMA	0	7	1	0	8	8.1	12.9	100.0	19.8	3.3	-	9.0	8.7	116	87.5
VI. KIDNEY	0	4	2	0	6	6.1	8.4	100.0	11.3	6.7	-	6.7	6.5	90	100.0
VII. LIVER	0	0	0	0	0	-	-	-	-	-	-	-	-	-	-
VIII. BONE	0	1	1	1	3	3.0	3.3	100.0	2.8	3.3	4.2	3.4	3.4	52	100.0
IX. SOFT TISSUE SARCOMAS	0	2	2	0	4	4.0	4.9	100.0	5.7	6.7	-	4.5	4.3	62	100.0
X. GONADAL & GERM CELL	0	0	0	1	1	1.0	0.9	100.0	-	-	4.2	1.1	1.2	21	100.0
XI. EPITHELIAL NEOPLASMS	0	0	0	3	3	3.0	2.6	100.0	-	-	12.6	3.4	3.7	63	100.0
XIII. OTHER	1	1	0	0	2	2.0	3.5	100.0	5.7	-	-	2.2	2.2	28	-

Commentary

Overall registration rates for 1960–1969 were very high compared with those for European countries. This was accounted for almost entirely by rates for lymphomas which were, for males and females respectively, 7.6 and 9.4 times those for England and Wales in 1971–1980. For 1960–1984, 83% of lymphomas, or 47% of all registrations were Burkitt's lymphoma. Rates for retinoblastoma were approximately double the corresponding British rates. Laterality was only recorded in seven of the 67 cases of retinoblastoma, but all of these were unilateral. Wilms' tumour and soft tissue sarcomas were also relatively frequent, but registration rates for all other diagnostic groups were lower than in western populations.

The ratios of male to female cases for lymphomas were very similar in 1960–1969 (1.82) and 1970–1984 (1.84). However, between these two periods there was a marked reduction in the sex ratio for the remainder of registrations, namely from 1.89 to 1.14. It is not known whether this reflects changes in patterns of ascertainment or in the underlying incidence rates.

References

Olisa, E.G., Chandra, R., Jackson, M.A., Kennedy, J. & Williams, A.O. (1975) Malignant tumours in American Black and Nigerian children: a comparative study. *J. natl Cancer Inst.*, *55*, 281-284

Williams, A.O. (1975) Tumours of childhood in Ibadan, Nigeria. *Cancer*, *36*, 370-378

Williams, C.K.O. & Bangboye, E.A. (1983) Estimation of human leukaemia subtypes in an urban African population. *Oncology*, *40*, 381-386

SUDAN

Registry of the Radiation and Isotope Centre, Khartoum, 1967–1984

A. Hidayatalla

The data presented here represent all cancer patients aged 0–14 seen at the Radiation and Isotope Centre, Khartoum, for treatment during the 18-year period since it was opened in 1967. The Centre is the only specialist hospital in the country for the treatment of cancer by radiotherapy and chemotherapy. It has 50 beds and is part of the Khartoum Teaching Hospital complex of 1200 beds. Cases are referred from all over the country, although cases from different geographical regions are not equally represented in the present series; for example, only 5.2% of cases came from the three southern provinces of the Sudan. The hospital registry records information on age, sex, residence, tribal group, tumour type and histology, and also clinical features.

The Sudan is the largest country in Africa (2.5 million square kilometres), with very diverse geographical and climatic conditions, from the desert bordering Egypt in the north to the swamp and jungle of Equatoria in the south. The population, estimated at 18.7 million in 1980, is of considerable ethnographic and cultural diversity; there are almost 600 different tribes belonging to three main ethnic groups: Arabs, Hamitic and Negroid.

The series has been divided into two broad ethnic groupings — Arabs (including Arabs, Mowalad, Nubians and Bejas) and Sudanics (including Nilotic and Sudanic tribes, and Beggara). However, it must be stressed that there is no clear demarcation between the two; there is, in fact, considerable sharing of characteristics between them.

A previous report (Abdel Rahman & Hidayatalla, 1969) described the 63 childhood cancer cases seen at the Centre in its first two years.

Commentary

Of the 789 cases reported, 558 were in the predominantly Arab subgroup and 217 in the Sudanic subgroup, the ethnicity of the remaining 14 being unknown. The registry is not population-based.

Both for the two groups taken together, and for the Arab subgroup, the commonest diagnostic category was the lymphomas, with 23% of all cases: for Hodgkin's disease, the relative frequencies were similar for Arabs and Sudanics, while Burkitt's lymphoma had a higher relative frequency for Sudanics and unspecified lymphomas for the Arabs. Leukaemia was uncommon in both groups, but particularly in the Sudanics; an exceptionally high proportion, 29%, of all leukaemias were classified as chronic myeloid.

The second largest category was the epithelial tumours (19% of the total), this proportion being even higher among the Sudanic subgroup. In both ethnic groups just over half these tumours were nasopharyngeal carcinomas.

The third largest category was retinoblastoma (15% of the total); however, among the Sudanic subgroup this tumour accounted for 23% of all cases and was more common than the lymphomas.

The proportion of brain tumours, neuroblastoma and Ewing's sarcoma was low in both ethnic groups.

Reference

Abdel Rahman, S. & Hidayatalla, A. (1969) The pattern of malignant disease in children seen at the Radiation and Isotope Centre, Khartoum. *Sudan med. J.*, 7, 7-12

Sudan, RICK, Arab

MALE

1967 – 1984

DIAGNOSTIC GROUP	NUMBER OF CASES				REL. FREQUENCY(%)			HV(%)
	0-4	5-9	10-14	All	Crude	Adj.	Group	
TOTAL	82	115	131	328	100.0	100.0	100.0	99.4
I. LEUKAEMIAS	7	16	9	32	9.8	9.6	100.0	100.0
Acute lymphocytic	5	11	4	20	6.1	6.2	62.5	100.0
Other lymphocytic	0	2	0	2	0.6	0.5	6.3	100.0
Acute non-lymphocytic	0	1	2	3	0.9	0.7	9.4	100.0
Chronic myeloid	2	2	3	7	2.1	2.2	21.9	100.0
Other and unspecified	0	0	0	0	-	-	-	-
II. LYMPHOMAS	19	47	29	95	29.0	28.2	100.0	100.0
Hodgkin's disease	6	18	18	42	12.8	11.7	44.2	100.0
Non-Hodgkin lymphoma	0	0	0	0	-	-	-	-
Burkitt's lymphoma	4	8	2	14	4.3	4.5	14.7	100.0
Unspecified lymphoma	9	19	8	36	11.0	11.2	37.9	100.0
Histiocytosis X	0	1	1	2	0.6	0.5	2.1	100.0
Other reticuloendothelial	0	1	0	1	0.3	0.3	1.1	100.0
III. BRAIN AND SPINAL	3	0	9	12	3.7	3.5	100.0	91.7
Ependymoma	0	0	0	0	-	-	-	-
Astrocytoma	0	0	0	0	-	-	-	-
Medulloblastoma	3	0	0	3	0.9	1.5	25.0	100.0
Other glioma	0	0	8	8	2.4	1.8	66.7	100.0
Other and unspecified *	0	0	1	1	0.3	0.2	8.3	-
IV. SYMPATHETIC N.S.	5	2	1	8	2.4	3.2	100.0	100.0
Neuroblastoma	5	2	1	8	2.4	3.2	100.0	100.0
Other	0	0	0	0	-	-	-	-
V. RETINOBLASTOMA	20	12	0	32	9.8	12.9	100.0	100.0
VI. KIDNEY	17	10	2	29	8.8	11.4	100.0	100.0
Wilms' tumour	14	8	2	24	7.3	9.4	82.8	100.0
Renal carcinoma	3	2	0	5	1.5	2.0	17.2	100.0
Other and unspecified	0	0	0	0	-	-	-	-
VII. LIVER	1	0	0	1	0.3	0.5	100.0	100.0
Hepatoblastoma	0	0	0	0	-	-	-	-
Hepatic carcinoma	1	0	0	1	0.3	0.5	100.0	100.0
Other and unspecified	0	0	0	0	-	-	-	-
VIII. BONE	1	3	22	26	7.9	6.3	100.0	100.0
Osteosarcoma	1	2	19	22	6.7	5.4	84.6	100.0
Chondrosarcoma	0	0	1	1	0.3	0.2	3.8	100.0
Ewing's sarcoma	0	1	2	3	0.9	0.7	11.5	100.0
Other and unspecified	0	0	0	0	-	-	-	-
IX. SOFT TISSUE SARCOMAS	7	8	12	27	8.2	8.2	100.0	100.0
Rhabdomyosarcoma	2	3	1	6	1.8	2.0	22.2	100.0
Fibrosarcoma	5	4	9	18	5.5	5.5	66.7	100.0
Other and unspecified	0	1	2	3	0.9	0.7	11.1	100.0
X. GONADAL & GERM CELL	0	0	5	5	1.5	1.1	100.0	100.0
Non-gonadal germ cell	0	0	2	2	0.6	0.5	40.0	100.0
Gonadal germ cell	0	0	3	3	0.9	0.7	60.0	100.0
Gonadal carcinoma	0	0	0	0	-	-	-	-
Other and unspecified	0	0	0	0	-	-	-	-
XI. EPITHELIAL NEOPLASMS	2	14	40	56	17.1	13.8	100.0	100.0
Adrenocortical carcinoma	0	0	0	0	-	-	-	-
Thyroid carcinoma	0	0	0	0	-	-	-	-
Nasopharyngeal carcinoma	0	5	26	31	9.5	7.3	55.4	100.0
Melanoma	0	0	1	1	0.3	0.2	1.8	100.0
Other carcinoma	2	9	13	24	7.3	6.3	42.9	100.0
XII. OTHER	0	3	2	5	1.5	1.2	100.0	80.0

* Specified as malignant | 0 | 0 | 1 | 1 | 0.3 | 0.2 | 100.0 | -

Sudan, RICK, Arab   1967 – 1984   FEMALE

DIAGNOSTIC GROUP	NUMBER OF CASES				REL. FREQUENCY(%)			HV(%)
	0-4	5-9	10-14	All	Crude	Adj.	Group	
TOTAL	85	75	70	230	100.0	100.0	100.0	97.8
I. LEUKAEMIAS	7	17	7	31	13.5	13.1	100.0	100.0
Acute lymphocytic	5	10	2	17	7.4	7.2	54.8	100.0
Other lymphocytic	1	0	1	2	0.9	0.9	6.5	100.0
Acute non-lymphocytic	0	1	0	1	0.4	0.4	3.2	100.0
Chronic myeloid	1	6	4	11	4.8	4.6	35.5	100.0
Other and unspecified	0	0	0	0	-	-	-	-
II. LYMPHOMAS	10	13	11	34	14.8	14.6	100.0	100.0
Hodgkin's disease	1	4	5	10	4.3	4.2	29.4	100.0
Non-Hodgkin lymphoma	0	0	0	0	-	-	-	-
Burkitt's lymphoma	2	0	0	2	0.9	0.9	5.9	100.0
Unspecified lymphoma	6	9	4	19	8.3	8.1	55.9	100.0
Histiocytosis X	0	0	2	2	0.9	0.9	5.9	100.0
Other reticuloendothelial	1	0	0	1	0.4	0.5	2.9	-
III. BRAIN AND SPINAL	1	6	6	13	5.7	5.4	100.0	84.6
Ependymoma	0	0	0	0	-	-	-	-
Astrocytoma	0	0	0	0	-	-	-	-
Medulloblastoma	1	1	0	2	0.9	0.9	15.4	100.0
Other glioma	0	3	3	6	2.6	2.5	46.2	100.0
Other and unspecified *	0	2	3	5	2.2	2.1	38.5	60.0
IV. SYMPATHETIC N.S.	3	1	0	4	1.7	1.8	100.0	100.0
Neuroblastoma	3	1	0	4	1.7	1.8	100.0	100.0
Other	0	0	0	0	-	-	-	-
V. RETINOBLASTOMA	36	4	0	40	17.4	18.5	100.0	100.0
VI. KIDNEY	16	10	0	26	11.3	11.5	100.0	100.0
Wilms' tumour	13	10	0	23	10.0	10.1	88.5	100.0
Renal carcinoma	3	0	0	3	1.3	1.4	11.5	100.0
Other and unspecified	0	0	0	0	-	-	-	-
VII. LIVER	2	1	0	3	1.3	1.3	100.0	100.0
Hepatoblastoma	0	0	0	0	-	-	-	-
Hepatic carcinoma	2	1	0	3	1.3	1.3	100.0	100.0
Other and unspecified	0	0	0	0	-	-	-	-
VIII. BONE	0	5	9	14	6.1	5.9	100.0	100.0
Osteosarcoma	0	3	9	12	5.2	5.1	85.7	100.0
Chondrosarcoma	0	1	0	1	0.4	0.4	7.1	100.0
Ewing's sarcoma	0	1	0	1	0.4	0.4	7.1	100.0
Other and unspecified	0	0	0	0	-	-	-	-
IX. SOFT TISSUE SARCOMAS	5	6	8	19	8.3	8.2	100.0	100.0
Rhabdomyosarcoma	1	1	0	2	0.9	0.9	10.5	100.0
Fibrosarcoma	4	4	7	15	6.5	6.5	78.9	100.0
Other and unspecified	0	1	1	2	0.9	0.8	10.5	100.0
X. GONADAL & GERM CELL	0	0	5	5	2.2	2.1	100.0	100.0
Non-gonadal germ cell	0	0	0	0	-	-	-	-
Gonadal germ cell	0	2	0	2	0.9	0.9	40.0	100.0
Gonadal carcinoma	0	0	3	3	1.3	1.3	60.0	100.0
Other and unspecified	0	0	0	0	-	-	-	-
XI. EPITHELIAL NEOPLASMS	4	10	21	35	15.2	14.9	100.0	100.0
Adrenocortical carcinoma	0	0	0	0	-	-	-	-
Thyroid carcinoma	0	2	0	2	0.9	0.8	5.7	100.0
Nasopharyngeal carcinoma	0	2	13	15	6.5	6.4	42.9	100.0
Melanoma	1	0	0	1	0.4	0.5	2.9	100.0
Other carcinoma	3	6	8	17	7.4	7.2	48.6	100.0
XII. OTHER	1	2	3	6	2.6	2.6	100.0	50.0
* Specified as malignant	0	1	1	2	0.9	0.8	100.0	-

Sudan, RICK, Sudanic   1967 - 1984   MALE

DIAGNOSTIC GROUP	NUMBER OF CASES				REL. FREQUENCY(%)			HV(%)
	0-4	5-9	10-14	All	Crude	Adj.	Group	
TOTAL	27	44	66	137	100.0	100.0	100.0	99.3
I. LEUKAEMIAS	1	0	5	6	4.4	3.8	100.0	100.0
Acute lymphocytic	0	0	2	2	1.5	0.9	33.3	100.0
Other lymphocytic	0	0	0	0	–	–	–	–
Acute non-lymphocytic	0	0	1	1	0.7	0.5	16.7	100.0
Chronic myeloid	1	0	2	3	2.2	2.4	50.0	100.0
Other and unspecified	0	0	0	0	–	–	–	–
II. LYMPHOMAS	2	18	16	36	26.3	22.5	100.0	100.0
Hodgkin's disease	0	7	9	16	11.7	8.9	44.4	100.0
Non-Hodgkin lymphoma	1	9	3	13	9.5	9.0	36.1	100.0
Burkitt's lymphoma	1	2	4	7	5.1	4.7	19.4	100.0
Unspecified lymphoma	0	0	0	0	–	–	–	–
Histiocytosis X	0	0	0	0	–	–	–	–
Other reticuloendothelial	0	0	0	0	–	–	–	–
III. BRAIN AND SPINAL	1	0	3	4	2.9	2.8	100.0	75.0
Ependymoma	0	0	0	0	–	–	–	–
Astrocytoma	0	0	0	0	–	–	–	–
Medulloblastoma	0	0	0	0	–	–	–	–
Other glioma	0	0	0	0	–	–	–	–
Other and unspecified *	1	0	3	4	2.9	2.8	100.0	75.0
IV. SYMPATHETIC N.S.	0	1	0	1	0.7	0.7	100.0	100.0
Neuroblastoma	0	1	0	1	0.7	0.7	100.0	100.0
Other	0	0	0	0	–	–	–	–
V. RETINOBLASTOMA	12	12	3	27	19.7	27.3	100.0	100.0
VI. KIDNEY	6	2	2	10	7.3	11.2	100.0	100.0
Wilms' tumour	5	1	1	7	5.1	8.5	70.0	100.0
Renal carcinoma	1	1	1	3	2.2	2.6	30.0	100.0
Other and unspecified	0	0	0	0	–	–	–	–
VII. LIVER	0	0	0	0	–	–	–	–
Hepatoblastoma	0	0	0	0	–	–	–	–
Hepatic carcinoma	0	0	0	0	–	–	–	–
Other and unspecified	0	0	0	0	–	–	–	–
VIII. BONE	1	1	3	5	3.6	3.5	100.0	100.0
Osteosarcoma	0	1	2	3	2.2	1.6	60.0	100.0
Chondrosarcoma	0	0	0	0	–	–	–	–
Ewing's sarcoma	0	0	1	1	0.7	0.5	20.0	100.0
Other and unspecified	1	0	0	1	0.7	1.5	20.0	100.0
IX. SOFT TISSUE SARCOMAS	1	3	5	9	6.6	5.8	100.0	100.0
Rhabdomyosarcoma	0	1	0	1	0.7	0.7	11.1	100.0
Fibrosarcoma	1	1	4	6	4.4	4.0	66.7	100.0
Other and unspecified	0	1	1	2	1.5	1.1	22.2	100.0
X. GONADAL & GERM CELL	0	0	2	2	1.5	0.9	100.0	100.0
Non-gonadal germ cell	0	0	1	1	0.7	0.5	50.0	100.0
Gonadal germ cell	0	0	1	1	0.7	0.5	50.0	100.0
Gonadal carcinoma	0	0	0	0	–	–	–	–
Other and unspecified	0	0	0	0	–	–	–	–
XI. EPITHELIAL NEOPLASMS	2	6	27	35	25.5	19.3	100.0	100.0
Adrenocortical carcinoma	0	0	0	0	–	–	–	–
Thyroid carcinoma	0	0	0	0	–	–	–	–
Nasopharyngeal carcinoma	1	2	20	23	16.8	11.9	65.7	100.0
Melanoma	0	0	0	0	–	–	–	–
Other carcinoma	1	4	7	12	8.8	7.4	34.3	100.0
XII. OTHER	1	1	0	2	1.5	2.2	100.0	100.0
* Specified as malignant	0	0	1	1	0.7	0.5	100.0	–

Sudan, RICK, Sudanic

1967 – 1984

FEMALE

DIAGNOSTIC GROUP	NUMBER OF CASES				REL. FREQUENCY(%)			HV(%)
	0-4	5-9	10-14	All	Crude	Adj.	Group	
TOTAL	34	18	28	80	100.0	100.0	100.0	
I. LEUKAEMIAS	1	1	0	2	2.5	2.8	100.0	100.0
Acute lymphocytic	1	1	0	2	2.5	2.8	100.0	100.0
Other lymphocytic	0	0	0	0	-	-	-	-
Acute non-lymphocytic	0	0	0	0	-	-	-	-
Chronic myeloid	0	0	0	0	-	-	-	-
Other and unspecified	0	0	0	0	-	-	-	-
II. LYMPHOMAS	3	2	5	10	12.5	12.2	100.0	100.0
Hodgkin's disease	0	0	3	3	3.8	3.2	30.0	100.0
Non-Hodgkin lymphoma	0	0	0	0	-	-	-	-
Burkitt's lymphoma	1	1	0	2	2.5	2.8	20.0	100.0
Unspecified lymphoma	2	1	2	5	6.3	6.2	50.0	100.0
Histiocytosis X	0	0	0	0	-	-	-	-
Other reticuloendothelial	0	0	0	0	-	-	-	-
III. BRAIN AND SPINAL	1	0	0	1	1.3	1.2	100.0	100.0
Ependymoma	0	0	0	0	-	-	-	-
Astrocytoma	0	0	0	0	-	-	-	-
Medulloblastoma	0	0	0	0	-	-	-	-
Other glioma	1	0	0	1	1.3	1.2	100.0	100.0
Other and unspecified *	0	0	0	0	-	-	-	-
IV. SYMPATHETIC N.S.	2	1	0	3	3.8	3.4	100.0	100.0
Neuroblastoma	2	1	0	3	3.8	3.4	100.0	100.0
Other	0	0	0	0	-	-	-	-
V. RETINOBLASTOMA	14	8	0	22	27.5	29.8	100.0	100.0
VI. KIDNEY	8	1	0	9	11.3	11.1	100.0	100.0
Wilms' tumour	7	1	0	8	10.0	9.9	88.9	100.0
Renal carcinoma	1	0	0	1	1.3	1.2	11.1	100.0
Other and unspecified	0	0	0	0	-	-	-	-
VII. LIVER	0	0	0	0	-	-	-	-
Hepatoblastoma	0	0	0	0	-	-	-	-
Hepatic carcinoma	0	0	0	0	-	-	-	-
Other and unspecified	0	0	0	0	-	-	-	-
VIII. BONE	0	0	4	4	5.0	4.3	100.0	100.0
Osteosarcoma	0	0	4	4	5.0	4.3	100.0	100.0
Chondrosarcoma	0	0	0	0	-	-	-	-
Ewing's sarcoma	0	0	0	0	-	-	-	-
Other and unspecified	0	0	0	0	-	-	-	-
IX. SOFT TISSUE SARCOMAS	1	4	1	6	7.5	8.9	100.0	100.0
Rhabdomyosarcoma	1	0	0	1	1.3	1.2	16.7	100.0
Fibrosarcoma	0	3	1	4	5.0	6.1	66.7	100.0
Other and unspecified	0	1	0	1	1.3	1.7	16.7	100.0
X. GONADAL & GERM CELL	0	0	0	0	-	-	-	-
Non-gonadal germ cell	0	0	0	0	-	-	-	-
Gonadal germ cell	0	0	0	0	-	-	-	-
Gonadal carcinoma	0	0	0	0	-	-	-	-
Other and unspecified	0	0	0	0	-	-	-	-
XI. EPITHELIAL NEOPLASMS	3	2	17	22	27.5	25.1	100.0	100.0
Adrenocortical carcinoma	0	0	0	0	-	-	-	-
Thyroid carcinoma	0	0	9	9	11.3	10.8	40.9	100.0
Nasopharyngeal carcinoma	0	2	7	9	1.3	1.1	4.5	100.0
Melanoma	0	0	1	1	1.3	1.1	4.5	100.0
Other carcinoma	3	0	9	12	15.0	13.2	54.5	100.0
XII. OTHER	1	0	0	1	1.3	1.2	100.0	-

* Specified as malignant

TANZANIA

Tanzania Cancer Registry, 1980–1981

J. Shaba

The Tanzania Cancer Registry was established in 1966. Before that time, analyses of histopathology diagnoses recorded in the Central Pathology Laboratory had been carried out (e.g., Linsell, 1967), but the establishment of a registry involved the collection of additional data on special forms for all cancer cases. The register is confined to histopathological specimens. An analysis of the data for the five-year period 1969–1973 has been published (Hiza, 1976).

The data presented here represent the cases of cancer in childhood diagnosed histologically in three government referral hospitals in 1980–1981, namely Muhimbili Medical Centre in Dar es Salaam, Mwanza hospital on the shores of Lake Victoria in the north of Tanzania, and the Kilimanjaro Christian Medical Centre at Moshi in the north-east. The data from Muhimbili Medical Centre have been supplemented by the inclusion of cases of haematological malignancy diagnosed by the Department of Haematology during the same period.

The Pathology Department of Muhimbili Medical Centre provides a diagnostic histopathology service for all the hospitals in central and southern Tanzania. The centre itself is a large, multispecialty hospital which acts as the major teaching hospital of the medical school. A Department of Radiology and Radiotherapy provides specialized treatment services for cancer patients.

Mwanza hospital is located in a densely populated region of Tanzania to the south of Lake Victoria, and acts as referral hospital for the north-eastern part of the country.

Kilimanjaro Christian Medical Centre is a 420-bed hospital including all the major specialties and providing specialist services for the north-western regions of the country. A cancer registry based on histologically diagnosed cases has been maintained in the Department of Pathology since 1974. Approximately half the workload of the Department derives from the hospital itself, the remainder coming from many other hospitals in the northern part of the country. The registry includes only histologically diagnosed cases, most of them biopsies, a few cytological specimens, and occasional autopsies without previous biopsy. The autopsy rate is low, and there is no system of death certification.

Commentary

Lymphomas accounted for 45% of all cases and were by far the largest diagnostic group. Burkitt's lymphoma accounted for 46% of lymphomas, 21% of all registrations, but there were also substantial numbers of registrations for Hodgkin's disease. The next largest diagnostic group was the soft-tissue sarcomas. Half of these, or 10% of all registrations, were Kaposi's sarcoma. Leukaemias and brain tumours were very rarely registered, but this probably reflects under-ascertainment rather than a truly low incidence rate, since tissue specimens from these cancers are unlikely to reach the histopathology services. Neuroblastoma was also extremely rare.

Overall, there was a high sex ratio (M/F = 1.8). However, the sex-ratio for retinoblastoma, which is close to unity in many population-based registries, was 3.33:1. It therefore seems possible that the high overall sex ratio can be partly accounted for by preferential referral for treatment rather than being entirely due to a higher incidence rate for childhood cancer in boys.

References

Hiza, P.R. (1976) Malignant disease in Tanzania. *East Afr. med. J.*, *53*, 82-95

Linsell, C.A. (1967) Cancer incidence in Kenya 1957-63. *Br. J. Cancer*, *21*, 465-473

Tanzania   MALE

1980 – 1981

DIAGNOSTIC GROUP	NUMBER OF CASES					REL. FREQUENCY(%)			HV(%)
	0	1-4	5-9	10-14	All	Crude	Adj.	Group	
TOTAL	3	35	65	56	166▫	100.0	100.0	100.0	100.0
I. LEUKAEMIAS	1	1	3	2	7	4.2	4.6	100.0	100.0
Acute lymphocytic	0	0	1	1	2	1.2	1.0	28.6	100.0
Other lymphocytic	0	1	0	0	1	0.6	1.1	14.3	100.0
Acute non-lymphocytic	1	0	1	1	3	1.8	2.0	42.9	100.0
Chronic myeloid	0	0	0	0	0	–	–	–	–
Other and unspecified	0	0	1	0	1	0.6	0.5	14.3	100.0
II. LYMPHOMAS	0	9	33	32	78▫	47.0	41.8	100.0	100.0
Hodgkin's disease	0	1	10	16	27▫	16.3	13.2	34.6	100.0
Non-Hodgkin lymphoma	0	1	7	1	10▫	6.0	4.8	12.8	100.0
Burkitt's lymphoma	0	7	16	11	36▫	21.7	20.6	46.2	100.0
Unspecified lymphoma	0	1	0	4	5	3.0	3.2	6.4	100.0
Histiocytosis X	0	0	0	0	0	–	–	–	–
Other reticuloendothelial	0	0	0	0	0	–	–	–	–
III. BRAIN AND SPINAL	0	0	0	0	0	–	–	–	–
Ependymoma	0	0	0	0	0	–	–	–	–
Astrocytoma	0	0	0	0	0	–	–	–	–
Medulloblastoma	0	0	0	0	0	–	–	–	–
Other glioma	0	0	0	0	0	–	–	–	–
Other and unspecified *	0	0	0	0	0	–	–	–	–
IV. SYMPATHETIC N.S.	0	0	1	0	1	0.6	0.5	100.0	100.0
Neuroblastoma	0	0	1	0	1	0.6	0.5	100.0	100.0
Other	0	0	0	0	0	–	–	–	–
V. RETINOBLASTOMA	0	11	6	0	20▫	12.0	14.3	100.0	100.0
VI. KIDNEY	1	2	2	1	6	3.6	4.6	100.0	100.0
Wilms' tumour	1	2	2	1	6	3.6	4.6	100.0	100.0
Renal carcinoma	0	0	0	0	0	–	–	–	–
Other and unspecified	0	0	0	0	0	–	–	–	–
VII. LIVER	0	0	0	0	0	–	–	–	–
Hepatoblastoma	0	0	0	0	0	–	–	–	–
Hepatic carcinoma	0	0	0	0	0	–	–	–	–
Other and unspecified	0	0	0	0	0	–	–	–	–
VIII. BONE	0	0	0	4	4	2.4	2.1	100.0	100.0
Osteosarcoma	0	0	0	4	4	2.4	2.1	100.0	100.0
Chondrosarcoma	0	0	0	0	0	–	–	–	–
Ewing's sarcoma	0	0	0	0	0	–	–	–	–
Other and unspecified	0	0	0	0	0	–	–	–	–
IX. SOFT TISSUE SARCOMAS	1	9	11	9	30	18.1	20.4	100.0	100.0
Rhabdomyosarcoma	0	1	4	2	7	4.2	4.0	23.3	100.0
Fibrosarcoma	0	1	1	1	3	1.8	2.0	10.0	100.0
Other and unspecified	1	7	6	6	20	12.0	14.4	66.7	100.0
X. GONADAL & GERM CELL	0	0	0	1	1	0.6	0.5	100.0	100.0
Non-gonadal germ cell	0	0	0	0	0	–	–	–	–
Gonadal germ cell	0	0	0	1	1	0.6	0.5	100.0	100.0
Gonadal carcinoma	0	0	0	0	0	–	–	–	–
Other and unspecified	0	0	0	0	0	–	–	–	–
XI. EPITHELIAL NEOPLASMS	0	2	5	6	13	7.8	7.6	100.0	100.0
Adrenocortical carcinoma	0	0	0	0	0	–	–	–	–
Thyroid carcinoma	0	0	0	0	0	–	–	–	–
Nasopharyngeal carcinoma	0	0	0	0	0	–	–	–	–
Melanoma	0	1	0	0	1	0.6	1.1	7.7	100.0
Other carcinoma	0	1	5	6	12	7.2	6.6	92.3	100.0
XII. OTHER	0	1	4	1	6	3.6	3.4	100.0	100.0
	0	0	0	0	0	–	–	–	–

* Specified as malignant
▫ Includes age unknown

Tanzania FEMALE

1980 – 1981

DIAGNOSTIC GROUP	NUMBER OF CASES					REL. FREQUENCY(%)			HV(%)
	0	1-4	5-9	10-14	All	Crude	Adj.	Group	
TOTAL	2	24	30	33	92¤	100.0	100.0	100.0	100.0
I. LEUKAEMIAS	0	0	3	2	5	5.4	4.8	100.0	100.0
Acute lymphocytic	0	0	1	1	2	2.2	1.9	40.0	100.0
Other lymphocytic	0	0	0	0	0	–	–	–	–
Acute non-lymphocytic	0	1	0	0	1	1.1	1.0	20.0	100.0
Chronic myeloid	0	0	0	1	1	1.1	0.9	20.0	100.0
Other and unspecified	0	0	1	0	1	1.1	1.0	20.0	100.0
II. LYMPHOMAS	0	6	12	19	37	40.2	38.5	100.0	100.0
Hodgkin's disease	0	0	0	6	6	6.5	5.5	16.2	100.0
Non-Hodgkin lymphoma	0	1	3	4	8	8.7	8.2	21.6	100.0
Burkitt's lymphoma	0	3	8	6	17	18.5	18.1	45.9	100.0
Unspecified lymphoma	0	2	1	3	6	6.5	6.8	16.2	100.0
Histiocytosis X	0	0	0	0	0	–	–	–	–
Other reticuloendothelial	0	0	0	0	0	–	–	–	–
III. BRAIN AND SPINAL	0	1	0	0	1	1.1	1.5	100.0	100.0
Ependymoma	0	1	0	0	1	1.1	1.5	100.0	100.0
Astrocytoma	0	0	0	0	0	–	–	–	–
Medulloblastoma	0	0	0	0	0	–	–	–	–
Other glioma	0	0	0	0	0	–	–	–	–
Other and unspecified *	0	0	0	0	0	–	–	–	–
IV. SYMPATHETIC N.S.	0	0	0	0	0	–	–	–	–
Neuroblastoma	0	0	0	0	0	–	–	–	–
Other	0	0	0	0	0	–	–	–	–
V. RETINOBLASTOMA	1	4	0	1	6	6.5	8.6	100.0	100.0
VI. KIDNEY	1	3	2	1	9¤	9.8	9.1	100.0	100.0
Wilms' tumour	1	3	2	1	9¤	9.8	9.1	100.0	100.0
Renal carcinoma	0	0	0	0	0	–	–	–	–
Other and unspecified	0	0	0	0	0	–	–	–	–
VII. LIVER	0	1	0	1	2	2.2	2.4	100.0	100.0
Hepatoblastoma	0	0	0	1	1	1.1	1.5	50.0	100.0
Hepatic carcinoma	0	1	0	0	1	1.1	0.9	50.0	100.0
Other and unspecified	0	0	0	0	0	–	–	–	–
VIII. BONE	0	0	0	3	3	3.3	2.7	100.0	100.0
Osteosarcoma	0	0	0	1	1	1.1	0.9	33.3	100.0
Chondrosarcoma	0	0	0	0	0	–	–	–	–
Ewing's sarcoma	0	0	0	2	2	2.2	1.8	66.7	100.0
Other and unspecified	0	0	0	0	0	–	–	–	–
IX. SOFT TISSUE SARCOMAS	0	7	10	3	21¤	22.8	23.5	100.0	100.0
Rhabdomyosarcoma	0	1	2	0	4¤	4.3	3.5	19.0	100.0
Fibrosarcoma	0	3	0	1	4	4.3	5.5	19.0	100.0
Other and unspecified	0	3	8	2	13	14.1	14.4	61.9	100.0
X. GONADAL & GERM CELL	0	1	0	0	1	1.1	1.5	100.0	100.0
Non-gonadal germ cell	0	0	0	0	0	–	–	–	–
Gonadal germ cell	0	0	0	0	0	–	–	–	–
Gonadal carcinoma	0	0	0	0	0	–	–	–	–
Other and unspecified	0	1	0	0	1	1.1	1.5	100.0	100.0
XI. EPITHELIAL NEOPLASMS	0	0	3	2	5	5.4	4.8	100.0	100.0
Adrenocortical carcinoma	0	0	0	0	0	–	–	–	–
Thyroid carcinoma	0	0	0	0	0	–	–	–	–
Nasopharyngeal carcinoma	0	0	0	0	0	–	–	–	–
Melanoma	0	0	0	0	0	–	–	–	–
Other carcinoma	0	0	3	2	5	5.4	4.8	100.0	100.0
XII. OTHER	0	1	0	1	2	2.2	2.4	100.0	100.0

* Specified as malignant
¤ Includes age unknown

TUNISIA

Institut Salah-Azaiz, 1969–1982

N. Mourali

The series consists of cases of childhood cancer seen at the Tunisian National Cancer Institute (Institut Salah-Azaiz) between 1969 and 1982. Only histopathologically diagnosed cases are included.

The hospital has 190 beds, and treats some 5000–6000 patients per year. Of the cases treated, 35% are from the city of Tunis itself, the remainder coming from the rest of the country. Several specialties, including radiotherapy and surgical and medical oncology, are available. Cases of childhood cancer may be diagnosed in many hospitals, but a large proportion will be referred to the Institut for adjuvant treatment. Cases of leukaemia are treated in the Haematology Centre in Tunis and in the paediatric departments of other hospitals and are thus not represented in the present series.

In 1975, the population of Tunisia was 5.6 million, of whom 43.9% were aged less than 15 years.

Commentary

The largest diagnostic group was the lymphomas, accounting for 36% of all cases. Within this group, there were large numbers of Hodgkin's disease, non-Hodgkin lymphoma and Burkitt's lymphoma. There was an apparent peak for Hodgkin's disease in the 5–9 age-group in males. The second largest group was the epithelial neoplasms; in this group there were very large numbers of carcinoma of skin and nasopharynx, accounting for 9% and 7% of all registrations respectively. The great majority of skin tumours (90%) were diagnosed in children with xeroderma pigmentosum; 79% were squamous-cell epitheliomas and 21% basal-cell carcinomas. Over two-thirds of brain tumours were medulloblastoma. The soft-tissue sarcomas included seven cases of liposarcoma, a tumour which is generally exceptionally rare in childhood.

Tunisia, Institut Salah-Azaiz   1969 – 1982   MALE

DIAGNOSTIC GROUP	NUMBER OF CASES					REL. FREQUENCY(%)			HV(%)
	0	1-4	5-9	10-14	All	Crude	Adj.	Group	
TOTAL	34	174	175	149	532	100.0	100.0	100.0	100.0
I. LEUKAEMIAS	0	0	0	0	0	-	-	-	-
Acute lymphocytic	0	0	0	0	0	-	-	-	-
Other lymphocytic	0	0	0	0	0	-	-	-	-
Acute non-lymphocytic	0	0	0	0	0	-	-	-	-
Chronic myeloid	0	0	0	0	0	-	-	-	-
Other and unspecified	0	0	0	0	0	-	-	-	-
II. LYMPHOMAS	4	71	94	53	222	41.7	41.2	100.0	100.0
Hodgkin's disease	1	21	51	27	100	18.8	18.4	45.0	100.0
Non-Hodgkin lymphoma	2	20	26	20	68	12.8	12.7	30.6	100.0
Burkitt's lymphoma	0	29	16	5	50	9.4	9.3	22.5	100.0
Unspecified lymphoma	0	0	0	0	0	-	-	-	-
Histiocytosis X	1	0	1	0	2	0.4	0.4	0.9	100.0
Other reticuloendothelial	0	1	0	1	2	0.4	0.4	0.9	100.0
III. BRAIN AND SPINAL	0	12	8	9	29	5.5	5.5	100.0	100.0
Ependymoma	0	0	0	1	1	0.2	0.2	3.4	100.0
Astrocytoma	0	3	2	1	6	1.1	1.1	20.7	100.0
Medulloblastoma	0	9	6	6	21	3.9	4.0	72.4	100.0
Other glioma	0	0	0	1	1	0.2	0.2	3.4	100.0
Other and unspecified *	0	0	0	0	0	-	-	-	-
IV. SYMPATHETIC N.S.	2	10	7	1	20	3.8	3.7	100.0	100.0
Neuroblastoma	2	10	6	1	19	3.6	3.5	95.0	100.0
Other	0	0	1	0	1	0.2	0.2	5.0	100.0
V. RETINOBLASTOMA	4	22	4	1	31	5.8	5.9	100.0	100.0
VI. KIDNEY	11	17	4	0	32	6.0	6.1	100.0	100.0
Wilms' tumour	11	17	4	0	32	6.0	6.1	100.0	100.0
Renal carcinoma	0	0	0	0	0	-	-	-	-
Other and unspecified	0	0	0	0	0	-	-	-	-
VII. LIVER	1	0	1	0	2	0.4	0.4	100.0	100.0
Hepatoblastoma	0	0	0	0	0	-	-	-	-
Hepatic carcinoma	1	0	1	0	2	0.4	0.4	100.0	100.0
Other and unspecified	0	0	0	0	0	-	-	-	-
VIII. BONE	1	3	7	23	34	6.4	6.6	100.0	100.0
Osteosarcoma	0	0	2	15	17	3.2	3.4	50.0	100.0
Chondrosarcoma	0	0	0	2	2	0.4	0.4	5.9	100.0
Ewing's sarcoma	1	3	4	5	13	2.4	2.5	38.2	100.0
Other and unspecified	0	0	1	1	2	0.4	0.4	5.9	100.0
IX. SOFT TISSUE SARCOMAS	7	18	20	14	59	11.1	11.1	100.0	100.0
Rhabdomyosarcoma	4	11	7	6	28	5.3	5.3	47.5	100.0
Fibrosarcoma	1	2	5	5	13	2.4	2.4	22.0	100.0
Other and unspecified	2	5	8	3	18	3.4	3.3	30.5	100.0
X. GONADAL & GERM CELL	2	5	1	0	8	1.5	1.5	100.0	100.0
Non-gonadal germ cell	1	2	1	0	4	0.8	0.7	50.0	100.0
Gonadal germ cell	1	3	0	0	4	0.8	0.8	50.0	100.0
Gonadal carcinoma	0	0	0	0	0	-	-	-	-
Other and unspecified	0	0	0	0	0	-	-	-	-
XI. EPITHELIAL NEOPLASMS	2	15	28	48	93	17.5	17.7	100.0	100.0
Adrenocortical carcinoma	0	1	0	0	1	0.2	0.2	1.1	100.0
Thyroid carcinoma	0	0	0	2	2	0.4	0.4	2.2	100.0
Nasopharyngeal carcinoma	0	0	8	36	44	8.3	8.6	47.3	100.0
Melanoma	0	0	0	0	0	-	-	-	-
Other carcinoma	2	14	20	10	46	8.6	8.5	49.5	100.0
XII. OTHER	0	1	1	0	2	0.4	0.4	100.0	100.0

* Specified as malignant   0 | 0 | 0 | 0 | 0 | - | - | - | -

Tunisia, Institut Salah-Azaiz 1969 – 1982 FEMALE

DIAGNOSTIC GROUP	0	1-4	5-9	10-14	All	Crude	Adj.	Group	HV(%)
TOTAL	22	137	98	111	368	100.0	100.0	100.0	100.0
I. LEUKAEMIAS	0	0	0	0	0	-	-	-	-
Acute lymphocytic	0	0	0	0	0	-	-	-	-
Other lymphocytic	0	0	0	0	0	-	-	-	-
Acute non-lymphocytic	0	0	0	0	0	-	-	-	-
Chronic myeloid	0	0	0	0	0	-	-	-	-
Other and unspecified	0	0	0	0	0	-	-	-	-
II. LYMPHOMAS	1	36	32	30	99	26.9	27.2	100.0	100.0
Hodgkin's disease	1	5	9	16	31	8.4	8.6	31.3	100.0
Non-Hodgkin lymphoma	0	7	16	9	32	8.7	9.1	32.3	100.0
Burkitt's lymphoma	0	23	7	4	34	9.2	9.0	34.3	100.0
Unspecified lymphoma	0	0	0	0	0	-	-	-	-
Histiocytosis X	0	1	0	0	1	0.3	0.3	1.0	100.0
Other reticuloendothelial	0	0	0	1	1	0.3	0.3	1.0	100.0
III. BRAIN AND SPINAL	1	3	3	6	13	3.5	3.5	100.0	100.0
Ependymoma	0	1	0	2	3	0.8	0.8	23.1	100.0
Astrocytoma	0	0	1	0	1	0.3	0.3	7.7	100.0
Medulloblastoma	1	2	2	3	8	2.2	2.2	61.5	100.0
Other glioma	0	0	0	1	1	0.3	0.3	7.7	100.0
Other and unspecified *	0	0	0	0	0	-	-	-	-
IV. SYMPATHETIC N.S.	4	12	5	0	21	5.7	5.6	100.0	100.0
Neuroblastoma	4	9	5	0	18	4.9	4.8	85.7	100.0
Other	0	3	0	0	3	0.8	0.8	14.3	100.0
V. RETINOBLASTOMA	1	27	2	0	30	8.2	7.7	100.0	100.0
VI. KIDNEY	6	23	10	0	39	10.6	10.4	100.0	100.0
Wilms' tumour	6	23	9	0	38	10.3	10.1	97.4	100.0
Renal carcinoma	0	0	1	0	1	0.3	0.3	2.6	100.0
Other and unspecified	0	0	0	0	0	-	-	-	-
VII. LIVER	0	0	0	0	0	-	-	-	-
Hepatoblastoma	0	0	0	0	0	-	-	-	-
Hepatic carcinoma	0	0	0	0	0	-	-	-	-
Other and unspecified	0	0	0	0	0	-	-	-	-
VIII.BONE	0	2	16	22	40	10.9	11.3	100.0	100.0
Osteosarcoma	0	1	4	18	23	6.3	6.3	57.5	100.0
Chondrosarcoma	0	0	1	0	1	0.3	0.3	2.5	100.0
Ewing's sarcoma	0	1	10	4	15	4.1	4.4	37.5	100.0
Other and unspecified	0	0	1	0	1	0.3	0.3	2.5	100.0
IX. SOFT TISSUE SARCOMAS	4	14	10	10	38	10.3	10.3	100.0	100.0
Rhabdomyosarcoma	3	10	5	7	25	6.8	6.7	65.8	100.0
Fibrosarcoma	1	2	2	0	5	1.4	1.4	13.2	100.0
Other and unspecified	0	2	3	3	8	2.2	2.2	21.1	100.0
X. GONADAL & GERM CELL	4	4	2	7	17	4.6	4.5	100.0	100.0
Non-gonadal germ cell	2	4	0	0	6	1.6	1.5	35.3	100.0
Gonadal germ cell	2	0	2	6	10	2.7	2.7	58.8	100.0
Gonadal carcinoma	0	0	0	1	1	0.3	0.3	5.9	100.0
Other and unspecified	0	0	0	0	0	-	-	-	-
XI. EPITHELIAL NEOPLASMS	1	14	16	36	67	18.2	18.4	100.0	100.0
Adrenocortical carcinoma	0	0	0	0	0	-	-	-	-
Thyroid carcinoma	0	0	2	1	3	0.8	0.9	4.5	100.0
Nasopharyngeal carcinoma	0	0	1	18	19	5.2	5.2	28.4	100.0
Melanoma	0	0	0	0	0	-	-	-	-
Other carcinoma	1	14	13	17	45	12.2	12.3	67.2	100.0
XII. OTHER	0	2	2	0	4	1.1	1.1	100.0	100.0
* Specified as malignant	0	0	0	0	0	-	-	-	-

NUMBER OF CASES — columns: 0, 1-4, 5-9, 10-14, All
REL. FREQUENCY(%) — columns: Crude, Adj., Group

UGANDA

Kampala Cancer Registry, 1968–1982

R. Owor

The Kampala Cancer Registry was established in 1951, and is based in the Department of Pathology of Makerere University School of Medicine, which is located in its main teaching hospital, Mulago Hospital. This is a large general hospital of some 960 beds, providing services for the residents of Kampala and acting as a referral centre for the whole country. In addition, the Department provides diagnostic histopathology services for the other government hospitals in Kampala (Mengo, Rubaga and Nsambya Hospitals), as well as for those elsewhere in the country. Specimens from private clinics are not dealt with. The great majority of specimens come from Kampala itself, and the tables presented here have been prepared for residents of Kyadondo County *only*.

The data presented here are for the period 1968–1982, and for histologically diagnosed cases only (including cytological and haematological specimens). No cases based on clinical diagnosis alone are included; however, cases of leukaemia diagnosed in the Department of Haematology from specimens of peripheral blood have been included. All of the children in this series are Africans, except for one Asian girl aged 1½ with a non-Hodgkin lymphoma.

The tables relating to Kyadondo give the relative frequencies of all tumour types and, for the major groups, the incidence rates also. The latter should be treated with considerable reserve since they are based on the population enumerated at the census of 1969, which is likely to be only the crudest approximation to the average annual population for the 15-year period covered here.

Several previous reports have been published describing the pattern of childhood cancer in Kampala: these include reports relating to 1952–1958 (O'Conor & Davies, 1960) and 1964–1968 (Davies, 1973).

Population

The population is that for Kyadondo County from the 1969 Uganda census (Templeton *et al.*, 1972). As already pointed out, this is unlikely to be more than a crude approximation to the population at risk over the period 1968-1982.

AVERAGE ANNUAL POPULATION: 1968-1982

Age	Male	Female
0–4	36013	36802
5–9	23989	26366
10–14	17355	17636
0–14	77357	80804

Commentary

In the Kampala Cancer Registry, 30% of all registrations for children were lymphomas; of these, 45% were non-Hodgkin lymphoma, 28% were Burkitt's lymphoma and 18% were Hodgkin's disease. Leukaemia accounted for 16% of registrations, and two-thirds of these were acute or other lymphocytic in type. Neuroblastoma and Ewing's sarcoma were very rare. Retinoblastoma was as common as Wilms' tumour and there were, in addition, three cases classified as eye carcinomas. There were few brain tumours.

Compared with the series from the Kampala Registry for 1964–1968 reported by Davies (1973), the present series contained markedly lower relative frequencies of lymphoma (especially Burkitt's) and relatively more leukaemias, brain tumours and epithelial tumours. Davies suggested that leukaemia and brain tumours were likely to have been under-ascertained, so it is possible that the position has improved in more recent years. It is not possible to say whether the underlying incidence of Burkitt's lymphoma has decreased, since the pre-

Contd p. 61

Uganda, Kampala   1968 – 1982   MALE

DIAGNOSTIC GROUP	NUMBER OF CASES					REL. FREQUENCY(%)			HV(%)
	0	1-4	5-9	10-14	All	Crude	Adj.	Group	
TOTAL	8	33	33	38	112	100.0	100.0	100.0	100.0
I. LEUKAEMIAS	0	7	7	5	19	17.0	17.1	100.0	100.0
Acute lymphocytic	0	6	3	1	10	8.9	9.4	52.6	100.0
Other lymphocytic	0	1	1	0	2	1.8	1.9	10.5	100.0
Acute non-lymphocytic	0	0	1	2	3	2.7	2.5	15.8	100.0
Chronic myeloid	0	0	0	1	1	0.9	0.6	5.3	100.0
Other and unspecified	0	0	2	1	3	2.7	2.6	15.8	100.0
II. LYMPHOMAS	0	6	14	15	35	31.3	30.4	100.0	100.0
Hodgkin's disease	0	1	0	4	5	4.5	4.1	14.3	100.0
Non-Hodgkin lymphoma	0	2	6	7	15	13.4	12.9	42.9	100.0
Burkitt's lymphoma	0	3	7	2	12	10.7	10.9	34.3	100.0
Unspecified lymphoma	0	0	1	2	3	2.7	2.5	8.6	100.0
Histiocytosis X	0	0	0	0	0	–	–	–	–
Other reticuloendothelial	0	0	0	0	0	–	–	–	–
III. BRAIN AND SPINAL	2	0	2	1	5	4.5	4.6	100.0	100.0
Ependymoma	1	0	0	0	1	0.9	1.0	20.0	100.0
Astrocytoma	1	0	1	0	2	1.8	1.9	40.0	100.0
Medulloblastoma	0	0	0	0	0	–	–	–	–
Other glioma	0	0	0	1	1	0.9	0.8	20.0	100.0
Other and unspecified *	0	0	1	0	1	0.9	0.9	20.0	100.0
IV. SYMPATHETIC N.S.	0	0	0	1	1	0.9	0.8	100.0	100.0
Neuroblastoma	0	0	0	1	1	0.9	0.8	100.0	100.0
Other	0	0	0	0	0	–	–	–	–
V. RETINOBLASTOMA	3	10	0	0	13	11.6	12.7	100.0	100.0
VI. KIDNEY	2	6	3	1	12	10.7	11.3	100.0	100.0
Wilms' tumour	2	6	3	1	12	10.7	11.3	100.0	100.0
Renal carcinoma	0	0	0	0	0	–	–	–	–
Other and unspecified	0	0	0	0	0	–	–	–	–
VII. LIVER	0	0	0	0	0	–	–	–	–
Hepatoblastoma	0	0	0	0	0	–	–	–	–
Hepatic carcinoma	0	0	0	0	0	–	–	–	–
Other and unspecified	0	0	0	0	0	–	–	–	–
VIII. BONE	0	0	1	4	5	4.5	4.1	100.0	100.0
Osteosarcoma	0	0	1	3	4	3.6	3.3	80.0	100.0
Chondrosarcoma	0	0	0	0	0	–	–	–	–
Ewing's sarcoma	0	0	0	1	1	0.9	0.8	20.0	100.0
Other and unspecified	0	0	0	0	0	–	–	–	–
IX. SOFT TISSUE SARCOMAS	0	3	4	5	12	10.7	10.5	100.0	100.0
Rhabdomyosarcoma	0	2	1	2	5	4.5	4.4	41.7	100.0
Fibrosarcoma	0	0	1	1	2	1.8	1.7	16.7	100.0
Other and unspecified	0	1	2	2	5	4.5	4.4	41.7	100.0
X. GONADAL & GERM CELL	1	0	1	0	2	1.8	1.9	100.0	100.0
Non-gonadal germ cell	0	0	1	0	1	0.9	0.9	50.0	100.0
Gonadal germ cell	1	0	0	0	1	0.9	1.0	50.0	100.0
Gonadal carcinoma	0	0	0	0	0	–	–	–	–
Other and unspecified	0	0	0	0	0	.	–	–	–
XI. EPITHELIAL NEOPLASMS	0	0	1	6	7	6.3	5.6	100.0	100.0
Adrenocortical carcinoma	0	0	0	0	0	–	–	–	–
Thyroid carcinoma	0	0	0	0	0	–	–	–	–
Nasopharyngeal carcinoma	0	0	0	3	3	2.7	2.4	42.9	100.0
Melanoma	0	0	1	0	1	0.9	0.9	14.3	100.0
Other carcinoma	0	0	0	3	3	2.7	2.4	42.9	100.0
XII. OTHER	0	1	0	0	1	0.9	1.0	100.0	100.0

* Specified as malignant

Uganda, Kampala   1968 - 1982   FEMALE

DIAGNOSTIC GROUP	NUMBER OF CASES					REL. FREQUENCY(%)			HV(%)
	0	1-4	5-9	10-14	All	Crude	Adj.	Group	
TOTAL	4	28	26	33	91	100.0	100.0	100.0	100.0
I. LEUKAEMIAS	2	2	7	3	14	15.4	15.8	100.0	100.0
Acute lymphocytic	2	2	3	3	10	11.0	11.2	71.4	100.0
Other lymphocytic	0	0	0	0	0	-	-	-	-
Acute non-lymphocytic	0	0	4	0	4	4.4	4.6	28.6	100.0
Chronic myeloid	0	0	0	0	0	-	-	-	-
Other and unspecified	0	0	0	0	0	-	-	-	-
II. LYMPHOMAS	1	6	9	9	25	27.5	27.3	100.0	100.0
Hodgkin's disease	0	1	2	3	6	6.6	6.4	24.0	100.0
Non-Hodgkin lymphoma	1	2	5	4	12	13.2	13.2	48.0	100.0
Burkitt's lymphoma	0	2	2	1	5	5.5	5.7	20.0	100.0
Unspecified lymphoma	0	0	0	1	1	1.1	1.2	4.0	100.0
Histiocytosis X	0	0	0	0	0	-	-	-	-
Other reticuloendothelial	0	0	0	1	1	1.1	0.9	4.0	-
III. BRAIN AND SPINAL	0	1	4	0	5	5.5	5.9	100.0	100.0
Ependymoma	0	0	1	0	1	1.1	1.2	20.0	100.0
Astrocytoma	0	1	0	0	1	1.1	1.3	20.0	100.0
Medulloblastoma	0	0	0	0	0	-	-	-	-
Other glioma	0	0	2	0	2	2.2	2.3	40.0	100.0
Other and unspecified *	0	0	1	0	1	1.1	1.2	20.0	100.0
IV. SYMPATHETIC N.S.	0	0	0	2	2	2.2	1.8	100.0	100.0
Neuroblastoma	0	0	0	1	1	1.1	0.9	50.0	100.0
Other	0	0	0	1	1	1.1	0.9	50.0	100.0
V. RETINOBLASTOMA	0	7	0	0	7	7.7	8.8	100.0	100.0
VI. KIDNEY	1	7	1	0	9	9.9	11.2	100.0	100.0
Wilms' tumour	1	7	1	0	9	9.9	11.2	100.0	100.0
Renal carcinoma	0	0	0	0	0	-	-	-	-
Other and unspecified	0	0	0	0	0	-	-	-	-
VII. LIVER	0	0	0	1	1	1.1	0.9	100.0	100.0
Hepatoblastoma	0	0	0	0	0	-	-	-	-
Hepatic carcinoma	0	0	1	0	1	1.1	0.9	100.0	100.0
Other and unspecified	0	0	0	0	0	-	-	-	-
VIII. BONE	0	0	1	8	9	9.9	8.4	100.0	100.0
Osteosarcoma	0	0	1	8	9	9.9	8.4	100.0	100.0
Chondrosarcoma	0	0	0	0	0	-	-	-	-
Ewing's sarcoma	0	0	0	0	0	-	-	-	-
Other and unspecified	0	0	0	0	0	-	-	-	-
IX. SOFT TISSUE SARCOMAS	0	1	1	3	5	5.5	5.1	100.0	100.0
Rhabdomyosarcoma	0	1	1	1	3	3.3	3.3	60.0	100.0
Fibrosarcoma	0	1	0	0	1	1.1	0.9	20.0	100.0
Other and unspecified	0	0	0	1	1	1.1	0.9	20.0	100.0
X. GONADAL & GERM CELL	0	1	1	1	3	3.3	3.3	100.0	100.0
Non-gonadal germ cell	0	1	1	0	2	2.2	2.4	66.7	100.0
Gonadal germ cell	0	0	0	1	1	1.1	0.9	33.3	100.0
Gonadal carcinoma	0	0	0	0	0	-	-	-	-
Other and unspecified	0	0	0	0	0	-	-	-	-
XI. EPITHELIAL NEOPLASMS	0	2	1	5	8	8.8	8.2	100.0	100.0
Adrenocortical carcinoma	0	0	0	0	0	-	-	-	-
Thyroid carcinoma	0	0	0	0	0	-	-	-	-
Nasopharyngeal carcinoma	0	0	0	0	0	-	-	-	-
Melanoma	0	0	0	1	1	1.1	0.9	12.5	100.0
Other carcinoma	0	2	1	4	7	7.7	7.3	87.5	100.0
XII. OTHER	0	1	1	1	3	3.3	3.3	100.0	100.0
* Specified as malignant	0	0	0	0	0	-	-	-	-

Uganda, Kampala

1968 – 1982

MALE

DIAGNOSTIC GROUP	NUMBER OF CASES					REL. FREQUENCY(%)			RATES PER MILLION						HV(%)
	0	1-4	5-9	10-14	All	Crude	Adj.	Group	0-4	5-9	10-14	Crude	Adj.	Cum	
TOTAL	8	33	33	38	112	100.0	100.0	100.0	75.9	91.7	146.0	96.5	101.3	1568	100.0
I. LEUKAEMIAS	0	7	7	5	19	17.0	17.1	100.0	13.0	19.5	19.2	16.4	16.9	258	100.0
II. LYMPHOMAS	0	6	14	15	35	31.3	30.4	100.0	11.1	38.9	57.6	30.2	33.6	538	100.0
III. BRAIN AND SPINAL	2	0	2	1	5	4.5	4.6	100.0	3.7	5.6	3.8	4.3	4.3	66	100.0
IV. SYMPATHETIC N.S.	0	0	0	1	1	0.9	0.8	100.0			3.8	0.9	1.1	19	100.0
V. RETINOBLASTOMA	3	10	0	0	13	11.6	12.7	100.0	24.1			11.2	9.3	120	100.0
VI. KIDNEY	2	6	3	1	12	10.7	11.3	100.0	14.8	8.3	3.8	10.3	9.5	135	100.0
VII. LIVER	0	0	0	0	0										–
VIII. BONE	0	0	1	4	5	4.5	4.1	100.0		2.8	15.4	4.3	5.4	91	100.0
IX. SOFT TISSUE SARCOMAS	0	3	4	5	12	10.7	10.5	100.0	5.6	11.1	19.2	10.3	11.3	179	100.0
X. GONADAL & GERM CELL	1	0	1	0	2	1.8	1.9	100.0	1.9	2.8		1.7	1.6	23	100.0
XI. EPITHELIAL NEOPLASMS	0	0	1	6	7	6.3	5.6	100.0		2.8	23.0	6.0	7.6	129	100.0
XII. OTHER	0	1	0	0	1	0.9	1.0	100.0	1.9			0.9	0.7	9	100.0

Uganda, Kampala

1968 – 1982

FEMALE

DIAGNOSTIC GROUP	NUMBER OF CASES					REL. FREQUENCY(%)			RATES PER MILLION						HV(%)
	0	1-4	5-9	10-14	All	Crude	Adj.	Group	0-4	5-9	10-14	Crude	Adj.	Cum	
TOTAL	4	28	26	33	91	100.0	100.0	100.0	58.0	65.7	124.7	75.1	79.9	1242	100.0
I. LEUKAEMIAS	2	2	7	3	14	15.4	15.8	100.0	7.2	17.7	11.3	11.6	11.8	181	100.0
II. LYMPHOMAS	1	6	9	9	25	27.5	27.3	100.0	12.7	22.8	34.0	20.6	22.1	347	100.0
III. BRAIN AND SPINAL	0	1	4	0	5	5.5	5.9	100.0	1.8	10.1		4.1	4.0	60	100.0
IV. SYMPATHETIC N.S.	0	0	0	2	2	2.2	1.8	100.0			7.6	1.7	2.2	38	100.0
V. RETINOBLASTOMA	0	7	0	0	7	7.7	8.8	100.0	12.7			5.8	4.9	63	100.0
VI. KIDNEY	1	7	1	0	9	9.9	11.2	100.0	14.5	2.5		7.4	6.4	85	100.0
VII. LIVER	0	0	0	1	1	1.1	0.9	100.0			3.8	0.8	1.1	19	100.0
VIII. BONE	0	0	1	8	9	9.9	8.4	100.0		2.5	30.2	7.4	9.6	164	100.0
IX. SOFT TISSUE SARCOMAS	0	1	1	3	5	5.5	5.1	100.0	1.8	2.5	11.3	4.1	4.8	78	100.0
X. GONADAL & GERM CELL	0	1	1	1	3	3.3	3.3	100.0	1.8	2.5	3.8	2.5	2.6	41	100.0
XI. EPITHELIAL NEOPLASMS	0	2	1	5	8	8.8	8.2	100.0	3.6	2.5	18.9	6.6	7.7	125	100.0
XII. OTHER	0	1	1	1	3	3.3	3.3	100.0	1.8	2.5	3.8	2.5	2.6	41	100.0

sent series is restricted to residents in Kyadondo County, and Davies pointed out that the frequency of Burkitt's lymphoma varied widely between different areas of the country.

References

Davies, J.N.P. (1973) Childhood tumours. In: Templeton, A.C., ed., *Tumours in a Tropical Country. A Survey in Uganda 1964-68*. Recent Results in Cancer Research, Vol. 41, Berlin, Heidelberg, New York, Springer, pp. 306-320

O'Conor, G.T. & Davies, J.N.P. (1960) Malignant tumours in African children. *J. Pediatr.*, *56*, 526-535

Templeton, A.C., Buxton, E. & Bianchi, A. (1972) Cancer in Kyadondo County, Uganda, 1968-70. *J. natl Cancer Inst.*, *48*, 865-874

Kuluva Hospital, West Nile District, 1961-1978

E.H. Williams

This series consists of all the cases of cancer in children aged 0–14 admitted to Kuluva Hospital in the West Nile District of Uganda during the 18 years between 1961 and 1978. A register of all the cancer cases seen over this period was created from the case records. No histopathology facilities were available in the hospital, and this service was provided by Makerere Medical School in Kampala; however, local cytological diagnosis was widely used to allow treatment to commence, and considerable experience with this technique developed.

Kuluva Hospital has about 75 beds, and is one of six hospitals serving the West Nile District (estimated population 551 000 in 1968); it is not possible to define a population from which the registered cases are drawn, so no incidence rates can be estimated.

A previous report (Williams, 1967) presented data from the early years of this registry.

Commentary

West Nile District is known to be an area with an exceptionally high incidence of Burkitt's lymphoma and a considerable amount of research has been carried out in this area on patterns of space-time clustering, and the relationship of this tumour to Epstein-Barr virus and malaria (Williams *et al.*, 1978; Geser *et al.*, 1983).

In the present series from West Nile District, 68% of all cases were Burkitt's lymphoma. Retinoblastoma accounted for 12/205 cases (5%) and there were a further six other and unspecified eye tumours. There was no other diagnosis in more than nine cases. There were no cases at all of brain tumours or neuroblastoma.

It may safely be concluded that Burkitt's lymphoma has a much higher incidence in West Nile than in Kyadondo. Small numbers and the unknown relationship between frequencies of ascertained cases and underlying incidence preclude any other meaningful comparisons between the two areas.

References

Geser, A., Lenoir, G.M., Anvret, M., Bornkamm, G., Klein, G., Williams, E.H., Wright, D.H. & de The, G. (1983) Epstein-Barr markers in a series of Burkitt's lymphomas from the West Nile District, Uganda. *Eur. J. Cancer clin. Oncol.*, *19*, 1393-1404

Williams, E.H. (1967) *Variations in tumour distribution in the West Nile District of Uganda.* In: Clifford, P., Linsell, C.A. & Timms, G.L., eds, *Cancer in Africa*, Nairobi, East African Publishing House, pp. 37-42

Williams, E.H., Smith, P.G., Day, N.E., Geser, A., Ellice, J. & Tukei, P. (1978) Space-time clustering of Burkitt's lymphoma in the West Nile District of Uganda 1961-75. *Br. J. Cancer, 37*, 109-122

Uganda, West Nile

MALE

1961 - 1978

DIAGNOSTIC GROUP	NUMBER OF CASES					REL. FREQUENCY(%)			HV(%)
	0	1-4	5-9	10-14	All	Crude	Adj.	Group	
TOTAL	4	28	66	23	121	100.0	100.0	100.0	88.4
I. LEUKAEMIAS	2	1	0	1	4	3.3	5.1	100.0	100.0
Acute lymphocytic	0	0	0	0	0	-	-	-	-
Other lymphocytic	0	0	0	0	0	-	-	-	-
Acute non-lymphocytic	0	0	0	1	1	0.8	1.3	25.0	100.0
Chronic myeloid	0	0	0	0	0	-	-	-	-
Other and unspecified	2	1	0	0	3	2.5	3.8	75.0	100.0
II. LYMPHOMAS	0	14	64	15	93	76.9	66.2	100.0	92.5
Hodgkin's disease	0	0	1	0	1	0.8	0.5	1.1	100.0
Non-Hodgkin lymphoma	0	1	2	2	5	4.1	4.8	5.4	100.0
Burkitt's lymphoma	0	13	61	10	84	69.4	57.0	90.3	91.7
Unspecified lymphoma	0	0	0	3	3	2.5	3.9	3.2	100.0
Histiocytosis X	0	0	0	0	0	-	-	-	-
Other reticuloendothelial	0	0	0	0	0	-	-	-	-
III. BRAIN AND SPINAL	0	0	0	0	0	-	-	-	-
Ependymoma	0	0	0	0	0	-	-	-	-
Astrocytoma	0	0	0	0	0	-	-	-	-
Medulloblastoma	0	0	0	0	0	-	-	-	-
Other glioma	0	0	0	0	0	-	-	-	-
Other and unspecified *	0	0	0	0	0	-	-	-	-
IV. SYMPATHETIC N.S.	0	0	0	0	0	-	-	-	-
Neuroblastoma	0	0	0	0	0	-	-	-	-
Other	0	0	0	0	0	-	-	-	-
V. RETINOBLASTOMA	0	5	1	0	6	5.0	6.7	100.0	100.0
VI. KIDNEY	0	3	1	0	4	3.3	4.2	100.0	100.0
Wilms' tumour	0	3	1	0	4	3.3	4.2	100.0	100.0
Renal carcinoma	0	0	0	0	0	-	-	-	-
Other and unspecified	0	0	0	0	0	-	-	-	-
VII. LIVER	0	0	0	1	1	0.8	1.3	100.0	100.0
Hepatoblastoma	0	0	0	0	0	-	-	-	-
Hepatic carcinoma	0	0	0	0	0	-	-	-	-
Other and unspecified	0	0	0	1	1	0.8	1.3	100.0	100.0
VIII.BONE	0	0	0	1	1	0.8	1.3	100.0	100.0
Osteosarcoma	0	0	0	1	1	0.8	1.3	100.0	100.0
Chondrosarcoma	0	0	0	0	0	-	-	-	-
Ewing's sarcoma	0	0	0	0	0	-	-	-	-
Other and unspecified	0	0	0	0	0	-	-	-	-
IX. SOFT TISSUE SARCOMAS	0	2	0	2	4	3.3	5.1	100.0	100.0
Rhabdomyosarcoma	0	1	0	0	1	0.8	1.3	25.0	100.0
Fibrosarcoma	0	0	0	0	0	-	-	-	-
Other and unspecified	0	1	0	2	3	2.5	3.9	75.0	100.0
X. GONADAL & GERM CELL	0	0	0	0	0	-	-	-	-
Non-gonadal germ cell	0	0	0	0	0	-	-	-	-
Gonadal germ cell	0	0	0	0	0	-	-	-	-
Gonadal carcinoma	0	0	0	0	0	-	-	-	-
Other and unspecified	0	0	0	0	0	-	-	-	-
XI. EPITHELIAL NEOPLASMS	0	0	0	1	1	0.8	1.3	100.0	100.0
Adrenocortical carcinoma	0	0	0	0	0	-	-	-	-
Thyroid carcinoma	0	0	0	0	0	-	-	-	-
Nasopharyngeal carcinoma	0	0	0	1	1	0.8	1.3	100.0	100.0
Melanoma	0	0	0	0	0	-	-	-	-
Other carcinoma	0	0	0	0	0	-	-	-	-
XII. OTHER	2	3	0	2	7	5.8	8.9	100.0	14.3

* Specified as malignant 0 0 0 0 0 - - - -

Uganda, West Nile

FEMALE

1961 - 1978

DIAGNOSTIC GROUP	NUMBER OF CASES					REL. FREQUENCY(%)			HV(%)
	0	1-4	5-9	10-14	All	Crude	Adj.	Group	
TOTAL	1	23	47	13	84	100.0	100.0	100.0	90.5
I. LEUKAEMIAS	1	1	2	0	4	4.8	4.6	100.0	100.0
Acute lymphocytic	0	0	0	0	0	-	-	-	-
Other lymphocytic	0	0	0	0	0	-	-	-	-
Acute non-lymphocytic	0	0	0	0	0	-	-	-	-
Chronic myeloid	0	0	0	0	0	-	-	-	-
Other and unspecified	1	1	2	0	4	4.8	4.6	100.0	100.0
II. LYMPHOMAS	0	11	42	9	62	73.8	65.9	100.0	88.7
Hodgkin's disease	0	0	0	0	0	-	-	-	-
Non-Hodgkin lymphoma	0	0	1	3	4	4.8	7.6	6.5	100.0
Burkitt's lymphoma	0	11	39	6	56	66.7	57.1	90.3	87.5
Unspecified lymphoma	0	0	2	0	2	2.4	1.3	3.2	100.0
Histiocytosis X	0	0	0	0	0	-	-	-	-
Other reticuloendothelial	0	0	0	0	0	-	-	-	-
III. BRAIN AND SPINAL	0	0	0	0	0	-	-	-	-
Ependymoma	0	0	0	0	0	-	-	-	-
Astrocytoma	0	0	0	0	0	-	-	-	-
Medulloblastoma	0	0	0	0	0	-	-	-	-
Other glioma	0	0	0	0	0	-	-	-	-
Other and unspecified *	0	0	0	0	0	-	-	-	-
IV. SYMPATHETIC N.S.	0	0	0	0	0	-	-	-	-
Neuroblastoma	0	0	0	0	0	-	-	-	-
Other	0	0	0	0	0	-	-	-	-
V. RETINOBLASTOMA	0	6	0	0	6	7.1	10.0	100.0	100.0
VI. KIDNEY	0	4	1	0	5	6.0	7.3	100.0	100.0
Wilms' tumour	0	4	1	0	5	6.0	7.3	100.0	100.0
Renal carcinoma	0	0	0	0	0	-	-	-	-
Other and unspecified	0	0	0	0	0	-	-	-	-
VII. LIVER	0	0	0	0	0	-	-	-	-
Hepatoblastoma	0	0	0	0	0	-	-	-	-
Hepatic carcinoma	0	0	0	0	0	-	-	-	-
Other and unspecified	0	0	0	0	0	-	-	-	-
VIII.BONE	0	0	0	1	1	1.2	2.3	100.0	100.0
Osteosarcoma	0	0	0	0	0	-	-	-	-
Chondrosarcoma	0	0	0	0	0	-	-	-	-
Ewing's sarcoma	0	0	0	0	0	-	-	-	-
Other and unspecified	0	0	0	1	1	1.2	2.3	100.0	100.0
IX. SOFT TISSUE SARCOMAS	0	0	1	1	2	2.4	2.9	100.0	100.0
Rhabdomyosarcoma	0	0	1	1	2	2.4	2.9	100.0	100.0
Fibrosarcoma	0	0	0	0	0	-	-	-	-
Other and unspecified	0	0	0	0	0	-	-	-	-
X. GONADAL & GERM CELL	0	0	1	1	2	2.4	2.9	100.0	100.0
Non-gonadal germ cell	0	0	0	0	0	-	-	-	-
Gonadal germ cell	0	0	1	1	2	2.4	2.9	100.0	100.0
Gonadal carcinoma	0	0	0	0	0	-	-	-	-
Other and unspecified	0	0	0	0	0	-	-	-	-
XI. EPITHELIAL NEOPLASMS	0	0	0	1	1	1.2	2.3	100.0	100.0
Adrenocortical carcinoma	0	0	0	0	0	-	-	-	-
Thyroid carcinoma	0	0	0	0	0	-	-	-	-
Nasopharyngeal carcinoma	0	0	0	0	0	-	-	-	-
Melanoma	0	0	0	0	0	-	-	-	-
Other carcinoma	0	0	0	1	1	1.2	2.3	100.0	100.0
XII. OTHER	0	1	0	0	1	1.2	1.7	100.0	-

* Specified as malignant

ZIMBABWE

Bulawayo Cancer Registry, 1963–1977

M.E.G. Skinner

Zimbabwe, until 1980 known as Rhodesia, is situated in southern Africa, between the northern border of the Transvaal and the Zambesi river. Its area is 390 000 square kilometres, and the population in 1982 was 7.5 million.

Bulawayo Cancer Registry was founded in 1963, and functioned as a population-based register for 15 years. It was based in Mpilo Central Hospital, a large regional hospital providing specialist services during that period for the African population of south-western Zimbabwe.

New cases of cancer were notified from all hospital wards and departments, pathology laboratories and the mortuary. Direct notification from other sources was unusual, but as Mpilo Hospital is the only hospital in the region with specialist cancer services, Africans with cancer diagnosed in the Bulawayo area were almost invariably referred for treatment and thus caught in the registration network. Notification was routine hospital procedure; hospital case notes with a diagnosis or suspected diagnosis of cancer were sent to the Registry on discharge or death. Copies of all histology and autopsy reports were submitted by both hospital and private laboratories. Death certificates were scrutinized monthly by the Registrar; however, initial notification from this source was rare and an attempt was made to obtain all information about the case prior to registration.

In the period under consideration, death certification prior to burial was mandatory in Bulawayo and the bodies of all persons dying outside hospital in the African townships of the city were brought to Mpilo Mortuary for autopsy prior to certification. Hence cancers in persons who did not seek medical attention during life were unlikely to be missed if those concerned died from cancer in the Bulawayo area. For most of the period considered here, the autopsy rate in the hospital was high and was in part responsible for the very high rate of histological proof of diagnosis.

All data were checked for duplication and error and coded before processing and computing at the Department of Social and Preventive Medicine of the Medical School.

The data presented here represent all cases of cancer in African children recorded by the registry for the 15-year period 1963–1977. These cases are drawn from the whole of south-western Zimbabwe.

In addition, a small table presents the results for children recorded as being residents of Bulawayo itself, and incidence rates have been calculated using as denominator a population based on data for 1965 and 1969. Some of the problems relating to the use made of medical services by the African population have been described previously (Skinner, 1976), particularly in relation to the habit of cancer patients returning 'home' to rural areas to invoke the aid of witchcraft or to die. However, it seems probable that a larger proportion of children than adults would be brought to hospital in the event of a serious illness, such as cancer, so that under-registration in this age-group may not be very great, at least until about 1973–1975. Towards the end of the period considered here, both registration processes and the stability of the population at risk were considerably disrupted by the civil war.

Population

The childhood population was estimated from the census of 1969 (Central Statistical Office) and from an estimate of the population for 1965, based in part on the census of 1962, and in part on a population sample survey (Mitchell, 1967).

AVERAGE ANNUAL POPULATION: 1963–1977
(Residents only)

Age	Male	Female
0–4	11121	10721
5–9	11744	11545
10–14	8638	9363
0–14	31503	31629

Contd p. 71

Zimbabwe, Bulawayo   1963 - 1977   MALE

DIAGNOSTIC GROUP	NUMBER OF CASES				REL. FREQUENCY(%)			HV(%)
	0-4	5-9	10-14	All	Crude	Adj.	Group	
TOTAL	137	84	77	298	100.0	100.0	100.0	95.6
I. LEUKAEMIAS	14	16	12	42	14.1	14.5	100.0	90.5
Acute lymphocytic	2	9	6	17	5.7	6.1	40.5	82.4
Other lymphocytic	1	0	1	2	0.7	0.7	4.8	100.0
Acute non-lymphocytic	4	3	3	10	3.4	3.4	23.8	100.0
Chronic myeloid	0	0	0	0	-	-	-	-
Other and unspecified	7	4	2	13	4.4	4.3	31.0	92.3
II. LYMPHOMAS	13	23	18	54	18.1	19.0	100.0	100.0
Hodgkin's disease	2	10	7	19	6.4	6.9	35.2	100.0
Non-Hodgkin lymphoma	7	9	10	26	8.7	9.2	48.1	100.0
Burkitt's lymphoma	4	2	1	7	2.3	2.3	13.0	100.0
Unspecified lymphoma	0	2	0	2	0.7	0.7	3.7	100.0
Histiocytosis X	0	0	0	0	-	-	-	-
Other reticuloendothelial	0	0	0	0	-	-	-	-
III. BRAIN AND SPINAL	9	8	4	21	7.0	7.0	100.0	90.5
Ependymoma	2	1	2	5	1.7	1.7	23.8	100.0
Astrocytoma	4	2	0	6	2.0	1.9	28.6	100.0
Medulloblastoma	1	1	0	2	0.7	0.6	9.5	100.0
Other glioma	0	1	1	2	0.7	0.7	9.5	100.0
Other and unspecified *	2	3	1	6	2.0	2.0	28.6	66.7
IV. SYMPATHETIC N.S.	8	2	1	11	3.7	3.4	100.0	100.0
Neuroblastoma	8	2	1	11	3.7	3.4	100.0	100.0
Other	0	0	0	0	-	-	-	-
V. RETINOBLASTOMA	36	6	0	42	14.1	12.7	100.0	100.0
VI. KIDNEY	34	6	0	40	13.4	12.1	100.0	90.0
Wilms' tumour	31	4	0	35	11.7	10.5	87.5	100.0
Renal carcinoma	0	1	0	1	0.3	0.4	2.5	100.0
Other and unspecified	3	1	0	4	1.3	1.2	10.0	-
VII. LIVER	0	2	15	17	5.7	6.6	100.0	100.0
Hepatoblastoma	0	1	0	1	0.3	0.4	5.9	100.0
Hepatic carcinoma	0	1	15	16	5.4	6.2	94.1	100.0
Other and unspecified	0	0	0	0	-	-	-	-
VIII. BONE	0	3	13	16	5.4	6.1	100.0	93.8
Osteosarcoma	0	2	7	9	3.0	3.4	56.3	100.0
Chondrosarcoma	0	0	4	4	1.3	1.6	25.0	100.0
Ewing's sarcoma	0	0	0	0	-	-	-	-
Other and unspecified	0	1	2	3	1.0	1.1	18.8	66.7
IX. SOFT TISSUE SARCOMAS	19	13	10	42	14.1	14.1	100.0	100.0
Rhabdomyosarcoma	5	3	0	8	2.7	2.5	19.0	100.0
Fibrosarcoma	4	4	3	11	3.7	3.8	26.2	100.0
Other and unspecified	10	6	7	23	7.7	7.8	54.8	100.0
X. GONADAL & GERM CELL	1	1	0	2	0.7	0.6	100.0	100.0
Non-gonadal germ cell	1	0	0	1	0.3	0.3	50.0	100.0
Gonadal germ cell	0	1	0	1	0.3	0.4	50.0	100.0
Gonadal carcinoma	0	0	0	0	-	-	-	-
Other and unspecified	0	0	0	0	-	-	-	-
XI. EPITHELIAL NEOPLASMS	2	3	3	8	2.7	2.8	100.0	100.0
Adrenocortical carcinoma	0	0	0	0	-	-	-	-
Thyroid carcinoma	0	0	1	1	0.3	0.4	12.5	100.0
Nasopharyngeal carcinoma	0	0	0	0	-	-	-	-
Melanoma	1	0	0	1	0.3	0.3	12.5	100.0
Other carcinoma	1	3	2	6	2.0	2.1	75.0	100.0
XII. OTHER	1	1	1	3	1.0	1.0	100.0	33.3
* Specified as malignant	1	2	0	3	1.0	1.0	100.0	33.3

Zimbabwe, Bulawayo

1963 - 1977

FEMALE

DIAGNOSTIC GROUP	NUMBER OF CASES				REL. FREQUENCY(%)			HV(%)
	0-4	5-9	10-14	All	Crude	Adj.	Group	
TOTAL	113	71	61	245	100.0	100.0	100.0	92.2
I. LEUKAEMIAS	9	20	7	36	14.7	15.1	100.0	86.1
Acute lymphocytic	3	9	1	13	5.3	5.4	36.1	76.9
Other lymphocytic	0	0	0	0	-	-	-	-
Acute non-lymphocytic	5	3	3	11	4.5	4.5	30.6	90.9
Chronic myeloid	0	1	0	1	0.4	0.4	2.8	100.0
Other and unspecified	1	7	3	11	4.5	4.8	30.6	90.9
II. LYMPHOMAS	7	12	10	29	11.8	12.5	100.0	100.0
Hodgkin's disease	1	4	7	12	4.9	5.5	41.4	100.0
Non-Hodgkin lymphoma	3	6	3	12	4.9	5.1	41.4	100.0
Burkitt's lymphoma	2	1	0	3	1.2	1.1	10.3	100.0
Unspecified lymphoma	1	1	0	2	0.8	0.8	6.9	100.0
Histiocytosis X	0	0	0	0	-	-	-	-
Other reticuloendothelial	0	0	0	0	-	-	-	-
III. BRAIN AND SPINAL	6	6	5	17	6.9	7.1	100.0	70.6
Ependymoma	0	1	0	1	0.4	0.4	5.9	100.0
Astrocytoma	1	2	2	5	2.0	2.2	29.4	100.0
Medulloblastoma	1	2	1	4	1.6	1.7	23.5	100.0
Other glioma	1	0	0	1	0.4	0.4	5.9	100.0
Other and unspecified *	3	1	2	6	2.4	2.5	35.3	16.7
IV. SYMPATHETIC N.S.	6	0	2	8	3.3	3.1	100.0	100.0
Neuroblastoma	6	0	2	8	3.3	3.1	100.0	100.0
Other	0	0	0	0	-	-	-	-
V. RETINOBLASTOMA	29	5	1	35	14.3	12.9	100.0	100.0
VI. KIDNEY	27	9	0	36	14.7	13.4	100.0	94.4
Wilms' tumour	26	8	0	34	13.9	12.6	94.4	100.0
Renal carcinoma	0	0	0	0	-	-	-	-
Other and unspecified	1	1	0	2	0.8	0.8	5.6	-
VII. LIVER	2	0	3	5	2.0	2.2	100.0	60.0
Hepatoblastoma	1	0	0	1	0.4	0.4	20.0	100.0
Hepatic carcinoma	1	0	1	2	0.8	0.8	40.0	100.0
Other and unspecified	0	0	2	2	0.8	1.0	40.0	-
VIII.BONE	0	0	6	6	2.4	3.0	100.0	83.3
Osteosarcoma	0	0	3	3	1.2	1.5	50.0	100.0
Chondrosarcoma	0	0	0	0	-	-	-	-
Ewing's sarcoma	0	0	1	1	0.4	0.5	16.7	100.0
Other and unspecified	0	0	2	2	0.8	1.0	33.3	50.0
IX. SOFT TISSUE SARCOMAS	18	7	8	33	13.5	13.3	100.0	100.0
Rhabdomyosarcoma	4	3	0	7	2.9	2.7	21.2	100.0
Fibrosarcoma	2	1	4	7	2.9	3.1	21.2	100.0
Other and unspecified	12	3	4	19	7.8	7.5	57.6	100.0
X. GONADAL & GERM CELL	4	7	5	16	6.5	6.8	100.0	100.0
Non-gonadal germ cell	4	0	0	4	1.6	1.4	25.0	100.0
Gonadal germ cell	0	4	2	6	2.4	2.7	37.5	100.0
Gonadal carcinoma	0	3	1	4	1.6	1.8	25.0	100.0
Other and unspecified	0	0	2	2	0.8	1.0	12.5	100.0
XI. EPITHELIAL NEOPLASMS	2	4	11	17	6.9	7.8	100.0	100.0
Adrenocortical carcinoma	0	0	1	1	0.4	0.5	5.9	100.0
Thyroid carcinoma	0	2	3	5	2.0	2.3	29.4	100.0
Nasopharyngeal carcinoma	0	0	0	0	-	-	-	-
Melanoma	0	0	1	1	0.4	0.5	5.9	100.0
Other carcinoma	2	2	6	10	4.1	4.5	58.8	100.0
XII. OTHER	3	1	3	7	2.9	3.0	100.0	42.9

* Specified as malignant | 3 | 0 | 2 | 5 | 2.0 | 2.0 | 100.0 | -

Zimbabwe, Bulawayo, Residents only　　　1963 - 1977　　　MALE

DIAGNOSTIC GROUP	NUMBER OF CASES				REL. FREQUENCY(%)			RATES PER MILLION						HV(%)
	0-4	5-9	10-14	All	Crude	Adj.	Group	0-4	5-9	10-14	Crude	Adj.	Cum	
TOTAL	26	11	3	40	100.0	100.0	100.0	155.9	62.4	23.2	84.6	87.2	1207	100.0
I. LEUKAEMIAS	4	2	1	7	17.5	21.6	100.0	24.0	11.4	7.7	14.8	15.2	215	100.0
II. LYMPHOMAS	5	3	0	8	20.0	15.9	100.0	30.0	17.0	-	16.9	17.1	235	100.0
III. BRAIN AND SPINAL	3	3	0	6	15.0	12.8	100.0	18.0	17.0	-	12.7	12.5	175	100.0
IV. SYMPATHETIC N.S.	4	1	0	5	12.5	8.9	100.0	24.0	5.7	-	10.6	11.1	148	100.0
V. RETINOBLASTOMA	2	0	0	2	5.0	3.1	100.0	12.0	-	-	4.2	4.6	60	100.0
VI. KIDNEY	5	0	0	5	12.5	7.7	100.0	30.0	-	-	10.6	11.6	150	100.0
VII. LIVER	0	0	0	0	-	-	-	-	-	-	-	-	-	-
VIII.BONE	0	1	0	1	2.5	2.7	100.0	-	5.7	-	2.1	1.8	28	100.0
IX. SOFT TISSUE SARCOMAS	2	1	2	5	12.5	25.8	100.0	12.0	5.7	15.4	10.6	11.0	166	100.0
X. GONADAL & GERM CELL	0	0	0	0	-	-	-	-	-	-	-	-	-	-
XI. EPITHELIAL NEOPLASMS	1	0	0	1	2.5	1.5	100.0	6.0	-	-	2.1	2.3	30	100.0
XII. OTHER	0	0	0	0	-	-	-	-	-	-	-	-	-	-

Zimbabwe, Bulawayo, Residents only　　　1963 - 1977　　　FEMALE

DIAGNOSTIC GROUP	NUMBER OF CASES				REL. FREQUENCY(%)			RATES PER MILLION						HV(%)
	0-4	5-9	10-14	All	Crude	Adj.	Group	0-4	5-9	10-14	Crude	Adj.	Cum	
TOTAL	17	11	10	38	100.0	100.0	100.0	105.7	63.5	71.2	80.1	82.1	1202	86.8
I. LEUKAEMIAS	3	3	2	8	21.1	21.2	100.0	18.7	17.3	14.2	16.9	16.9	251	87.5
II. LYMPHOMAS	1	4	1	6	15.8	16.3	100.0	6.2	23.1	7.1	12.6	11.9	182	100.0
III. BRAIN AND SPINAL	3	3	2	8	21.1	21.2	100.0	18.7	17.3	14.2	16.9	16.9	251	62.5
IV. SYMPATHETIC N.S.	2	0	0	2	5.3	4.7	100.0	12.4	-	-	4.2	4.8	62	100.0
V. RETINOBLASTOMA	3	0	0	3	7.9	7.1	100.0	18.7	-	-	6.3	7.2	93	100.0
VI. KIDNEY	2	0	0	2	5.3	4.7	100.0	12.4	-	-	4.2	4.8	62	50.0
VII. LIVER	0	0	0	0	-	-	-	-	-	-	-	-	-	-
VIII.BONE	0	0	1	1	2.6	3.0	100.0	-	-	7.1	2.1	2.1	36	100.0
IX. SOFT TISSUE SARCOMAS	1	1	1	3	7.9	8.1	100.0	6.2	5.8	7.1	6.3	6.3	96	100.0
X. GONADAL & GERM CELL	1	0	1	2	5.3	5.4	100.0	6.2	-	7.1	4.2	4.5	67	100.0
XI. EPITHELIAL NEOPLASMS	1	0	2	3	7.9	8.4	100.0	6.2	-	14.2	6.3	6.5	102	100.0
XIII. OTHER	0	0	0	0	-	-	-	-	-	-	-	-	-	-

Commentary

Lymphomas were the most numerous diagnostic group, accounting for 15% of all cases. These included substantial numbers of Hodgkin's disease and non-Hodgkin lymphoma, but Burkitt's lymphoma was comparatively rare. Leukaemia, retinoblastoma, kidney tumours and soft-tissue sarcomas each accounted for 14% of the series. Acute lymphocytic leukaemia appeared to be slightly more common than acute non-lymphocytic leukaemia but there were also a considerable number of unspecified leukaemias; the highest number of cases of acute lymphocytic leukaemia occurred in the 5—9 age-group. A quarter of soft-tissue sarcomas were Kaposi's sarcoma. Liver tumours, nearly always hepatic carcinoma, had a high relative frequency in boys. Only one case of Ewing's sarcoma was found. Neuroblastoma had a low relative frequency overall, but accounted for the same number of cases as Wilms' tumour in Bulawayo residents. This observation is based on small numbers and so may well be due to chance. However, it may also indicate under-ascertainment of neuroblastoma outside Bulawayo or a real difference in incidence between urban and rural areas. There were no other major differences between the Bulawayo residents and the main series.

References

Mitchell, F.H. (1967) Sociological aspects of cancer rate surveys in Africa. *Natl Cancer Inst. Monogr.*, 25, 151-170

Skinner, M.E.G. (1976) *Rhodesia, Bulawayo*. In: Waterhouse, J.A.H., Muir, C., Correa, P. & Powell, J., eds, *Cancer Incidence in Five Continents*, Vol. III (*IARC Scientific Publications No. 15*), Lyon, International Agency for Research on Cancer, pp. 120-123

NORTH AMERICA

CANADA

Two sets of data from Canada, covering eight of the ten provinces, are presented in this volume, one for the Western Provinces — British Columbia, Alberta, Saskatchewan and Manitoba — and one for the Atlantic Provinces — New Brunswick, Nova Scotia, Prince Edward Island and Newfoundland.

In 1969 a National Cancer Incidence Reporting System (NCIRS) was established as a co-operative undertaking by Statistics Canada, Canada's central statistical agency, and the provincial and territorial cancer registries. The system now covers the entire Canadian population. The development of this system was fostered and co-ordinated by the National Cancer Institute of Canada. The objectives of the NCIRS are to build a large data base for use in cancer surveillance of the Canadian population and for epidemiological research, and to determine survival rates through linkage with death records. Participating provinces send Statistics Canada a notification, together with basic patient and diagnostic information, for each new primary malignant neoplasm.

Diagnostic information was classified in accordance with the Eighth Revision of the *International Classification of Diseases* from 1969 to 1978; since 1979, the majority of registries have used the *International Classification of Diseases for Oncology*.

Canada has a total area of 9.98 million square kilometres and is a country of great regional diversity, ranging from the temperate areas of the Great Lakes peninsula and the south-west Pacific coast to wide fertile prairies, great areas of mountain and lake, northern wilderness and arctic tundra. Most of Canada's population lives along the southern border in a corridor about 300 kilometres in width.

At the latest census in June 1981, the population of Canada was just over 24 million; of these, 23% were under 15 years of age. The data presented here cover a total population of about 2 300 000 children. The population is very heterogeneous with respect to ethnic origin. Major groups include British (40%), French (27%), German (4.7%), Italian (3.1%), Ukrainian (2.2%) and Chinese (1.2%). The native population of Canada consists of native Indians, Métis and Inuit; together they account for 2% of the population. The great majority of Canadians are Christians by heritage. Approximately 75% lives in urban areas and 41% lives in urban centres with populations of half a million and over.

Atlantic Provinces, 1970–1979

R. Nimmagadda & D. Robb (New Brunswick)
T. Croucher & D.H. Thomson (Nova Scotia)
D.E. Dryer (Prince Edward Island)
S.K. Buehler (Newfoundland)

(i) **New Brunswick**. The Registry was set up in 1955 to register all malignant disease in the Province. Sources of data are the radiotherapy department, pathology laboratories, operation reports, X-rays and death certificates. All reporting is voluntary.

The area covered by the Registry is 73 437 square kilometres. There are five cities, none of which has more than 100 000 inhabitants. The population in 1981 was 696 400, of whom 57% are classed as urban, 39% are in non-farming rural areas and 4% are in areas classed as farming. The main occupations are manufacturing, services, fishing and farming. The majority of the population are of British or French extraction, with a small percentage of German and Dutch extraction and of native Indians.

(ii) **Nova Scotia**. The Cancer Registry of Nova Scotia was established in 1964. In 1981, responsibility for its operation was transferred to the Cancer Treatment and Research Foundation of Nova Scotia, which, in turn, is supported by the Department of Health.

The Province is covered by a provincially funded comprehensive health insurance scheme. Cancer patients diagnosed in all hospitals, clinics, physicians' offices and the Cancer Foundation are registered. Copies of the pathology reports from all hospitals in the Province, with a diagnosis of the neoplasm, are used as a basis for registration after appropriate inquiries have been made. The Department of Vital Statistics supplies lists of all deaths in the Province and these are used to obtain information on death for those patients already registered. Registration of a cancer patient is a legal requirement. Annual reports of the incidence of cancer are published.

Nova Scotia has an area of 55 491 square kilometres; in 1981 the population was 847 430, of whom 77% are of British stock, 10% French and 5% German. The predominant occupations are manufac-turing, services, mining and construction. Fishing and ship-building, formerly of substantial importance, still occupy a sizeable proportion of the work force. Some 57% of the population live in areas designated as urban, 25% in conurbations of 100 000 or more, while 43% live in rural areas.

(iii) **Prince Edward Island**. The Registry of the Province of Prince Edward Island is operated by the Division of Oncology of the Provincial Department of Health and Social Services. This Division has been in existence since 1951. Participation in the national cancer reporting scheme commenced in 1969.

Registration is voluntary. The main source of data is pathology reports with a diagnosis of cancer. Additional data necessary for cancer registration may be obtained either from the patient or from hospital records. Only a small number of registrations are based on death certificates as the sole source of information.

Hospital organization and practice are based on a comprehensive government-organized health insurance scheme.

The Registry covers the whole of Prince Edward Island, the smallest province in Canada, and with an area of 5657 square kilometres. At the 1981 census, the population was 121 225, of whom 25% were under the age of 15. Most are of European origin. The major occupations are farming, fishing and tourism. There is no heavy industry. Approximately 36% of the population live in areas designated as urban while 64% live in rural areas.

(iv) **Newfoundland**. The Newfoundland Cancer Treatment and Research Foundation is responsible for the Provincial Tumour Registry. Registration is voluntary. The Registry obtains data from sources which include pathology laboratories in the Province, haematology reports, hospital discharge information, copies of death certificates with mention of cancer, and records from the Department of Radiotherapy of the General Hospital.

Contd p. 76

Canada, Atlantic Provinces   1970 - 1979   MALE

DIAGNOSTIC GROUP	NUMBER OF CASES 0	1-4	5-9	10-14	All	REL. FREQUENCY(%) Crude	Adj.	Group	RATES PER MILLION 0	1-4	5-9	10-14	Crude	Adj.	Cum	HV(%)
TOTAL	15	118	94	97	324	100.0	100.0	100.0	77.5	148.7	84.1	80.7	98.0	102.6	1497	83.0
I. LEUKAEMIAS	3	55	37	29	124	38.3	38.2	100.0	15.5	69.3	33.1	24.1	37.5	40.4	579	79.0
Acute lymphocytic	1	32	17	11	61	18.8	18.8	49.2	5.2	40.3	15.2	9.2	18.4	20.5	288	86.9
Other lymphocytic	1	7	4	6	18	5.6	5.5	14.5	5.2	8.8	3.6	5.0	5.5	5.7	83	100.0
Acute non-lymphocytic	0	2	2	9	13	4.0	4.0	10.5	-	2.5	1.8	7.5	3.9	3.5	56	69.2
Chronic myeloid	0	0	1	0	1	0.3	0.3	0.8	-	-	0.9	-	0.3	0.3	4	100.0
Other and unspecified	1	14	13	3	31	9.6	9.6	25.0	5.2	17.6	11.6	2.5	9.4	10.3	146	54.8
II. LYMPHOMAS	0	11	12	13	36	11.1	11.2	100.0	-	13.9	10.7	10.8	10.9	10.9	163	100.0
Hodgkin's disease	0	2	4	8	14	4.3	4.4	38.9	-	2.5	3.6	6.7	4.2	3.9	61	100.0
Non-Hodgkin lymphoma	0	8	8	5	21	6.5	6.5	58.3	-	10.1	7.2	4.2	6.4	6.6	97	100.0
Burkitt's lymphoma	0	0	0	0	0	-	-	-	-	-	-	-	-	-	-	-
Unspecified lymphoma	0	0	0	0	0	-	-	-	-	-	-	-	-	-	-	-
Histiocytosis X	0	0	0	0	0	-	-	-	-	-	-	-	-	-	-	-
Other reticuloendothelial	0	1	0	0	1	0.3	0.3	2.8	-	1.3	-	-	0.3	0.4	5	100.0
III. BRAIN AND SPINAL	3	16	25	29	73	22.5	22.7	100.0	15.5	20.2	22.4	24.1	22.1	21.7	329	71.2
Ependymoma	0	6	4	0	10	3.1	3.1	13.7	-	7.6	3.6	-	3.0	3.5	48	90.0
Astrocytoma	3	1	6	14	24	7.4	7.4	32.9	15.5	1.3	5.4	11.6	7.3	6.7	106	87.5
Medulloblastoma	0	5	4	5	14	4.3	4.3	19.2	-	6.3	3.6	4.2	4.2	4.3	64	92.9
Other glioma	0	1	5	4	10	3.1	3.1	13.7	-	1.3	4.5	3.3	3.0	2.8	44	50.0
Other and unspecified *	0	3	6	6	15	4.6	4.7	20.5	-	3.8	5.4	5.0	4.5	4.4	67	26.7
IV. SYMPATHETIC N.S.	6	8	6	2	22	6.8	6.7	100.0	31.0	10.1	5.4	1.7	6.7	7.7	106	95.5
Neuroblastoma	6	8	6	1	21	6.5	6.4	95.5	31.0	10.1	5.4	0.8	6.4	7.5	102	95.2
Other	0	0	0	1	1	0.3	0.3	4.5	-	-	-	0.8	0.3	0.2	4	100.0
V. RETINOBLASTOMA	1	4	0	0	5	1.5	1.5	100.0	5.2	5.0	-	-	1.5	2.0	25	80.0
VI. KIDNEY	0	14	4	1	19	5.9	5.8	100.0	-	17.6	3.6	0.8	5.7	6.6	93	89.5
Wilms' tumour	0	14	4	0	18	5.6	5.5	94.7	-	17.6	3.6	-	5.4	6.6	88	88.9
Renal carcinoma	0	0	0	1	1	0.3	0.3	5.3	-	-	-	0.8	0.3	0.2	4	100.0
Other and unspecified	0	0	0	0	0	-	-	-	-	-	-	-	-	-	-	-
VII. LIVER	0	2	1	0	3	0.9	0.9	100.0	-	2.5	0.9	-	0.9	1.1	15	33.3
Hepatoblastoma	0	1	0	0	1	0.3	0.3	33.3	-	1.3	-	-	0.3	0.4	5	-
Hepatic carcinoma	0	0	1	0	1	0.3	0.3	33.3	-	-	0.9	-	0.3	0.4	4	100.0
Other and unspecified	0	1	0	0	1	0.3	0.3	33.3	-	1.3	-	-	0.3	0.4	5	-
VIII. BONE	0	1	1	14	16	4.9	4.9	100.0	-	1.3	0.9	11.6	4.8	4.1	68	100.0
Osteosarcoma	0	0	0	5	5	1.5	1.5	31.3	-	-	-	4.2	1.5	1.2	21	100.0
Chondrosarcoma	0	0	0	0	0	-	-	-	-	-	-	-	-	-	-	-
Ewing's sarcoma	0	1	1	8	10	3.1	3.1	62.5	-	1.3	0.9	6.7	3.0	2.6	43	100.0
Other and unspecified	0	0	0	1	1	0.3	0.3	6.3	-	-	-	0.8	0.3	0.2	4	100.0
IX. SOFT TISSUE SARCOMAS	1	3	7	4	15	4.6	4.7	100.0	5.2	3.8	6.3	3.3	4.5	4.6	68	93.3
Rhabdomyosarcoma	1	3	6	1	11	3.4	3.4	73.3	5.2	3.8	5.4	1.7	3.3	3.4	50	90.9
Fibrosarcoma	1	0	1	1	3	0.9	0.9	20.0	5.2	-	0.9	0.8	0.9	0.8	14	100.0
Other and unspecified	0	0	0	1	1	0.3	0.3	6.7	-	-	-	0.8	0.3	0.2	4	100.0
X. GONADAL & GERM CELL	1	3	0	0	4	1.2	1.2	100.0	5.2	3.8	-	-	1.2	1.6	20	100.0
Non-gonadal germ cell	0	0	0	0	0	-	-	-	-	-	-	-	-	-	-	-
Gonadal germ cell	1	2	0	0	3	0.9	0.9	75.0	5.2	2.5	-	-	0.9	1.2	15	100.0
Gonadal carcinoma	0	1	0	0	1	0.3	0.3	25.0	-	1.3	-	-	0.3	0.4	5	100.0
Other and unspecified	0	0	0	0	0	-	-	-	-	-	-	-	-	-	-	-
XI. EPITHELIAL NEOPLASMS	0	1	0	5	6	1.9	1.8	100.0	-	1.3	-	4.2	1.8	1.6	26	83.3
Adrenocortical carcinoma	0	0	0	0	0	-	-	-	-	-	-	-	-	-	-	-
Thyroid carcinoma	0	0	0	0	0	-	-	-	-	-	-	-	-	-	-	-
Nasopharyngeal carcinoma	0	0	0	0	0	-	-	-	-	-	-	-	-	-	-	-
Melanoma	0	1	0	3	4	1.2	1.2	66.7	-	1.3	-	2.5	1.2	1.1	18	100.0
Other carcinoma	0	0	0	2	2	0.6	0.6	33.3	-	-	-	1.7	0.6	0.5	8	50.0
XII. OTHER	0	0	1	0	1	0.3	0.3	100.0	-	-	0.9	-	0.3	0.3	4	100.0
* Specified as malignant	0	3	4	5	12	3.7	3.7		-	3.8	3.6	4.2	3.6	3.5	54	25.0

Canada, Atlantic Provinces 1970 – 1979 FEMALE

DIAGNOSTIC GROUP	N 0	N 1-4	N 5-9	N 10-14	N All	Crude	Adj.	Group	R 0	R 1-4	R 5-9	R 10-14	R Crude	R Adj.	Cum	HV(%)
TOTAL	13	108	70	76	267	100.0	100.0	100.0	70.9	143.1	66.0	66.4	84.9	90.4	1305	82.4
I. LEUKAEMIAS	4	50	29	17	100	37.5	37.0	100.0	21.8	66.2	27.4	14.8	31.8	35.3	498	76.0
Acute lymphocytic	0	26	18	4	48	18.0	17.9	48.0	-	34.4	17.0	3.5	15.3	17.2	240	85.4
Other lymphocytic	0	10	1	2	13	4.9	4.5	13.0	-	13.2	0.9	1.7	4.1	4.9	66	100.0
Acute non-lymphocytic	2	3	1	2	8	3.0	2.9	8.0	10.9	4.0	0.9	1.7	2.5	2.9	40	100.0
Chronic myeloid	0	0	1	0	1	0.4	0.4	1.0	-	-	0.9	-	0.3	0.3	5	100.0
Other and unspecified	2	11	8	9	30	11.2	11.3	30.0	10.9	14.6	7.5	7.9	9.5	10.1	146	43.3
II. LYMPHOMAS	1	5	7	9	22	8.2	8.5	100.0	5.5	6.6	6.6	7.9	7.0	6.9	104	95.5
Hodgkin's disease	0	1	1	6	8	3.0	3.1	36.4	-	1.3	0.9	5.2	2.5	2.2	36	100.0
Non-Hodgkin lymphoma	1	2	3	2	8	3.0	3.1	36.4	5.5	2.6	2.8	1.7	2.5	2.7	39	100.0
Burkitt's lymphoma	0	1	1	0	2	0.7	0.8	9.1	-	1.3	0.9	-	0.6	0.7	10	100.0
Unspecified lymphoma	0	1	2	1	4	1.5	1.6	18.2	-	1.3	1.9	0.9	1.3	1.3	19	75.0
Histiocytosis X	0	0	0	0	0	-	-	-	-	-	-	-	-	-	-	-
Other reticuloendothelial	0	0	0	0	0	-	-	-	-	-	-	-	-	-	-	-
III. BRAIN AND SPINAL	1	21	17	14	53	19.9	20.1	100.0	5.5	27.8	16.0	12.2	16.9	17.8	258	73.6
Ependymoma	0	3	3	1	7	2.6	2.7	13.2	-	4.0	2.8	0.9	2.2	2.4	34	100.0
Astrocytoma	1	6	4	5	16	6.0	6.0	30.2	5.5	7.9	4.7	4.4	5.1	5.4	78	93.8
Medulloblastoma	0	3	5	1	9	3.4	3.5	17.0	-	4.0	2.8	0.9	2.9	3.0	44	100.0
Other glioma	0	5	3	3	11	4.1	4.1	20.8	-	6.6	1.9	2.6	3.5	3.7	54	36.4
Other and unspecified *	0	4	2	4	10	3.7	3.8	18.9	-	5.3	2.8	3.5	3.2	3.3	48	40.0
IV. SYMPATHETIC N.S.	4	7	3	1	15	5.6	5.3	100.0	21.8	9.3	2.8	0.9	4.8	5.7	77	100.0
Neuroblastoma	4	7	3	1	15	5.6	5.3	100.0	21.8	9.3	2.8	0.9	4.8	5.7	77	100.0
Other	0	0	0	0	0	-	-	-	-	-	-	-	-	-	-	-
V. RETINOBLASTOMA	1	4	0	0	5	1.9	1.7	100.0	5.5	5.3	-	-	1.6	2.1	27	100.0
VI. KIDNEY	0	13	2	1	16	6.0	5.5	100.0	-	17.2	1.9	0.9	5.1	6.2	83	100.0
Wilms' tumour	0	13	2	0	15	5.6	5.2	93.8	-	17.2	1.9	-	4.8	5.9	78	100.0
Renal carcinoma	0	0	0	1	1	0.4	0.4	6.3	-	-	-	0.9	0.3	0.3	4	100.0
Other and unspecified	0	0	0	0	0	-	-	-	-	-	-	-	-	-	-	-
VII. LIVER	1	2	0	0	3	1.1	1.0	100.0	5.5	2.6	-	-	1.0	1.2	16	33.3
Hepatoblastoma	1	0	0	0	1	0.4	0.3	33.3	5.5	-	-	-	0.3	0.4	5	100.0
Hepatic carcinoma	0	1	0	0	1	0.4	0.3	33.3	-	1.3	-	-	0.3	0.4	5	-
Other and unspecified	0	1	0	0	1	0.4	0.3	33.3	-	1.3	-	-	0.3	0.4	5	-
VIII. BONE	0	1	6	12	19	7.1	7.6	100.0	-	1.3	5.7	10.5	6.0	5.3	86	89.5
Osteosarcoma	0	0	3	8	11	4.1	4.4	57.9	-	-	2.8	7.0	3.5	2.9	49	100.0
Chondrosarcoma	0	0	0	0	0	-	-	-	-	-	-	-	-	-	-	-
Ewing's sarcoma	0	1	2	3	6	2.2	2.4	31.6	-	1.3	1.9	2.6	1.9	1.8	28	66.7
Other and unspecified	0	0	1	1	2	0.7	0.8	10.5	-	-	0.9	0.9	0.6	0.6	9	100.0
IX. SOFT TISSUE SARCOMAS	1	2	2	6	11	4.1	4.2	100.0	5.5	2.6	1.9	5.2	3.5	3.4	52	90.9
Rhabdomyosarcoma	0	2	2	4	8	3.0	3.1	72.7	-	2.6	1.9	3.5	2.4	2.5	37	87.5
Fibrosarcoma	0	0	0	2	2	0.7	0.8	18.2	-	-	-	1.7	0.6	0.5	9	100.0
Other and unspecified	1	0	0	0	1	0.4	0.3	9.1	5.5	-	-	-	0.3	0.4	5	100.0
X. GONADAL & GERM CELL	0	2	1	2	5	1.9	1.9	100.0	-	2.6	0.9	1.7	1.6	1.6	24	80.0
Non-gonadal germ cell	0	2	1	0	3	1.1	1.1	60.0	-	2.6	0.9	-	1.0	1.1	15	66.7
Gonadal germ cell	0	0	0	2	2	0.7	0.8	40.0	-	-	-	1.7	0.6	0.5	9	100.0
Gonadal carcinoma	0	0	0	0	0	-	-	-	-	-	-	-	-	-	-	-
Other and unspecified	0	0	0	0	0	-	-	-	-	-	-	-	-	-	-	-
XI. EPITHELIAL NEOPLASMS	0	1	3	14	18	6.7	7.1	100.0	-	1.3	2.8	12.2	5.7	4.9	81	88.9
Adrenocortical carcinoma	0	0	0	1	1	0.4	0.4	5.6	-	-	-	0.9	0.3	0.3	4	100.0
Thyroid carcinoma	0	0	0	5	5	1.9	2.0	27.8	-	-	-	4.4	1.6	1.6	22	100.0
Nasopharyngeal carcinoma	0	0	0	2	2	0.7	0.8	11.1	-	-	-	1.7	0.6	0.5	9	100.0
Melanoma	0	0	2	1	3	1.1	1.3	16.7	-	-	1.9	0.9	1.0	0.9	14	100.0
Other carcinoma	0	1	1	5	7	2.6	2.7	38.9	-	1.3	0.9	4.4	2.2	2.0	32	71.4
XII. OTHER	0	0	0	0	0	-	-	-	-	-	-	-	-	-	-	-
* Specified as malignant	0	4	1	4	9	3.4	3.3	100.0	-	5.3	0.9	3.5	2.9	3.0	43	33.3

The Province is covered by a comprehensive provincially-funded health insurance plan.

The Registry covers the island of Newfoundland and the whole of Labrador on the mainland of Canada; the total area is 371 634 square kilometres. At the 1981 census, the population was 566 739, more than 95% of whom are descendants of migrants from the United Kingdom and Ireland. The majority live in small communities along the coastline. The predominant occupations are in the fishing, pulp and paper, and mining industries.

AVERAGE ANNUAL POPULATION: 1970–1979

Age	Male	Female
0	19358	18344
1–4	79333	75479
5–9	111729	106024
10–14	120215	114530
0–14	330635	314377

Population

The average population at risk for each of the provinces has been calculated using the results from the censuses of 1971, 1976 and 1981 (Statistics Canada).

Commentary

The rate for 'All cancers' is among the lowest for white North American and European populations. The rates for individual diagnostic groups are generally low. That for acute lymphocytic leukaemia is particularly low; this is largely explained by the fact that many leukaemias are classified as 'Other lymphocytic' or 'Other and unspecified'. The low rate for CNS tumours may be partly explained by the fact that three of the provinces register only malignant CNS tumours.

Western Provinces, 1970–1979

M. McBride & P. Hayles (British Columbia)
M. Koch & G.B. Hill (Alberta)
D. Robson (Saskatchewan)
N.W. Choi (Manitoba)

(i) **British Columbia**. The British Columbia Cancer Registry is now part of a computerized on-line patient information system for cancer cases in the Province and is the responsibility of the Cancer Control Agency of British Columbia, a non-profit-making society responsible for cancer care, control, and research.

Reporting of cancer by private physicians has been required since 1935. In 1966, a register of all known live cancer cases was instituted within the Provincial Division of Vital Statistics. A register of deceased cases has been kept since 1969. Over 80% of cases are registered either by submission of copies of pathology reports, or via attendance at a Cancer Control Agency clinic. Death certificates now account for approximately 13% of registrations, and many of these are later confirmed by diagnostic reports. Other sources of notification are exploited whenever possible.

The Registry produces annual reports and provides data to the NCIRS. The data have been used in a study of cancer incidence trends and in geographical mapping of cancer incidence in the Province.

The Registry covers the whole of British Columbia (948 600 square kilometres). The population at the 1981 census was 2 744 465, of whom 21% were less than 15 years of age. The main ethnic groups are: British, 51%, other European, 27%, Oriental, 4.5% and native Indian 2.2%. Approximately 78% of the population is urban. The largest component of the working population is employed in manufacturing industries (20%) and in independent business and service industries (20%). Other important industries include: construction, transport and communications, forestry, agriculture, mining, and fishing.

(ii) **Alberta**. The Alberta Cancer Registry was established in 1942. Cancer Registry personnel are located in the three main treatment centres in the province. All pathological reports and death certificates with a malignant diagnosis in the entire Province are forwarded to the Registry, and completeness of registration is estimated at 97% if non-melanoma skin cancer and *in situ* cancers at any site are excluded. The data are used extensively for regional comparisons within the Province, epidemiological studies, treatment reviews, health care planning, etc.

The Alberta Cancer Registry covers an area of 653 530 square kilometres and a population of 2.2 million, of whom approximately 1 million reside in the two main urban centres (Edmonton and Calgary), another 0.6 million in smaller towns and the remaining 0.6 million are rural. The population is mostly Caucasian, with a high proportion of descendants of immigrants originating from eastern and northern Europe. More recent immigrants originate from all parts of the world, including Asia, South America, western Europe, etc.

Traditionally, farming has been the main occupation in Alberta, but in the past 40 years, since large deposits of petroleum and natural gas have been found, exploration, extraction and processing of these products have been a very important part of the economy. This has led to a steady increase in population, especially in the urban centres.

(iii) **Saskatchewan**. Registration dates from 1932. The Saskatchewan Cancer Foundation maintains two treatment centres (the Allan Blair Memorial Clinic in Regina and the Saskatoon Cancer Clinic) and registry services are an integral part of each clinic.

Data on 60–70% of all patients with cancer are drawn from clinic records and for the remainder are obtained from sources such as pathology, operative and autopsy reports, and correspondence with specialists and family physicians. Cases ascertained only through a death certificate account for approximately 5% of all registrations. The province is covered by a universal comprehensive health insu-

Contd p. 80

Canada, Western Provinces   1970 - 1979   MALE

DIAGNOSTIC GROUP	NUMBER OF CASES					REL. FREQUENCY(%)			RATES PER MILLION							HV(%)
	0	1-4	5-9	10-14	All	Crude	Adj.	Group	0	1-4	5-9	10-14	Crude	Adj.	Cum	
TOTAL	99	436	331	303	1169	100.0	100.0	100.0	194.8	216.1	117.8	98.8	139.1	148.7	2142	85.4
I. LEUKAEMIAS	15	175	118	55	363	31.1	30.3	100.0	29.5	86.7	42.0	17.9	43.2	47.9	676	91.2
Acute lymphocytic	4	133	80	32	249	21.3	20.7	68.6	7.9	65.9	28.5	10.4	29.6	33.2	466	91.5
Other lymphocytic	0	0	1	0	1	0.1	0.1	0.3	–	–	0.4	–	0.1	0.1	2	100.0
Acute non-lymphocytic	1	15	16	8	40	3.4	3.4	11.0	2.0	7.4	5.7	2.6	4.8	5.0	73	92.3
Chronic myeloid	1	4	2	4	11	0.9	1.0	3.0	2.0	2.0	0.7	1.3	1.4	1.4	20	75.0
Other and unspecified	9	23	19	11	62	5.3	5.2	17.1	17.7	11.4	6.8	3.6	7.4	8.1	115	91.5
II. LYMPHOMAS	9	44	65	64	182	15.6	16.2	100.0	17.7	21.8	23.1	20.9	21.7	21.6	325	87.6
Hodgkin's disease	0	3	13	28	44	3.8	4.2	24.2	–	1.5	4.3	9.1	5.2	4.6	75	90.9
Non-Hodgkin lymphoma	2	20	33	24	79	6.8	7.0	43.4	3.9	9.5	11.7	7.8	9.4	9.4	141	90.9
Burkitt's lymphoma	0	4	1	0	5	0.4	0.5	2.7	–	2.0	0.4	–	0.6	0.6	9	80.0
Unspecified lymphoma	1	4	14	8	27	2.3	2.4	14.8	2.0	2.0	5.0	2.6	3.2	3.1	48	88.5
Histiocytosis X	4	11	1	1	17	1.5	1.3	9.3	7.9	5.5	0.4	0.3	2.0	2.5	33	76.5
Other reticuloendothelial	2	6	1	1	10	0.9	0.8	5.5	3.9	3.0	0.4	0.3	1.2	1.4	19	66.7
III. BRAIN AND SPINAL	11	63	73	76	223	19.1	19.7	100.0	21.6	31.2	26.0	24.8	26.5	26.9	400	77.4
Ependymoma	5	12	3	2	22	1.9	1.7	9.9	9.8	5.9	1.1	0.7	2.6	3.1	42	85.7
Astrocytoma	4	24	36	53	117	10.0	10.6	52.5	7.9	11.9	12.8	17.3	13.9	13.4	206	82.6
Medulloblastoma	2	15	22	10	49	4.2	4.3	22.0	3.9	7.4	7.8	3.6	5.8	6.0	89	91.3
Other glioma	0	5	6	8	19	1.6	1.7	8.5	–	2.5	2.1	2.6	2.3	2.2	34	42.1
Other and unspecified *	0	7	6	3	16	1.4	1.3	7.2	–	3.5	2.1	1.9	1.9	2.1	30	31.3
IV. SYMPATHETIC N.S.	20	43	10	5	78	6.7	6.1	100.0	39.4	21.3	3.6	1.6	9.3	11.3	151	74.4
Neuroblastoma	20	43	10	3	76	6.5	5.9	97.4	39.4	21.3	3.6	1.0	9.0	11.1	147	73.7
Other	0	0	0	2	2	0.2	0.2	2.6	–	–	–	0.7	0.2	0.2	3	100.0
V. RETINOBLASTOMA	9	20	1	1	31	2.7	2.4	100.0	17.7	9.9	0.4	0.3	3.7	4.7	61	90.0
VI. KIDNEY	7	38	9	3	57	4.9	4.5	100.0	13.8	18.8	3.2	1.0	6.8	8.2	110	91.1
Wilms' tumour	7	36	9	2	54	4.6	4.2	94.7	13.8	17.8	3.2	0.7	6.4	7.8	104	90.7
Renal carcinoma	0	2	0	1	3	0.3	0.2	5.3	–	1.0	–	0.3	0.4	0.4	6	100.0
Other and unspecified	0	0	0	0	0	–	–	–	–	–	–	–	–	–	–	–
VII. LIVER	5	6	4	0	15	1.3	1.2	100.0	9.8	3.0	1.4	–	1.8	2.1	29	92.9
Hepatoblastoma	4	3	0	0	7	0.6	0.5	46.7	7.9	1.5	–	–	0.8	1.0	14	83.3
Hepatic carcinoma	0	3	4	0	7	0.6	0.6	46.7	–	1.5	1.4	–	0.8	0.9	13	100.0
Other and unspecified	1	0	0	0	1	0.1	0.1	6.7	2.0	–	–	–	0.1	0.2	2	100.0
VIII. BONE	0	4	13	35	52	4.4	4.9	100.0	–	2.0	4.6	11.4	6.2	5.4	88	90.2
Osteosarcoma	0	0	4	22	26	2.2	2.5	50.0	–	–	1.4	7.2	3.1	2.5	43	80.8
Chondrosarcoma	0	0	1	1	2	0.2	0.2	3.8	–	–	0.4	0.3	0.2	0.2	4	100.0
Ewing's sarcoma	0	4	7	10	21	1.8	1.9	40.4	–	2.0	2.5	3.3	2.5	2.4	37	100.0
Other and unspecified	0	0	1	2	3	0.3	0.3	5.8	–	–	0.4	0.7	0.3	0.3	6	100.0
IX. SOFT TISSUE SARCOMAS	8	16	20	25	69	5.9	6.1	100.0	15.7	7.9	7.1	8.2	8.2	8.3	124	89.9
Rhabdomyosarcoma	1	11	12	11	35	3.0	3.1	50.7	2.0	5.5	4.3	3.6	4.2	4.3	63	85.7
Fibrosarcoma	4	2	4	9	19	1.6	1.7	27.5	7.9	1.0	1.4	2.9	2.3	2.2	34	89.5
Other and unspecified	3	3	4	5	15	1.3	1.3	21.7	5.9	1.5	1.4	1.6	1.8	1.8	27	100.0
X. GONADAL & GERM CELL	6	11	0	7	24	2.1	2.0	100.0	11.8	5.5	–	2.3	2.9	3.3	45	70.8
Non-gonadal germ cell	2	6	0	3	11	0.9	1.0	45.8	3.9	3.0	–	1.0	1.3	1.3	20	63.6
Gonadal germ cell	2	3	0	4	9	0.8	0.7	37.5	3.9	1.5	–	1.3	1.1	1.3	17	66.7
Gonadal carcinoma	1	2	0	0	3	0.3	0.2	12.5	2.0	1.0	–	–	0.3	0.2	6	66.7
Other and unspecified	1	0	0	0	1	0.1	0.1	4.2	2.0	–	–	–	0.1	0.2	2	100.0
XI. EPITHELIAL NEOPLASMS	8	7	15	27	57	4.9	5.2	100.0	15.7	3.5	5.3	8.8	6.8	6.6	100	83.3
Adrenocortical carcinoma	0	1	0	0	1	0.1	0.1	1.8	–	0.5	–	–	0.1	0.1	2	100.0
Thyroid carcinoma	0	0	3	3	6	0.5	0.6	10.5	–	–	1.1	1.0	0.7	0.6	10	66.7
Nasopharyngeal carcinoma	0	0	0	1	1	0.1	0.1	1.8	–	–	–	0.3	0.1	0.2	2	100.0
Melanoma	0	2	5	4	11	0.9	1.0	19.3	–	1.0	1.8	1.3	1.3	1.2	19	90.0
Other carcinoma	8	4	7	19	38	3.3	3.4	66.7	15.7	2.0	2.5	6.2	4.5	4.4	67	83.8
XII. OTHER	1	9	3	5	18	1.5	1.5	100.0	2.0	4.5	1.1	1.6	2.1	2.4	33	64.7
* Specified as malignant	1	5	7	1	14	1.2	1.2		2.0	2.5	2.5	0.3	1.7	1.8	26	28.6

Canada, Western Provinces

FEMALE

1970 - 1979

DIAGNOSTIC GROUP	NUMBER OF CASES					REL. FREQUENCY(%)			RATES PER MILLION						Cum	HV(%)
	0	1-4	5-9	10-14	All	Crude	Adj.	Group	0	1-4	5-9	10-14	Crude	Adj.		
TOTAL	82	336	205	280	903	100.0	100.0	100.0	169.2	174.8	76.2	95.2	112.3	119.4	1725	86.2
I. LEUKAEMIAS	19	138	74	55	286	31.7	31.7	100.0	39.2	71.8	27.5	18.7	35.6	39.6	557	92.0
Acute lymphocytic	9	99	55	28	191	21.2	21.4	66.8	18.6	51.5	20.4	9.5	23.8	26.7	374	92.3
Other lymphocytic	0	5	3	0	8	0.9	0.9	2.8	-	2.6	1.1	-	1.0	1.2	16	100.0
Acute non-lymphocytic	3	8	8	14	33	3.7	3.7	11.5	6.2	4.2	3.0	4.8	4.1	4.1	61	96.7
Chronic myeloid	0	1	1	3	5	0.6	0.6	1.7	-	0.5	0.4	1.0	0.6	0.6	9	100.0
Other and unspecified	7	25	7	10	49	5.4	5.2	17.1	14.4	13.0	2.6	3.4	6.1	7.0	96	85.4
II. LYMPHOMAS	2	16	20	50	88	9.7	10.0	100.0	4.1	8.3	7.4	17.0	10.9	10.2	160	89.8
Hodgkin's disease	0	1	5	30	36	4.0	4.0	40.9	-	0.5	1.9	10.2	4.5	3.7	62	94.4
Non-Hodgkin lymphoma	1	7	11	14	33	3.7	3.9	37.5	2.1	3.6	4.1	4.8	4.1	4.0	61	90.9
Burkitt's lymphoma	0	0	0	0	0											
Unspecified lymphoma	0	0	2	5	7	0.8	0.8	8.0	-	-	0.7	1.7	0.9	0.7	12	100.0
Histiocytosis X	1	4	0	0	5	0.6	0.5	5.7	2.1	2.1	-	-	0.6	0.8	10	40.0
Other reticuloendothelial	0	4	2	1	7	0.8	0.8	8.0	-	2.1	0.7	0.3	0.9	1.0	14	85.7
III. BRAIN AND SPINAL	6	61	55	57	179	19.8	20.6	100.0	12.4	31.7	20.4	19.4	22.3	23.0	338	68.6
Ependymoma	0	7	4	5	16	1.8	1.8	8.9	-	3.6	1.5	1.7	2.0	2.1	30	81.3
Astrocytoma	1	35	25	32	93	10.3	10.5	52.0	2.1	18.2	9.3	10.9	11.6	12.0	176	76.1
Medulloblastoma	3	10	11	7	31	3.4	3.6	17.3	6.2	5.2	4.1	2.4	3.9	4.1	59	76.7
Other glioma	1	7	9	7	24	2.7	2.8	13.4	2.1	3.6	3.3	2.4	3.0	3.1	45	40.9
Other and unspecified *	1	2	6	6	15	1.7	1.8	8.4	2.1	1.0	2.2	2.0	1.9	1.8	28	33.3
IV. SYMPATHETIC N.S.	19	36	7	4	66	7.3	6.7	100.0	39.2	18.7	2.6	1.4	8.2	10.1	134	86.4
Neuroblastoma	19	36	7	3	65	7.2	6.6	98.5	39.2	18.7	2.6	1.0	8.1	10.0	132	86.2
Other	0	0	0	1	1	0.1	0.1	1.5	-	-	-	0.3	0.1	0.1		100.0
V. RETINOBLASTOMA	7	16	5	0	28	3.1	2.9	100.0	14.4	8.3	1.9	-	3.5	4.3	57	89.3
VI. KIDNEY	8	28	9	5	50	5.5	5.3	100.0	16.5	14.6	3.3	1.7	6.2	7.4	100	94.0
Wilms' tumour	8	28	9	4	49	5.4	5.2	98.0	16.5	14.6	3.3	1.4	6.1	7.3	98	93.9
Renal carcinoma	0	0	0	1	1	0.1	0.1	2.0	-	-	-	0.3	0.1	0.1	2	100.0
Other and unspecified	0	0	0	0	0											
VII. LIVER	0	4	2	0	6	0.7	0.7	100.0	-	2.1	0.7	-	0.7	0.9	12	83.3
Hepatoblastoma	0	1	0	0	3	0.3	0.4	50.0	-	0.5	0.7	-	0.4	0.4	6	66.7
Hepatic carcinoma	0	3	0	0	3	0.3	0.3	50.0	-	1.6	-	-	-	0.5	6	100.0
Other and unspecified	0	0	0	0	0											
VIII. BONE	1	2	6	29	38	4.2	4.3	100.0	2.1	1.0	2.2	9.9	4.7	4.1	67	100.0
Osteosarcoma	0	0	2	13	15	1.7	1.7	39.5	-	-	0.7	4.4	1.9	1.5	26	100.0
Chondrosarcoma	0	0	0	1	1	0.1	0.1	2.6	-	-	-	0.3	0.1	0.1	2	100.0
Ewing's sarcoma	1	2	3	14	20	2.2	2.2	52.6	2.1	1.0	1.1	4.8	2.5	2.2	36	100.0
Other and unspecified	0	0	1	1	2	0.2	0.3	5.3	-	-	0.4	0.3	0.2	0.2	4	100.0
IX. SOFT TISSUE SARCOMAS	6	14	12	27	59	6.5	6.6	100.0	12.4	7.3	4.5	9.2	7.3	7.3	110	94.6
Rhabdomyosarcoma	1	10	7	8	26	2.9	2.9	44.1	2.1	5.2	2.6	2.7	3.2	3.4	49	96.0
Fibrosarcoma	3	2	3	7	15	1.7	1.7	25.4	6.2	1.0	1.1	2.4	1.9	1.7	27	92.9
Other and unspecified	2	2	2	12	18	2.0	1.9	30.5	4.1	1.0	0.7	4.1	2.2	2.2	33	94.1
X. GONADAL & GERM CELL	4	12	2	18	36	4.0	3.8	100.0	8.3	6.2	0.7	6.1	4.5	4.6	68	83.3
Non-gonadal germ cell	4	10	1	4	19	2.1	1.9	52.8	8.3	5.2	0.4	1.4	2.4	2.8	38	78.9
Gonadal germ cell	0	1	1	11	12	1.3	1.3	33.3	-	0.5	0.4	3.7	1.5	1.4	21	83.3
Gonadal carcinoma	0	0	0	2	3	0.3	0.4	8.3	-	-	-	0.7	0.4	0.3	5	100.0
Other and unspecified	0	1	0	1	2	0.2	0.2	5.6	-	0.5	-	0.3	0.2	0.3	4	100.0
XI. EPITHELIAL NEOPLASMS	8	7	11	35	61	6.8	6.1	100.0	16.5	3.6	4.1	11.9	7.6	7.2	111	86.9
Adrenocortical carcinoma	0	1	0	0	1	0.1	0.1	1.6	-	0.5	-	-	0.1	0.2	2	100.0
Thyroid carcinoma	0	0	3	11	14	1.6	1.6	23.0	-	-	1.1	3.7	1.7	1.4	24	92.9
Nasopharyngeal carcinoma	0	0	0	0	0											
Melanoma	0	0	0	6	6	0.7	0.6	9.8	-	-	-	2.0	0.7	0.6	10	100.0
Other carcinoma	8	6	8	18	40	4.4	4.4	65.6	16.5	3.1	3.0	6.1	5.0	5.0	74	85.0
XII. OTHER	2	2	2	0	6	0.7	0.7	100.0	4.1	1.0	0.7	-	0.7	0.9	12	60.0
* Specified as malignant	0	2	5	3	10	1.1	1.2	100.0	-	1.0	1.9	1.0	1.2	1.2	19	30.0

rance scheme and, to be eligible for payment under this plan, physicians are required to report all cases of cancer to the Registry. Incidence rates are computed annually.

The total area is 651 903 square kilometres. At the 1981 census the population was 968 310, of whom 25% were under 15 years of age. Approximately 63% of the population live in urban areas, with 31% in the two largest cities (Regina and Saskatoon); 31% of the total population live in rural areas and 4% live on reservations.

Agriculture is a main occupation, accounting for approximately 25% of the male work force involved; industry, commerce and construction each account for a further 10%.

(iv) **Manitoba**. In 1937 the Province of Manitoba established a central registry to enumerate cancer cases. In 1950 it was re-organized on a population basis. The registry is situated in and administered by the Manitoba Cancer Treatment and Research Foundation.

Essentially all the cancer cases are reported to the Registry in accordance with the Public Health Act. Information sources include: pathology, cytology, and autopsy records; hospital admission/-separation information; vital statistics information; and letters and report of malignant neoplasm forms from physicians.

Incidence and mortality rates are published annually in the Manitoba Cancer Foundation annual report.

The registry covers the whole of Manitoba, the most central province of Canada, with an area of 650 000 square kilometres. The population in 1981 was 1 026 240, of whom 23% were under 15 years of age. The population includes approximately 42% of British extraction; 12.5% German; 12% Ukrainian; 9% French; 4% Dutch; 4% Polish; 3% Scandinavian; 2% Jewish and 4% native Indian Eskimo. Of the total population, 71% reside in the urban areas and 29% in the rural areas of the Province.

Predominant occupations include clerical, service occupations, construction and production work and farming.

Population

The average population at risk for each of the provinces has been calculated using the results from the censuses of 1971, 1976 and 1981 (Statistics Canada).

AVERAGE ANNUAL POPULATION: 1970-1979

Age	Male	Female
0	50811	48475
1–4	201731	192242
5–9	281053	269193
10–14	306726	294104
0–14	840321	804014

Commentary

The rates for 'All cancers' and for the major tumour groups were in general above the average for white North American and European populations and, in particular, usually greater than those for the Atlantic Provinces. The rate given for acute lymphocytic leukaemia is probably lower than the true value because of the proportion of leukaemias classified as 'Other and unspecified', though the effect is not as great as for the Atlantic Provinces, and only nine cases were classified as 'Other lymphocytic'. The high rate for 'Other carcinoma' is at least partly attributable to the numbers of skin cancers registered; this accounts for nearly half the cases in this group.

UNITED STATES OF AMERICA

Greater Delaware Valley Pediatric Tumor Registry, 1970–1979

G.R. Bunin, P. Jarrett & A.T. Meadows

The Children's Hospital of Philadelphia established the Greater Delaware Valley Pediatric Tumor Registry (GDVPTR) in 1972 in order to facilitate research on the distribution and causes of childhood cancer and the survival of the affected children. Eligibility criteria for inclusion in the GDVPTR are: (1) diagnosis of a malignant tumour on or after 1 January 1970; (2) age 0–14 at the time of diagnosis; and (3) residence in the 31-county region at the time of diagnosis.

Although GDVPTR began operation in 1972, systematic collection of data for all cases diagnosed as far back as 1970 began in 1975. Ascertainment of cases is done through the area's hospitals, as children with cancer are always seen in a hospital in order to make or confirm the diagnosis.

Reporting by hospitals is voluntary, but co-operation is excellent. All the 150 hospitals in the area, as well as 10 major referral centres outside the region, co-operate in ascertainment of eligible cases. Cases are reported by the hospitals as they occur. In hospitals identified as under-reporting or where there are staff changes, GDVPTR personnel survey in-patient medical records as well as key hospital departments, such as pathology, radiotherapy, surgery and haematology. Of the hospitals contributing to the GDVPTR, 72% have active tumour registries. A GDVPTR staff member reviews medical records to abstract details of clinical and disease characteristics, therapy, other significant conditions and demographic information. In addition to hospital surveillance, death certificates from all counties covered by the Registry and contiguous areas for individuals less than 20 years of age for whom a neoplasm is listed as a cause of death are reviewed. Cases initially identified through the death certificate review for whom no supporting clinical information is located are not considered eligible for the Registry. About 3% of the cases diagnosed in 1970-1979 were first ascertained by death certificate review. Diagnoses are made histologically in almost all cases.

The Registry covers a 31-county region that includes parts of Pennsylvania, New Jersey, Maryland, and the entire State of Delaware (see Fig. 1). This region, the Greater Delaware Valley, has a population of approximately 2.2 million people aged 0–14 years. The population has been relatively stable over the last 15 years. Racial distribution is similar to that of the USA as a whole, with approximately 16% non-Whites, 90% of whom are Blacks. The GDV includes urban and suburban communities, as well as rural, agricultural areas. Manufacturing industries are well represented and include petrochemical refineries.

The GDVPTR data have been used to describe the incidence of childhood cancer by histological type and racial differences in incidence patterns. The Registry has also made possible studies of referral patterns and the relationship between treatment and type of hospital (community or university).

The data presented here have been discussed in detail by Kramer *et al.* (1983).

Population

The population at risk has been calculated from the census data of 1970 and 1980 for the 31 counties covered by the Registry (US Bureau of the Census).

AVERAGE ANNUAL POPULATION: 1970–1979

Age	Male	Female
White		
0–4	246759	235991
5–9	281944	268483
10–14	309721	296084
0–14	838424	800558
Non-White		
0–4	57239	56757
5–9	62400	61421
10–14	65813	65955
0–14	185452	184133

Contd. p. 86

USA, Greater Delaware Valley, White   1970 – 1979   MALE

DIAGNOSTIC GROUP	NUMBER OF CASES					REL. FREQUENCY(%)			RATES PER MILLION						HV(%)
	0	1-4	5-9	10-14	All	Crude	Adj.	Group	0-4	5-9	10-14	Crude	Adj.	Cum	
TOTAL	102	360	313	330	1105	100.0	100.0	100.0	187.2	111.0	106.5	131.8	139.2	2024	
I. LEUKAEMIAS	20	146	118	86	370	33.5	33.5	100.0	67.3	41.9	27.8	44.1	47.6	684	
Acute lymphocytic	11	131	95	55	292	26.4	26.4	78.9	57.5	33.7	17.8	34.8	38.3	545	
Other lymphocytic	0	0	0	1	1	0.1	0.1	0.3	-	-	0.3	0.1	0.1	2	
Acute non-lymphocytic	7	9	17	20	53	4.8	4.8	14.3	6.5	6.0	6.5	6.3	6.3	95	
Chronic myeloid	1	2	0	5	8	0.7	0.7	2.2	1.2	-	1.6	1.0	0.9	14	
Other and unspecified	1	4	6	5	16	1.4	1.5	4.3	2.0	2.1	1.6	1.4	1.9	29	
II. LYMPHOMAS	5	20	48	80	153	13.8	14.0	100.0	10.1	17.0	25.8	18.2	16.9	265	
Hodgkin's disease	0	3	15	48	66	6.0	6.1	43.1	1.2	5.3	15.5	7.9	6.7	110	
Non-Hodgkin lymphoma	0	6	20	23	49	4.4	4.5	32.0	2.4	7.1	7.4	5.8	5.4	85	
Burkitt's lymphoma	0	2	5	3	10	0.9	0.9	6.5	0.8	1.8	1.0	0.9	1.2	18	
Unspecified lymphoma	0	3	5	5	13	1.2	1.2	8.5	1.6	1.8	1.6	1.6	1.5	23	
Histiocytosis X	1	3	1	0	5	0.5	0.4	3.3	1.6	0.4	-	0.6	0.7	10	
Other reticuloendothelial	4	3	2	1	10	0.9	0.9	6.5	2.8	0.7	0.3	1.2	1.4	19	
III. BRAIN AND SPINAL	8	53	81	74	216	19.5	19.8	100.0	24.7	28.7	23.9	25.8	25.8	387	
Ependymoma	0	16	7	4	27	2.4	2.4	12.5	6.5	1.4	2.3	3.2	3.6	51	
Astrocytoma	3	15	36	38	92	8.3	8.5	42.6	7.3	12.8	12.3	11.0	10.5	162	
Medulloblastoma	3	14	23	11	51	4.6	4.7	23.6	6.9	8.2	3.6	6.1	6.3	93	
Other glioma	1	6	9	7	23	2.1	2.1	10.6	2.8	3.2	2.3	2.7	2.8	41	
Other and unspecified *	1	2	9	11	23	2.1	2.1	10.6	1.2	3.2	3.6	2.7	2.5	40	
IV. SYMPATHETIC N.S.	31	40	13	2	86	7.8	7.6	100.0	28.8	4.6	0.6	10.3	12.8	170	
Neuroblastoma	31	40	13	2	86	7.8	7.6	100.0	28.8	4.6	0.6	10.3	12.8	170	
Other	0	0	0	0	0	-	-	-	-	-	-	-	-	-	
V. RETINOBLASTOMA	11	25	3	0	39	3.5	3.4	100.0	14.6	1.1	-	4.7	6.0	78	
VI. KIDNEY	14	29	9	4	56	5.1	4.9	100.0	17.4	3.2	1.3	6.7	8.2	110	
Wilms' tumour	14	29	8	3	54	4.9	4.8	96.4	17.4	2.8	1.0	6.4	7.9	106	
Renal carcinoma	0	0	1	1	2	0.2	0.2	3.6	-	0.4	0.3	0.2	0.2	3	
Other and unspecified	0	0	0	0	0	-	-	-	-	-	-	-	-	-	
VII. LIVER	2	5	2	2	11	1.0	1.0	100.0	2.8	0.7	0.6	1.3	1.5	21	
Hepatoblastoma	1	4	0	2	7	0.6	0.6	63.6	2.0	0.7	0.6	0.8	1.0	14	
Hepatic carcinoma	1	0	2	0	3	0.3	0.3	27.3	0.4	-	-	0.4	0.3	5	
Other and unspecified	0	1	0	0	1	0.1	0.1	9.1	-	-	-	0.1	0.2	2	
VIII. BONE	0	0	14	34	48	4.3	4.4	100.0	-	5.0	11.0	5.7	4.8	80	
Osteosarcoma	0	0	5	20	25	2.3	2.3	52.1	-	1.8	6.5	3.0	2.4	41	
Chondrosarcoma	0	0	1	0	1	0.1	0.1	2.1	-	0.4	-	0.1	0.1	2	
Ewing's sarcoma	0	0	8	13	21	1.9	1.9	43.8	-	2.8	4.2	2.5	2.1	35	
Other and unspecified	0	0	0	1	1	0.1	0.1	2.1	-	-	0.3	0.1	0.1	2	
IX. SOFT TISSUE SARCOMAS	7	24	15	25	71	6.4	6.4	100.0	12.6	5.3	8.1	8.5	8.9	130	
Rhabdomyosarcoma	3	20	8	9	40	3.6	3.6	56.3	9.3	2.8	2.9	4.8	4.8	75	
Fibrosarcoma	0	1	3	8	12	1.1	1.1	16.9	0.4	1.1	2.6	1.4	1.3	20	
Other and unspecified	4	3	4	8	19	1.7	1.7	26.8	2.8	1.4	2.6	2.3	2.3	34	
X. GONADAL & GERM CELL	4	15	4	7	30	2.7	2.7	100.0	7.7	1.4	2.3	3.6	4.1	57	
Non-gonadal germ cell	0	7	3	3	13	1.2	1.2	43.3	2.8	1.1	1.0	1.6	1.7	24	
Gonadal germ cell	4	7	1	4	16	1.4	1.4	53.3	4.5	0.4	1.3	1.9	2.2	31	
Gonadal carcinoma	0	1	0	0	1	0.1	0.1	3.3	0.4	-	-	0.1	0.2	2	
Other and unspecified	0	0	0	0	0	-	-	-	-	-	-	-	-	-	
XI. EPITHELIAL NEOPLASMS	0	3	5	16	24	2.2	2.2	100.0	1.2	1.8	5.2	2.9	2.5	41	
Adrenocortical carcinoma	0	1	0	0	1	0.1	0.1	4.2	0.4	-	-	0.1	0.1	2	
Thyroid carcinoma	0	0	4	3	7	0.6	0.6	29.2	-	1.1	1.0	0.8	0.6	12	
Nasopharyngeal carcinoma	0	0	0	2	2	0.2	0.2	8.3	-	-	0.6	0.2	0.2	3	
Melanoma	0	1	0	5	6	0.5	0.5	25.0	0.4	-	1.6	0.7	0.6	10	
Other carcinoma	0	1	1	6	8	0.7	0.7	33.3	0.4	0.4	1.9	1.0	0.8	13	
XII. OTHER	0	0	1	0	1	0.1	0.1	100.0	-	0.4	-	0.1	0.1	2	
* Specified as malignant	0	1	2	3	6	0.5	0.6	100.0	0.4	0.7	1.0	0.7	0.7	10	

USA, Greater Delaware Valley, White   1970 - 1979   FEMALE

DIAGNOSTIC GROUP	NUMBER OF CASES					REL. FREQUENCY(%)			RATES PER MILLION						HV(%)
	0	1-4	5-9	10-14	All	Crude	Adj.	Group	0-4	5-9	10-14	Crude	Adj.	Cum	
TOTAL	67	288	245	265	865	100.0	100.0	100.0	150.4	91.3	89.5	108.0	113.7	1656	
I. LEUKAEMIAS	9	127	81	58	275	31.8	31.8	100.0	57.6	30.2	19.6	34.4	37.7	537	
Acute lymphocytic	6	100	64	38	208	24.0	24.1	75.6	44.9	23.8	12.8	26.0	28.8	408	
Other lymphocytic	0	1	0	0	1	0.1	0.1	0.4	0.4	-	-	0.1	0.2	2	
Acute non-lymphocytic	1	16	15	16	48	5.5	5.6	17.5	7.2	5.6	5.4	6.0	6.2	91	
Chronic myeloid	0	4	0	2	6	0.7	0.7	2.2	1.7	-	0.7	0.7	0.9	12	
Other and unspecified	2	6	2	2	12	1.4	1.4	4.4	3.4	0.7	0.7	1.5	1.7	24	
II. LYMPHOMAS	4	10	16	46	76	8.8	8.7	100.0	5.9	6.0	15.5	9.5	8.7	137	
Hodgkin's disease	0	1	5	34	40	4.6	4.6	52.6	0.4	1.9	11.5	5.0	4.1	69	
Non-Hodgkin lymphoma	1	7	6	9	23	2.7	2.7	30.3	3.4	2.2	3.0	2.9	2.9	43	
Burkitt's lymphoma	0	0	1	0	1	0.1	0.1	1.3	-	0.4	-	0.1	0.1	2	
Unspecified lymphoma	0	0	2	3	5	0.6	0.6	6.6	-	0.7	1.0	0.6	0.5	9	
Histiocytosis X	2	1	1	0	4	0.5	0.5	5.3	1.3	0.4	-	0.5	0.6	8	
Other reticuloendothelial	1	1	1	0	3	0.3	0.3	3.9	0.8	0.4	-	0.4	0.4	6	
III. BRAIN AND SPINAL	12	49	82	65	208	24.0	24.3	100.0	25.8	30.5	22.0	26.0	26.2	392	
Ependymoma	3	4	9	2	18	2.1	2.1	8.7	3.0	3.4	0.7	2.2	2.4	35	
Astrocytoma	5	23	33	39	100	11.6	11.6	48.1	11.9	12.3	13.2	12.5	12.4	187	
Medulloblastoma	2	5	14	10	31	3.6	3.6	14.9	3.0	5.2	3.4	3.9	3.8	58	
Other glioma	1	8	13	4	26	3.0	3.1	12.5	3.8	4.8	1.4	3.2	3.4	50	
Other and unspecified *	1	9	13	10	33	3.8	3.9	15.9	4.2	4.8	3.4	4.1	4.2	62	
IV. SYMPATHETIC N.S.	17	26	12	2	57	6.6	6.5	100.0	18.2	4.5	0.7	7.1	8.7	117	
Neuroblastoma	17	26	12	2	57	6.6	6.5	100.0	18.2	4.5	0.7	7.1	8.7	117	
Other	0	0	0	0	0	-	-	-	-	-	-	-	-	-	
V. RETINOBLASTOMA	6	17	1	0	24	2.8	2.7	100.0	9.7	0.4	-	3.0	3.9	51	
VI. KIDNEY	7	25	13	2	47	5.4	5.4	100.0	13.6	4.8	0.7	5.9	7.0	95	
Wilms' tumour	7	25	12	2	46	5.3	5.3	97.9	13.6	4.5	0.7	5.7	6.9	94	
Renal carcinoma	0	0	1	0	1	0.1	0.1	2.1	-	0.4	-	0.1	0.1	2	
Other and unspecified	0	0	0	0	0	-	-	-	-	-	-	-	-	-	
VII. LIVER	1	3	0	1	5	0.6	0.6	100.0	1.7	-	0.3	0.6	0.8	10	
Hepatoblastoma	1	1	0	0	2	0.2	0.2	40.0	0.8	-	-	0.2	0.3	4	
Hepatic carcinoma	0	2	0	1	3	0.3	0.3	60.0	0.8	-	0.3	0.4	0.4	6	
Other and unspecified	0	0	0	0	0	-	-	-	-	-	-	-	-	-	
VIII. BONE	0	4	16	28	48	5.5	5.6	100.0	1.7	6.0	9.5	6.0	5.3	86	
Osteosarcoma	0	2	9	10	21	2.4	2.5	43.8	0.8	3.4	3.4	2.6	2.4	38	
Chondrosarcoma	0	0	1	3	4	0.5	0.5	8.3	-	0.4	1.0	0.5	0.4	7	
Ewing's sarcoma	0	2	5	12	19	2.2	2.2	39.6	0.8	1.9	4.1	2.4	2.1	34	
Other and unspecified	0	0	1	3	4	0.5	0.5	8.3	-	0.4	1.0	0.5	0.4	7	
IX. SOFT TISSUE SARCOMAS	5	18	15	23	61	7.1	7.0	100.0	9.7	5.6	7.8	7.6	7.8	116	
Rhabdomyosarcoma	3	13	7	8	31	3.6	3.6	50.8	6.8	2.6	2.7	3.9	4.2	60	
Fibrosarcoma	1	3	4	6	14	1.6	1.8	23.0	1.7	1.5	2.0	1.7	1.7	26	
Other and unspecified	1	2	4	9	16	1.8	1.8	26.2	1.3	1.5	3.0	2.0	1.9	29	
X. GONADAL & GERM CELL	6	7	3	20	36	4.2	4.1	100.0	5.5	1.1	6.8	4.5	4.5	67	
Non-gonadal germ cell	6	7	0	6	19	2.2	2.1	52.8	5.5	-	2.0	2.4	2.7	38	
Gonadal germ cell	0	0	2	10	12	1.4	1.4	33.3	-	0.7	3.4	1.5	1.2	21	
Gonadal carcinoma	0	0	0	3	3	0.3	0.3	8.3	-	-	1.0	0.4	0.3	5	
Other and unspecified	0	0	1	1	2	0.2	0.2	5.6	-	0.4	0.3	0.2	0.2	4	
XI. EPITHELIAL NEOPLASMS	0	1	4	19	24	2.8	2.8	100.0	0.4	1.5	6.4	3.0	2.5	42	
Adenocortical carcinoma	0	0	0	0	0	-	-	-	-	-	-	-	-	-	
Thyroid carcinoma	0	1	2	9	12	1.4	1.4	50.0	0.4	0.7	3.0	1.5	1.3	21	
Nasopharyngeal carcinoma	0	0	0	1	1	0.1	0.1	4.2	-	-	0.3	0.1	0.1	2	
Melanoma	0	0	1	2	3	0.3	0.3	12.5	-	0.4	0.7	0.4	0.3	5	
Other carcinoma	0	0	1	7	8	0.9	0.9	33.3	-	0.4	2.4	1.0	0.8	14	
XII. OTHER	0	1	2	1	4	0.5	0.5	100.0	0.4	0.7	0.3	0.5	0.5	8	
* Specified as malignant	0	5	2	2	9	1.0	1.0	100.0	2.1	0.7	0.7	1.1	1.3	18	

MALE

USA, Greater Delaware Valley, non White   1970 – 1979

DIAGNOSTIC GROUP	0	1-4	5-9	10-14	All	Crude	Adj.	Group	0-4	5-9	10-14	Crude	Adj.	Cum
	\<NUMBER OF CASES\>					\<REL. FREQUENCY (%)\>			\<RATES PER MILLION\>					
TOTAL	10	62	73	63	208	100.0	100.0	100.0	125.8	117.0	95.7	112.2	114.2	1693
I. LEUKAEMIAS	1	16	27	13	57	27.4	26.7	100.0	29.7	43.3	19.8	30.7	31.2	464
Acute lymphocytic	1	14	20	7	42	20.2	19.9	73.7	26.2	32.1	10.6	22.6	23.6	344
Other lymphocytic	0	0	0	0	0	-	-	-	-	-	-	-	-	-
Acute non-lymphocytic	0	2	3	5	10	4.8	4.7	17.5	3.5	4.8	7.6	5.4	5.1	79
Chronic myeloid	0	0	1	1	2	1.0	0.9	3.5	-	1.6	1.5	1.1	1.0	16
Other and unspecified	0	0	3	0	3	1.4	1.2	5.3	-	4.8	-	1.6	1.6	24
II. LYMPHOMAS	0	7	9	13	29	13.9	13.8	100.0	12.2	14.4	19.8	15.6	15.1	232
Hodgkin's disease	0	2	5	8	15	7.2	7.0	51.7	3.5	8.0	12.2	8.1	7.5	118
Non-Hodgkin lymphoma	0	1	2	3	6	2.9	2.8	20.7	1.7	3.2	4.6	3.2	3.0	48
Burkitt's lymphoma	0	1	0	1	2	1.0	1.0	6.9	1.7	-	1.5	1.1	1.1	16
Unspecified lymphoma	0	0	1	0	1	0.5	0.4	3.4	-	1.6	-	0.5	0.5	8
Histiocytosis X	0	2	1	1	4	1.9	2.0	13.8	3.5	1.6	1.5	2.2	2.3	33
Other reticuloendothelial	0	1	0	0	1	0.5	0.6	3.4	1.7	-	-	0.5	0.7	9
III. BRAIN AND SPINAL	1	14	19	11	45	21.6	21.4	100.0	26.2	30.4	16.7	24.3	24.8	367
Ependymoma	0	2	2	0	4	1.9	1.9	8.9	3.5	3.2	-	2.2	2.4	33
Astrocytoma	1	5	5	7	18	8.7	8.7	40.0	10.5	8.0	10.6	9.7	9.7	146
Medulloblastoma	0	6	3	2	11	5.3	5.5	24.4	10.5	4.8	3.0	5.9	6.5	92
Other glioma	0	1	5	1	7	3.4	3.1	15.6	1.7	8.0	1.5	3.8	3.7	56
Other and unspecified *	0	0	4	1	5	2.4	2.1	11.1	-	6.4	1.5	2.7	2.5	40
IV. SYMPATHETIC N.S.	0	6	4	0	10	4.8	5.0	100.0	10.5	6.4	-	5.4	6.1	84
Neuroblastoma	0	6	4	0	10	4.8	5.0	100.0	10.5	6.4	-	5.4	6.1	84
Other	0	0	0	0	0	-	-	-	-	-	-	-	-	-
V. RETINOBLASTOMA	2	6	0	0	8	3.8	4.4	100.0	14.0	-	-	4.3	5.4	70
VI. KIDNEY	4	9	2	2	17	8.2	9.0	100.0	22.7	3.2	3.0	9.2	10.7	145
Wilms' tumour	4	9	2	2	17	8.2	9.0	100.0	22.7	3.2	3.0	9.2	10.7	145
Renal carcinoma	0	0	0	0	0	-	-	-	-	-	-	-	-	-
Other and unspecified	0	0	0	0	0	-	-	-	-	-	-	-	-	-
VII. LIVER	0	0	1	0	1	0.5	0.4	100.0	-	1.6	-	0.5	0.5	8
Hepatoblastoma	0	0	0	0	0	-	-	-	-	-	-	-	-	-
Hepatic carcinoma	0	0	1	0	1	0.5	0.4	100.0	-	1.6	-	0.5	0.5	8
Other and unspecified	0	0	0	0	0	-	-	-	-	-	-	-	-	-
VIII. BONE	0	0	4	7	11	5.3	5.0	100.0	-	6.4	10.6	5.9	5.2	85
Osteosarcoma	0	0	4	6	10	4.8	4.5	90.9	-	6.4	9.1	5.4	4.7	78
Chondrosarcoma	0	0	0	1	1	0.5	0.5	9.1	-	-	1.5	0.5	0.4	8
Ewing's sarcoma	0	0	0	0	0	-	-	-	-	-	-	-	-	-
Other and unspecified	0	0	0	0	0	-	-	-	-	-	-	-	-	-
IX. SOFT TISSUE SARCOMAS	1	4	6	12	23	11.1	11.0	100.0	8.7	9.6	18.2	12.4	11.8	183
Rhabdomyosarcoma	0	3	3	4	10	4.8	4.8	43.5	5.2	4.8	6.1	5.4	5.3	81
Fibrosarcoma	1	0	1	4	6	2.9	2.9	26.1	1.7	1.6	6.1	3.2	3.0	47
Other and unspecified	0	1	2	4	7	3.4	3.3	30.4	1.7	3.2	6.1	3.8	3.5	55
X. GONADAL & GERM CELL	1	0	0	1	2	1.0	1.0	100.0	1.7	-	1.5	1.1	1.1	16
Non-gonadal germ cell	0	0	0	1	1	0.5	0.5	50.0	-	-	1.5	0.5	0.5	8
Gonadal germ cell	1	0	0	0	1	0.5	0.6	50.0	1.7	-	-	0.5	0.7	9
Gonadal carcinoma	0	0	0	0	0	-	-	-	-	-	-	-	-	-
Other and unspecified	0	0	0	0	0	-	-	-	-	-	-	-	-	-
XI. EPITHELIAL NEOPLASMS	0	0	1	4	5	2.4	2.3	100.0	-	1.6	6.1	2.7	2.3	38
Adrenocortical carcinoma	0	0	1	0	1	0.5	0.4	20.0	-	1.6	-	0.5	0.4	8
Thyroid carcinoma	0	0	0	0	0	-	-	-	-	-	-	-	-	-
Nasopharyngeal carcinoma	0	0	0	2	2	1.0	1.0	40.0	-	-	3.0	1.1	0.9	15
Melanoma	0	0	0	0	0	-	-	-	-	-	-	-	-	-
Other carcinoma	0	0	0	2	2	1.0	1.0	40.0	-	-	3.0	1.1	1.0	15
XII. OTHER	0	0	0	0	0	-	-	-	-	-	-	-	-	-
* Specified as malignant	0	0	0	1	1	0.5	0.5	100.0	-	-	1.5	0.5	0.4	8

USA, Greater Delaware Valley, non White · 1970 - 1979 · FEMALE

DIAGNOSTIC GROUP	NUMBER OF CASES 0	1-4	5-9	10-14	All	REL. FREQUENCY(%) Crude	Adj.	Group	RATES PER MILLION 0-4	5-9	10-14	Crude	Adj.	Cum	HV(%)
TOTAL	15	54	54	48	171	100.0	100.0	100.0	121.6	87.9	72.8	92.9	96.5	1411	
I. LEUKAEMIAS	1	9	6	8	24	14.0	14.1	100.0	17.6	9.8	12.1	13.0	13.5	198	
Acute lymphocytic	0	7	1	7	15	8.8	9.0	62.5	12.3	1.6	10.6	8.1	8.4	123	
Other lymphocytic	0	0	0	0	0										
Acute non-lymphocytic	1	1	4	1	7	4.1	4.0	29.2	3.5	6.5	1.5	3.8	3.9	58	
Chronic myeloid	0	0	0	0	0										
Other and unspecified	0	1	1	0	2	1.2	1.1	8.3	1.8	1.6		1.1	1.2	17	
II. LYMPHOMAS	1	3	7	6	17	9.9	10.0	100.0	7.0	11.4	9.1	9.2	9.0	138	
Hodgkin's disease	0	0	3	5	8	4.7	4.8	47.1		4.9	7.6	4.3	3.8	62	
Non-Hodgkin lymphoma	0	2	4	1	7	4.1	4.0	41.2	3.5	6.5	1.5	3.8	3.9	58	
Burkitt's lymphoma	0	0	0	0	0										
Unspecified lymphoma	0	0	0	0	0										
Histiocytosis X	0	0	0	0	1	0.6	0.6	5.9	1.8			0.5	0.7	9	
Other reticuloendothelial	0	1	0	0	1	0.6	0.6	5.9	1.8			0.5	0.7	9	
III. BRAIN AND SPINAL	0	11	14	16	41	24.0	24.2	100.0	19.4	22.8	24.3	22.3	21.9	332	
Ependymoma	0	2	2	0	4	2.3	2.3	9.8	3.5	3.3		2.2	2.4	34	
Astrocytoma	0	2	4	6	12	7.0	7.1	29.3	3.5	6.5	9.1	6.5	6.1	96	
Medulloblastoma	0	3	2	4	9	5.3	5.4	22.0	5.3	3.3	6.1	4.9	4.9	73	
Other glioma	0	2	2	4	8	4.7	4.8	19.5	3.5	3.3	6.1	4.3	4.2	64	
Other and unspecified *	0	2	4	2	8	4.7	4.6	19.5	3.5	6.5	3.0	4.3	4.3	65	
IV. SYMPATHETIC N.S.	2	3	4	0	9	5.3	5.1	100.0	8.8	6.5		4.9	5.5	77	
Neuroblastoma	2	3	4	0	9	5.3	5.1	100.0	8.8	6.5		4.9	5.5	77	
Other	0	0	0	0	0										
V. RETINOBLASTOMA	6	4	1	0	11	6.4	6.4	100.0	17.6	1.6		6.0	7.3	96	
VI. KIDNEY	3	17	6	0	26	15.2	14.9	100.0	35.2	9.8		14.1	16.8	225	
Wilms' tumour	3	17	6	0	26	15.2	14.9	100.0	35.2	9.8		14.1	16.8	225	
Renal carcinoma	0	0	0	0	0										
Other and unspecified	0	0	0	0	0										
VII. LIVER	0	1	0	0	1	0.6	0.6	100.0	1.8			0.5	0.7	9	
Hepatoblastoma	0	1	0	0	1	0.6	0.6	100.0	1.8			0.5	0.7	9	
Hepatic carcinoma	0	0	0	0	0										
Other and unspecified	0	0	0	0	0										
VIII. BONE	0	0	4	6	10	5.8	6.0	100.0		6.5	9.1	5.4	4.7	78	
Osteosarcoma	0	0	2	6	8	4.7	4.9	80.0		3.3	9.1	4.3	3.7	62	
Chondrosarcoma	0	0	1	0	1	0.6	0.6	10.0		1.6		0.5	0.5	8	
Ewing's sarcoma	0	0	1	0	1	0.6	0.6	10.0		1.6		0.5	0.5	8	
Other and unspecified	0	0	0	0	0										
IX. SOFT TISSUE SARCOMAS	1	4	3	4	12	7.0	7.1	100.0	8.8	4.9	6.1	6.5	6.7	99	
Rhabdomyosarcoma	0	2	1	1	5	2.9	2.9	41.7	5.3	1.6	1.5	2.7	3.0	42	
Fibrosarcoma	0	1	0	1	2	1.2	1.2	16.7	1.8		1.5	1.1	1.1	16	
Other and unspecified	0	1	2	2	5	2.9	2.9	41.7	1.8	3.3	3.0	2.7	2.6	40	
X. GONADAL & GERM CELL	1	1	7	3	12	7.0	6.9	100.0	3.5	11.4	4.5	6.5	6.4	97	
Non-gonadal germ cell	1	0	2	1	4	2.3	2.3	33.3	1.8	3.3	1.5	2.2	2.2	33	
Gonadal germ cell	0	1	3	1	5	2.9	2.9	41.7	1.8	4.9	1.5	2.7	2.7	41	
Gonadal carcinoma	0	0	0	0	1	0.6	0.6	8.3			1.5	0.5	0.4	8	
Other and unspecified	0	0	2	0	2	1.2	1.1	16.7		3.3		1.1	1.1	16	
XI. EPITHELIAL NEOPLASMS	0	1	2	5	8	4.7	4.8	100.0	1.8	3.3	7.6	4.3	3.9	63	
Adrenocortical carcinoma	0	0	0	0	0										
Thyroid carcinoma	0	0	0	3	3	1.8	1.8	37.5			3.0	1.6	1.4	23	
Nasopharyngeal carcinoma	0	0	1	0	1	0.6	0.6	12.5		1.6		0.5	0.7	9	
Melanoma	0	0	0	0	0										
Other carcinoma	0	0	1	3	4	2.3	2.4	50.0	1.8	1.6	4.5	2.2	1.8	31	
XII. OTHER	0	0	0	0	0										
* Specified as malignant	0	0	1	0	1	0.6	0.6	100.0		1.6		0.5	0.5	8	

Figure 1. Area covered by the Greater Delaware Valley Registry

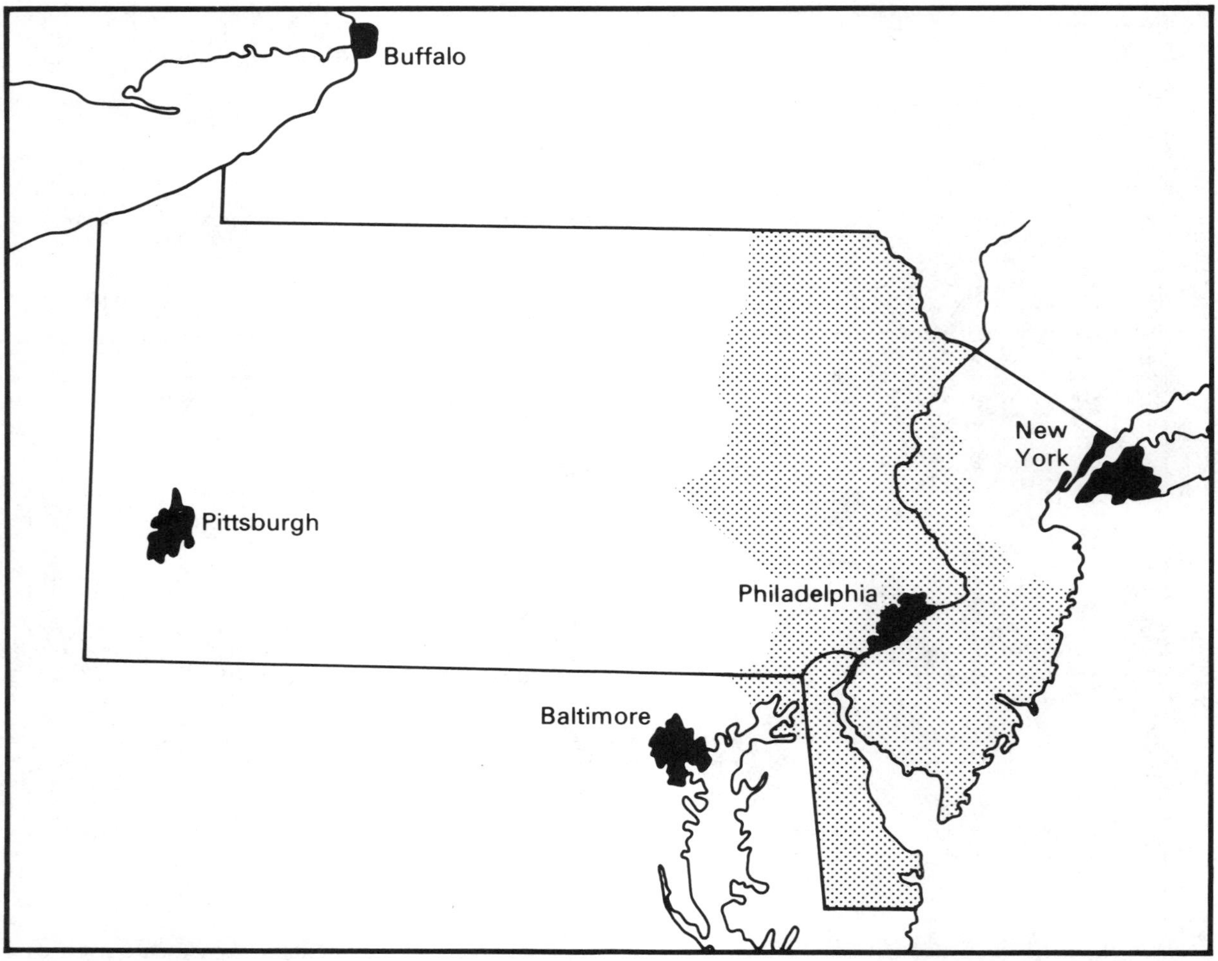

Commentary

Among Whites, the total rate for the population and the rates for individual tumour types are similar to those for European and other North American series.

For non-Whites, the total rates, and those for both acute lymphocytic and acute non-lymphocytic leukaemia are lower than for Whites, and the early age-peak for acute lymphocytic leukaemia observed in both Whites and Blacks in other United States registries is missing. Neuroblastoma rates are lower, and Wilms' tumour rates higher than for Whites; similar higher rates for the latter tumour in non-Whites are also found in the SEER Program

and Los Angeles. Ewing's sarcoma is rare (only one case was recorded), as for other black populations in the United States and in many other African and Asian populations. Osteosarcoma rates are higher for non-Whites than for Whites; this difference is also found for the other US data presented here. The rate for nasopharyngeal carcinoma was high, though this was based on only five cases.

Reference

Kramer, S., Meadows, A.T., Jarrett, P. & Evans, A.E. (1983) Incidence of childhood cancer: experience of a decade in a population-based registry. *J. natl Cancer Inst.*, 70, 49-55

Los Angeles County Cancer Surveillance Program, 1972–1983

H.R. Menck & R.L. Philipps

The Cancer Surveillance Program (CSP) of Los Angeles County was started at the University of Southern California in 1970 as part of an epidemiology and biostatistics programme. The CSP was designed explicitly for purposes of etiological research. Complete ascertainment began in 1972.

Cases of cancer in Los Angeles County residents are actively sought and abstracted by CSP personnel from 195 hospitals within the county, and from 42 in adjacent counties. Case identification depends primarily on the screening of pathology files. All other files that contain reports of microscopically verified malignancy, such as autopsy, cytology and haematology files, are included in the regular review. Files on out-patients, if separate, are similarly screened. All death certificates of Los Angeles County are examined to pick up cases with clinical evidence of cancer but in which a pathological confirmation was deemed unnecessary or impossible, and to provide feedback on efficiency of the case-ascertainment procedures. Follow-up data are not routinely collected.

For each case, 55 data items, made up of 23 disease or medical care items, 26 demographic items and six administrative items, are coded and computerized. Data regarding race, nationality, birthplace, religion, surname and first name are collected to allow classification by ethnicity, religion and migrant status.

Manual and computerized record-linkage is performed separately using surname and social security numbers. Multiple primaries are noted by tumour sequence number. Validity and selected inter-data-item checks are performed.

Los Angeles County is a large urban area with approximately 7 495 000 inhabitants. Since 1972, incidence rates have been calculated separately for the three largest ethnic groups: Spanish-surnamed Whites, Other Whites and Blacks, and also for four smaller groups, Japanese, Chinese, Korean and Filipino. The numbers of cancers in children aged under 15 in these last four groups (28, 24, 19 and 26,

respectively) were too small to permit the calculation of reliable rates.

The primary use of the CSP is in the identification of representative cases for analytical studies. The population-based surveillance also allows computation of incidence rates for subgroups of the population defined by the demographic data available.

Population

The population, by race, is available from the censuses of 1970 and 1980 (US Bureau of the Census). Adjustments for under-counting at censuses have been made, according to estimates of their coverage by sex, race, and age. The 'Other White' populations are obtained by subtracting the Hispanic population from the total of all Whites.

AVERAGE ANNUAL POPULATION: 1972–1983

Age	Male	Female
Black		
0	8808	8644
1–4	33237	31084
5–9	42211	41455
10–14	48199	46938
0–14	132455	128121
Hispanic		
0	22843	20982
1–4	77579	74669
5–9	91835	88860
10–14	79483	77823
0–14	271740	262334
Other White		
0	26945	26411
1–4	99305	96214
5–9	133751	126709
10–14	151705	147308
0–14	411706	396642

Contd. p. 94

USA, Los Angeles, Black

1972 – 1983   MALE

DIAGNOSTIC GROUP	NUMBER OF CASES					REL. FREQUENCY(%)			RATES PER MILLION							
	'0	1-4	5-9	10-14	All	Crude	Adj.	Group	0	1-4	5-9	10-14	Crude	Adj.	Cum	HV(%)
TOTAL	21	55	53	53	182	100.0	100.0	100.0	198.7	137.9	104.6	91.6	114.5	118.4	1732	97.3
I. LEUKAEMIAS	4	16	16	12	48	26.4	26.4	100.0	37.8	40.1	31.6	20.7	30.2	31.6	460	100.0
Acute lymphocytic	3	11	13	8	35	19.2	19.3	72.9	28.4	27.6	25.7	13.8	22.0	23.0	336	100.0
Other lymphocytic	0	0	0	0	0	-	-	-	-	-	-	-	-	-	-	-
Acute non-lymphocytic	1	2	2	4	9	4.9	5.0	18.8	9.5	5.0	3.9	6.9	5.7	5.6	84	100.0
Chronic myeloid	0	1	1	0	2	1.1	1.1	4.2	-	2.5	2.0	-	1.3	1.4	20	100.0
Other and unspecified	0	2	0	0	2	1.1	1.1	4.2	-	5.0	-	-	1.3	1.6	20	100.0
II. LYMPHOMAS	0	1	12	9	22	12.1	12.4	100.0	-	2.5	23.7	15.6	13.8	12.9	206	100.0
Hodgkin's disease	0	0	5	6	11	6.0	6.2	50.0	-	-	9.9	10.4	6.9	6.2	101	100.0
Non-Hodgkin lymphoma	0	0	6	2	8	4.4	4.5	36.4	-	-	11.8	3.5	5.0	4.8	77	100.0
Burkitt's lymphoma	0	0	1	0	1	0.5	0.5	4.5	-	-	-	1.7	0.6	0.5	9	100.0
Unspecified lymphoma	0	0	0	1	1	0.5	0.6	4.5	-	-	-	-	0.6	0.6	10	100.0
Histiocytosis X	0	1	0	0	1	0.5	0.5	4.5	-	2.5	-	-	0.6	0.8	10	100.0
Other reticuloendothelial	0	0	0	0	0	-	-	-	-	-	-	-	-	-	-	-
III. BRAIN AND SPINAL	1	14	8	9	32	17.6	17.5	100.0	9.5	35.1	15.8	15.6	20.1	21.2	307	90.6
Ependymoma	0	4	0	0	4	2.2	2.1	12.5	-	10.0	-	-	2.5	3.1	40	100.0
Astrocytoma	0	5	5	6	16	8.8	8.9	50.0	-	12.5	9.9	10.4	10.1	10.1	151	100.0
Medulloblastoma	1	2	1	1	5	2.7	2.7	15.6	9.5	5.0	2.0	1.7	3.1	3.4	48	100.0
Other glioma	0	1	0	0	1	0.5	0.5	3.1	-	2.5	-	-	0.6	0.8	10	100.0
Other and unspecified *	0	2	2	2	6	3.3	3.3	18.8	-	5.0	3.9	3.5	3.8	3.8	57	50.0
IV. SYMPATHETIC N.S.	7	4	3	1	15	8.2	8.1	100.0	66.2	10.0	5.9	1.7	9.4	10.6	145	100.0
Neuroblastoma	7	4	3	1	15	8.2	8.1	100.0	66.2	10.0	5.9	1.7	9.4	10.6	145	100.0
Other	0	0	0	0	0	-	-	-	-	-	-	-	-	-	-	-
V. RETINOBLASTOMA	3	4	0	0	7	3.8	3.7	100.0	28.4	10.0	-	-	4.4	5.3	68	100.0
VI. KIDNEY	2	7	5	0	14	7.7	7.6	100.0	18.9	17.6	9.9	-	8.8	10.1	138	100.0
Wilms' tumour	2	7	5	0	14	7.7	7.6	100.0	18.9	17.6	9.9	-	8.8	10.1	138	100.0
Renal carcinoma	0	0	0	0	0	-	-	-	-	-	-	-	-	-	-	-
Other and unspecified	0	0	0	0	0	-	-	-	-	-	-	-	-	-	-	-
VII. LIVER	2	0	0	1	3	1.6	1.6	100.0	18.9	-	-	1.7	1.9	2.0	28	100.0
Hepatoblastoma	2	0	0	0	2	1.1	1.1	66.7	18.9	-	-	-	1.3	1.5	19	100.0
Hepatic carcinoma	0	0	0	1	1	0.5	0.6	33.3	-	-	-	1.7	0.6	0.5	9	100.0
Other and unspecified	0	0	0	0	0	-	-	-	-	-	-	-	-	-	-	-
VIII. BONE	0	0	3	7	10	5.5	5.7	100.0	-	-	5.9	12.1	6.3	5.4	90	90.0
Osteosarcoma	0	0	3	6	9	4.9	5.1	90.0	-	-	5.9	10.4	5.7	4.9	81	88.9
Chondrosarcoma	0	0	0	1	1	0.5	0.6	10.0	-	-	-	1.7	0.6	0.5	9	100.0
Ewing's sarcoma	0	0	0	0	0	-	-	-	-	-	-	-	-	-	-	-
Other and unspecified	0	0	0	0	0	-	-	-	-	-	-	-	-	-	-	-
IX. SOFT TISSUE SARCOMAS	1	4	5	4	14	7.7	7.7	100.0	-	10.0	9.9	6.9	8.8	9.0	134	100.0
Rhabdomyosarcoma	1	3	4	1	9	4.9	4.9	64.3	-	7.5	7.9	1.7	5.7	6.1	88	100.0
Fibrosarcoma	0	0	0	2	2	1.1	1.1	14.3	-	-	-	3.5	1.3	1.3	17	100.0
Other and unspecified	0	1	1	1	3	1.6	1.7	21.4	-	2.5	2.0	1.7	1.9	1.9	29	100.0
X. GONADAL & GERM CELL	1	3	0	1	5	2.7	2.7	100.0	9.5	7.5	-	1.7	3.1	3.6	48	100.0
Non-gonadal germ cell	1	3	0	0	4	2.2	2.1	80.0	9.5	7.5	-	-	2.5	3.1	40	100.0
Gonadal germ cell	0	0	0	1	1	0.5	0.6	20.0	-	-	-	1.7	0.6	0.5	9	100.0
Gonadal carcinoma	0	0	0	0	0	-	-	-	-	-	-	-	-	-	-	-
Other and unspecified	0	0	0	0	0	-	-	-	-	-	-	-	-	-	-	-
XI. EPITHELIAL NEOPLASMS	0	0	0	8	8	4.4	4.5	100.0	-	-	-	13.8	5.0	4.0	69	100.0
Adrenocortical carcinoma	0	0	0	0	0	-	-	-	-	-	-	-	-	-	-	-
Thyroid carcinoma	0	0	0	1	1	0.5	0.6	12.5	-	-	-	1.7	0.6	0.5	9	100.0
Nasopharyngeal carcinoma	0	0	0	3	3	1.6	1.7	37.5	-	-	-	5.2	1.9	1.5	26	100.0
Melanoma	0	0	0	0	0	-	-	-	-	-	-	-	-	-	-	-
Other carcinoma	0	0	0	4	4	2.2	2.3	50.0	-	-	-	6.9	2.5	2.0	35	100.0
XII. OTHER	0	2	1	1	4	2.2	2.2	100.0	-	5.0	2.0	1.7	2.5	2.7	39	75.0
* Specified as malignant	0	0	1	1	2	1.1	1.1	100.0	-	-	2.0	1.7	1.3	1.1	19	-

USA, Los Angeles, Black 1972 - 1983 FEMALE

DIAGNOSTIC GROUP	NUMBER OF CASES					REL. FREQUENCY(%)			RATES PER MILLION						Cum	HV(%)
	0	1-4	5-9	10-14	All	Crude	Adj.	Group	0	1-4	5-9	10-14	Crude	Adj.		
TOTAL	13	43	42	54	152	100.0	100.0	100.0	125.3	115.3	84.4	95.9	98.9	100.5	1488	98.0
I. LEUKAEMIAS	3	13	12	6	34	22.4	23.3	100.0	28.9	34.9	24.1	10.7	22.1	23.9	342	100.0
Acute lymphocytic	2	10	6	3	21	13.8	14.5	61.8	19.3	26.8	12.1	5.3	13.7	15.2	213	100.0
Other lymphocytic	0	0	0	0	0	-	-	-	-	-	-	-	-	-	-	-
Acute non-lymphocytic	0	2	5	1	8	5.3	5.6	23.5	-	5.4	10.1	1.8	5.2	5.4	81	100.0
Chronic myeloid	0	0	0	0	0	-	-	-	-	-	-	-	-	-	-	-
Other and unspecified	1	1	1	2	5	3.3	3.3	14.7	9.6	2.7	2.0	3.6	3.3	3.3	48	100.0
II. LYMPHOMAS	0	3	1	13	17	11.2	10.1	100.0	-	8.0	2.0	23.1	11.1	9.8	158	100.0
Hodgkin's disease	0	1	1	11	13	8.6	7.5	76.5	-	2.7	2.0	19.5	8.5	7.1	118	100.0
Non-Hodgkin lymphoma	0	0	0	2	2	1.3	1.1	11.8	-	-	-	3.6	1.3	1.0	18	100.0
Burkitt's lymphoma	0	0	0	0	0	-	-	-	-	-	-	-	-	-	-	-
Unspecified lymphoma	0	0	0	0	0	-	-	-	-	-	-	-	-	-	-	-
Histiocytosis X	0	1	0	0	1	0.7	0.7	5.9	-	2.7	-	-	0.7	0.8	11	100.0
Other reticuloendothelial	0	1	0	0	1	0.7	0.7	5.9	-	2.7	-	-	0.7	0.8	11	100.0
III. BRAIN AND SPINAL	0	6	13	8	27	17.8	18.0	100.0	-	16.1	26.1	14.2	17.6	17.5	266	88.9
Ependymoma	0	0	0	0	0	-	-	-	-	-	-	-	-	-	-	-
Astrocytoma	0	4	6	4	14	9.2	9.4	51.9	-	10.7	12.1	7.1	9.1	9.3	139	100.0
Medulloblastoma	0	2	4	1	7	4.6	4.8	25.9	-	5.4	8.0	1.8	4.6	4.8	71	100.0
Other glioma	0	0	1	1	2	1.3	1.3	7.4	-	-	2.0	1.8	1.3	1.2	19	100.0
Other and unspecified *	0	0	2	2	4	2.6	2.5	14.8	-	-	4.0	3.6	2.6	2.3	38	25.0
IV. SYMPATHETIC N.S.	3	6	2	1	12	7.9	8.4	100.0	28.9	16.1	4.0	1.8	7.8	9.0	122	100.0
Neuroblastoma	3	6	2	1	12	7.9	8.4	100.0	28.9	16.1	4.0	1.8	7.8	9.0	122	100.0
Other	0	0	0	0	0	-	-	-	-	-	-	-	-	-	-	-
V. RETINOBLASTOMA	1	4	0	1	6	3.9	4.1	100.0	9.6	10.7	-	1.8	3.9	4.6	61	100.0
VI. KIDNEY	3	9	6	0	18	11.8	12.9	100.0	28.9	24.1	12.1	-	11.7	13.6	186	100.0
Wilms' tumour	3	9	6	0	18	11.8	12.9	100.0	28.9	24.1	12.1	-	11.7	13.6	186	100.0
Renal carcinoma	0	0	0	0	0	-	-	-	-	-	-	-	-	-	-	-
Other and unspecified	0	0	0	0	0	-	-	-	-	-	-	-	-	-	-	-
VII. LIVER	0	1	0	1	2	1.3	1.3	100.0	-	2.7	-	1.8	1.3	0.8	20	100.0
Hepatoblastoma	0	1	0	0	1	0.7	0.7	50.0	-	2.7	-	-	0.7	0.3	11	100.0
Hepatic carcinoma	0	0	0	1	1	0.7	0.6	50.0	-	-	-	1.8	0.7	0.5	9	100.0
Other and unspecified	0	0	0	0	0	-	-	-	-	-	-	-	-	-	-	-
VIII. BONE	1	0	1	9	11	7.2	6.4	100.0	9.6	-	2.0	16.0	7.2	6.0	100	100.0
Osteosarcoma	0	0	1	7	8	5.3	4.6	72.7	-	-	2.0	12.4	5.2	4.3	72	100.0
Chondrosarcoma	0	0	0	1	1	0.7	0.6	9.1	-	-	-	1.8	0.7	0.5	9	100.0
Ewing's sarcoma	1	0	0	1	2	1.3	1.3	18.2	9.6	-	-	1.8	1.3	1.3	19	100.0
Other and unspecified	0	0	0	0	0	-	-	-	-	-	-	-	-	-	-	-
IX. SOFT TISSUE SARCOMAS	1	1	2	5	9	5.9	5.6	100.0	9.6	2.7	4.0	8.9	5.9	5.5	85	100.0
Rhabdomyosarcoma	0	1	2	0	3	2.0	2.1	33.3	-	2.7	4.0	-	2.0	2.1	31	100.0
Fibrosarcoma	0	0	0	2	2	1.3	1.1	22.2	-	-	-	3.6	1.3	1.0	18	100.0
Other and unspecified	1	0	0	3	4	2.6	2.4	44.4	9.6	-	-	5.3	2.6	2.3	36	100.0
X. GONADAL & GERM CELL	0	0	1	3	4	2.6	2.4	100.0	-	-	2.0	5.3	2.6	2.2	37	100.0
Non-gonadal germ cell	0	0	0	0	0	-	-	-	-	-	-	-	-	-	-	-
Gonadal germ cell	0	0	1	2	3	2.0	1.8	75.0	-	-	2.0	3.6	2.0	1.7	28	100.0
Gonadal carcinoma	0	0	0	1	1	0.7	0.6	25.0	-	-	-	1.8	0.7	0.5	9	100.0
Other and unspecified	0	0	0	0	0	-	-	-	-	-	-	-	-	-	-	-
XI. EPITHELIAL NEOPLASMS	1	0	3	7	11	7.2	6.7	100.0	9.6	-	6.0	12.4	7.2	6.3	102	100.0
Adrenocortical carcinoma	0	0	0	0	0	-	-	-	-	-	-	-	-	-	-	-
Thyroid carcinoma	0	0	2	3	5	3.3	3.1	45.5	-	-	4.0	5.3	3.3	2.8	47	100.0
Nasopharyngeal carcinoma	0	0	0	3	3	2.0	1.7	27.3	-	-	-	5.3	2.0	1.5	27	100.0
Melanoma	1	0	0	0	1	0.7	0.7	9.1	9.6	-	-	-	0.7	0.7	10	100.0
Other carcinoma	0	0	1	1	2	1.3	1.3	18.2	-	-	2.0	1.8	1.3	1.2	19	100.0
XII. OTHER	0	0	1	0	1	0.7	0.7	100.0	-	-	2.0	-	0.7	0.6	10	100.0
* Specified as malignant	0	0	1	1	2	1.3	1.3	100.0	-	-	2.0	1.8	1.3	1.2	19	-

USA, Los Angeles, Hispanic   1972 - 1983   MALE

DIAGNOSTIC GROUP	NUMBER OF CASES					REL. FREQUENCY(%)			RATES PER MILLION						Cum	HV(%)
	0	1-4	5-9	10-14	All	Crude	Adj.	Group	0	1-4	5-9	10-14	Crude	Adj.		
TOTAL	59	195	127	104	485	100.0	100.0	-	215.2	209.5	115.2	109.0	148.7	150.4	2174	99.0
I. LEUKAEMIAS	15	85	47	32	179	36.9	36.1	100.0	54.7	91.3	42.6	33.5	54.9	56.0	801	100.0
Acute lymphocytic	8	76	40	21	145	29.9	28.7	81.0	29.2	81.6	36.3	22.0	44.5	45.6	647	100.0
Other lymphocytic	0	1	0	0	1	0.2	0.2	0.6	-	1.1	-	-	0.3	0.2	4	100.0
Acute non-lymphocytic	7	5	6	10	28	5.8	6.2	15.6	25.5	5.4	5.4	10.5	8.6	8.4	127	100.0
Chronic myeloid	0	2	0	1	3	0.6	0.6	1.7	-	2.1	-	1.0	0.9	1.0	14	100.0
Other and unspecified	0	1	1	0	2	0.4	0.4	1.1	-	1.1	0.9	-	0.6	0.6	9	100.0
II. LYMPHOMAS	3	24	30	31	88	18.1	20.3	100.0	10.9	25.8	27.2	32.5	27.0	27.0	413	100.0
Hodgkin's disease	0	6	18	15	39	8.0	9.5	44.3	-	6.4	16.3	15.7	12.0	11.8	186	100.0
Non-Hodgkin lymphoma	0	9	8	12	29	6.0	6.8	33.0	-	9.7	7.3	12.6	8.9	9.0	138	100.0
Burkitt's lymphoma	0	3	2	1	6	1.2	1.2	6.8	-	3.2	1.8	1.0	1.8	1.9	27	100.0
Unspecified lymphoma	1	4	2	3	10	2.1	2.1	11.4	3.6	4.3	1.8	3.1	3.1	3.1	46	100.0
Histiocytosis X	1	1	0	0	2	0.4	0.3	2.3	3.6	1.1	-	-	0.6	0.6	8	100.0
Other reticuloendothelial	1	1	0	0	2	0.4	0.3	2.3	3.6	1.1	-	-	0.6	0.6	8	100.0
III. BRAIN AND SPINAL	4	29	34	18	85	17.5	18.4	100.0	14.6	31.2	30.9	18.9	26.1	26.2	388	95.3
Ependymoma	3	5	2	2	12	2.5	2.3	14.1	10.9	5.4	1.8	2.1	3.7	3.7	52	100.0
Astrocytoma	0	4	15	7	26	5.4	6.2	30.6	-	4.3	13.6	7.3	8.0	7.9	122	100.0
Medulloblastoma	1	13	9	5	28	5.8	5.8	32.9	3.6	14.0	8.2	5.2	8.6	8.8	127	100.0
Other glioma	0	3	0	1	4	0.8	0.8	4.7	-	3.2	-	1.0	1.2	1.3	18	100.0
Other and unspecified *	0	4	8	3	15	3.1	3.4	17.6	-	4.3	7.3	3.1	4.6	4.6	69	73.3
IV. SYMPATHETIC N.S.	9	5	0	0	14	2.9	2.2	100.0	32.8	5.4	-	-	4.3	4.2	54	100.0
Neuroblastoma	9	5	0	0	14	2.9	2.2	100.0	32.8	5.4	-	-	4.3	4.2	54	100.0
Other	0	0	0	0	0	-	-	-	-	-	-	-	-	-	-	-
V. RETINOBLASTOMA	5	12	1	0	18	3.7	2.9	100.0	18.2	12.9	0.9	-	5.5	5.7	74	100.0
VI. KIDNEY	6	9	3	1	19	3.9	3.4	100.0	21.9	9.7	2.7	1.0	5.8	5.9	79	100.0
Wilms' tumour	6	9	3	0	18	3.7	3.1	94.7	21.9	9.7	2.7	-	5.5	5.6	74	100.0
Renal carcinoma	0	0	0	1	1	0.2	0.3	5.3	-	-	-	1.0	0.3	0.3	5	100.0
Other and unspecified	0	0	0	0	0	-	-	-	-	-	-	-	-	-	-	-
VII. LIVER	4	3	1	2	10	2.1	1.9	100.0	14.6	3.2	0.9	2.1	3.1	3.0	43	100.0
Hepatoblastoma	3	2	1	0	6	1.2	1.0	60.0	10.9	2.1	0.9	-	1.8	1.8	24	100.0
Hepatic carcinoma	1	1	0	2	4	0.8	0.9	40.0	3.6	1.1	-	2.1	1.2	1.2	18	100.0
Other and unspecified	0	0	0	0	0	-	-	-	-	-	-	-	-	-	-	-
VIII. BONE	0	1	3	5	9	1.9	2.3	100.0	-	1.1	2.7	5.2	2.8	2.7	44	100.0
Osteosarcoma	0	0	0	4	4	0.8	1.2	44.4	-	-	-	4.2	1.2	1.2	21	100.0
Chondrosarcoma	0	0	0	0	0	-	-	-	-	-	-	-	-	-	-	-
Ewing's sarcoma	0	1	3	1	5	1.0	1.2	55.6	-	1.1	2.7	1.0	1.5	1.5	23	100.0
Other and unspecified	0	0	0	0	0	-	-	-	-	-	-	-	-	-	-	-
IX. SOFT TISSUE SARCOMAS	4	16	5	9	34	7.0	6.9	100.0	14.6	17.2	4.5	9.4	10.4	10.7	153	100.0
Rhabdomyosarcoma	2	9	4	6	21	4.3	4.4	61.8	7.3	9.7	3.6	6.3	6.4	6.6	96	100.0
Fibrosarcoma	0	2	0	0	2	0.4	0.3	5.9	-	2.1	-	-	0.6	0.7	9	100.0
Other and unspecified	2	5	1	3	11	2.3	2.2	32.4	7.3	5.4	0.9	3.1	3.4	3.4	49	100.0
X. GONADAL & GERM CELL	7	11	1	1	20	4.1	3.4	100.0	25.5	11.8	0.9	1.0	6.1	6.2	83	95.0
Non-gonadal germ cell	1	0	1	1	3	0.6	0.7	15.0	3.6	-	0.9	1.0	0.9	0.9	13	100.0
Gonadal germ cell	6	11	0	0	17	3.5	2.7	85.0	21.9	11.8	-	-	5.2	5.4	69	94.1
Gonadal carcinoma	0	0	0	0	0	-	-	-	-	-	-	-	-	-	-	-
Other and unspecified	0	0	0	0	0	-	-	-	-	-	-	-	-	-	-	-
XI. EPITHELIAL NEOPLASMS	1	0	0	4	5	1.0	1.3	100.0	3.6	-	-	4.2	1.5	1.5	25	100.0
Adrenocortical carcinoma	0	0	0	1	1	0.2	0.3	20.0	-	-	-	1.0	0.3	0.3	-	100.0
Thyroid carcinoma	0	0	0	1	1	0.2	0.3	20.0	-	-	-	1.0	0.3	0.3	5	100.0
Nasopharyngeal carcinoma	0	0	0	0	0	-	-	-	-	-	-	-	-	-	-	-
Melanoma	0	0	0	0	0	-	-	-	-	-	-	-	-	-	-	-
Other carcinoma	1	0	0	3	4	0.8	1.0	80.0	3.6	-	-	3.1	1.2	1.2	19	100.0
XII. OTHER	1	0	2	1	4	0.8	0.9	100.0	3.6	-	1.8	1.0	1.2	1.2	18	100.0
* Specified as malignant	0	3	1	2	6	1.2	1.3	100.0	-	3.2	0.9	2.1	1.8	1.9	28	33.3

USA, Los Angeles, Hispanic

1972 – 1983

FEMALE

DIAGNOSTIC GROUP	NUMBER OF CASES 0	1-4	5-9	10-14	All	REL. FREQUENCY(%) Crude	Adj.	Group	RATES PER MILLION 0	1-4	5-9	10-14	Crude	Adj.	Cum	HV(%)
TOTAL	42	148	103	113	406	100.0	100.0	100.0	166.8	165.2	96.6	121.0	129.0	130.4	1915	98.5
I. LEUKAEMIAS	11	64	38	23	136	33.5	33.0	100.0	43.7	71.4	35.6	24.6	43.2	44.1	631	100.0
Acute lymphocytic	3	49	26	15	93	22.9	22.5	68.4	11.9	54.7	24.4	16.1	29.5	30.4	433	100.0
Other lymphocytic	0	0	0	0	0	-	-	-	-	-	-	-	-	-	-	-
Acute non-lymphocytic	3	11	10	6	30	7.4	7.5	22.1	11.9	12.3	9.4	6.4	9.5	9.6	140	100.0
Chronic myeloid	1	1	2	0	4	1.0	1.0	2.9	4.0	1.1	1.9	-	1.3	1.3	18	100.0
Other and unspecified	4	3	0	2	9	2.2	2.0	6.6	15.9	3.3	-	2.1	2.9	2.9	40	100.0
II. LYMPHOMAS	1	6	7	17	31	7.6	8.0	100.0	4.0	6.7	6.6	18.2	9.8	9.8	155	100.0
Hodgkin's disease	0	0	3	14	17	4.2	4.6	54.8	-	-	2.8	15.0	5.4	5.3	89	100.0
Non-Hodgkin lymphoma	0	1	4	1	6	1.5	1.6	19.4	-	1.1	3.8	1.1	1.9	1.9	29	100.0
Burkitt's lymphoma	0	0	0	0	0	-	-	-	-	-	-	-	-	-	-	-
Unspecified lymphoma	0	3	0	2	5	1.2	1.2	16.1	-	3.3	-	2.1	1.6	1.7	24	100.0
Histiocytosis X	1	1	0	0	2	0.5	0.4	6.5	4.0	1.1	-	-	0.6	0.7	8	100.0
Other reticuloendothelial	0	1	0	0	1	0.2	0.2	3.2	-	1.1	-	-	0.3	0.3	4	100.0
III. BRAIN AND SPINAL	2	25	25	18	70	17.2	17.7	100.0	7.9	27.9	23.4	19.3	22.2	22.4	333	95.7
Ependymoma	0	3	2	3	8	2.0	2.0	11.4	-	3.3	1.9	2.1	2.5	2.6	37	100.0
Astrocytoma	1	14	14	8	37	9.1	9.4	52.9	4.0	15.6	14.1	8.6	11.8	11.9	176	100.0
Medulloblastoma	1	3	3	2	9	2.2	2.2	12.9	4.0	3.3	2.8	2.1	2.9	3.2	43	100.0
Other glioma	0	0	3	2	5	1.2	1.4	7.1	-	-	2.8	3.2	1.6	1.5	25	100.0
Other and unspecified *	0	5	3	3	11	2.7	2.7	15.7	-	5.6	2.8	3.2	3.5	3.6	52	72.7
IV. SYMPATHETIC N.S.	8	11	3	0	22	5.4	4.9	100.0	31.8	12.3	2.8	-	7.0	7.2	95	100.0
Neuroblastoma	7	11	3	0	21	5.2	4.7	95.5	27.8	12.3	2.8	-	6.7	6.9	91	100.0
Other	1	0	0	0	1	0.2	0.2	4.5	4.0	-	-	-	0.3	0.3	4	100.0
V. RETINOBLASTOMA	5	15	0	0	20	4.9	4.2	100.0	19.9	16.7	-	-	6.4	6.7	87	100.0
VI. KIDNEY	5	16	9	2	32	7.9	7.6	100.0	19.9	17.9	8.4	2.1	10.2	10.4	144	100.0
Wilms' tumour	5	16	9	2	32	7.9	7.6	100.0	19.9	17.9	8.4	2.1	10.2	10.4	144	100.0
Renal carcinoma	0	0	0	0	0	-	-	-	-	-	-	-	-	-	-	-
Other and unspecified	0	0	0	0	0	-	-	-	-	-	-	-	-	-	-	-
VII. LIVER	0	2	1	1	4	1.0	1.0	100.0	-	2.2	0.9	1.1	1.3	1.3	19	100.0
Hepatoblastoma	0	2	0	0	2	0.5	0.4	50.0	-	2.2	-	-	0.6	0.7	9	100.0
Hepatic carcinoma	0	0	1	1	2	0.5	0.6	50.0	-	-	0.9	1.1	0.6	0.6	10	100.0
Other and unspecified	0	0	0	0	0	-	-	-	-	-	-	-	-	-	-	-
VIII. BONE	0	0	7	17	24	5.9	6.6	100.0	-	-	6.6	18.2	7.6	7.4	124	95.8
Osteosarcoma	0	0	5	13	18	4.4	4.9	75.0	-	-	4.7	13.9	5.7	5.6	93	94.4
Chondrosarcoma	0	0	0	0	0	-	-	-	-	-	-	-	-	-	-	-
Ewing's sarcoma	0	0	2	3	5	1.2	1.4	20.8	-	-	1.9	3.2	1.6	1.5	25	100.0
Other and unspecified	0	0	0	1	1	0.3	0.3	4.2	-	-	-	1.1	0.3	0.3	5	100.0
IX. SOFT TISSUE SARCOMAS	6	7	5	13	31	7.6	7.6	100.0	23.8	7.8	4.7	13.9	9.8	9.8	148	100.0
Rhabdomyosarcoma	3	4	3	4	14	3.4	3.4	45.2	11.9	4.5	2.8	4.3	4.4	4.5	65	100.0
Fibrosarcoma	2	0	0	5	7	1.7	1.7	22.6	7.9	-	-	5.4	2.2	2.3	35	100.0
Other and unspecified	1	3	2	4	10	2.5	2.5	32.3	4.0	3.3	1.9	4.3	3.2	3.2	48	100.0
X. GONADAL & GERM CELL	3	0	4	9	16	3.9	4.2	100.0	11.9	-	3.8	9.6	5.1	4.9	79	100.0
Non-gonadal germ cell	3	0	0	1	4	1.0	0.9	25.0	11.9	-	-	1.1	1.3	1.2	17	100.0
Gonadal germ cell	0	0	4	8	12	3.0	3.3	75.0	-	-	3.8	8.6	3.8	3.7	62	100.0
Gonadal carcinoma	0	0	0	0	0	-	-	-	-	-	-	-	-	-	-	-
Other and unspecified	0	0	0	0	0	-	-	-	-	-	-	-	-	-	-	-
XI. EPITHELIAL NEOPLASMS	0	0	3	11	14	3.4	3.8	100.0	-	-	2.8	11.8	4.4	4.3	73	100.0
Adrenocortical carcinoma	0	0	0	0	0	-	-	-	-	-	-	-	-	-	-	-
Thyroid carcinoma	0	0	2	6	8	2.0	2.2	57.1	-	-	1.9	6.4	2.5	2.5	42	100.0
Nasopharyngeal carcinoma	0	0	0	0	0	-	-	-	-	-	-	-	-	-	-	-
Melanoma	0	0	0	0	0	-	-	-	-	-	-	-	-	-	-	-
Other carcinoma	0	0	1	5	6	1.5	1.6	42.9	-	-	0.9	5.4	1.9	1.9	31	100.0
XII. OTHER	1	2	1	2	6	1.5	1.5	100.0	4.0	2.2	0.9	2.1	1.9	1.9	28	66.7
* Specified as malignant	0	3	2	0	5	1.2	1.2	100.0	-	3.3	1.9	-	1.6	1.6	23	40.0

USA, Los Angeles, Other White   1972 – 1983   MALE

DIAGNOSTIC GROUP	NUMBER OF CASES					REL. FREQUENCY(%)			RATES PER MILLION							HV(%)
	0	1-4	5-9	10-14	All	Crude	Adj.	Group	0	1-4	5-9	10-14	Crude	Adj.	Cum	
TOTAL	50	264	196	231	741	100.0	100.0	100.0	154.6	221.5	122.1	126.9	150.0	156.8	2286	98.2
I. LEUKAEMIAS	10	114	63	50	237	32.0	31.9	100.0	30.9	95.7	39.3	27.5	48.0	52.7	747	99.6
Acute lymphocytic	3	103	52	33	191	25.8	25.7	80.6	9.3	86.4	32.4	18.1	38.7	43.2	608	99.5
Other lymphocytic	0	0	0	0	0											
Acute non-lymphocytic	5	9	8	15	37	5.0	5.0	15.6	15.5	7.6	5.0	8.2	7.5	7.5	112	100.0
Chronic myeloid	0	0	1	0	1	0.1	0.1	0.4	-	-	-	0.5	0.2	0.2	3	100.0
Other and unspecified	2	2	3	1	8	1.1	1.1	3.4	6.2	1.7	1.9	0.5	1.6	1.8	25	100.0
II. LYMPHOMAS	2	15	34	61	112	15.1	15.3	100.0	6.2	12.6	21.2	33.5	22.7	20.9	330	100.0
Hodgkin's disease	0	1	15	36	52	7.0	7.1	46.4	-	0.8	9.3	19.8	10.5	9.0	149	100.0
Non-Hodgkin lymphoma	0	8	11	21	40	5.4	5.4	35.7	-	6.7	6.9	11.5	8.1	7.6	119	100.0
Burkitt's lymphoma	0	0	4	0	4	1.1	1.1	7.1	-	0.8	2.5	1.6	1.6	1.6	24	100.0
Unspecified lymphoma	0	1	2	1	4	0.5	0.6	3.6	-	0.8	1.2	0.5	0.8	0.8	12	100.0
Histiocytosis X	2	3	2	0	7	0.9	0.9	6.3	6.2	2.5	1.2	-	1.4	1.7	22	100.0
Other reticuloendothelial	0	1	0	0	1	0.1	0.1	0.9	-	0.8	-	-	0.2	0.3	3	100.0
III. BRAIN AND SPINAL	4	47	52	49	152	20.5	20.8	100.0	12.4	39.4	32.4	26.9	30.8	31.4	467	95.4
Ependymoma	2	8	3	3	16	2.2	2.1	10.5	6.2	6.7	1.9	1.6	3.2	3.6	51	100.0
Astrocytoma	0	18	24	28	70	9.4	9.6	46.1	-	15.1	15.0	15.4	14.2	14.0	212	100.0
Medulloblastoma	1	14	14	11	40	5.4	5.5	26.3	3.1	11.7	8.7	6.0	8.1	8.4	124	97.5
Other glioma	0	1	3	5	9	1.2	1.3	5.9	-	0.8	3.1	1.6	1.8	1.7	27	100.0
Other and unspecified *	1	6	6	4	17	2.3	2.3	11.2	3.1	5.0	3.7	2.2	3.4	3.6	53	64.7
IV. SYMPATHETIC N.S.	17	15	6	1	39	5.3	5.1	100.0	52.6	12.6	3.7	0.5	7.9	9.3	124	100.0
Neuroblastoma	17	14	6	1	38	5.1	5.0	97.4	52.6	11.7	3.7	0.5	7.7	9.1	121	100.0
Other	0	1	0	0	1	0.1	0.1	2.6	-	0.8	-	-	0.2	0.3	3	100.0
V. RETINOBLASTOMA	2	19	2	0	23	3.1	3.0	100.0	6.2	15.9	1.2	-	4.7	5.8	76	100.0
VI. KIDNEY	5	26	7	0	38	5.1	5.0	100.0	15.5	21.8	4.4	-	7.7	9.4	125	100.0
Wilms' tumour	5	26	7	0	38	5.1	5.0	100.0	15.5	21.8	4.4	-	7.7	9.4	125	100.0
Renal carcinoma	0	0	0	0	0											
Other and unspecified	0	0	0	0	0											
VII. LIVER	0	3	2	1	6	0.8	0.8	100.0	-	2.5	1.2	0.5	1.2	1.3	19	100.0
Hepatoblastoma	0	3	1	1	5	0.7	0.7	83.3	-	2.5	0.6	0.5	1.0	1.1	16	100.0
Hepatic carcinoma	0	0	1	0	1	0.1	0.2	16.7	-	-	0.6	-	0.2	0.2	3	100.0
Other and unspecified	0	0	0	0	0											
VIII. BONE	0	4	6	22	32	4.3	4.3	100.0	-	3.4	3.7	12.1	6.5	5.8	93	100.0
Osteosarcoma	0	2	2	10	14	1.9	1.9	43.8	-	1.7	1.2	5.5	2.8	2.5	40	100.0
Chondrosarcoma	0	0	0	3	3	0.4	0.4	9.4	-	-	-	1.6	0.6	0.5	8	100.0
Ewing's sarcoma	0	1	4	9	14	1.9	1.9	43.8	-	0.8	2.5	4.9	2.8	2.5	41	100.0
Other and unspecified	0	1	0	0	1	0.1	0.1	3.1	-	0.8	-	-	0.2	0.3	3	100.0
IX. SOFT TISSUE SARCOMAS	3	11	16	29	59	8.0	8.0	100.0	9.3	9.2	10.0	15.9	11.9	11.4	176	100.0
Rhabdomyosarcoma	2	7	8	12	29	3.9	3.9	49.2	6.2	5.9	5.0	6.6	5.9	5.8	88	100.0
Fibrosarcoma	0	1	4	9	14	1.9	1.9	23.7	-	0.8	2.5	4.9	2.8	2.5	41	100.0
Other and unspecified	1	3	4	8	16	2.2	2.2	27.1	3.1	2.5	2.5	4.4	3.2	3.1	48	100.0
X. GONADAL & GERM CELL	4	7	1	3	15	2.0	1.9	100.0	12.4	5.9	0.6	1.6	3.0	3.5	47	100.0
Non-gonadal germ cell	3	2	1	2	8	1.1	1.0	53.3	9.3	1.7	0.6	1.1	1.6	1.8	25	100.0
Gonadal germ cell	1	4	0	1	6	0.8	0.8	40.0	3.1	3.4	-	0.5	1.2	1.4	19	100.0
Gonadal carcinoma	0	0	0	0	0											
Other and unspecified	0	1	0	0	1	0.1	0.1	6.7	-	0.8	-	-	0.2	0.3	3	100.0
XI. EPITHELIAL NEOPLASMS	1	1	5	12	19	2.6	2.6	100.0	3.1	0.8	3.1	6.6	3.8	3.4	55	100.0
Adrenocortical carcinoma	0	0	0	0	0											
Thyroid carcinoma	0	0	1	2	3	0.3	0.4	15.8	-	-	0.6	1.1	0.6	0.5	9	100.0
Nasopharyngeal carcinoma	0	0	0	2	2	0.3	0.3	10.5	-	-	-	1.1	0.4	0.3	5	100.0
Melanoma	0	0	3	5	8	1.1	1.1	42.1	-	-	1.9	2.7	1.6	1.4	23	100.0
Other carcinoma	1	1	1	3	6	0.8	0.8	31.6	3.1	0.8	0.6	1.6	1.2	1.2	18	100.0
XII. OTHER	2	2	2	3	9	1.2	1.2	100.0	6.2	1.7	1.2	1.6	1.8	1.9	27	44.4
* Specified as malignant	1	3	4	1	9	1.2	1.3	100.0	3.1	2.5	2.5	0.5	1.8	2.0	28	55.6

USA, Los Angeles, Other White

1972 - 1983

FEMALE

DIAGNOSTIC GROUP	NUMBER OF CASES					REL. FREQUENCY(%)			RATES PER MILLION						Cum	HV(%)
	0	1-4	5-9	10-14	All	Crude	Adj.	Group	0	1-4	5-9	10-14	Crude	Adj.		
TOTAL	69	193	160	205	627	100.0	100.0	100.0	217.7	167.2	105.2	116.0	131.7	136.2	1992	97.3
I. LEUKAEMIAS	11	82	59	39	191	30.5	31.0	100.0	34.7	71.0	38.8	22.1	40.1	43.6	623	100.0
Acute lymphocytic	5	73	50	25	153	24.4	24.9	80.1	15.8	63.2	32.9	14.1	32.1	35.5	504	100.0
Other lymphocytic	0	0	0	0	0	-	-	-	-	-	-	-	-	-	-	
Acute non-lymphocytic	4	4	6	12	26	4.1	4.1	13.6	12.6	3.5	3.9	6.8	5.5	5.3	80	100.0
Chronic myeloid	0	2	1	2	5	0.8	0.8	2.6	-	1.7	0.7	1.1	1.1	1.1	16	100.0
Other and unspecified	2	3	2	0	7	1.1	1.1	3.7	6.3	2.6	1.3	-	1.5	1.7	23	100.0
II. LYMPHOMAS	2	5	11	40	58	9.3	9.0	100.0	6.3	4.3	7.2	22.6	12.2	10.7	173	100.0
Hodgkin's disease	0	0	3	26	29	4.6	4.4	50.0	-	-	2.0	14.7	6.1	4.9	83	100.0
Non-Hodgkin lymphoma	2	2	6	11	21	3.3	3.3	36.2	6.3	1.7	3.9	6.2	4.4	4.1	64	100.0
Burkitt's lymphoma	0	1	1	0	2	0.3	0.3	3.4	-	0.9	0.7	-	0.4	0.5	7	100.0
Unspecified lymphoma	0	1	0	1	2	0.3	0.3	3.4	-	0.9	-	0.6	0.4	0.4	6	100.0
Histiocytosis X	0	1	1	1	3	0.5	0.5	5.2	-	0.9	0.7	0.6	0.6	0.6	10	100.0
Other reticuloendothelial	0	0	0	1	1	0.2	0.1	1.7	-	-	-	0.6	0.2	0.2	3	-
III. BRAIN AND SPINAL	9	32	47	39	127	20.3	20.8	100.0	28.4	27.7	30.9	22.1	26.7	27.2	404	89.8
Ependymoma	3	2	0	3	8	1.3	1.2	6.3	9.5	1.7	-	1.7	1.7	1.8	25	100.0
Astrocytoma	2	16	23	23	64	10.2	10.4	50.4	6.3	13.9	15.1	13.0	13.4	13.4	202	98.4
Medulloblastoma	4	7	9	3	23	3.7	3.8	18.1	12.6	6.1	5.9	1.7	4.8	5.3	75	100.0
Other glioma	0	2	6	3	11	1.8	1.9	8.7	-	1.7	3.9	1.7	2.3	2.3	35	90.9
Other and unspecified *	0	5	9	7	21	3.3	3.5	16.5	-	4.3	5.9	4.0	4.4	4.4	67	47.6
IV. SYMPATHETIC N.S.	21	15	2	2	40	6.4	6.2	100.0	66.3	13.0	1.3	1.1	8.4	9.9	130	100.0
Neuroblastoma	21	15	2	1	39	6.2	6.0	97.5	66.3	13.0	1.3	0.6	8.2	9.7	128	100.0
Other	0	0	0	1	1	0.2	0.1	2.5	-	-	-	0.6	0.2	0.2	3	100.0
V. RETINOBLASTOMA	6	8	1	1	16	2.6	2.5	100.0	18.9	6.9	0.7	0.6	3.4	4.0	53	100.0
VI. KIDNEY	7	22	12	3	44	7.0	7.1	100.0	22.1	19.1	7.9	1.7	9.2	10.6	146	97.7
Wilms' tumour	6	22	12	2	42	6.7	6.8	95.5	18.9	19.1	7.9	1.1	8.8	10.2	140	100.0
Renal carcinoma	0	0	0	1	1	0.2	0.1	2.3	-	-	-	0.6	0.2	0.2	3	100.0
Other and unspecified	1	0	0	0	1	0.2	0.2	2.3	3.2	-	-	-	0.2	0.2	3	-
VII. LIVER	1	1	1	4	7	1.1	1.1	100.0	3.2	0.9	0.7	2.3	1.5	1.4	21	100.0
Hepatoblastoma	0	1	0	2	3	0.5	0.4	42.9	-	0.9	-	1.1	0.6	0.6	9	100.0
Hepatic carcinoma	1	0	1	2	4	0.6	0.6	57.1	3.2	-	0.7	1.1	0.8	0.8	12	100.0
Other and unspecified	0	0	0	0	0	-	-	-	-	-	-	-	-	-	-	-
VIII. BONE	0	3	10	20	33	5.3	5.3	100.0	-	2.6	6.6	11.3	6.9	6.2	100	100.0
Osteosarcoma	0	1	3	7	11	1.8	1.7	33.3	-	0.9	2.0	4.0	2.3	2.1	33	100.0
Chondrosarcoma	0	0	0	2	3	0.5	0.5	9.1	-	-	0.7	1.1	0.6	0.5	9	100.0
Ewing's sarcoma	0	0	5	9	14	2.2	2.3	42.4	-	-	3.3	5.1	2.9	2.5	42	100.0
Other and unspecified	0	2	1	2	5	0.8	0.8	15.2	-	1.7	0.7	1.1	1.1	1.1	16	100.0
IX. SOFT TISSUE SARCOMAS	6	14	8	21	49	7.8	7.6	100.0	18.9	12.1	5.3	11.9	10.3	10.4	153	100.0
Rhabdomyosarcoma	4	6	4	6	20	3.2	3.2	40.8	12.6	5.2	2.6	3.4	4.2	4.4	64	100.0
Fibrosarcoma	0	3	2	4	9	1.4	1.4	18.4	-	2.6	1.3	2.3	1.9	1.9	28	100.0
Other and unspecified	2	5	2	11	20	3.2	3.1	40.8	6.3	4.3	1.3	6.2	4.2	4.1	61	100.0
X. GONADAL & GERM CELL	2	6	3	14	25	4.0	3.8	100.0	6.3	5.2	2.0	7.9	5.3	5.0	77	100.0
Non-gonadal germ cell	2	6	0	2	10	1.6	1.5	40.0	6.3	5.2	-	1.1	2.1	2.4	33	100.0
Gonadal germ cell	0	0	2	11	13	2.1	2.0	52.0	-	-	1.3	6.2	2.7	2.2	38	100.0
Gonadal carcinoma	0	0	1	0	1	0.2	0.2	4.0	-	-	0.7	-	0.2	0.2	3	100.0
Other and unspecified	0	0	0	1	1	0.2	0.1	4.0	-	-	-	0.6	0.2	0.2	3	100.0
XI. EPITHELIAL NEOPLASMS	0	4	6	22	32	5.1	5.0	100.0	-	3.5	3.9	12.4	6.7	6.0	96	96.9
Adrenocortical carcinoma	0	1	0	0	1	0.2	0.2	3.1	-	0.9	-	-	0.2	0.3	3	100.0
Thyroid carcinoma	0	1	2	11	14	2.2	2.1	43.8	-	0.9	1.3	6.2	2.9	2.5	41	92.9
Nasopharyngeal carcinoma	0	0	0	1	1	0.2	0.1	3.1	-	-	-	0.6	0.2	0.2	3	100.0
Melanoma	0	1	1	6	8	1.3	1.2	25.0	-	0.9	0.7	3.4	1.7	1.5	24	100.0
Other carcinoma	0	1	3	4	8	1.3	1.3	25.0	-	0.9	2.0	2.3	1.7	1.6	25	100.0
XII. OTHER	4	1	0	0	5	0.8	0.8	100.0	12.6	0.9	-	-	1.1	1.2	16	60.0
* Specified as malignant	0	2	4	2	8	1.3	1.3	100.0	-	1.7	2.6	1.1	1.7	1.7	26	12.5

The average population for the period 1972–1983 has been obtained by linear interpolation of the age-sex-race-specific populations of 1970 and 1980.

Commentary

The overall incidence rate for non-Hispanic Whites was one of the highest recorded in the present volume. In general, the patterns of incidence rates for non-Hispanic Whites and for Blacks were similar to those observed for Whites and Blacks in the SEER Program.

Incidence rates for Hispanics were mostly similar to or slightly lower than those for other Whites. However, Hispanics had markedly higher rates for acute non-lymphocytic leukaemia, retinoblastoma, liver tumours and gonadal germ-cell tumours. The rate for neuroblastoma was about 60% of that in other Whites. There was a high ratio of osteosarcoma to Ewing's sarcoma, though Ewing's sarcoma was not as rare as in Blacks.

New York Cancer Registry, 1976–1982

W. Burnett

The reporting of cancer in New York State, excluding New York City, began on 1 January 1940, and was extended to include New York City on 1 January 1973. The law requires the reporting of every cancer case encountered by physicians, laboratories and medical care institutions, both public and private. The original intent was to make available accurate information on: (*a*) the magnitude of the cancer problem; (*b*) the incidence of cancer in different parts of the State and among various social and economic groups; (*c*) the relation between cancer and such factors as occupation; (*d*) the extent of the alleged increase in cancer above that due to the ageing of the population; (*e*) the accuracy of mortality statistics; and (*f*) the true incidence of the various forms of cancer. In addition, it was felt that registration would help to establish priorities for such control measures as education and the establishment of detection, diagnostic and treatment facilities. From its inception, cancer morbidity reporting in New York State has had the active support of the medical profession.

Reports are now received from five sources, namely physicians, hospitals, pathology laboratories, death certificates, and through reciprocal inter-state reporting agreements. Because almost all patients with a diagnosis of cancer are admitted to a hospital, the Registry relies for reporting primarily on hospitals or, where they exist, hospital-based tumour registries. Nearly 300 acute care hospitals report to the Registry. Many hospitals have specialist paediatric oncology facilities. Completeness of reporting, based on a variety of special studies, is estimated to be at least 90% for New York City and over 95% for the rest of the State.

The Registry covers the whole of New York State, which is located in the north-eastern part of the United States between Canada and the Atlantic Ocean. The climate is temperate, with a temperature range of 10 to 27° C in summer and −12 to 5° C in winter. The altitude ranges from sea level to over 1520 m; the geology varies and includes limestone and sandy soil; rainfall varies from 65 to 150 cm. The total area is 124 164 square kilometres.

The State is one of great diversity, with large urban areas, particularly in the vicinity of New York City; in contrast, the Alleghany Plateau and the Catskill and Adirondack Mountains remain extremely rural.

The population of New York State in 1980 was 17 539 100, of whom 7 050 300 (40.2%) resided in New York City. The black population of the State is 13.7% of the total, about three-quarters living in New York City. There are about 300 000 residents in the Asian and Pacific Islander categories, including about 150 000 Chinese and 60 000 Asian Indians. Just under 10% of the population is of Hispanic origin; of these, 85% reside in New York City. More than 13.6% of the population is foreign-born; about 45% of these were born in Europe, including the USSR.

The Registry regularly publishes tabulations of incidence rates for New York City and upstate New York, and of numbers of cases, by sex and site, for each county. It is also used extensively as a source of cases for specific analytical epidemiological studies. Although most studies are carried out within the Cancer Control Program, many collaborative studies with research workers in other institutions are under way.

The tables show data for the whole of New York (City plus State) for the period 1976–1982.

Population

The population for the period 1976–1982 has been estimated by linear interpolation of census data by sex, race, and age (single year) for 1970 and 1980 (US Bureau of the Census). Because the definition of 'white' was different at the two censuses, the 1980 'White' population was recalculated to correspond to the definition used in 1970. This population includes children of Hispanic origin, but excludes those described as of Asian or Pacific origin, as well as American Indians, Eskimos and Aleuts.

Contd p. 100

USA, New York (City and State), White   1976 – 1982   MALE

DIAGNOSTIC GROUP	NUMBER OF CASES					REL. FREQUENCY(%)			RATES PER MILLION						Cum	HV(%)
	0	1-4	5-9	10-14	All	Crude	Adj.	Group	0	1-4	5-9	10-14	Crude	Adj.		
TOTAL	114	491	450	508	1563	100.0	100.0	100.0	162.6	185.1	125.6	121.0	140.3	145.5	2136	95.8
I. LEUKAEMIAS	16	215	156	120	507	32.4	32.8	100.0	22.8	81.0	43.5	28.6	45.5	49.2	708	97.5
Acute lymphocytic	4	163	118	78	363	23.2	23.5	71.6	5.7	61.4	32.9	18.6	32.6	35.5	509	96.9
Other lymphocytic	1	10	8	5	24	1.6	1.6	4.7	1.4	3.8	2.2	1.2	2.2	2.3	34	100.0
Acute non-lymphocytic	4	24	19	20	67	4.3	4.3	13.2	5.7	9.0	5.3	4.8	6.0	6.3	92	100.0
Chronic myeloid	1	9	1	5	16	1.0	1.0	3.2	1.4	3.4	0.3	1.2	1.4	1.6	22	93.3
Other and unspecified	6	9	10	12	37	2.4	2.4	7.3	8.6	3.4	2.8	2.9	3.3	3.4	50	100.0
II. LYMPHOMAS	3	25	81	140	249	15.9	15.5	100.0	4.3	9.4	22.6	33.3	22.4	20.2	322	99.2
Hodgkin's disease	0	6	21	80	107	6.8	6.5	43.0	-	2.3	5.9	19.0	9.6	8.1	134	99.0
Non-Hodgkin lymphoma	0	9	38	33	80	5.1	5.1	32.1	-	3.4	10.6	7.9	7.2	6.8	106	100.0
Burkitt's lymphoma	1	2	8	9	20	1.3	1.3	8.0	1.4	0.8	2.2	2.1	1.8	1.7	26	100.0
Unspecified lymphoma	0	5	14	15	34	2.2	2.1	13.7	-	1.9	3.9	3.6	3.1	2.9	45	96.8
Histiocytosis X	1	0	0	0	1	0.1	0.1	0.4	1.4	-	-	-	0.1	0.1	1	100.0
Other reticuloendothelial	1	3	0	3	7	0.4	0.4	2.8	1.4	1.1	-	0.7	0.6	0.7	10	100.0
III. BRAIN AND SPINAL	12	85	126	119	342	21.9	21.8	100.0	17.1	32.0	35.2	28.3	30.7	30.8	463	89.3
Ependymoma	1	10	10	6	27	1.7	1.7	7.9	1.4	3.8	2.8	1.4	2.4	2.6	38	100.0
Astrocytoma	4	32	54	59	149	9.5	9.5	43.6	5.7	12.1	15.1	14.0	13.4	13.1	200	93.2
Medulloblastoma	3	23	23	17	66	4.2	4.3	19.3	4.3	8.7	6.4	4.0	5.9	6.3	91	98.4
Other glioma	2	12	17	11	42	2.7	2.7	12.3	2.9	4.5	4.7	2.6	3.8	3.9	58	73.2
Other and unspecified *	2	8	22	26	58	3.7	3.7	17.0	2.9	3.0	6.1	6.2	5.2	4.9	77	68.4
IV. SYMPATHETIC N.S.	30	53	14	9	106	6.8	7.0	100.0	42.8	20.0	3.9	2.1	9.5	11.4	153	98.1
Neuroblastoma	30	53	13	8	104	6.7	6.8	98.1	42.8	20.0	3.6	1.9	9.3	11.2	150	98.1
Other	0	0	1	1	2	0.1	0.1	1.9	-	-	0.3	0.2	0.2	0.2	3	100.0
V. RETINOBLASTOMA	9	13	1	0	23	1.5	1.5	100.0	12.8	4.9	0.3	-	2.1	2.6	34	85.7
VI. KIDNEY	11	42	13	6	72	4.6	4.7	100.0	15.7	15.8	3.6	1.4	6.5	7.7	104	94.4
Wilms' tumour	10	41	11	3	65	4.2	4.3	90.3	14.3	15.5	3.1	0.7	5.8	7.1	95	96.9
Renal carcinoma	1	1	2	3	7	0.4	0.4	9.7	1.4	0.4	0.6	0.7	0.6	0.6	9	71.4
Other and unspecified	0	0	0	0	0	-	-	-	-	-	-	-	-	-	-	-
VII. LIVER	3	3	1	5	12	0.8	0.8	100.0	4.3	1.1	0.3	1.2	1.1	1.1	16	100.0
Hepatoblastoma	3	3	0	3	9	0.6	0.6	75.0	4.3	1.1	-	0.7	0.8	0.9	13	100.0
Hepatic carcinoma	0	0	0	2	2	0.1	0.1	16.7	-	-	-	0.5	0.2	0.1	2	100.0
Other and unspecified	0	0	1	0	1	0.1	0.1	8.3	-	-	0.3	-	0.1	0.1	1	-
VIII. BONE	0	3	20	50	73	4.7	4.5	100.0	-	1.1	5.6	11.9	6.6	5.6	92	100.0
Osteosarcoma	0	2	7	22	31	2.0	1.9	42.5	-	0.8	2.0	5.2	2.8	2.4	39	100.0
Chondrosarcoma	0	0	1	2	3	0.2	0.2	4.1	-	-	0.3	0.5	0.3	0.2	4	100.0
Ewing's sarcoma	0	1	12	22	35	2.2	2.2	47.9	-	0.4	3.3	5.2	3.1	2.7	44	100.0
Other and unspecified	0	0	0	4	4	0.3	0.2	5.5	-	-	-	1.0	0.4	0.3	5	100.0
IX. SOFT TISSUE SARCOMAS	12	28	25	31	96	6.1	6.1	100.0	17.1	10.6	7.0	7.4	8.6	9.0	131	96.9
Rhabdomyosarcoma	6	21	18	16	61	3.9	3.9	63.5	8.6	7.9	5.0	3.8	5.5	5.8	84	98.4
Fibrosarcoma	2	4	4	8	18	1.2	1.2	18.8	2.9	1.5	1.1	1.9	1.6	1.6	24	100.0
Other and unspecified	4	3	3	7	17	1.1	1.1	17.7	5.7	1.1	0.8	1.7	1.5	1.5	23	88.2
X. GONADAL & GERM CELL	10	13	4	9	36	2.3	2.3	100.0	14.3	4.9	1.1	2.1	3.2	3.6	50	100.0
Non-gonadal germ cell	8	2	4	0	14	0.9	0.9	38.9	11.4	0.8	1.1	-	1.3	1.2	19	100.0
Gonadal germ cell	2	11	0	8	21	1.3	1.4	58.3	2.9	4.1	-	1.9	1.9	2.3	30	100.0
Gonadal carcinoma	0	0	0	1	1	0.1	0.1	2.8	-	-	-	0.2	0.1	0.1	1	100.0
Other and unspecified	0	0	0	0	0	-	-	-	-	-	-	-	-	-	-	-
XI. EPITHELIAL NEOPLASMS	3	0	7	14	24	1.5	1.5	100.0	4.3	-	2.0	3.3	2.2	1.9	31	91.3
Adenocortical carcinoma	0	0	0	0	0	-	-	-	-	-	-	-	-	-	-	-
Thyroid carcinoma	0	0	2	3	5	0.3	0.3	20.8	-	-	0.6	0.7	0.4	0.4	6	100.0
Nasopharyngeal carcinoma	0	0	0	0	0	-	-	-	-	-	-	-	-	-	-	-
Melanoma	1	0	1	3	5	0.3	0.3	20.8	1.4	-	0.3	0.7	0.4	0.4	6	100.0
Other carcinoma	2	0	4	8	14	0.9	0.9	58.3	2.9	-	1.1	1.9	1.3	1.1	18	84.6
XII. OTHER	5	11	2	5	23	1.5	1.5	100.0	7.1	4.1	0.6	1.2	2.1	2.4	32	100.0
* Specified as malignant	2	7	14	13	36	2.3	2.3	100.0	2.9	2.6	3.9	3.1	3.2	3.2	48	55.6

USA, New York (City and State), White   1976 – 1982   FEMALE

DIAGNOSTIC GROUP	NUMBER OF CASES					REL. FREQUENCY(%)			RATES PER MILLION							HV(%)
	0	1-4	5-9	10-14	All	Crude	Adj.	Group	0	1-4	5-9	10-14	Crude	Adj.	Cum	
TOTAL	125	431	302	432	1290	100.0	100.0	100.0	186.7	171.4	88.7	107.8	121.7	127.4	1855	95.3
I. LEUKAEMIAS	25	194	112	90	421	32.6	33.1	100.0	37.3	77.1	32.9	22.5	39.7	43.9	623	98.0
Acute lymphocytic	14	145	78	55	292	22.6	23.0	69.4	20.9	57.7	22.9	13.7	27.6	30.8	435	97.9
Other lymphocytic	1	15	8	4	28	2.2	2.2	6.7	1.5	6.0	2.3	1.0	2.6	3.0	42	95.7
Acute non-lymphocytic	4	15	19	21	59	4.6	4.7	14.0	6.0	6.0	5.6	5.2	5.6	5.6	84	100.0
Chronic myeloid	2	3	2	3	10	0.8	0.8	2.4	3.0	1.2	0.6	0.7	0.9	1.0	14	100.0
Other and unspecified	4	16	5	7	32	2.5	2.4	7.6	6.0	6.4	1.5	1.7	3.0	3.4	47	96.4
II. LYMPHOMAS	2	13	21	85	121	9.4	9.1	100.0	3.0	5.2	6.2	21.2	11.4	10.0	161	100.0
Hodgkin's disease	0	1	5	61	67	5.2	4.8	55.4	-	0.4	1.5	15.2	6.3	5.0	85	100.0
Non-Hodgkin lymphoma	1	5	7	13	26	2.0	2.0	21.5	1.5	2.0	2.1	3.2	2.5	2.3	36	100.0
Burkitt's lymphoma	0	3	3	4	10	0.8	0.8	8.3	-	1.2	0.9	1.0	0.9	0.9	14	100.0
Unspecified lymphoma	0	4	6	6	16	1.2	1.3	13.2	-	1.6	1.8	1.5	1.5	1.5	23	100.0
Histiocytosis X	1	0	0	0	1	0.1	0.1	0.8	1.5	-	-	-	0.1	0.1	1	100.0
Other reticuloendothelial	0	0	0	1	1	0.1	0.1	0.8	-	-	-	0.2	0.1	0.1	1	-
III. BRAIN AND SPINAL	9	80	83	88	260	20.2	20.8	100.0	13.4	31.8	24.4	22.0	24.5	25.1	372	86.6
Ependymoma	2	7	4	1	14	1.1	1.1	5.4	3.0	2.8	1.2	0.2	1.3	1.5	21	100.0
Astrocytoma	4	26	41	45	116	9.0	9.4	44.6	6.0	10.3	12.0	11.2	10.9	10.8	164	96.5
Medulloblastoma	1	19	11	11	42	3.3	3.3	16.2	1.5	7.6	3.2	2.7	4.0	4.3	62	100.0
Other glioma	0	13	9	12	34	2.6	2.6	13.1	-	5.2	2.6	3.0	3.2	3.3	49	41.9
Other and unspecified *	2	15	18	19	54	4.2	4.3	20.8	3.0	6.0	5.3	4.7	5.1	5.2	77	74.4
IV. SYMPATHETIC N.S.	37	40	13	5	95	7.4	7.2	100.0	55.3	15.9	3.8	1.2	9.0	10.8	144	94.5
Neuroblastoma	37	40	13	5	95	7.4	7.2	100.0	55.3	15.9	3.8	1.2	9.0	10.8	144	94.5
Other	0	0	0	0	0	-	-	-	-	-	-	-	-	-	-	-
V. RETINOBLASTOMA	10	12	1	0	23	1.8	1.7	100.0	14.9	4.8	0.3	-	2.2	2.7	35	91.3
VI. KIDNEY	13	41	20	4	78	6.0	6.1	100.0	19.4	16.3	5.9	1.0	7.4	8.7	119	96.0
Wilms' tumour	13	40	20	2	75	5.8	5.9	96.2	19.4	15.9	5.9	0.5	7.1	8.5	115	95.9
Renal carcinoma	0	0	0	2	2	0.2	0.1	2.6	-	-	-	0.5	0.2	0.1	2	100.0
Other and unspecified	0	1	0	0	1	0.1	0.1	1.3	-	0.4	-	-	0.1	0.1	2	-
VII. LIVER	3	6	1	2	12	0.9	0.9	100.0	4.5	2.4	0.3	0.5	1.1	1.3	18	100.0
Hepatoblastoma	3	6	0	2	11	0.9	0.8	91.7	4.5	2.4	-	0.5	1.0	1.2	17	100.0
Hepatic carcinoma	0	0	1	0	1	0.1	0.1	8.3	-	-	0.3	-	0.1	0.1	1	100.0
Other and unspecified	0	0	0	0	0	-	-	-	-	-	-	-	-	-	-	-
VIII. BONE	0	4	14	52	70	5.4	5.3	100.0	-	1.6	4.1	13.0	6.6	5.6	92	98.5
Osteosarcoma	0	2	5	30	37	2.9	2.7	52.9	-	0.8	1.5	7.5	3.5	2.9	48	100.0
Chondrosarcoma	0	0	0	1	1	0.1	0.1	1.4	-	-	-	0.2	0.1	0.1	1	100.0
Ewing's sarcoma	0	2	7	17	26	2.0	2.0	37.1	-	0.8	2.1	4.2	2.5	2.1	35	96.2
Other and unspecified	0	0	2	4	6	0.5	0.5	8.6	-	-	0.6	1.0	0.6	0.5	8	100.0
IX. SOFT TISSUE SARCOMAS	10	27	21	32	90	7.0	7.0	100.0	14.9	10.7	6.2	8.0	8.5	8.8	129	97.8
Rhabdomyosarcoma	9	21	12	12	54	4.2	4.2	60.0	13.4	8.4	3.5	3.0	5.1	5.6	79	98.1
Fibrosarcoma	0	6	4	4	14	1.1	1.1	15.6	-	2.4	1.5	1.0	1.3	1.3	20	100.0
Other and unspecified	1	0	5	16	22	1.7	1.7	24.4	1.5	-	1.5	4.0	2.1	1.7	29	95.5
X. GONADAL & GERM CELL	10	5	6	30	51	4.0	3.8	100.0	14.9	2.0	1.8	7.5	4.8	4.5	69	100.0
Non-gonadal germ cell	9	4	1	4	18	1.4	1.3	35.3	13.4	1.6	0.3	1.0	1.7	1.9	26	100.0
Gonadal germ cell	0	0	5	22	27	2.1	1.7	52.9	-	-	1.5	5.5	2.5	2.1	35	100.0
Gonadal carcinoma	0	0	0	2	2	0.2	0.2	3.9	-	-	-	0.5	0.3	0.3	4	100.0
Other and unspecified	1	1	0	2	4	0.3	0.2	7.8	1.5	0.4	-	0.5	0.3	0.3	4	100.0
XI. EPITHELIAL NEOPLASMS	3	6	10	33	52	4.0	3.9	100.0	4.5	2.4	2.9	8.2	4.9	4.4	70	96.1
Adrenocortical carcinoma	0	1	0	1	2	0.2	0.1	3.8	-	0.4	-	0.2	0.2	0.2	3	100.0
Thyroid carcinoma	0	0	5	20	25	1.9	1.9	48.1	-	-	1.5	5.0	2.4	1.9	32	100.0
Nasopharyngeal carcinoma	0	0	0	1	1	0.1	0.1	1.9	-	-	-	0.2	0.1	0.1	2	100.0
Melanoma	1	2	2	6	11	0.9	0.8	21.2	1.5	0.8	0.6	1.2	1.0	1.0	15	100.0
Other carcinoma	2	3	3	5	13	1.0	1.0	25.0	3.0	1.2	0.9	1.2	1.2	1.2	18	84.6
XII. OTHER	3	3	0	11	17	1.3	1.2	100.0	4.5	1.2	-	2.7	1.6	1.5	23	77.8
* Specified as malignant	2	8	9	12	31	2.4	2.4	100.0	3.0	3.2	2.6	3.0	2.9	2.9	44	50.0

USA, New York (City and State), Black   1976 - 1982   MALE

DIAGNOSTIC GROUP	NUMBER OF CASES 0	1-4	5-9	10-14	All	REL. FREQUENCY(%) Crude	Adj.	Group	RATES PER MILLION 0	1-4	5-9	10-14	Crude	Adj.	Cum	HV(%)
TOTAL	22	79	76	96	273	100.0	100.0	100.0	141.2	138.3	104.6	115.4	119.4	121.0	1794	94.5
I. LEUKAEMIAS	5	27	22	24	78	28.6	28.9	100.0	32.1	47.3	30.3	28.8	34.1	35.3	517	94.4
Acute lymphocytic	4	19	9	14	46	16.8	17.0	59.0	25.7	33.3	12.4	16.8	20.1	21.2	305	97.7
Other lymphocytic	0	1	1	0	2	0.7	0.8	2.6	-	1.8	1.4	-	0.9	1.0	14	100.0
Acute non-lymphocytic	0	4	5	6	15	5.5	5.4	19.2	-	7.0	6.9	7.2	6.6	6.5	98	78.6
Chronic myeloid	0	2	1	1	4	1.5	1.5	5.1	-	3.5	1.4	1.2	1.7	1.9	27	100.0
Other and unspecified	1	1	6	3	11	4.0	4.1	14.1	6.4	1.8	8.3	3.6	4.8	4.7	73	100.0
II. LYMPHOMAS	2	3	17	19	41	15.0	14.6	100.0	12.8	5.3	23.4	22.8	17.9	16.8	265	100.0
Hodgkin's disease	0	1	8	12	21	7.7	7.3	51.2	-	1.8	11.0	14.4	9.2	8.3	134	100.0
Non-Hodgkin lymphoma	0	1	7	5	13	4.8	4.7	31.7	-	1.8	9.6	6.0	5.7	5.4	85	100.0
Burkitt's lymphoma	0	0	1	1	2	0.7	0.7	4.9	-	-	1.4	1.2	0.9	0.8	13	100.0
Unspecified lymphoma	0	1	1	1	3	1.1	1.1	7.3	-	1.8	1.4	1.2	1.3	1.3	20	100.0
Histiocytosis X	0	0	0	0	0	-	-	-	-	-	-	-	-	-	-	-
Other reticuloendothelial	2	0	0	0	2	0.7	0.8	4.9	12.8	-	-	-	0.9	1.0	13	100.0
III. BRAIN AND SPINAL	3	18	17	14	52	19.0	19.4	100.0	19.3	31.5	23.4	16.8	22.7	23.7	346	92.2
Ependymoma	1	2	0	1	4	1.5	1.5	7.7	6.4	3.5	-	1.2	1.7	1.9	26	100.0
Astrocytoma	1	8	9	8	26	9.5	9.6	50.0	6.4	14.0	12.4	9.6	11.4	11.6	172	96.2
Medulloblastoma	1	4	0	0	5	1.8	2.0	9.6	6.4	7.0	-	-	2.2	2.7	34	100.0
Other glioma	0	2	5	3	10	3.7	3.7	19.2	-	3.5	6.9	3.6	4.4	4.4	66	77.8
Other and unspecified *	0	2	3	2	7	2.6	2.6	13.5	-	3.5	4.1	2.4	3.1	3.1	47	85.7
IV. SYMPATHETIC N.S.	3	10	4	0	17	6.2	6.7	100.0	19.3	17.5	5.5	-	7.4	8.7	117	94.1
Neuroblastoma	3	10	4	0	17	6.2	6.7	100.0	19.3	17.5	5.5	-	7.4	8.7	117	94.1
Other	0	0	0	0	0	-	-	-	-	-	-	-	-	-	-	-
V. RETINOBLASTOMA	2	4	0	0	6	2.2	2.4	100.0	12.8	7.0	-	-	2.6	3.2	41	83.3
VI. KIDNEY	2	14	4	1	21	7.7	8.2	100.0	12.8	24.5	5.5	1.2	9.2	10.7	144	94.1
Wilms' tumour	2	13	2	0	17	6.2	6.7	81.0	12.8	22.8	2.8	-	7.4	8.9	118	94.1
Renal carcinoma	0	0	0	0	0	-	-	-	-	-	-	-	-	-	-	-
Other and unspecified	0	1	2	1	4	1.5	1.5	19.0	-	1.8	2.8	1.2	1.7	1.8	27	-
VII. LIVER	2	0	0	3	5	1.8	1.7	100.0	12.8	-	-	3.6	2.2	2.0	31	80.0
Hepatoblastoma	2	0	0	0	2	0.7	0.8	40.0	12.8	-	-	-	0.9	1.0	13	100.0
Hepatic carcinoma	0	0	0	3	3	1.1	0.9	60.0	-	-	-	3.6	1.3	1.0	18	66.7
Other and unspecified	0	0	0	0	0	-	-	-	-	-	-	-	-	-	-	-
VIII. BONE	0	1	3	7	11	4.0	3.8	100.0	-	1.8	4.1	8.4	4.8	4.3	70	100.0
Osteosarcoma	0	0	2	4	6	2.2	2.0	54.5	-	-	2.8	4.8	2.6	2.3	38	100.0
Chondrosarcoma	0	0	0	0	0	-	-	-	-	-	-	-	-	-	-	-
Ewing's sarcoma	0	0	1	0	1	0.4	0.4	9.1	-	-	1.4	-	0.4	0.4	7	100.0
Other and unspecified	0	1	0	3	4	1.5	1.3	36.4	-	1.8	-	3.6	1.7	1.6	25	100.0
IX. SOFT TISSUE SARCOMAS	1	1	7	10	19	7.0	6.7	100.0	6.4	1.8	9.6	12.0	8.3	7.6	122	89.5
Rhabdomyosarcoma	1	1	4	5	11	4.0	3.9	57.9	6.4	1.8	5.5	6.0	4.8	4.6	71	90.9
Fibrosarcoma	0	0	2	2	4	1.5	1.4	21.1	-	-	2.8	2.4	1.7	1.6	26	75.0
Other and unspecified	0	0	1	3	4	1.5	1.3	21.1	-	-	1.4	3.6	1.7	1.5	25	100.0
X. GONADAL & GERM CELL	1	0	1	1	3	1.1	1.1	100.0	6.4	-	1.4	1.2	1.3	1.3	19	100.0
Non-gonadal germ cell	1	0	0	1	2	0.7	0.7	66.7	6.4	-	-	1.2	0.9	0.8	12	100.0
Gonadal germ cell	0	0	1	0	1	0.4	0.4	33.3	-	-	1.4	-	0.4	0.4	7	100.0
Gonadal carcinoma	0	0	0	0	0	-	-	-	-	-	-	-	-	-	-	-
Other and unspecified	0	0	0	0	0	-	-	-	-	-	-	-	-	-	-	-
XI. EPITHELIAL NEOPLASMS	0	1	0	13	14	5.1	4.5	100.0	-	1.8	-	15.6	6.1	5.1	85	100.0
Adrenocortical carcinoma	0	1	0	0	1	0.4	0.4	7.1	-	1.8	-	-	0.4	0.5	7	100.0
Thyroid carcinoma	0	0	0	5	5	1.8	1.6	35.7	-	-	-	6.0	2.2	1.6	30	100.0
Nasopharyngeal carcinoma	0	0	0	4	4	1.5	1.3	28.6	-	-	-	4.8	1.7	1.4	24	100.0
Melanoma	0	0	0	0	0	-	-	-	-	-	-	-	-	-	-	-
Other carcinoma	0	0	0	4	4	1.5	1.3	28.6	-	-	-	4.8	1.7	1.4	24	100.0
XII. OTHER	1	0	1	4	6	2.2	2.0	100.0	6.4	-	1.4	4.8	2.6	2.3	37	100.0
* Specified as malignant	0	1	0	1	2	0.7	0.7	100.0	-	1.8	-	4.8	0.9	0.9	13	50.0

USA, New York (City and State), Black   1976 - 1982   FEMALE

DIAGNOSTIC GROUP	NUMBER OF CASES					REL. FREQUENCY(%)			RATES PER MILLION						Cum	HV(%)
	0	1-4	5-9	10-14	All	Crude	Adj.	Group	0	1-4	5-9	10-14	Crude	Adj.		
TOTAL	12	66	43	60	181	100.0	100.0	100.0	77.3	116.7	59.8	72.3	79.8	82.4	1205	96.3
I. LEUKAEMIAS	3	22	10	8	43	23.8	23.8	100.0	19.3	38.9	13.9	9.6	18.9	20.8	293	97.4
Acute lymphocytic	3	14	6	6	29	16.0	15.9	67.4	19.3	24.8	8.3	7.2	12.8	14.0	196	96.2
Other lymphocytic	0	3	1	0	4	2.2	2.2	9.3	–	5.3	1.4	–	1.8	2.1	28	100.0
Acute non-lymphocytic	0	5	2	2	9	5.0	5.0	20.9	–	8.8	2.8	2.4	4.0	4.3	61	100.0
Chronic myeloid	0	0	1	0	1	0.6	0.7	2.3	–	–	1.4	–	0.4	0.4	7	100.0
Other and unspecified	0	0	0	0	0	–	–	–	–	–	–	–	–	–	–	–
II. LYMPHOMAS	1	0	7	11	19	10.5	10.9	100.0	6.4	–	9.7	13.3	8.4	7.5	121	100.0
Hodgkin's disease	0	0	4	5	9	5.0	5.3	47.4	–	–	5.6	6.0	4.0	3.5	58	100.0
Non-Hodgkin lymphoma	0	0	2	2	4	2.2	2.4	21.1	–	–	2.8	2.4	1.8	1.6	26	100.0
Burkitt's lymphoma	0	0	0	0	0	–	–	–	–	–	–	–	–	–	–	–
Unspecified lymphoma	0	0	1	4	5	2.8	2.7	26.3	–	–	1.4	4.8	2.2	1.8	31	100.0
Histiocytosis X	0	0	0	0	0	–	–	–	–	–	–	–	–	–	–	–
Other reticuloendothelial	1	0	0	0	1	0.6	0.5	5.3	6.4	–	–	–	0.4	0.5	6	100.0
III. BRAIN AND SPINAL	2	17	9	14	42	23.2	23.0	100.0	12.9	30.1	12.5	16.9	18.5	19.2	280	94.1
Ependymoma	0	2	0	0	2	1.1	1.0	4.8	–	3.5	–	–	0.9	1.1	14	100.0
Astrocytoma	1	7	3	6	17	9.4	9.2	40.5	6.4	12.4	4.2	7.2	7.5	7.8	113	100.0
Medulloblastoma	0	5	1	1	7	3.9	3.8	16.7	–	8.8	1.4	1.2	3.1	3.5	48	100.0
Other glioma	0	3	2	4	9	5.0	4.9	21.4	–	5.3	2.8	4.8	4.0	3.9	59	83.3
Other and unspecified *	1	0	3	3	7	3.9	4.1	16.7	6.4	–	4.2	3.6	3.1	2.9	45	75.0
IV. SYMPATHETIC N.S.	0	9	2	1	12	6.6	6.5	100.0	–	15.9	2.8	1.2	5.3	6.2	84	100.0
Neuroblastoma	0	9	2	1	12	6.6	6.5	100.0	–	15.9	2.8	1.2	5.3	6.2	84	100.0
Other	0	0	0	0	0	–	–	–	–	–	–	–	–	–	–	–
V. RETINOBLASTOMA	1	2	1	0	4	2.2	2.2	100.0	6.4	3.5	1.4	–	1.8	2.0	28	100.0
VI. KIDNEY	1	9	3	1	14	7.7	7.7	100.0	6.4	15.9	4.2	1.2	6.2	7.1	97	92.3
Wilms' tumour	1	9	2	1	13	7.2	7.0	92.9	6.4	15.9	2.8	1.2	5.7	6.7	90	92.3
Renal carcinoma	0	0	0	0	0	–	–	–	–	–	–	–	–	–	–	–
Other and unspecified	0	0	1	0	1	0.6	0.7	7.1	–	–	1.4	–	0.4	0.4	7	–
VII. LIVER	0	0	2	2	4	2.2	2.4	100.0	–	–	2.8	2.4	1.8	1.6	26	100.0
Hepatoblastoma	0	0	1	0	1	0.6	0.7	25.0	–	–	1.4	–	0.4	0.4	7	100.0
Hepatic carcinoma	0	0	0	1	1	0.6	0.5	25.0	–	–	–	1.2	0.4	0.4	6	100.0
Other and unspecified	0	0	1	1	2	1.1	1.2	50.0	–	–	1.4	1.2	0.9	0.8	13	–
VIII. BONE	0	0	4	7	11	6.1	6.3	100.0	–	–	5.6	8.4	4.8	4.2	70	100.0
Osteosarcoma	0	0	4	6	10	5.5	5.8	90.9	–	–	5.6	7.2	4.4	3.9	64	100.0
Chondrosarcoma	0	0	0	1	1	0.6	0.5	9.1	–	–	–	1.2	0.4	0.4	6	100.0
Ewing's sarcoma	0	0	0	0	0	–	–	–	–	–	–	–	–	–	–	–
Other and unspecified	0	0	0	0	0	–	–	–	–	–	–	–	–	–	–	–
IX. SOFT TISSUE SARCOMAS	1	3	2	3	9	5.0	4.9	100.0	6.4	5.3	2.8	3.6	4.0	4.1	60	100.0
Rhabdomyosarcoma	0	2	1	2	5	2.8	2.7	55.6	–	3.5	1.4	2.4	2.2	2.2	33	100.0
Fibrosarcoma	1	1	0	1	3	1.7	1.7	33.3	6.4	1.8	–	1.2	1.3	1.5	20	100.0
Other and unspecified	0	0	1	0	1	0.6	0.5	11.1	–	–	1.4	–	0.4	0.4	6	100.0
X. GONADAL & GERM CELL	2	1	2	6	11	6.1	5.9	100.0	12.9	1.8	2.8	7.2	4.8	4.5	70	100.0
Non-gonadal germ cell	2	1	0	1	4	2.2	2.2	36.4	12.9	1.8	–	1.2	1.8	1.9	26	100.0
Gonadal germ cell	0	0	1	4	5	2.8	2.7	45.5	–	–	1.4	4.8	2.2	1.8	31	100.0
Gonadal carcinoma	0	0	1	1	2	1.1	1.2	18.2	–	–	1.4	1.2	0.9	0.8	13	100.0
Other and unspecified	0	0	0	0	0	–	–	–	–	–	–	–	–	–	–	–
XI. EPITHELIAL NEOPLASMS	0	2	1	7	10	5.5	5.2	100.0	–	3.5	1.4	8.4	4.4	4.0	63	90.0
Adrenocortical carcinoma	0	0	0	0	0	–	–	–	–	–	–	–	–	–	–	–
Thyroid carcinoma	0	0	1	1	2	1.1	1.2	20.0	–	–	1.4	1.2	0.9	0.8	13	100.0
Nasopharyngeal carcinoma	0	0	0	1	1	0.6	0.5	10.0	–	–	–	1.2	0.4	0.4	6	100.0
Melanoma	0	1	0	1	2	1.1	1.0	20.0	–	1.8	–	1.2	0.9	0.9	13	100.0
Other carcinoma	0	1	0	4	5	2.8	2.5	50.0	–	1.8	–	4.8	2.2	1.9	31	80.0
XII. OTHER	1	1	0	0	2	1.1	1.0	100.0	6.4	1.8	–	–	0.9	1.0	14	–
* Specified as malignant	1	0	2	2	5	2.8	2.9	100.0	6.4	–	2.8	2.4	2.2	2.1	32	50.0

AVERAGE ANNUAL POPULATION: 1976-1982

Age	Male	Female
White		
0	100166	95659
1–4	379005	359243
5–9	511781	486422
10–14	600011	572511
0–14	1590963	1513835
Black		
0	22262	22185
1–4	81587	80764
5–9	103835	102769
10–14	118881	118494
0–14	326565	324212

Commentary

Whites. The general pattern of rates is similar to that for European and other North American registries.

Blacks. The total rates and those for leukaemia and brain and spinal tumours are lower than those for Whites. Only one case of Ewing's sarcoma was recorded. The rate for nasopharyngeal carcinoma (though based on only five cases) was high. As in the Greater Delaware Valley (GDV) and SEER registries, the rate for neuroblastoma is considerably lower than that for the white population; however, unlike those registries, the rates for Wilms' tumour are similar in Blacks and Whites. In contrast to many other non-white populations reported in this volume, the rate for retinoblastoma is not high.

The SEER Program, 1973–1982

D.F. Austin, J. Flannery, R. Greenberg, P. Isaacson, C. Key,
L.N. Kolonel, C. Platz, G.M. Swanson, D. Thomas, D. West & J.L. Young

The Surveillance, Epidemiology and End Results (SEER) Program is a continuing project of the Biometry Branch of the National Cancer Institute (NCI). The Program was initiated in 1972 as an outgrowth of two earlier NCI programmes: the End Results Program and the three National Cancer Surveys.

Participants in the SEER Program were selected on the basis of their ability to operate and maintain a population-based cancer reporting system, and for their population subgroups, which were of special epidemiological interest rather than representative of the demographic characteristics of the US population. Eight participants began collecting data for cases diagnosed in 1973, one began with 1974 and another with 1975 diagnoses. We report here the data from the nine participants in the USA proper, that is excluding Puerto Rico, which is presented elsewhere (page 135). The nine participants (Connecticut; Detroit, Michigan; Iowa; Atlanta, Georgia; New Mexico; Utah; Seattle, Washington; San Francisco – Oakland, California; and Hawaii) cover approximately 10% of the total population of the USA and are fairly representative with respect to age. Blacks are under-represented whereas other minority populations (Chinese, Japanese, Hawaiians and American Indians) are over-represented. Rural populations, especially rural Blacks, are also under-represented.

Each participant is required to maintain a cancer information reporting system in their geographical area; to utilize standardized abstracts of records for resident cancer patients seen in every hospital inside and outside the area; to abstract all death certificates on which cancer is mentioned of residents dying within or outside the area, as well as those for any case listed in the reporting system; to utilize the records of private laboratories and radiotherapy units to ensure complete coverage of cases; to use the records of nursing homes which provide the services of diagnostic physicians and/or laboratories to patients; and to maintain reporting and data processing procedures so as to produce valid incidence rates within 11 months after the end of each calendar year.

All participants are required to report all malignant and *in situ* neoplasms listed in ICD-O, except papillary, squamous-cell, basal-cell and histologically unspecified carcinomas of skin. The data they collect must include sufficient detail for each cancer to be classified according to the variables described in the Code Manual of the SEER Program. Participants also collaborate in a variety of quality-control activities. Each participant is responsible for consolidating all data concerning an individual cancer case, with the exception of any identifying information, into a single record. The total file for each area is then submitted to the NCI via computer tape. Data are computer-edited for legitimate codes and internal consistency both by the participant and the NCI.

Mortality tapes containing data on all deaths occurring within the USA and Puerto Rico are obtained annually from the National Center for Health Statistics. From these tapes, a file of all cancer deaths classifiable by age, sex, race and cancer site is extracted so that cancer mortality for the entire USA and each SEER area can be determined.

The location of the nine participating registries within the United States is shown in Fig. 2. Their combined population at the 1980 census was 21.7 million, of whom 22.6% were aged less than 15. The racial composition of this population includes 83.2% White, 10.3% Black, 1.3% Japanese, 1.1% Filipino, 1.0% Chinese, 0.8% Hawaiian and 0.7% American Indian.

The objectives of the SEER Program are to monitor incidence and survival rates and trends in relation to demographic and social characteristics of the population, and to identify etiological factors and determinants of survival. A large number of

Contd p. 106

USA, SEER, White   1973 – 1982   MALE

DIAGNOSTIC GROUP	NUMBER OF CASES					REL. FREQUENCY(%)			RATES PER MILLION					Cum	HV(%)
	0	1-4	5-9	10-14	All	Crude	Adj.	Group	0-4	5-9	10-14	Crude	Adj.		
TOTAL	247	943	752	850	2792	100.0	100.0	100.0	190.8	114.5	113.9	137.8	143.9	2096	97.1
I. LEUKAEMIAS	42	411	235	208	896	32.1	31.9	100.0	72.6	35.8	27.9	44.2	47.8	681	99.1
Acute lymphocytic	22	329	180	136	667	23.9	23.8	74.4	56.3	27.4	18.2	32.9	35.9	510	98.9
Other lymphocytic		7	1	2	10	0.4	0.3	1.1	1.1	0.2	0.3	0.5	0.6	8	100.0
Acute non-lymphocytic	8	29	31	47	115	4.1	4.1	12.8	5.9	4.7	6.3	5.7	5.6	85	99.1
Chronic myeloid	1	3	6	3	13	0.5	0.5	1.5	0.6	0.9	0.4	0.6	0.7	10	100.0
Other and unspecified	11	43	17	20	91	3.3	3.2	10.2	8.7	2.6	2.7	4.5	5.0	70	100.0
II. LYMPHOMAS	10	65	149	215	439	15.7	16.1	100.0	12.0	22.7	28.8	21.7	20.3	318	99.1
Hodgkin's disease		4	45	103	152	5.4	5.6	34.6	0.6	6.9	13.8	7.5	6.5	106	100.0
Non-Hodgkin lymphoma	2	29	51	64	146	5.2	5.3	33.3	5.0	7.8	8.6	7.2	6.9	107	100.0
Burkitt's lymphoma		17	29	27	73	2.6	2.7	16.6	2.7	4.4	3.6	3.6	3.5	54	97.3
Unspecified lymphoma		11	19	18	48	1.7	1.8	10.9	1.8	2.9	2.4	2.4	2.3	35	95.8
Histiocytosis X	4	3			7	0.2	0.2	1.6	1.1	-	-	0.3	0.4	6	100.0
Other reticuloendothelial	4	1	5	3	13	0.5	0.5	3.0	0.8	0.8	0.4	0.6	0.7	10	100.0
III. BRAIN AND SPINAL	30	140	185	174	529	18.9	19.2	100.0	27.3	28.2	23.3	26.1	26.4	394	89.5
Ependymoma	7	26	6	12	51	1.8	1.8	9.6	5.3	0.9	1.6	2.5	2.8	39	98.0
Astrocytoma	11	57	92	92	252	9.0	9.2	47.6	10.9	14.0	12.3	12.4	12.3	186	95.2
Medulloblastoma	5	39	52	41	137	4.9	5.0	25.9	7.1	7.9	5.5	6.8	6.9	102	100.0
Other glioma	3	15	30	23	71	2.5	2.6	13.4	2.9	4.6	3.1	3.5	3.5	53	49.3
Other and unspecified *	4	3	5	6	18	0.6	0.6	3.4	1.1	0.8	0.8	0.9	0.9	13	61.1
IV. SYMPATHETIC N.S.	70	108	28	10	216	7.7	7.5	100.0	28.5	4.3	1.3	10.7	12.8	171	98.1
Neuroblastoma	70	107	28	7	212	7.6	7.3	98.1	28.4	4.3	0.9	10.5	12.6	168	98.1
Other		1		3	4	0.1	0.1	1.9	0.2	-	0.4	0.2	0.2	3	100.0
V. RETINOBLASTOMA	26	30	4		60	2.1	2.0	100.0	9.0	0.6	-	3.0	3.7	48	95.0
VI. KIDNEY	24	76	31	8	139	5.0	4.9	100.0	16.0	4.7	1.1	6.9	8.0	109	100.0
Wilms' tumour	24	75	31	6	136	4.9	4.8	97.8	15.9	4.7	0.8	6.7	7.9	107	100.0
Renal carcinoma		1		1	2	0.1	0.1	1.4	0.2	-	0.3	0.1	0.1	1	100.0
Other and unspecified				1	1	-	-	0.7	0.2	-	-	0.1	0.1	1	100.0
VII. LIVER	15	13	3	6	37	1.3	1.3	100.0	4.5	0.5	0.8	1.8	2.1	29	94.6
Hepatoblastoma	13	11			24	0.9	0.8	64.9	3.8	-	-	1.2	1.5	19	95.8
Hepatic carcinoma	2	2	3	5	12	0.4	0.4	32.4	0.6	0.5	0.7	0.6	0.6	9	100.0
Other and unspecified				1	1	-	-	2.7	-	-	0.1	-	-	1	-
VIII. BONE		4	25	91	126	4.5	4.5	100.0	1.6	3.8	12.2	6.2	5.4	88	98.4
Osteosarcoma		1	10	40	54	1.9	1.9	42.9	0.6	1.5	5.4	2.7	2.3	38	98.1
Chondrosarcoma				6	6	0.2	0.2	4.8	0.2	-	0.8	0.3	0.3	5	100.0
Ewing's sarcoma		4	12	43	59	2.1	2.1	46.8	0.6	1.8	5.8	2.9	2.5	41	98.2
Other and unspecified		1	3	2	6	0.2	0.2	4.8	0.2	0.5	0.3	0.3	0.3	4	100.0
IX. SOFT TISSUE SARCOMAS	15	42	60	65	182	6.5	6.6	100.0	9.1	9.1	8.7	9.0	9.0	135	100.0
Rhabdomyosarcoma	8	28	37	25	98	3.5	3.6	53.8	5.8	5.6	3.3	4.8	5.0	74	100.0
Fibrosarcoma	3	6	8	19	36	1.3	1.3	19.8	1.4	1.2	2.5	1.8	1.7	26	100.0
Other and unspecified	4	8	15	21	48	1.7	1.7	26.4	1.9	-	2.8	2.4	2.3	35	100.0
X. GONADAL & GERM CELL	13	38	9	18	78	2.8	2.7	100.0	8.2	1.4	2.4	3.8	4.3	60	98.7
Non-gonadal germ cell	4	14	7	10	35	1.3	1.2	44.9	2.9	1.1	1.3	1.7	1.9	26	97.1
Gonadal germ cell	9	24	1	8	42	1.5	1.4	53.8	5.3	0.2	1.1	2.1	2.4	33	100.0
Gonadal carcinoma			1		1	-	-	1.3	-	0.2	-	-	-	1	100.0
Other and unspecified						-	-	-	-	-	-	-	-	-	-
XI. EPITHELIAL NEOPLASMS	1	5	17	51	74	2.7	2.7	100.0	1.0	2.6	6.8	3.7	3.2	52	98.6
Adrenocortical carcinoma		2	2	2	6	0.2	0.2	8.1	0.3	0.3	0.3	0.3	0.3	4	100.0
Thyroid carcinoma			7	14	21	0.8	0.8	28.4	-	1.1	1.9	1.0	0.9	15	95.2
Nasopharyngeal carcinoma			1	4	5	0.2	0.2	6.8	-	0.2	0.5	0.2	0.2	3	100.0
Melanoma		2	6	11	19	0.7	0.7	25.7	0.3	0.9	1.5	0.9	0.8	14	100.0
Other carcinoma	1	1	1	20	23	0.8	0.8	31.1	0.3	0.2	2.7	1.1	1.0	16	100.0
XII. OTHER	1	5	6	4	16	0.6	0.6	100.0	1.0	0.9	0.5	0.8	0.8	12	100.0
* Specified as malignant	4	3	5	6	18	0.6	0.6	100.0	1.1	0.8	0.8	0.9	0.9	13	61.1

USA, SEER, White

1973 - 1982

FEMALE

DIAGNOSTIC GROUP	NUMBER OF CASES					REL. FREQUENCY(%)			RATES PER MILLION						HV(%)
	0	1-4	5-9	10-14	All	Crude	Adj.	Group	0-4	5-9	10-14	Crude	Adj.	Cum	
TOTAL	272	754	573	751	2350	100.0	100.0	100.0	172.9	91.3	105.4	121.5	126.9	1848	97.2
I. LEUKAEMIAS	53	315	206	121	695	29.6	30.0	100.0	62.0	32.8	17.0	35.9	39.5	559	100.0
Acute lymphocytic	30	254	158	74	516	22.0	22.3	74.2	47.8	25.2	10.4	26.7	29.7	417	100.0
Other lymphocytic	0	0	1	2	3	0.1	0.1	0.4	-	0.2	0.3	0.2	0.1	2	100.0
Acute non-lymphocytic	16	38	27	40	121	5.1	5.1	17.4	9.1	4.3	5.6	6.3	6.5	95	100.0
Chronic myeloid	1	1	4	2	8	0.3	0.4	1.2	0.3	0.6	0.3	0.4	0.4	6	100.0
Other and unspecified	6	22	16	3	47	2.0	2.0	6.8	4.7	2.5	0.4	2.4	2.8	38	100.0
II. LYMPHOMAS	11	34	40	160	245	10.4	10.2	100.0	7.6	6.4	22.4	12.7	11.5	182	98.4
Hodgkin's disease	0	4	16	119	139	5.9	5.7	56.7	0.7	2.5	16.7	7.2	5.8	100	99.3
Non-Hodgkin lymphoma	2	14	16	22	54	2.3	2.3	22.0	2.7	2.5	3.1	2.8	2.9	42	98.1
Burkitt's lymphoma	0	4	1	3	8	0.3	0.3	3.3	0.7	0.2	0.4	0.4	0.4	6	100.0
Unspecified lymphoma	0	6	7	13	26	1.1	1.1	10.6	1.0	1.1	1.8	1.3	1.3	20	92.0
Histiocytosis X	1	2	0	0	3	0.1	0.1	1.2	0.5	-	-	0.2	0.2	3	100.0
Other reticuloendothelial	8	4	0	3	15	0.6	0.6	6.1	2.0	-	0.4	0.8	0.9	12	100.0
III. BRAIN AND SPINAL	34	115	143	154	446	19.0	19.4	100.0	25.1	22.8	21.6	23.1	23.3	347	89.3
Ependymoma	3	15	7	10	35	1.5	1.5	7.8	3.0	1.1	1.4	1.8	1.9	28	100.0
Astrocytoma	18	42	80	103	243	10.3	10.6	54.5	10.1	12.7	14.4	12.6	12.2	187	96.7
Medulloblastoma	8	27	29	16	80	3.4	3.5	17.9	5.9	4.6	2.2	4.1	4.4	64	98.8
Other glioma	4	25	20	22	71	3.0	3.5	15.9	4.9	3.2	3.1	3.7	3.8	56	52.9
Other and unspecified *	1	6	7	3	17	0.7	0.8	3.8	1.2	1.1	0.4	0.9	0.9	14	62.5
IV. SYMPATHETIC N.S.	78	93	18	13	202	8.6	8.1	100.0	28.8	2.9	1.8	10.4	12.6	168	98.0
Neuroblastoma	76	92	18	11	197	8.4	7.9	97.5	28.3	2.9	1.5	10.2	12.3	164	98.0
Other	2	1	0	2	5	0.2	0.2	2.5	0.7	-	0.3	0.3	0.3	4	100.0
V. RETINOBLASTOMA	28	37	3	0	68	2.9	2.7	100.0	11.0	0.5	-	3.5	4.4	57	94.1
VI. KIDNEY	32	84	42	8	166	7.1	7.0	100.0	19.5	6.7	1.1	8.6	10.0	137	98.2
Wilms' tumour	32	84	42	7	165	7.0	7.0	99.4	19.5	6.7	1.0	8.5	10.0	136	98.2
Renal carcinoma	0	0	0	1	1	-	-	0.6	-	-	0.1	0.1	-	1	100.0
Other and unspecified	0	0	0	0	0	-	-	-	-	-	-	-	-	-	-
VII. LIVER	6	5	5	4	20	0.9	0.9	100.0	1.9	0.8	0.6	1.0	1.1	16	95.0
Hepatoblastoma	5	4	1	0	10	0.4	0.4	50.0	1.5	0.2	-	0.5	0.6	8	100.0
Hepatic carcinoma	1	1	4	4	10	0.4	0.4	50.0	0.3	0.6	0.6	0.5	0.5	8	90.0
Other and unspecified	0	0	0	0	0	-	-	-	-	-	-	-	-	-	-
VIII. BONE	1	9	28	86	124	5.3	5.3	100.0	1.7	4.5	12.1	6.4	5.6	91	100.0
Osteosarcoma	0	2	8	52	62	2.6	2.6	50.0	0.2	1.3	7.3	3.2	2.7	45	100.0
Chondrosarcoma	0	1	0	6	7	0.3	0.3	5.6	-	-	0.8	0.4	0.3	5	100.0
Ewing's sarcoma	1	6	18	24	49	2.1	2.2	39.5	1.2	2.9	3.4	2.5	2.4	37	100.0
Other and unspecified	0	0	2	4	6	0.3	0.3	4.8	-	0.3	0.6	0.3	0.3	5	100.0
IX. SOFT TISSUE SARCOMAS	16	37	45	60	158	6.7	6.8	100.0	8.9	7.2	8.4	8.2	8.2	123	98.7
Rhabdomyosarcoma	9	21	32	20	82	3.5	3.6	51.9	5.1	5.1	2.8	4.2	4.4	65	98.8
Fibrosarcoma	4	5	2	19	30	1.3	1.2	19.0	1.5	0.3	2.7	1.6	1.5	23	100.0
Other and unspecified	3	11	11	21	46	2.0	2.0	29.1	2.4	1.8	2.9	2.4	2.4	35	97.8
X. GONADAL & GERM CELL	5	11	21	49	86	3.7	3.7	100.0	2.7	3.3	6.9	4.4	4.1	65	100.0
Non-gonadal germ cell	5	10	0	14	29	1.2	1.2	33.7	2.5	0.8	1.3	1.5	1.6	23	100.0
Gonadal germ cell	0	0	14	34	48	2.0	2.1	55.8	-	2.2	4.8	2.5	2.1	35	100.0
Gonadal carcinoma	0	0	0	3	3	0.1	0.1	3.5	-	-	0.4	0.1	-	2	100.0
Other and unspecified	0	1	2	3	6	0.3	0.3	7.0	0.2	0.3	0.4	0.3	0.3	5	100.0
XI. EPITHELIAL NEOPLASMS	6	8	22	92	128	5.4	5.4	100.0	2.4	3.5	12.9	6.6	5.8	94	99.2
Adrenocortical carcinoma	1	4	0	2	7	0.3	0.3	5.5	0.8	-	0.3	0.4	0.4	6	100.0
Thyroid carcinoma	0	0	13	37	50	2.1	2.2	39.1	-	2.1	5.2	2.6	2.2	36	100.0
Nasopharyngeal carcinoma	0	1	0	0	1	-	-	0.8	0.2	-	-	0.1	0.1	1	100.0
Melanoma	3	1	6	22	32	1.4	1.3	25.0	0.7	1.0	3.1	1.7	1.5	24	96.9
Other carcinoma	2	2	3	31	38	1.6	1.6	29.7	0.7	0.5	4.3	2.0	1.7	28	100.0
XII. OTHER	2	6	0	4	12	0.5	0.5	100.0	1.3	-	0.6	0.6	0.7	10	100.0
* Specified as malignant	1	6	7	3	17	0.7	0.8	100.0	1.2	1.1	0.4	0.9	0.9	14	62.5

USA, SEER, Black   MALE   1973 – 1982

DIAGNOSTIC GROUP	NUMBER OF CASES 0	1-4	5-9	10-14	All	REL. FREQUENCY(%) Crude	Adj.	Group	RATES PER MILLION 0-4	5-9	10-14	Crude	Adj.	Cum	HV(%)
TOTAL	28	99	83	96	306	100.0	100.0	100.0	135.2	85.9	93.6	104.4	107.2	1573	95.7
I. LEUKAEMIAS	3	29	18	17	67	21.9	21.9	100.0	34.1	18.6	16.6	22.9	24.0	346	100.0
Acute lymphocytic	1	18	12	9	40	13.1	13.1	59.7	20.2	12.4	8.8	13.6	14.4	207	100.0
Other lymphocytic	0	0	0	0	0	–	–	–	–	–	–	–	–	–	–
Acute non-lymphocytic	0	3	5	5	13	4.2	4.3	19.4	3.2	5.2	4.9	4.4	4.3	66	100.0
Chronic myeloid	0	1	1	1	3	1.0	1.0	4.5	1.1	1.0	1.0	1.0	1.0	15	100.0
Other and unspecified	2	7	0	2	11	3.6	3.5	16.4	9.6	–	1.9	3.8	4.3	58	100.0
II. LYMPHOMAS	1	9	10	24	44	14.4	14.3	100.0	10.6	10.4	23.4	15.0	14.3	222	100.0
Hodgkin's disease	0	3	6	15	24	7.8	7.8	54.5	3.2	6.2	14.6	8.2	7.5	120	100.0
Non-Hodgkin lymphoma	0	3	3	6	12	3.9	3.9	27.3	3.2	3.1	5.8	4.1	3.9	61	100.0
Burkitt's lymphoma	0	0	1	1	2	0.7	0.7	4.5	–	1.0	1.0	0.7	0.6	10	100.0
Unspecified lymphoma	1	1	0	2	4	1.3	1.3	9.1	2.1	–	1.9	1.4	1.4	20	100.0
Histiocytosis X	0	1	0	0	1	0.3	0.3	2.3	1.1	–	–	0.3	0.4	5	100.0
Other reticuloendothelial	0	1	0	0	1	0.3	0.3	2.3	1.1	–	–	0.3	0.4	5	100.0
III. BRAIN AND SPINAL	3	12	29	18	62	20.3	20.8	100.0	16.0	30.0	17.5	21.1	21.0	318	79.0
Ependymoma	0	1	0	3	4	1.3	1.3	6.5	1.1	–	2.9	1.4	1.3	20	100.0
Astrocytoma	1	4	12	11	28	9.2	9.3	45.2	5.3	12.4	10.7	9.6	9.2	142	92.9
Medulloblastoma	1	4	9	1	15	4.9	5.1	24.2	5.3	9.3	1.0	5.1	5.3	78	100.0
Other glioma	0	2	8	3	13	4.2	4.5	21.0	2.1	8.3	2.9	4.4	4.3	67	23.1
Other and unspecified *	1	1	0	0	2	0.7	0.6	3.2	2.1	–	–	0.7	0.8	11	50.0
IV. SYMPATHETIC N.S.	5	17	2	1	25	8.2	8.0	100.0	23.4	2.1	1.0	8.5	10.0	132	100.0
Neuroblastoma	5	16	2	1	24	7.8	7.6	96.0	22.4	2.1	1.0	8.2	9.6	127	100.0
Other	0	1	0	0	1	0.3	0.3	4.0	1.1	–	–	0.3	0.4	5	100.0
V. RETINOBLASTOMA	3	8	0	1	12	3.9	3.8	100.0	11.7	–	1.0	4.1	4.8	63	100.0
VI. KIDNEY	5	14	7	4	30	9.8	9.8	100.0	20.2	7.2	3.9	10.2	11.3	157	100.0
Wilms' tumour	5	13	5	3	26	8.5	8.4	86.7	19.2	5.2	2.9	8.9	9.9	136	100.0
Renal carcinoma	0	0	2	1	3	1.0	1.0	10.0	–	2.1	1.0	1.0	1.0	15	100.0
Other and unspecified	0	1	0	0	1	0.3	0.3	3.3	1.1	–	–	0.3	0.4	5	100.0
VII. LIVER	1	0	1	1	3	1.0	1.0	100.0	1.1	1.0	1.0	1.0	1.0	15	100.0
Hepatoblastoma	1	0	1	0	2	0.7	0.7	66.7	1.1	1.0	–	0.7	0.7	10	100.0
Hepatic carcinoma	0	0	0	1	1	0.3	0.3	33.3	–	–	1.0	0.3	0.3	5	100.0
Other and unspecified	0	0	0	0	0	–	–	–	–	–	–	–	–	–	–
VIII. BONE	0	1	2	11	14	4.6	4.5	100.0	1.1	2.1	10.7	4.8	4.2	69	100.0
Osteosarcoma	0	1	1	8	10	3.3	3.2	71.4	1.1	1.0	7.8	3.4	3.0	49	100.0
Chondrosarcoma	0	0	0	0	0	–	–	–	–	–	–	–	–	–	–
Ewing's sarcoma	0	0	1	0	1	0.3	0.3	7.1	–	1.0	–	0.3	0.3	5	100.0
Other and unspecified	0	0	0	3	3	1.0	1.0	21.4	–	–	1.9	1.0	0.9	15	100.0
IX. SOFT TISSUE SARCOMAS	2	5	11	10	28	9.2	9.3	100.0	7.5	11.4	9.7	9.6	9.4	143	100.0
Rhabdomyosarcoma	1	4	7	3	15	4.9	5.0	53.6	5.3	7.2	2.9	5.1	5.1	77	100.0
Fibrosarcoma	1	0	3	4	8	2.6	2.6	28.6	1.1	3.1	3.9	2.7	2.5	40	100.0
Other and unspecified	0	1	1	3	5	1.6	1.6	17.9	1.1	1.0	2.9	1.7	1.6	25	100.0
X. GONADAL & GERM CELL	4	3	0	1	8	2.6	2.5	100.0	7.5	–	1.0	2.7	3.2	42	100.0
Non-gonadal germ cell	2	0	0	1	3	1.0	0.9	37.5	3.2	–	1.0	1.0	1.0	16	100.0
Gonadal germ cell	2	2	0	0	4	1.3	1.3	50.0	4.3	–	–	1.4	1.6	21	100.0
Gonadal carcinoma	0	0	0	0	0	–	–	–	–	–	–	–	–	–	–
Other and unspecified	0	1	0	0	1	0.3	0.3	12.5	–	1.0	–	0.3	0.3	5	100.0
XI. EPITHELIAL NEOPLASMS	1	1	3	8	13	4.2	4.2	100.0	2.1	3.1	7.8	4.4	4.1	65	100.0
Adrenocortical carcinoma	0	0	0	1	1	0.3	0.3	7.7	–	–	1.0	0.3	0.3	5	100.0
Thyroid carcinoma	0	0	1	0	1	0.3	0.4	7.7	–	1.0	–	0.3	0.3	5	100.0
Nasopharyngeal carcinoma	1	0	0	3	4	1.3	1.3	30.8	1.1	–	2.9	1.4	1.3	20	100.0
Melanoma	0	1	0	0	1	0.3	0.3	7.7	1.1	–	–	0.3	0.4	5	100.0
Other carcinoma	0	0	2	4	6	2.0	2.0	46.2	–	2.1	3.9	2.0	1.8	30	100.0
XII. OTHER	0	0	0	0	0	–	–	–	–	–	–	–	–	–	–
* Specified as malignant	1	1	0	0	2	0.7	0.6	100.0	2.1	–	–	0.7	0.8	11	50.0

USA, SEER, Black 1973 – 1982 FEMALE

DIAGNOSTIC GROUP	NUMBER OF CASES 0	1-4	5-9	10-14	All	REL. FREQUENCY(%) Crude	Adj.	Group	RATES PER MILLION 0-4	5-9	10-14	Crude	Adj.	Cum	HV(%)
TOTAL	31	93	82	98	304	100.0	100.0	100.0	134.8	86.2	96.4	105.2	107.9	1587	96.0
I. LEUKAEMIAS	5	26	19	24	74	24.3	24.3	100.0	33.7	20.0	23.6	25.6	26.3	386	100.0
Acute lymphocytic	3	18	8	13	42	13.8	13.7	56.8	22.8	8.4	12.8	14.5	15.3	220	100.0
Other lymphocytic	0	0	1	0	1	0.3	0.4	1.4	-	1.1	-	0.3	0.3	5	100.0
Acute non-lymphocytic	2	3	7	6	18	5.9	6.0	24.3	5.4	7.4	5.9	6.2	6.2	93	100.0
Chronic myeloid	0	0	1	3	4	1.3	1.3	5.4	-	1.1	2.9	1.4	1.2	20	100.0
Other and unspecified	0	5	2	2	9	3.0	3.4	12.2	5.4	2.1	2.0	3.1	3.4	48	100.0
II. LYMPHOMAS	1	4	4	9	18	5.9	5.8	100.0	5.4	4.2	8.8	6.2	6.0	92	100.0
Hodgkin's disease	0	1	1	4	6	2.0	1.9	33.3	1.1	1.1	3.9	2.1	1.9	30	100.0
Non-Hodgkin lymphoma	0	2	1	1	4	1.3	1.3	22.2	2.2	1.1	1.0	1.4	1.5	21	100.0
Burkitt's lymphoma	0	0	0	0	0	-	-	-	-	-	-	-	-	-	-
Unspecified lymphoma	0	1	2	2	5	1.6	1.7	27.8	1.1	2.1	2.0	1.7	1.7	26	100.0
Histiocytosis X	0	0	0	0	0	-	-	-	-	-	-	-	-	-	-
Other reticuloendothelial	1	0	0	2	3	1.0	0.9	16.7	1.1	-	2.0	1.0	1.0	15	100.0
III. BRAIN AND SPINAL	2	19	30	14	65	21.4	22.0	100.0	22.8	31.5	13.8	22.5	23.0	341	84.4
Ependymoma	0	4	4	0	8	2.6	2.8	12.3	4.3	4.2	-	2.8	3.0	43	87.5
Astrocytoma	2	7	12	4	25	8.2	8.5	38.5	9.8	12.6	3.9	8.7	9.0	132	96.0
Medulloblastoma	0	6	3	4	13	4.3	4.4	20.0	4.3	6.3	2.9	4.5	4.6	68	100.0
Other glioma	0	2	7	7	16	5.3	5.3	24.6	2.2	7.4	6.9	5.5	5.2	82	50.0
Other and unspecified *	0	2	1	0	3	1.0	1.0	4.6	2.2	1.1	-	1.0	1.2	16	100.0
IV. SYMPATHETIC N.S.	10	11	5	1	27	8.9	8.9	100.0	22.8	5.3	1.0	9.3	10.8	145	96.3
Neuroblastoma	10	11	5	1	27	8.9	8.9	100.0	22.8	5.3	1.0	9.3	10.8	145	96.3
Other	0	0	0	0	0	-	-	-	-	-	-	-	-	-	-
V. RETINOBLASTOMA	5	8	0	0	13	4.3	4.2	100.0	14.1	-	-	4.5	5.5	71	91.7
VI. KIDNEY	5	15	11	5	36	11.8	12.0	100.0	21.7	11.6	4.9	12.5	13.6	191	100.0
Wilms' tumour	5	15	9	3	32	10.5	10.7	88.9	21.7	9.5	2.9	11.1	12.3	171	100.0
Renal carcinoma	0	0	1	1	2	0.7	0.7	5.6	-	1.1	1.0	0.7	0.6	10	100.0
Other and unspecified	0	0	1	1	2	0.7	0.7	5.6	-	1.1	1.0	0.7	0.6	10	100.0
VII. LIVER	0	4	0	0	4	1.3	1.3	100.0	4.3	-	-	1.4	1.7	22	100.0
Hepatoblastoma	0	3	0	0	3	1.0	1.0	75.0	3.3	-	-	1.0	1.3	16	100.0
Hepatic carcinoma	0	1	0	0	1	0.3	0.3	25.0	1.1	-	-	0.3	0.4	5	100.0
Other and unspecified	0	0	0	0	0	-	-	-	-	-	-	-	-	-	-
VIII. BONE	0	1	1	13	15	4.9	4.7	100.0	1.1	1.1	12.8	5.2	4.5	75	100.0
Osteosarcoma	0	0	1	12	13	4.3	4.0	86.7	-	1.1	11.8	4.5	3.8	64	100.0
Chondrosarcoma	0	0	0	1	1	0.3	0.3	6.7	-	-	1.0	0.3	0.4	5	100.0
Ewing's sarcoma	0	0	0	1	1	0.3	0.3	6.7	-	-	1.0	0.3	0.4	5	100.0
Other and unspecified	0	0	0	0	0	-	-	-	-	-	-	-	-	-	-
IX. SOFT TISSUE SARCOMAS	2	1	9	10	22	7.2	7.3	100.0	3.3	9.5	9.8	7.6	7.2	113	100.0
Rhabdomyosarcoma	0	1	2	2	5	1.6	1.7	22.7	1.1	2.1	2.0	1.7	1.7	26	100.0
Fibrosarcoma	2	0	3	5	10	3.3	3.3	45.5	2.2	3.2	4.9	3.5	3.3	51	100.0
Other and unspecified	0	0	4	3	7	2.3	2.4	31.8	-	4.2	2.9	2.4	2.2	36	100.0
X. GONADAL & GERM CELL	1	3	1	11	16	5.3	5.0	100.0	4.3	1.1	10.8	5.5	5.2	81	100.0
Non-gonadal germ cell	1	3	0	3	7	2.3	2.2	43.8	4.3	-	2.9	2.4	2.5	36	100.0
Gonadal germ cell	0	0	1	7	8	2.6	2.5	50.0	-	1.1	6.9	2.8	2.3	40	100.0
Gonadal carcinoma	0	0	0	1	1	0.3	0.3	6.3	-	-	1.0	0.3	0.3	5	100.0
Other and unspecified	0	0	0	0	0	-	-	-	-	-	-	-	-	-	-
XI. EPITHELIAL NEOPLASMS	0	1	2	9	12	3.9	3.8	100.0	1.1	2.1	8.8	4.2	3.7	60	100.0
Adrenocortical carcinoma	0	0	0	0	0	-	-	-	-	-	-	-	-	-	-
Thyroid carcinoma	0	0	0	4	4	1.3	1.2	33.3	-	-	3.9	1.4	1.1	20	100.0
Nasopharyngeal carcinoma	0	0	0	0	0	-	-	-	-	-	-	-	-	-	-
Melanoma	0	0	0	0	0	-	-	-	-	-	-	-	-	-	-
Other carcinoma	0	1	2	5	8	2.6	2.6	66.7	1.1	2.1	4.9	2.8	2.5	41	100.0
XII. OTHER	0	0	0	2	2	0.7	0.6	100.0	-	-	2.0	0.7	0.6	10	100.0
* Specified as malignant	0	2	1	0	3	1.0	1.0	100.0	2.2	1.1	-	1.0	1.2	16	100.0

Figure 2. Location of registries included in the SEER Program

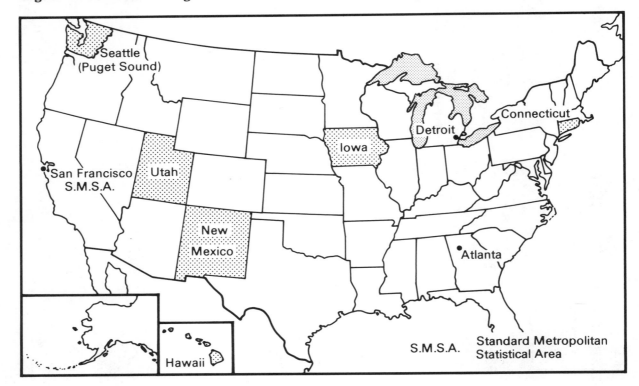

publications, both from the SEER Program as a whole and from participant registries, appear each year. Recent descriptive studies of childhood cancer include those by Young and Miller (1975), Bader and Miller (1979), Breslow and Langholz (1983) and Young *et al.* (1986).

The results in the tables relate to the incidence of childhood cancer in the white and black populations of the nine SEER registries within the United States (i.e., excluding Puerto Rico).

AVERAGE ANNUAL POPULATION: 1973–1982

Age	Male	Female
White		
0–4	623630	593578
5–9	656845	627596
10–14	746279	712812
0–14	2026754	1933986
Black		
0–4	93945	91988
5–9	96602	95179
10–14	102611	101697
0–14	293158	288864

Population

The SEER Program makes annual estimates of the populations of the participant registry areas, which are derived from the results of the censuses of 1970 and 1980 (US Bureau of the Census). The populations shown are the average annual population in the participating registries during the 10-year period 1973–1982.

Commentary

The data from the SEER Program constitute one of the largest population-based series in the present volume. The incidence rates for Whites were broadly similar to those observed in many other Western populations. The commonest diagnostic group was leukaemia, accounting for 31% of registrations. Of these, 74% were acute lymphocytic in type, and this subgroup exhibited a characteristic excess of males and a peak incidence in the 1–4 age-group for both sexes. The next largest diagnostic groups were brain and spinal tumours (19%) and lymphomas (13%).

For Blacks, incidence rates overall and in most diagnostic groups were lower than for Whites. Unsually, the incidence of acute lymphocytic leukaemia was similar in females and in males.

Ewing's sarcoma and malignant melanoma were extremely rare. Carcinoma of the thyroid occurred less than half as frequently as in Whites. Retinoblastoma had a higher incidence in Blacks than in Whites. Wilms' tumour, osteosarcoma and fibrosarcoma also had a higher incidence in Blacks.

References

Bader, J.L. & Miller, R.W. (1979) US Cancer incidence and mortality in the first year of life. *Am. J. Dis. Child.*, *133*, 157-159

Breslow, N.E. & Langholz, B. (1983) Childhood cancer incidence: geographical and temporal variations. *Int. J. Cancer*, *32*, 703-716

Young, J.L., Gloekler-Ries, L., Silverberg, E., Horm, J.W. & Miller, R.W. (1986) Cancer incidence, survival and mortality for children under 15 years of age. *Cancer*, *58*, 598-602

Young, J.L. & Miller, R.W. (1975) Incidence of malignant tumours in US children. *J. Pediatr.*, *86*, 254-258

CENTRAL AND SOUTH AMERICA AND CARIBBEAN

BRAZIL

Data are presented from three population-based cancer registries, Ceara (Fortaleza) and Pernambuco (Recife) in the north-east, and São Paulo in the south.

Cancer Registry of Ceara (Fortaleza), 1978–1980

Marcelo Gurgel Carlos da Silva

The Cancer Registry of Ceara was established in 1971 by the Cancer Institute of Ceara in Fortaleza, with the main purpose of developing epidemiological studies on cancer in the State. The Registry is located within the Institute, and is funded by it; special donations are received also from the Federal Government, through the National Campaign for Cancer Control. Coverage is restricted to the urbanized county of Fortaleza, which is 336 square kilometres in area.

Notification of cancer cases is not compulsory in Brazil. The Registry collects data actively and is responsible for the process of notification in the State. The data are collated on standardized filing cards by medical students, who receive special training in data collection. The sources are as follows: hospitals, clinics, anatomo-pathological laboratories, autopsy services, radiotherapy departments, institutes for cancer prevention and the Division of Epidemiology and Statistics of the Secretary of Health of the State (death certificates).

The neoplasms are classified and coded topographically according to ICD-9, and morphologically in accordance with the *Manual of Tumor Nomenclature and Coding* of the American Cancer Society.

Data on the methods and techniques of diagnosis are also collected, namely, clinical examination, radiology, surgery, cytology, histology, autopsy and other methods.

The filing cards are collated and inspected to ensure that there is only one for each case. The maximum amount of information on place of residence is included to avoid registering cases coming from inland and from other states. New registrations are matched with the archive index to avoid duplication of cases already registered. The whole process is entirely manual.

Fortaleza is the capital of the state of Ceara in the north-east of Brazil. It has about 1 400 000 inhabitants — more than one-fourth of the total population of the State. There is a very high rate of demographic growth, chiefly due to migration from the hinterland. According to the 1980 census, the distribution of the population by colour was as follows: white (31.7%), black (2.5%), yellow (0.1%), mixed (65.2%). More than 95% of the population are Catholics, followed by Protestants with 2%. Among those aged over five years the literacy rate is 72%.

Apart from increasing urbanization, the city is undergoing rapid industrialization on account of the implantation of the so-called Third Pole of Economic Development, which emphasizes medium-size enterprises. The main economic activities are those related to commerce, the export of raw materials, the production of vegetable oils, fishing and metallurgy.

Fortaleza has severe deficiencies in the social infrastructure; the piped water supply reaches only 14% of homes and the sewerage system even fewer — namely around 3%.

The public health services are well established, and consist of posts and health centres operated by the Government; the majority of hospitals are private institutions.

AVERAGE ANNUAL POPULATION: 1978–1980

Age	Male	Female
0	19766	19553
1–4	73316	72404
5–9	87861	86752
10–14	70090	77715
0–14	251033	256424

Population

The population is an estimate for 1 July 1979, based on the results of the censuses of 1970 and 1980 (Fundação Instituto Brasileiro de Geografica e Estadistica — IBGE).

Cancer Registry of Pernambuco (Recife), 1967–1979

Manoel Ricardo da Costa Carvalho

The cancer registry of Pernambuco started operation in 1967. It is located in the School of Medicine, and works in co-operation with the Bureau of Health of the State of Pernambuco, and the Ministry of Health. Registration is an active process, data collectors (medical students) paying regular visits to all potential sources of information on cancer patients. These comprise some 32 hospitals and clinics in the city of Recife (with a total of about 6000 beds) and including the Hospital for Cancer (220 beds), pathology laboratories in the University and major hospitals, and 24 private laboratories. Copies of death certificates are sent to the Registry by the State Department of Health.

The Registry reporting forms completed by the data-collectors contain a relatively small amount of information for each cancer case, including number, name, age, sex, marital status, occupation, source of information, date and basis of diagnosis, site and histology of tumour and the name of the pathologist or laboratory. However, information is often not well recorded in the source documents. Place of residence of all cases is recorded and, for Recife residents, the duration of stay. It is thus possi-

ble to restrict analysis to Recife residents, and calculate rates of incidence for the population of the city.

Recife has a population of 1.2 million (1980 census), and is the capital of Pernambuco State and the largest city in north-east Brazil. The population density is around 8250 per square kilometre and the area is an industrial one with many immigrants from other regions, and areas of poor housing, sanitation and health. Temperatures range from 20° C to 30° C.

Population

The population at risk for the 13-year period has been estimated from the census populations of 1970 and 1980 (Fundação Instituto Brasileiro de Geographica e Estadistica - IBGE)

AVERAGE ANNUAL POPULATION: 1967–1979

Age	Male	Female
0–4	78409	76076
5–9	75085	74298
10–14	64813	68432
0–14	218307	218806

Cancer Registry of São Paulo, 1969–1978

A.P. Mirra, J.P.A. de Freitas, C. Marigo, R. Laurenti
E.F. Pastorelo, J.M.P. de Souza & S.L. Gotlieb

The São Paulo Cancer Registry was established in January 1969, with the support of the Ministry of Health (National Cancer Division), the State Health Department and the County and University of São Paulo, to study cancer incidence and mortality in São Paulo County and provide a base for etiological studies.

The Registry is part of the Department of Epidemiology of the School of Public Health, University of São Paulo. There is a Board of Technical Advisers and an executive staff headed by a Programme Coordinator.

Data are actively collected in a standard format from 199 hospitals (145 general and surgical, 51 specialized and 3 cancer), 66 clinics (including 12 radiotherapy clinics), 17 homes for the aged, the drug control services, 12 radiotherapy clinics, 48 pathology laboratories and three autopsy services. The State Department of Statistics provides all death certificates mentioning cancer. Notification of cancer is not compulsory but registration is nonetheless active.

Registrations are filed by first name, last name and registration number. Classification by first and last name facilitates manual checking for duplication. Each neoplasm (if there is more than one neoplasm in one person) is registered separately, the unit being the cancer case and not the cancer patient. The Registry transfers coded data to magnetic tape. The University computer is used. The 9th Revision of the *International Classification of Diseases* is used for coding the site and the *Manual of Tumor Nomenclature and Coding* of the American Cancer Society for histology.

The area covered by the Registry is the County of São Paulo, capital of the State of São Paulo, located at 731 m above sea level on the plateau of Serra do Mar. The climate is temperate (average annual maximum temperature 25.6° C, with a minimum of 16.1° C). The total area of São Paulo County is 1516 square kilometres or 0.6% of the total area of São Paulo State.

The population of São Paulo County in 1978 (6 856 000) accounted for 40% of the total population of São Paulo State. The population is essentially urban, with many migrant groups: Portuguese, Italian, Spanish, Japanese and others. Nearly 90% are Roman Catholics.

In the registration area of São Paulo County there are four medical schools, 30 830 beds in 199 private, official or social security hospitals (4.5 beds per 1000 inhabitants) and 18 000 physicians (2.6 physicians per 1000 inhabitants).

Population

The population has been estimated by linear interpolation using the census populations of São Paulo for 1970 and 1980 (Fundação Instituto Brasileiro de Geografica e Estadistica — IBGE).

AVERAGE ANNUAL POPULATION: 1969–1978

Age	Male	Female
0	74320	71902
1–4	276637	271168
5–9	331401	325172
10–14	299449	303240
0–14	981807	971482

Commentary

Incidence rates for all cancers were high in Fortaleza and São Paulo, both of which had high rates for lymphomas. The rates for acute lymphocytic leukaemia were rather low, except for Fortaleza, but many cases were in the 'Other and unspecified' category; the peak in incidence in the age-group 1–4 seen in many registries is less marked or absent in the Brazilian registries. The ratio of acute lymphocytic to acute non-lymphocytic leukaemia is relatively low, but again this ratio is distorted by the number of unclassified cases. The high lymphoma rate is seen particularly for non-Hodgkin lymphoma below age 10. Retinoblastoma rates are high but there is no information on laterality for any of the registries. The rates could be rather higher than those given here, since there were additional eye tumours in the 'Other and unspecified' category (12 in São Paulo, two in Recife). High incidence rates for bone tumours are found in São Paulo, and there is also a surprisingly high incidence of adrenocortical carcinoma.

Reference

Marigo, C., Muller, H. & Davies, J.N.P. (1969) Survey of cancer in children admitted to a Brazilian charity hospital. *J. natl Cancer Inst.*, 43, 1231-1240

Brazil, Fortaleza   1978 – 1980   MALE

DIAGNOSTIC GROUP	NUMBER OF CASES 0	1-4	5-9	10-14	All	REL. FREQUENCY(%) Crude	Adj.	Group	RATES PER MILLION 0	1-4	5-9	10-14	Crude	Adj.	Cum	HV(%)
TOTAL	4	32	30	37	103	100.0	100.0	100.0	67.5	145.5	113.8	176.0	136.8	138.1	2098	96.6
I. LEUKAEMIAS	2	7	8	16	33	32.0	31.0	100.0	33.7	31.8	30.4	76.1	43.8	44.3	693	100.0
Acute lymphocytic	0	5	6	10	21	20.4	19.7	63.6	16.9	22.7	22.8	47.6	27.9	28.2	443	100.0
Other lymphocytic	1	0	0	0	2	1.9	1.9	6.1				4.8	2.7	2.7	41	100.0
Acute non-lymphocytic	0	1	2	4	7	6.8	6.4	21.2		4.5	7.6	19.0	9.3	9.4	151	100.0
Chronic myeloid	0	0	0	0	0	–	–	–	–	–	–	–	–	–	–	–
Other and unspecified	1	1	0	1	3	2.9	3.0	9.1	16.9	4.5		4.8	4.0	4.1	59	100.0
II. LYMPHOMAS	0	8	14	8	30	29.1	29.4	100.0		36.4	53.1	38.0	39.8	39.4	601	100.0
Hodgkin's disease	0	2	4	1	7	6.8	7.0	23.3		9.1	15.2	4.8	9.3	9.1	136	100.0
Non-Hodgkin lymphoma	0	5	7	6	18	17.5	17.4	60.0		22.7	26.6	28.5	23.9	23.9	366	100.0
Burkitt's lymphoma	0	1	1	0	2	1.0		3.3			3.8		1.3	1.2	19	100.0
Unspecified lymphoma	0	0	2	1	3	2.9	2.8	10.0			7.6	4.8	4.0	3.8	62	100.0
Histiocytosis X	0	1	0	0	1	1.0	1.1	3.3		4.5			1.3	1.4	18	100.0
Other reticuloendothelial	0	0	0	0	0	–	–	–	–	–	–	–	–	–	–	–
III. BRAIN AND SPINAL	0	1	4	4	9	8.7	8.4	100.0		4.5	15.2	19.0	12.0	11.8	189	66.7
Ependymoma	0	0	0	0	0	–	–	–	–	–	–	–	–	–	–	–
Astrocytoma	0	0	0	1	1	1.0	0.8	11.1				4.8	1.3	1.4	24	100.0
Medulloblastoma	0	0	0	0	0	–	–	–	–	–	–	–	–	–	–	–
Other glioma	0	1	0	0	1	1.0	1.1	11.1		4.5			1.3	1.4	18	100.0
Other and unspecified *	0	0	4	3	7	6.8	6.4	77.8			15.2	14.3	9.3	9.0	147	–
IV. SYMPATHETIC N.S.	2	3	0	0	5	4.9	5.6	100.0	33.7	13.6			6.6	6.8	88	100.0
Neuroblastoma	2	3	0	0	5	4.9	5.6	100.0	33.7	13.6			6.6	6.8	88	100.0
Other	0	0	0	0	0	–	–	–	–	–	–	–	–	–	–	–
V. RETINOBLASTOMA	0	4	0	0	4	3.9	4.4	100.0		18.2			5.3	5.6	73	100.0
VI. KIDNEY	0	2	1	0	3	2.9	3.2	100.0		9.1	3.8		4.0	4.0	55	100.0
Wilms' tumour	0	2	1	0	3	2.9	3.2	100.0		9.1	3.8		4.0	4.0	55	100.0
Renal carcinoma	0	0	0	0	0	–	–	–	–	–	–	–	–	–	–	–
Other and unspecified	0	0	0	0	0	–	–	–	–	–	–	–	–	–	–	–
VII. LIVER	0	1	0	0	1	1.0	1.1	100.0		4.5			1.3	1.4	18	100.0
Hepatoblastoma	0	1	0	0	1	1.0	1.1	100.0		4.5			1.3	1.4	18	100.0
Hepatic carcinoma	0	0	0	0	0	–	–	–	–	–	–	–	–	–	–	–
Other and unspecified	0	0	0	0	0	–	–	–	–	–	–	–	–	–	–	–
VIII. BONE	0	1	1	2	4	3.9	3.7	100.0		4.5	3.8	9.5	5.3	5.4	85	75.0
Osteosarcoma	0	0	0	2	2	1.9	1.6	50.0				9.5	2.7	2.8	48	100.0
Chondrosarcoma	0	0	0	0	0	–	–	–	–	–	–	–	–	–	–	–
Ewing's sarcoma	0	0	1	0	1	1.0	1.0	25.0			3.8		1.3	1.2	19	–
Other and unspecified	0	1	0	0	1	1.0	1.1	25.0		4.5			1.3	1.4	18	100.0
IX. SOFT TISSUE SARCOMAS	0	1	1	2	4	3.9	3.7	100.0		4.5	3.8	9.5	5.3	5.4	85	100.0
Rhabdomyosarcoma	0	1	0	0	1	1.0	1.0	25.0		4.5			1.3	1.2	19	100.0
Fibrosarcoma	0	0	1	2	3	2.9	2.7	75.0			3.8	9.5	4.0	4.2	66	100.0
Other and unspecified	0	0	0	0	0	–	–	–	–	–	–	–	–	–	–	–
X. GONADAL & GERM CELL	0	0	0	0	0	–	–	–	–	–	–	–	–	–	–	–
Non-gonadal germ cell	0	0	0	0	0	–	–	–	–	–	–	–	–	–	–	–
Gonadal germ cell	0	0	0	0	0	–	–	–	–	–	–	–	–	–	–	–
Gonadal carcinoma	0	0	0	0	0	–	–	–	–	–	–	–	–	–	–	–
Other and unspecified	0	0	0	0	0	–	–	–	–	–	–	–	–	–	–	–
XI. EPITHELIAL NEOPLASMS	0	0	0	4	4	3.9	3.2	100.0				19.0	5.3	5.5	95	100.0
Adrenocortical carcinoma	0	0	0	0	0	–	–	–	–	–	–	–	–	–	–	–
Thyroid carcinoma	0	0	0	0	0	–	–	–	–	–	–	–	–	–	–	–
Nasopharyngeal carcinoma	0	0	0	0	0	–	–	–	–	–	–	–	–	–	–	–
Melanoma	0	0	0	0	0	–	–	–	–	–	–	–	–	–	–	–
Other carcinoma	0	0	0	4	4	3.9	3.2	100.0				19.0	5.3	5.5	95	100.0
XII. OTHER	0	4	1	1	6	5.8	6.3	100.0		18.2	3.8	4.8	8.0	8.2	115	50.0
* Specified as malignant	0	0	4	3	7	6.8	6.4	100.0			15.2	14.3	9.3	9.0	147	–

Brazil, Fortaleza

1978 - 1980

FEMALE

DIAGNOSTIC GROUP	NUMBER OF CASES					REL. FREQUENCY(%)			RATES PER MILLION							HV(%)
	0	1-4	5-9	10-14	All	Crude	Adj.	Group	0	1-4	5-9	10-14	Crude	Adj.	Cum	
TOTAL	6	36	27	35	104	100.0	100.0	100.0	102.3	165.7	103.7	150.1	135.2	136.3	2035	94.3
I. LEUKAEMIAS	1	8	13	9	31	29.8	30.7	100.0	17.0	36.8	50.0	38.6	40.3	40.0	607	96.2
Acute lymphocytic	0	6	10	6	22	21.2	22.0	71.0	-	27.6	38.4	25.7	28.6	28.4	431	100.0
Other lymphocytic	0	0	0	0	0	-	-	-	-	-	-	-	-	-	-	-
Acute non-lymphocytic	0	1	0	1	2	1.9	2.1	6.5	-	4.6	-	4.3	2.6	2.7	38	100.0
Chronic myeloid	0	0	1	0	1	1.0	0.9	3.2	-	-	3.8	-	1.3	1.2	21	100.0
Other and unspecified	1	1	2	2	6	5.8	5.8	19.4	17.0	4.6	7.7	8.6	7.8	7.7	117	-
II. LYMPHOMAS	0	5	5	2	12	11.5	12.0	100.0	-	23.0	19.2	8.6	15.6	15.8	231	100.0
Hodgkin's disease	0	1	2	0	3	2.9	3.2	25.0	-	4.6	7.7	-	3.9	3.9	57	100.0
Non-Hodgkin lymphoma	0	4	3	2	9	8.7	8.9	75.0	-	18.4	11.5	8.6	11.7	11.9	174	100.0
Burkitt's lymphoma	0	0	0	0	0	-	-	-	-	-	-	-	-	-	-	-
Unspecified lymphoma	0	0	0	0	0	-	-	-	-	-	-	-	-	-	-	-
Histiocytosis X	0	0	0	0	0	-	-	-	-	-	-	-	-	-	-	-
Other reticuloendothelial	0	0	0	0	0	-	-	-	-	-	-	-	-	-	-	-
III. BRAIN AND SPINAL	0	2	2	7	11	10.6	10.1	100.0	-	9.2	7.7	30.0	14.3	14.0	225	100.0
Ependymoma	0	0	0	0	0	-	-	-	-	-	-	-	-	-	-	-
Astrocytoma	0	0	0	0	0	-	-	-	-	-	-	-	-	-	-	-
Medulloblastoma	0	0	0	0	0	-	-	-	-	-	-	-	-	-	-	-
Other glioma	0	0	1	1	2	1.9	2.0	18.2	-	-	3.8	4.3	2.6	2.5	41	100.0
Other and unspecified *	0	2	1	6	9	8.7	8.2	81.8	-	9.2	3.8	25.7	11.7	11.6	185	100.0
IV. SYMPATHETIC N.S.	1	1	2	0	4	3.8	4.1	100.0	17.0	4.6	7.7	-	5.2	5.2	74	100.0
Neuroblastoma	1	1	2	0	4	3.8	4.1	100.0	17.0	4.6	7.7	-	5.2	5.2	74	100.0
Other	0	0	0	0	0	-	-	-	-	-	-	-	-	-	-	-
V. RETINOBLASTOMA	0	6	2	0	8	7.7	7.9	100.0	-	27.6	7.7	-	10.4	11.0	149	100.0
VI. KIDNEY	0	9	1	2	12	11.5	11.4	100.0	-	41.4	3.8	8.6	15.6	16.6	228	100.0
Wilms' tumour	0	9	1	2	12	11.5	11.4	100.0	-	41.4	3.8	8.6	15.6	16.6	228	100.0
Renal carcinoma	0	0	0	0	0	-	-	-	-	-	-	-	-	-	-	-
Other and unspecified	0	0	0	0	0	-	-	-	-	-	-	-	-	-	-	-
VII. LIVER	0	0	0	0	0	-	-	-	-	-	-	-	-	-	-	-
Hepatoblastoma	0	0	0	0	0	-	-	-	-	-	-	-	-	-	-	-
Hepatic carcinoma	0	0	0	0	0	-	-	-	-	-	-	-	-	-	-	-
Other and unspecified	0	0	0	0	0	-	-	-	-	-	-	-	-	-	-	-
VIII. BONE	1	0	0	6	7	6.7	6.1	100.0	-	-	-	25.7	9.1	8.8	146	85.7
Osteosarcoma	1	0	0	4	5	4.8	4.4	71.4	-	-	-	17.2	6.5	6.3	103	100.0
Chondrosarcoma	0	0	0	0	0	-	-	-	-	-	-	-	-	-	-	-
Ewing's sarcoma	0	0	0	2	2	1.9	1.7	28.6	-	-	-	8.6	2.6	2.5	43	50.0
Other and unspecified	0	0	0	0	0	-	-	-	-	-	-	-	-	-	-	-
IX. SOFT TISSUE SARCOMAS	0	0	0	5	5	4.8	4.3	100.0	-	-	-	21.4	6.5	6.2	107	100.0
Rhabdomyosarcoma	0	0	0	1	1	1.0	0.9	20.0	-	-	-	4.3	1.3	1.2	21	100.0
Fibrosarcoma	0	0	0	4	4	3.8	3.4	80.0	-	-	-	17.2	5.2	5.0	86	100.0
Other and unspecified	0	0	0	0	0	-	-	-	-	-	-	-	-	-	-	-
X. GONADAL & GERM CELL	0	4	2	1	7	6.7	6.9	100.0	-	18.4	7.7	4.3	9.1	9.4	134	100.0
Non-gonadal germ cell	0	2	2	1	5	4.8	5.0	71.4	-	9.2	7.7	4.3	6.5	6.6	97	100.0
Gonadal germ cell	0	1	0	0	1	1.0	1.0	14.3	-	4.6	-	-	1.3	1.4	18	100.0
Gonadal carcinoma	0	1	0	0	1	1.0	1.0	14.3	-	4.6	-	-	1.3	1.4	18	100.0
Other and unspecified	0	0	0	0	0	-	-	-	-	-	-	-	-	-	-	-
XI. EPITHELIAL NEOPLASMS	0	0	0	1	1	1.0	0.9	100.0	-	-	-	4.3	1.3	1.2	21	100.0
Adrenocortical carcinoma	0	0	0	0	0	-	-	-	-	-	-	-	-	-	-	-
Thyroid carcinoma	0	0	0	0	0	-	-	-	-	-	-	-	-	-	-	-
Nasopharyngeal carcinoma	0	0	0	0	0	-	-	-	-	-	-	-	-	-	-	-
Melanoma	0	0	0	0	0	-	-	-	-	-	-	-	-	-	-	-
Other carcinoma	0	0	0	1	1	1.0	0.9	100.0	-	-	-	4.3	1.3	1.2	21	100.0
XII. OTHER	3	1	0	2	6	5.8	5.5	100.0	51.1	4.6	-	8.6	7.8	7.9	112	-
* Specified as malignant	0	2	1	6	9	8.7	8.2	100.0	-	9.2	3.8	25.7	11.7	11.6	185	-

Brazil, Recife   MALE

1967 – 1979

DIAGNOSTIC GROUP	NUMBER OF CASES 0	1-4	5-9	10-14	All	REL. FREQUENCY(%) Crude	Adj.	Group	RATES PER MILLION 0-4	5-9	10-14	Crude	Adj.	Cum	HV(%)
TOTAL	19	96	107	81	303	100.0	100.0	100.0	112.8	109.6	96.1	106.8	106.9	1593	96.0
I. LEUKAEMIAS	3	29	27	20	79	26.1	26.1	100.0	31.4	27.7	23.7	27.8	28.0	414	100.0
Acute lymphocytic	1	10	11	4	26	8.6	8.4	32.9	10.8	11.3	4.7	9.2	9.2	134	100.0
Other lymphocytic	0	1	2	2	5	1.7	1.6	6.3	1.0	2.0	2.4	1.8	1.7	27	100.0
Acute non-lymphocytic	0	1	2	5	8	2.6	2.8	10.1	1.0	2.0	5.9	2.8	2.8	45	100.0
Chronic myeloid	0	0	0	1	1	0.3	0.4	1.3	-	-	1.2	0.4	0.3	6	100.0
Other and unspecified	2	17	12	8	39	12.9	12.9	49.4	18.6	12.3	9.5	13.7	13.9	202	100.0
II. LYMPHOMAS	2	13	27	17	59	19.5	19.1	100.0	14.7	27.7	20.2	20.8	20.5	313	98.3
Hodgkin's disease	1	0	12	10	23	7.6	7.4	39.0	1.0	12.3	11.9	8.1	7.8	126	100.0
Non-Hodgkin lymphoma	0	10	14	4	28	9.2	8.9	47.5	9.8	14.3	4.7	9.9	9.8	145	100.0
Burkitt's lymphoma	0	0	0	0	0	-	-	-	-	-	-	-	-	-	-
Unspecified lymphoma	1	3	1	2	7	2.3	2.4	11.9	3.9	1.0	2.4	2.5	2.5	37	85.7
Histiocytosis X	0	0	0	0	0	-	-	-	-	-	-	-	-	-	-
Other reticuloendothelial	0	0	0	1	1	0.3	0.4	1.7	-	-	1.2	0.4	0.3	6	100.0
III. BRAIN AND SPINAL	1	11	21	13	46	15.2	14.9	100.0	11.8	21.5	15.4	16.2	16.0	244	89.1
Ependymoma	0	0	2	2	4	1.3	1.3	8.7	-	2.0	2.4	1.4	1.4	22	100.0
Astrocytoma	0	3	6	3	12	4.0	3.8	26.1	2.9	6.1	3.6	4.2	4.2	63	100.0
Medulloblastoma	0	3	4	6	13	4.3	4.4	28.3	2.9	4.1	7.1	4.6	4.5	71	100.0
Other glioma	0	0	1	0	1	0.3	0.3	2.2	-	1.0	-	0.4	0.5	5	100.0
Other and unspecified *	1	5	8	2	16	5.3	5.1	34.8	5.9	8.2	2.4	5.6	5.6	82	68.8
IV. SYMPATHETIC N.S.	2	10	6	1	19	6.3	6.2	100.0	11.8	6.1	1.2	6.7	6.9	96	100.0
Neuroblastoma	2	10	6	1	19	6.3	6.2	100.0	11.8	6.1	1.2	6.7	6.9	96	100.0
Other	0	0	0	0	0	-	-	-	-	-	-	-	-	-	-
V. RETINOBLASTOMA	2	10	3	0	15	5.0	5.0	100.0	11.8	3.1	-	5.3	5.5	74	100.0
VI. KIDNEY	2	7	3	1	13	4.3	4.3	100.0	8.8	3.1	1.2	4.6	4.8	65	100.0
Wilms' tumour	2	7	3	0	12	4.0	4.0	92.3	8.8	3.1	-	4.2	4.4	60	100.0
Renal carcinoma	0	0	0	1	1	0.3	0.4	7.7	-	-	1.2	0.4	0.3	6	100.0
Other and unspecified	0	0	0	0	0	-	-	-	-	-	-	-	-	-	-
VII. LIVER	1	1	0	0	2	0.7	0.7	100.0	2.0	-	-	0.7	0.8	10	100.0
Hepatoblastoma	0	1	0	0	1	0.3	0.3	50.0	1.0	-	-	0.4	0.4	5	100.0
Hepatic carcinoma	1	0	0	0	1	0.3	0.3	50.0	1.0	-	-	0.4	0.4	5	100.0
Other and unspecified	0	0	0	0	0	-	-	-	-	-	-	-	-	-	-
VIII. BONE	0	1	3	5	9	3.0	3.0	100.0	1.0	3.1	5.9	3.2	3.1	50	100.0
Osteosarcoma	0	0	2	1	3	1.0	0.9	33.3	-	2.0	1.2	1.1	1.0	16	100.0
Chondrosarcoma	0	0	0	2	2	0.7	0.7	22.2	-	-	2.4	0.7	0.7	12	100.0
Ewing's sarcoma	0	0	1	2	3	1.0	1.0	33.3	-	1.0	2.4	1.1	1.0	17	100.0
Other and unspecified	0	1	0	0	1	0.3	0.3	11.1	1.0	-	-	0.4	0.4	5	100.0
IX. SOFT TISSUE SARCOMAS	1	6	4	11	22	7.3	7.6	100.0	6.9	4.1	13.1	7.8	7.8	120	100.0
Rhabdomyosarcoma	1	3	3	0	7	2.3	2.2	31.8	3.9	3.1	-	2.5	2.5	35	100.0
Fibrosarcoma	0	0	0	3	3	1.1	1.1	13.6	-	-	3.6	1.1	1.0	18	100.0
Other and unspecified	0	3	1	8	12	4.0	4.3	54.5	2.9	1.0	9.5	4.2	4.2	67	100.0
X. GONADAL & GERM CELL	2	1	0	0	3	1.0	1.0	100.0	2.9	-	-	1.1	1.1	15	100.0
Non-gonadal germ cell	1	1	0	0	2	0.7	0.7	66.7	2.0	-	-	0.7	0.8	10	100.0
Gonadal germ cell	0	0	0	0	0	-	-	-	-	-	-	-	-	-	-
Gonadal carcinoma	0	0	0	0	0	-	-	-	-	-	-	-	-	-	-
Other and unspecified	1	0	0	0	1	0.3	0.3	33.3	1.0	-	-	0.4	0.3	5	100.0
XI. EPITHELIAL NEOPLASMS	0	2	7	5	14	4.6	4.5	100.0	2.0	7.2	5.9	4.9	4.8	75	100.0
Adrenocortical carcinoma	0	0	0	0	0	-	-	-	-	-	-	-	-	-	-
Thyroid carcinoma	0	0	0	0	0	-	-	-	-	-	-	-	-	-	-
Nasopharyngeal carcinoma	0	0	0	0	0	-	-	-	-	-	-	-	-	-	-
Melanoma	0	0	1	0	1	0.3	0.3	7.1	-	1.0	-	0.4	0.3	5	100.0
Other carcinoma	0	2	6	5	13	4.3	4.2	92.9	2.0	6.1	5.9	4.6	4.5	70	100.0
XII. OTHER	3	5	6	8	22	7.3	7.4	100.0	7.8	6.1	9.5	7.8	7.8	117	72.7
* Specified as malignant	1	5	7	1	14	4.6	4.4	100.0	5.9	7.2	1.2	4.9	4.9	71	64.3

Brazil, Recife   1967 – 1979   FEMALE

DIAGNOSTIC GROUP	NUMBER OF CASES					REL. FREQUENCY(%)			RATES PER MILLION					Cum	HV(%)
	0	1-4	5-9	10-14	All	Crude	Adj.	Group	0-4	5-9	10-14	Crude	Adj.		
TOTAL	17	90	88	104	299	100.0	100.0	100.0	108.2	91.1	116.9	105.1	105.2	1581	93.6
I. LEUKAEMIAS	2	25	15	22	64	21.4	21.6	100.0	27.3	15.5	24.7	22.5	22.8	338	100.0
Acute lymphocytic	0	7	9	5	21	7.0	7.1	32.8	7.1	9.3	5.6	7.4	7.4	110	100.0
Other lymphocytic	0	2	1	0	3	1.0	1.1	4.7	2.0	1.0	-	1.1	1.1	15	100.0
Acute non-lymphocytic	0	2	1	2	5	1.7	1.7	7.8	2.0	1.0	2.2	1.8	1.8	27	100.0
Chronic myeloid	0	0	0	0	0	-	-	-	-	-	-	-	-	-	-
Other and unspecified	2	14	4	15	35	11.7	11.7	54.7	16.2	4.1	16.9	12.3	12.5	186	100.0
II. LYMPHOMAS	1	7	15	15	38	12.7	12.4	100.0	8.1	15.5	16.9	13.4	13.0	202	100.0
Hodgkin's disease	0	0	5	8	13	4.3	4.0	34.2	-	5.2	9.0	4.6	4.3	71	100.0
Non-Hodgkin lymphoma	1	4	7	6	18	6.0	6.0	47.4	5.1	7.2	6.7	6.3	6.3	95	100.0
Burkitt's lymphoma	0	0	0	0	0	-	-	-	-	-	-	-	-	-	-
Unspecified lymphoma	0	3	2	1	6	2.0	2.1	15.8	3.0	2.1	1.1	2.1	2.2	31	100.0
Histiocytosis X	0	0	0	0	0	-	-	-	-	-	-	-	-	-	-
Other reticuloendothelial	0	0	1	0	1	0.3	0.3	2.6	-	1.0	-	0.4	0.3	5	100.0
III. BRAIN AND SPINAL	1	10	18	13	42	14.0	14.0	100.0	11.1	18.6	14.6	14.8	14.6	222	83.3
Ependymoma	0	1	4	0	5	1.7	1.7	11.9	1.0	4.1	-	1.8	1.7	26	100.0
Astrocytoma	0	2	6	5	13	4.3	4.2	31.0	2.0	6.2	5.6	4.6	4.4	69	100.0
Medulloblastoma	0	2	4	1	7	2.3	2.4	16.7	2.0	4.1	1.1	2.5	2.4	36	100.0
Other glioma	0	0	0	0	0	-	-	-	-	-	-	-	-	-	-
Other and unspecified *	1	5	4	7	17	5.7	5.6	40.5	6.1	4.1	7.9	6.0	6.0	90	58.8
IV. SYMPATHETIC N.S.	1	7	4	3	15	5.0	5.2	100.0	8.1	4.1	3.4	5.3	5.4	78	100.0
Neuroblastoma	1	7	4	3	15	5.0	5.2	100.0	8.1	4.1	3.4	5.3	5.4	78	100.0
Other	0	0	0	0	0	-	-	-	-	-	-	-	-	-	-
V. RETINOBLASTOMA	1	9	2	0	12	4.0	4.4	100.0	10.1	2.1	-	4.2	4.6	61	100.0
VI. KIDNEY	3	16	4	2	25	8.4	9.0	100.0	19.2	4.1	2.2	8.8	9.4	128	92.0
Wilms' tumour	3	14	4	0	21	7.0	7.7	84.0	17.2	4.1	-	7.4	8.0	107	95.2
Renal carcinoma	0	0	0	2	2	0.7	0.6	8.0	-	-	2.2	0.7	0.7	11	100.0
Other and unspecified	0	2	0	0	2	0.7	0.7	8.0	2.0	-	-	0.7	0.8	10	50.0
VII. LIVER	1	1	0	1	3	1.0	1.0	100.0	2.0	-	1.1	1.1	1.1	16	100.0
Hepatoblastoma	1	1	0	0	2	0.7	0.7	66.7	2.0	-	-	0.7	0.8	10	100.0
Hepatic carcinoma	0	0	0	0	0	-	-	-	-	-	-	-	-	-	-
Other and unspecified	0	0	0	1	1	0.3	0.3	33.3	-	-	1.1	0.4	0.3	6	100.0
VIII. BONE	0	0	6	15	21	7.0	6.4	100.0	-	6.2	16.9	7.4	6.9	115	95.2
Osteosarcoma	0	0	3	10	13	4.3	3.9	61.9	-	3.1	11.2	4.6	4.3	72	92.3
Chondrosarcoma	0	0	1	0	1	0.3	0.3	4.8	-	1.0	-	0.4	0.3	5	100.0
Ewing's sarcoma	0	0	2	4	6	2.0	1.8	28.6	-	2.1	4.5	2.1	2.0	33	100.0
Other and unspecified	0	0	0	1	1	0.3	0.3	4.8	-	-	1.1	0.4	0.3	6	100.0
IX. SOFT TISSUE SARCOMAS	3	5	4	7	19	6.4	6.4	100.0	8.1	4.1	7.9	6.7	6.8	100	94.7
Rhabdomyosarcoma	2	3	1	2	8	2.7	2.8	42.1	5.1	1.0	2.2	2.8	2.7	42	100.0
Fibrosarcoma	0	1	1	1	3	1.0	0.6	10.5	-	1.0	1.1	0.7	0.7	11	100.0
Other and unspecified	1	2	2	4	9	3.0	3.0	47.4	3.0	2.1	4.5	3.2	3.1	48	88.9
X. GONADAL & GERM CELL	1	2	3	6	12	4.0	3.9	100.0	3.0	3.1	6.7	4.2	4.1	64	91.7
Non-gonadal germ cell	1	2	0	0	3	1.0	1.1	25.0	3.0	-	-	1.1	1.2	15	100.0
Gonadal germ cell	0	0	2	1	3	1.0	1.0	25.0	-	2.1	1.1	1.1	1.0	16	100.0
Gonadal carcinoma	0	0	1	2	3	1.0	1.0	25.0	-	1.0	2.2	1.1	1.0	16	100.0
Other and unspecified	0	0	0	3	3	1.0	0.9	25.0	-	-	3.4	1.1	1.0	17	66.7
XI. EPITHELIAL NEOPLASMS	1	4	10	12	27	9.0	8.7	100.0	5.1	10.4	13.5	9.5	9.2	144	96.3
Adrenocortical carcinoma	0	0	1	0	1	0.3	0.3	3.7	-	1.0	-	0.4	0.3	5	100.0
Thyroid carcinoma	0	0	2	2	4	1.3	1.3	14.8	-	2.1	2.2	1.4	1.3	22	100.0
Nasopharyngeal carcinoma	0	0	0	0	0	-	-	-	-	-	-	-	-	-	-
Melanoma	0	0	0	0	0	-	-	-	-	-	-	-	-	-	-
Other carcinoma	1	4	7	10	22	7.4	7.1	81.5	5.1	7.2	11.2	7.7	7.6	118	95.5
XII. OTHER	2	4	7	8	21	7.0	6.9	100.0	6.1	7.2	9.0	7.4	7.3	112	71.4
* Specified as malignant	1	5	4	6	16	5.4	5.3	100.0	6.1	4.1	6.7	5.6	5.6	85	56.3

Brazil, Sao Paulo

1969 – 1978　　　　　　　　MALE

DIAGNOSTIC GROUP	NUMBER OF CASES					REL. FREQUENCY(%)			RATES PER MILLION						Cum	HV(%)
	0	1-4	5-9	10-14	All	Crude	Adj.	Group	0	1-4	5-9	10-14	Crude	Adj.		
TOTAL	106	591	490	404	1594¤	100.0	100.0	100.0	142.6	213.6	147.9	134.9	162.4	164.1	2411	79.8
I. LEUKAEMIAS	17	151	111	84	363	22.8	22.7	100.0	22.9	54.6	33.5	28.1	37.0	37.6	549	60.6
Acute lymphocytic	5	64	55	30	154	9.7	9.6	42.4	6.7	23.1	16.6	10.0	15.7	15.9	232	62.3
Other lymphocytic	2	10	5	6	23	1.4	1.4	6.3	2.7	3.6	1.5	2.0	2.3	2.4	35	65.2
Acute non-lymphocytic	4	20	22	21	67	4.2	4.3	18.5	5.4	7.2	6.6	7.0	6.8	6.8	103	64.2
Chronic myeloid	1	3	1	4	9	0.6	0.6	2.5	1.3	1.1	0.3	1.3	0.9	0.9	14	77.8
Other and unspecified	5	54	28	23	110	6.9	6.8	30.3	6.7	19.5	8.4	7.7	11.2	11.5	165	53.6
II. LYMPHOMAS	5	110	152	112	379	23.8	24.2	100.0	6.7	39.8	45.9	37.4	38.6	38.5	582	98.4
Hodgkin's disease	0	21	55	47	123	7.7	8.1	32.5	–	7.6	16.6	15.7	12.5	12.3	192	96.7
Non-Hodgkin lymphoma	3	79	87	52	221	13.9	13.9	58.3	4.0	28.6	26.3	17.4	22.5	22.7	336	99.5
Burkitt's lymphoma	1	2	3	2	8	0.5	0.5	2.1	1.3	0.7	0.9	0.7	0.8	0.8	12	100.0
Unspecified lymphoma	1	7	6	11	25	1.6	1.6	6.6	1.3	2.5	1.8	3.7	2.5	2.5	39	96.0
Histiocytosis X	0	0	1	0		–	–	–	–	–	–	–	–	–	–	–
Other reticuloendothelial	0	1	0	0	2	0.1	0.1	0.5	–	0.4	–	–	0.2	0.2	3	100.0
III. BRAIN AND SPINAL	9	58	83	65	215	13.5	13.8	100.0	12.1	21.0	25.0	21.7	21.9	21.8	330	63.3
Ependymoma	0	6	6	8	20	1.3	1.3	9.3	–	2.2	1.8	2.7	2.0	2.0	31	100.0
Astrocytoma	0	11	25	14	50	3.1	3.0	23.3	–	4.0	7.5	4.7	5.1	5.0	77	100.0
Medulloblastoma	1	18	18	11	48	3.0	3.0	23.3	1.3	6.5	5.4	3.7	4.9	4.9	73	100.0
Other glioma	0	1	4	2	7	0.4	0.5	3.3	–	0.4	1.2	0.7	0.7	0.7	11	100.0
Other and unspecified *	8	22	30	30	90	5.6	5.8	41.9	10.8	8.0	9.1	10.0	9.2	9.1	138	12.2
IV. SYMPATHETIC N.S.	7	45	25	8	86¤	5.4	5.1	100.0	9.4	16.3	7.5	2.7	8.8	9.0	126	98.8
Neuroblastoma	7	45	25	8	86¤	5.4	5.1	100.0	9.4	16.3	7.5	2.7	8.8	9.0	126	98.8
Other	0	0	0	0	0	–	–	–	–	–	–	–	–	–	–	–
V. RETINOBLASTOMA	5	38	7	0	51¤	3.2	2.9	100.0	6.7	13.7	2.1	–	5.2	5.5	72	100.0
VI. KIDNEY	14	50	19	3	87¤	5.5	5.1	100.0	18.8	18.1	5.7	1.0	8.9	9.2	125	83.9
Wilms' tumour	10	38	15	2	66¤	4.1	3.8	75.9	13.5	13.7	4.5	0.7	6.7	6.9	94	100.0
Renal carcinoma	2	4	0	0	6	0.4	0.3	6.9	2.7	1.4	–	–	0.6	0.7	8	100.0
Other and unspecified	2	8	4	1	15	0.9	0.9	17.2	2.7	2.9	1.2	0.3	1.5	1.6	22	6.7
VII. LIVER	5	9	2	3	19	1.2	1.1	100.0	6.7	3.3	0.6	1.0	1.9	2.0	28	89.5
Hepatoblastoma	2	4	2	0	8	0.5	0.5	42.1	2.7	1.4	0.6	–	0.8	0.9	11	100.0
Hepatic carcinoma	2	4	0	3	9	0.6	0.6	47.4	2.7	1.4	–	1.0	0.9	0.9	13	100.0
Other and unspecified	1	1	0	0	2	0.1	0.1	10.5	1.3	0.4	–	–	0.2	0.2	3	–
VIII. BONE	0	6	19	63	88	5.5	6.2	100.0	–	2.2	5.7	21.0	9.0	8.6	143	93.2
Osteosarcoma	0	1	9	33	43	2.7	3.1	48.9	–	0.4	2.7	11.0	4.4	4.2	70	100.0
Chondrosarcoma	0	0	2	1	3	0.2	0.2	3.4	–	–	0.6	0.3	0.3	0.3	5	100.0
Ewing's sarcoma	0	3	8	23	34	2.1	2.4	38.6	–	1.1	2.4	7.7	3.5	3.3	55	100.0
Other and unspecified	0	1	2	5	8	0.5	0.6	9.1	–	0.4	0.6	1.7	0.8	0.8	13	25.0
IX. SOFT TISSUE SARCOMAS	13	36	22	20	91	5.7	5.6	100.0	17.5	13.0	6.6	6.7	9.3	9.5	136	100.0
Rhabdomyosarcoma	5	16	10	3	34	2.1	2.0	37.4	6.7	5.8	3.0	1.0	3.5	3.6	50	100.0
Fibrosarcoma	3	9	3	4	19	1.2	1.2	20.9	4.0	3.3	0.9	1.3	1.9	2.0	28	100.0
Other and unspecified	5	11	9	13	38	2.4	2.4	41.8	6.7	4.0	2.7	4.3	3.9	3.9	58	100.0
X. GONADAL & GERM CELL	11	32	3	4	50	3.1	2.9	100.0	14.8	11.6	0.9	1.3	5.1	5.4	72	90.0
Non-gonadal germ cell	5	5	1	3	14	0.9	0.9	28.0	6.7	1.8	0.3	1.0	1.4	1.5	20	100.0
Gonadal germ cell	4	14	0	0	18	1.1	1.0	36.0	5.4	5.1	–	–	1.8	2.0	26	100.0
Gonadal carcinoma	1	4	1	1	7	0.4	0.4	14.0	1.3	1.4	0.3	0.3	0.7	0.7	10	100.0
Other and unspecified	1	9	1	0	11	0.7	0.6	22.0	1.3	3.3	0.3	–	1.1	1.2	16	54.5
XI. EPITHELIAL NEOPLASMS	3	30	22	23	78	4.9	4.9	100.0	4.0	10.8	6.6	7.7	7.9	8.0	119	100.0
Adrenocortical carcinoma	0	5	2	3	10	0.6	0.6	12.8	–	1.8	0.6	1.0	1.0	1.0	15	100.0
Thyroid carcinoma	0	0	0	1	1	0.1	0.1	1.3	–	–	–	0.3	0.1	0.1	3	100.0
Nasopharyngeal carcinoma	0	0	1	2	2	0.1	0.1	2.6	–	–	0.3	0.7	0.2	0.2	3	100.0
Melanoma	0	3	2	1	6	0.4	0.4	7.7	–	1.1	0.6	0.3	0.6	0.6	9	100.0
Other carcinoma	3	22	18	16	59	3.7	3.7	75.6	4.0	8.0	5.4	5.3	6.0	6.1	90	100.0
XII. OTHER	17	26	25	19	87	5.5	5.4	100.0	22.9	9.4	7.5	6.3	8.9	9.0	130	24.1
* Specified as malignant	8	22	26	27	83	5.2	5.3	100.0	10.8	8.0	7.8	9.0	8.5	8.4	127	4.8

¤ Includes age unknown

Brazil, Sao Paulo

1969 - 1978

FEMALE

Column groups: **NUMBER OF CASES** (0, 1-4, 5-9, 10-14, All) · **REL. FREQUENCY (%)** (Crude, Adj., Group) · **RATES PER MILLION** (0, 1-4, 5-9, 10-14, Crude, Adj., Cum) · **HV (%)**

DIAGNOSTIC GROUP	0	1-4	5-9	10-14	All	Crude	Adj.	Group	0	1-4	5-9	10-14	Crude	Adj.	Cum	HV(%)
TOTAL	79	463	316	352	1212¤	100.0	100.0	100.0	109.9	170.7	97.2	116.1	124.8	126.4	1859	78.3
I. LEUKAEMIAS	17	114	79	70	280	23.1	23.1	100.0	23.6	42.0	24.3	23.1	28.8	29.4	429	65.4
Acute lymphocytic	6	46	36	31	119	9.8	9.9	42.5	8.3	17.0	11.1	10.2	12.2	12.4	183	64.7
Other lymphocytic	2	10	10	3	25	2.1	2.1	8.9	2.8	3.7	3.1	1.0	2.6	2.6	38	84.0
Acute non-lymphocytic	1	18	14	14	47	3.9	3.9	16.8	1.4	6.6	4.3	4.6	4.8	4.9	73	68.1
Chronic myeloid	0	2	0	1	3	0.2	0.2	1.1	-	0.7	-	0.3	0.3	0.3	5	100.0
Other and unspecified	8	38	19	21	86	7.1	7.0	30.7	11.1	14.0	5.8	6.9	8.9	9.1	131	58.1
II. LYMPHOMAS	4	65	58	61	188	15.5	15.8	100.0	5.6	24.0	17.8	20.1	19.4	19.4	291	97.3
Hodgkin's disease	0	7	16	27	50	4.1	4.3	26.6	-	2.6	4.6	8.9	5.1	5.0	79	100.0
Non-Hodgkin lymphoma	3	49	37	30	119	9.8	9.3	63.3	4.2	18.1	11.4	9.9	12.2	12.5	183	98.3
Burkitt's lymphoma	0	0	1	0	1	0.1	0.1	0.5	-	-	0.3	-	0.1	0.1	2	100.0
Unspecified lymphoma	1	8	3	4	16	1.3	1.3	8.5	1.4	3.0	0.9	1.3	1.6	1.7	24	81.3
Histiocytosis X	0	0	0	0	0	-	-	-	-	-	-	-	-	-	-	-
Other reticuloendothelial	0	1	1	0	2	0.2	0.2	1.1	-	0.4	0.3	-	0.2	0.2	3	100.0
III. BRAIN AND SPINAL	8	59	68	70	205	16.9	17.4	100.0	11.1	21.8	20.9	23.1	21.1	21.0	318	53.7
Ependymoma	0	5	5	1	11	0.9	0.9	5.4	-	1.8	1.5	1.6	1.1	1.1	17	100.0
Astrocytoma	1	10	15	17	43	3.5	3.7	21.0	1.4	3.7	4.6	5.6	4.4	4.4	67	100.0
Medulloblastoma	1	8	19	9	37	3.1	3.2	18.0	1.4	3.0	5.8	3.0	3.8	3.8	57	100.0
Other glioma	2	4	4	2	12	1.0	1.0	5.9	2.8	1.5	1.2	1.3	1.2	1.3	18	100.0
Other and unspecified *	4	32	31	35	102	8.4	8.6	49.8	5.6	11.8	9.5	11.5	10.5	10.5	158	6.9
IV. SYMPATHETIC N.S.	13	31	15	2	62¤	5.1	4.8	100.0	18.1	11.4	4.6	0.7	6.4	6.6	90	100.0
Neuroblastoma	13	31	15	1	61¤	5.0	4.8	98.4	18.1	11.4	4.6	0.3	6.3	6.5	89	100.0
Other	0	0	0	1	1	0.1	0.2	1.6	-	-	-	0.3	0.1	0.2	2	100.0
V. RETINOBLASTOMA	3	47	3	3	57¤	4.7	4.2	100.0	4.2	17.3	0.9	1.0	5.9	6.3	83	100.0
VI. KIDNEY	11	47	20	7	85	7.0	6.8	100.0	15.3	17.3	6.2	2.3	8.7	9.2	127	87.1
Wilms' tumour	8	40	16	4	68	5.6	5.4	80.0	11.1	14.8	4.9	1.3	7.0	7.4	101	100.0
Renal carcinoma	0	0	1	3	4	0.3	0.4	4.7	-	-	0.3	1.0	0.4	0.4	6	100.0
Other and unspecified	3	7	3	0	13	1.1	1.0	15.3	4.2	2.6	0.9	-	1.3	1.4	19	15.4
VII. LIVER	1	1	0	1	3	0.2	0.2	100.0	1.4	0.4	-	0.3	0.3	0.3	5	100.0
Hepatoblastoma	1	1	0	0	2	0.1	0.1	33.3	1.4	0.4	-	-	0.1	0.1	1	100.0
Hepatic carcinoma	0	0	0	1	1	0.2	0.2	66.7	-	-	-	0.3	0.2	0.2	3	100.0
Other and unspecified	0	0	0	0	0	-	-	-	-	-	-	-	-	-	-	-
VIII. BONE	1	6	14	47	68	5.6	5.9	100.0	1.4	2.2	4.3	15.5	7.0	6.7	109	89.7
Osteosarcoma	0	2	5	31	38	3.1	3.3	55.9	-	0.7	1.5	10.2	3.9	3.7	62	100.0
Chondrosarcoma	0	0	0	5	5	0.4	0.3	7.4	-	-	-	1.6	0.5	0.5	8	100.0
Ewing's sarcoma	0	2	8	6	16	1.3	1.4	23.5	-	0.7	2.5	2.0	1.6	1.6	25	100.0
Other and unspecified	1	2	1	5	9	0.7	0.9	13.2	1.4	0.7	0.3	1.6	0.9	0.9	14	22.2
IX. SOFT TISSUE SARCOMAS	2	25	10	26	63	5.2	5.2	100.0	2.8	9.2	3.1	8.6	6.5	6.6	98	100.0
Rhabdomyosarcoma	0	16	5	4	25	2.1	2.0	39.7	-	5.9	1.5	1.3	2.6	2.7	38	100.0
Fibrosarcoma	0	4	2	8	14	1.2	1.1	22.2	-	1.5	0.6	2.6	1.4	1.4	22	100.0
Other and unspecified	2	5	3	14	24	2.0	2.0	38.1	2.8	1.8	0.9	4.6	2.5	2.4	38	100.0
X. GONADAL & GERM CELL	3	15	10	17	45	3.7	3.7	100.0	4.2	5.5	3.1	5.6	4.6	4.7	70	91.1
Non-gonadal germ cell	2	11	0	1	14	1.2	1.0	31.1	2.8	4.1	-	0.3	1.4	1.6	21	100.0
Gonadal germ cell	0	1	8	8	17	1.2	1.5	37.8	-	0.4	2.5	2.6	1.7	1.7	27	100.0
Gonadal carcinoma	0	2	2	5	9	0.7	0.7	20.0	-	0.7	0.6	1.6	0.9	0.9	14	100.0
Other and unspecified	1	1	0	3	5	0.4	0.4	11.1	1.4	0.4	-	1.0	0.5	0.5	8	20.0
XI. EPITHELIAL NEOPLASMS	9	28	23	29	89	7.3	7.4	100.0	12.5	10.3	7.1	9.6	9.2	9.2	137	100.0
Adrenocortical carcinoma	3	13	2	0	18	1.5	1.4	20.2	4.2	4.8	0.6	-	1.9	2.0	26	100.0
Thyroid carcinoma	0	0	3	4	7	0.6	0.6	7.9	-	-	0.9	1.3	0.7	0.7	11	100.0
Nasopharyngeal carcinoma	0	0	1	1	2	0.2	0.2	2.2	-	-	0.3	0.3	0.3	0.2	3	100.0
Melanoma	0	0	0	7	7	0.6	0.6	7.9	-	-	-	2.3	0.7	0.7	12	100.0
Other carcinoma	6	15	17	17	55	4.5	4.6	61.8	8.3	5.5	5.2	5.6	5.7	5.7	85	100.0
XII. OTHER	7	25	16	19	67	5.5	5.5	100.0	9.7	9.2	4.9	6.3	6.9	7.0	103	34.3
	3	32	30	33	98	8.1	8.2		4.2	11.8	9.2	10.9	10.1	10.1	152	3.1

* Specified as malignant
¤ Includes age unknown

COLOMBIA

Cali Cancer Registry, 1977–1981

C. Cuello

The Registry has been in continuous operation since 1962. It is located in the Department of Pathology of the Medical School in the Universidad del Valle. The staff includes a Director, who is the professor of pathology, an experienced records officer, a statistician and three record clerks.

Case reports are received routinely from the major hospitals and pathology laboratories, and from the X-ray, haematology and radiotherapy departments mainly through the secretarial and clerical staff. Once a year, to supplement these data, a field survey of all sources of cases (including private physicians) is made by a group of medical students given special training for this work. Every month information from death certificates is obtained from the Municipal Office of Vital Statistics, to check against cancer registrations. Data are not recorded for all deaths during the period but deaths with mention of cancer that have not been previously registered are traced through the certifying doctor for further details. For sites such as pancreas and liver, surgical or pathological evidence is required before inclusion on the register. Doubtful cases are either excluded, or described as site unspecified. There is no follow-up of cases, on grounds of cost.

Site and histology are coded according to ICD-O. A computer-based system is in process of being established. Data are stored on tape and duplicate entries are identified manually and by computer. Subsequent primaries in the same patient are registered.

In 1985, Cali had 2070 hospital beds and 1400 medical practitioners. The Registry is population-based and covers the urban area of the city, between the Cauca River to the east and the chain of the Andes to the west. The city is 1000 m above sea level. The total registration area is 98.4 square kilometres. The great majority of the people are mestizos (mixture of Spanish and Indian). There is a minority of pure negroes and whites. More than half of the population are migrants from other areas of Colombia and from other countries, mainly Lebanon, Italy, Germany and Central Europe.

From information on family income, the census tracts (neighbourhoods) have been assigned to one of four socioeconomic classes. This system of classification of the population at risk makes it feasible to calculate and present incidence rates by socioeconomic class.

Registry data have been used to obtain cancer incidence rates for the city of Cali, and for sub-groups of the population defined by birthplace and social class, etc. They have also been used for case-control studies of etiological factors and for the investigation of precursor lesions.

Population

The population is an estimate for mid-1979, prepared from a linear projection, by age and sex, of the 1964 and 1973 census figures (Departamento Administrario Nacional de Estadistica).

AVERAGE ANNUAL POPULATION: 1977–1981

Age	Male	Female
0–4	68453	67373
5–9	74071	73861
10–14	73853	76411
0–14	216377	217645

Commentary

Few of the rates observed in this registry were remarkable. The rate for Burkitt's lymphoma is one of the highest for a non-African population but is based on only 12 cases, all occurring in boys.

Colombia, Cali   1977 - 1981   MALE

DIAGNOSTIC GROUP	NUMBER OF CASES 0	1-4	5-9	10-14	All	REL. FREQUENCY(%) Crude	Adj.	Group	RATES PER MILLION 0-4	5-9	10-14	Crude	Adj.	Cum	HV(%)
TOTAL	4	50	45	38	137	100.0	100.0	100.0	157.8	121.5	102.9	126.6	130.1	1911	96.1
I. LEUKAEMIAS	3	22	14	16	55	40.1	40.5	100.0	73.0	37.8	43.3	50.8	53.0	771	100.0
Acute lymphocytic	2	18	10	11	41	29.9	30.2	74.5	58.4	27.0	29.8	37.9	40.0	576	100.0
Other lymphocytic	0	0	0	0	0										-
Acute non-lymphocytic	0	0	2	1	3	2.2	2.1	5.5	-	5.4	2.7	2.8	2.5	41	100.0
Chronic myeloid	0	1	0	1	2	1.5	1.5	3.6	2.9	-	2.7	1.8	1.9	28	100.0
Other and unspecified	1	3	2	3	9	6.6	6.7	16.4	11.7	5.4	8.1	8.3	8.6	126	100.0
II. LYMPHOMAS	0	8	15	6	29	21.2	20.7	100.0	23.4	40.5	16.2	26.8	26.8	401	100.0
Hodgkin's disease	0	1	5	3	9	6.6	6.4	31.0	2.9	13.5	8.1	8.3	7.8	123	100.0
Non-Hodgkin lymphoma	0	0	3	1	4	2.9	2.8	13.8	-	8.1	2.7	3.7	3.4	54	100.0
Burkitt's lymphoma	0	6	5	1	12	8.8	8.6	41.4	17.5	13.5	2.7	11.1	11.9	169	100.0
Unspecified lymphoma	0	1	2	1	4	2.9	2.9	13.8	2.9	5.4	2.7	3.7	3.7	55	100.0
Histiocytosis X	0	0	0	0	0										-
Other reticuloendothelial	0	0	0	0	0										-
III. BRAIN AND SPINAL	0	3	10	6	19	13.9	13.6	100.0	8.8	27.0	16.2	17.6	16.8	260	78.6
Ependymoma	0	1	4	3	8	5.8	5.8	42.1	2.9	10.8	8.1	7.4	7.0	109	100.0
Astrocytoma	0	0	1	1	2	1.5	1.5	10.5	-	2.7	2.7	1.8	1.7	27	100.0
Medulloblastoma	0	0	1	0	1	0.7	0.7	5.3	-	2.7	-	0.9	0.9	14	100.0
Other glioma	0	0	0	0	0										-
Other and unspecified *	0	2	4	2	8	5.8	5.7	42.1	5.8	10.8	5.4	7.4	7.3	110	-
IV. SYMPATHETIC N.S.	0	5	0	0	5	3.6	3.7	100.0	14.6	-	-	4.6	5.7	73	100.0
Neuroblastoma	0	5	0	0	5	3.6	3.7	100.0	14.6	-	-	4.6	5.7	73	100.0
Other	0	0	0	0	0										-
V. RETINOBLASTOMA	1	3	0	0	4	2.9	3.0	100.0	11.7	-	-	3.7	4.5	58	100.0
VI. KIDNEY	0	2	2	0	4	2.9	2.8	100.0	5.8	5.4	-	3.7	4.0	56	100.0
Wilms' tumour	0	2	2	0	4	2.9	2.8	100.0	5.8	5.4	-	3.7	4.0	56	100.0
Renal carcinoma	0	0	0	0	0										-
Other and unspecified	0	0	0	0	0										-
VII. LIVER	0	0	0	1	1	0.7	0.8	100.0	-	-	2.7	0.9	0.8	14	100.0
Hepatoblastoma	0	0	0	0	0										-
Hepatic carcinoma	0	0	0	1	1	0.7	0.8	100.0	-	-	2.7	0.9	0.8	14	100.0
Other and unspecified	0	0	0	0	0										-
VIII. BONE	0	0	0	4	4	2.9	3.2	100.0	-	-	10.8	3.7	3.1	54	100.0
Osteosarcoma	0	0	0	3	3	2.2	2.4	75.0	-	-	8.1	2.8	2.4	41	100.0
Chondrosarcoma	0	0	0	0	0										-
Ewing's sarcoma	0	0	0	1	1	0.7	0.8	25.0	-	-	2.7	0.9	0.8	14	100.0
Other and unspecified	0	0	0	0	0										-
IX. SOFT TISSUE SARCOMAS	0	4	1	1	6	4.4	4.4	100.0	11.7	2.7	2.7	5.5	6.2	85	100.0
Rhabdomyosarcoma	0	2	0	0	2	1.5	1.5	33.3	5.8	-	-	1.8	2.3	29	100.0
Fibrosarcoma	0	1	0	0	1	0.7	0.7	16.7	2.9	-	-	0.9	1.1	15	100.0
Other and unspecified	0	1	1	1	3	2.2	2.2	50.0	2.9	2.7	2.7	2.8	2.8	42	100.0
X. GONADAL & GERM CELL	0	0	0	0	0										-
Non-gonadal germ cell	0	0	0	0	0										-
Gonadal germ cell	0	0	0	0	0										-
Gonadal carcinoma	0	0	0	0	0										-
Other and unspecified	0	0	0	0	0										-
XI. EPITHELIAL NEOPLASMS	0	1	3	3	7	5.1	5.1	100.0	2.9	8.1	8.1	6.5	6.1	96	100.0
Adrenocortical carcinoma	0	0	0	0	0										-
Thyroid carcinoma	0	0	0	0	0										-
Nasopharyngeal carcinoma	0	0	0	0	0										-
Melanoma	0	0	1	1	2	1.5	1.5	28.6	-	2.7	2.7	1.8	1.7	27	100.0
Other carcinoma	0	1	2	2	5	3.6	3.7	71.4	2.9	5.4	5.4	4.6	4.4	69	100.0
XII. OTHER	0	2	0	1	3	2.2	2.3	100.0	5.8	-	2.7	2.8	3.0	43	-
* Specified as malignant	0	2	4	2	8	5.8	5.7	100.0	5.8	10.8	5.4	7.4	7.3	110	-

Colombia, Cali

1977 - 1981

FEMALE

DIAGNOSTIC GROUP	NUMBER OF CASES					REL. FREQUENCY(%)			RATES PER MILLION					Cum	HV(%)
	0	1-4	5-9	10-14	All	Crude	Adj.	Group	0-4	5-9	10-14	Crude	Adj.		
TOTAL	6	43	33	30	112	100.0	100.0	100.0	145.5	89.4	78.5	102.9	107.9	1567	96.2
I. LEUKAEMIAS	1	11	14	12	38	33.9	34.5	100.0	35.6	37.9	31.4	34.9	35.1	525	100.0
Acute lymphocytic	1	7	10	7	25	22.3	22.6	65.8	23.7	27.1	18.3	23.0	23.2	346	100.0
Other lymphocytic	0	0	0	0	0	—	—	—	—	—	—	—	—	—	—
Acute non-lymphocytic	0	2	3	3	8	7.1	7.4	21.1	5.9	8.1	7.9	7.4	7.2	110	100.0
Chronic myeloid	0	1	0	0	1	0.9	0.8	2.6	3.0	—	—	0.9	1.1	15	100.0
Other and unspecified	0	1	1	2	4	3.6	3.7	10.5	3.0	2.7	5.2	3.7	3.5	55	100.0
II. LYMPHOMAS	2	4	2	6	14	12.5	12.7	100.0	17.8	5.4	15.7	12.9	13.2	195	100.0
Hodgkin's disease	0	1	1	3	5	4.5	4.7	35.7	3.0	2.7	7.9	4.6	4.3	68	100.0
Non-Hodgkin lymphoma	0	2	1	3	6	5.4	5.5	42.9	5.9	2.7	7.9	5.5	5.5	82	100.0
Burkitt's lymphoma	0	0	0	0	0	—	—	—	—	—	—	—	—	—	—
Unspecified lymphoma	0	0	0	0	0	—	—	—	—	—	—	—	—	—	—
Histiocytosis X	0	0	0	0	0	—	—	—	—	—	—	—	—	—	—
Other reticuloendothelial	2	1	0	0	3	2.7	2.4	21.4	8.9	—	—	2.8	3.4	45	100.0
III. BRAIN AND SPINAL	0	6	8	4	18	16.1	16.2	100.0	17.8	21.7	10.5	16.5	16.9	250	75.0
Ependymoma	0	1	1	0	2	1.8	1.7	11.1	3.0	2.7	—	1.8	2.0	28	100.0
Astrocytoma	0	1	2	2	5	4.5	4.6	27.8	3.0	5.4	5.2	4.6	4.4	68	80.0
Medulloblastoma	0	1	3	0	4	3.6	3.5	22.2	3.0	8.1	—	3.7	3.8	55	100.0
Other glioma	0	0	0	0	0	—	—	—	—	—	—	—	—	—	—
Other and unspecified *	0	3	2	2	7	6.3	6.3	38.9	8.9	5.4	5.2	6.4	6.7	98	40.0
IV. SYMPATHETIC N.S.	0	4	2	0	6	5.4	5.1	100.0	11.9	5.4	—	5.5	6.3	86	100.0
Neuroblastoma	0	3	2	0	5	4.5	4.3	83.3	8.9	5.4	—	4.6	5.2	72	100.0
Other	0	1	0	0	1	0.9	0.8	16.7	3.0	—	—	0.9	1.1	15	100.0
V. RETINOBLASTOMA	0	7	1	0	8	7.1	6.6	100.0	20.8	2.7	—	7.4	8.9	117	100.0
VI. KIDNEY	2	5	0	0	7	6.3	5.7	100.0	20.8	—	—	6.4	8.0	104	100.0
Wilms' tumour	2	5	0	0	7	6.3	5.7	100.0	20.8	—	—	6.4	8.0	104	100.0
Renal carcinoma	0	0	0	0	0	—	—	—	—	—	—	—	—	—	—
Other and unspecified	0	0	0	0	0	—	—	—	—	—	—	—	—	—	—
VII. LIVER	0	1	0	0	1	0.9	0.8	100.0	3.0	—	—	0.9	1.1	15	100.0
Hepatoblastoma	0	1	0	0	1	0.9	0.8	100.0	3.0	—	—	0.9	1.1	15	100.0
Hepatic carcinoma	0	0	0	0	0	—	—	—	—	—	—	—	—	—	—
Other and unspecified	0	0	0	0	0	—	—	—	—	—	—	—	—	—	—
VIII. BONE	0	0	0	4	4	3.6	4.0	100.0	—	—	10.5	3.7	3.0	52	100.0
Osteosarcoma	0	0	0	4	4	3.6	4.0	100.0	—	—	10.5	3.7	3.0	52	100.0
Chondrosarcoma	0	0	0	0	0	—	—	—	—	—	—	—	—	—	—
Ewing's sarcoma	0	0	0	0	0	—	—	—	—	—	—	—	—	—	—
Other and unspecified	0	0	0	0	0	—	—	—	—	—	—	—	—	—	—
IX. SOFT TISSUE SARCOMAS	0	1	3	1	5	4.5	4.5	100.0	3.0	8.1	2.6	4.6	4.5	69	100.0
Rhabdomyosarcoma	0	0	2	1	3	2.7	2.8	60.0	—	5.4	2.6	2.8	2.5	40	100.0
Fibrosarcoma	0	1	1	0	2	1.8	1.7	40.0	3.0	2.7	—	1.8	2.0	28	100.0
Other and unspecified	0	0	0	0	0	—	—	—	—	—	—	—	—	—	—
X. GONADAL & GERM CELL	0	2	0	2	4	3.6	3.6	100.0	5.9	—	5.2	3.7	3.8	56	100.0
Non-gonadal germ cell	0	2	0	0	2	1.8	1.6	50.0	5.9	—	—	1.8	2.3	30	100.0
Gonadal germ cell	0	0	0	0	0	—	—	—	—	—	—	—	—	—	—
Gonadal carcinoma	0	0	0	2	2	1.8	2.0	50.0	—	—	5.2	1.8	1.5	26	100.0
Other and unspecified	0	0	0	0	0	—	—	—	—	—	—	—	—	—	—
XI. EPITHELIAL NEOPLASMS	0	2	2	1	5	4.5	4.5	100.0	5.9	5.4	2.6	4.6	4.8	70	100.0
Adrenocortical carcinoma	0	0	0	0	0	—	—	—	—	—	—	—	—	—	—
Thyroid carcinoma	0	0	0	0	0	—	—	—	—	—	—	—	—	—	—
Nasopharyngeal carcinoma	0	0	0	0	0	—	—	—	—	—	—	—	—	—	—
Melanoma	0	2	1	1	4	3.6	3.5	80.0	5.9	2.7	2.6	3.7	3.9	56	100.0
Other carcinoma	0	0	1	0	1	0.9	0.9	20.0	—	2.7	—	0.9	0.9	14	100.0
XII. OTHER	1	0	1	0	2	1.8	1.7	100.0	3.0	2.7	—	1.8	2.0	28	100.0
* Specified as malignant	0	3	2	2	7	6.3	6.3	100.0	8.9	5.4	5.2	6.4	6.7	98	40.0

COSTA RICA

National Cancer Registry, 1980–1983

G. Muñoz & R. Sierra

Legislation making cancer a notifiable disease was introduced in Costa Rica in 1976. At the same time, a National Tumour Registry was established, and collection of data commenced in March 1977. The aims of the National Tumour Registry, specified by legislation, were to collect data which would permit assessment of:

(1) the incidence and prevalence of cancer by anatomical site, sex, age, occupation and geographical area;

(2) the distribution and quality of medical services provided to persons suffering from cancer;

(3) all new cases of malignant cancer diagnosed within the national boundaries, and any other relevant problems.

The Cancer Registry of Costa Rica obtains data on cancer cases from hospital records, death certificates, biopsies and autopsies.

For every patient who leaves hospital with a diagnosis of malignant cancer, the following information is given to the Cancer Registry: hospital and locality, clinical record number, name, sex and civil status, date and place of birth, age, occupation, habitual place of residence, diagnosis, basis of diagnosis, histological diagnosis and previous history of cancer.

This information is collected on a standard form and used by the Registry to establish a patient index which permits the unequivocal identification of every person presenting with cancer. This index includes the patient's full name, identification number and registration number.

Since 1980, the Registry has received a copy of all histological diagnoses of cancer from both public and private laboratories.

The Pan American Health Organization has, since 1979, given technical support to the work of the Registry by arranging seminars in which Registry personnel, as well as personnel from all hospitals in the area, can take part, and by sending consultants to visit and evaluate the Registry.

In 1978, an Administrative Board was established for the Registry, with the participation of pathologists, oncologists and statisticians of the Ministry of Health and of the Social Security System.

Costa Rica is a small country (51 000 square kilometres) situated in Central America. The central mountains divide the country into Caribbean and Pacific zones. The country is predominantly agricultural, the major crops being coffee, bananas and sugar cane. Cattle breeding is also an important industry. Costa Rica has one of the highest levels of education and health in Latin America — in 1983 the infant mortality rate was 18.6 per 1000 live births, and average expectation of life at birth was 73.7 years. Health services cover 98% of the population. There is one doctor and seven nurses per 1000 inhabitants, 29 hospitals and 184 clinics.

Population

The population at risk has been calculated from annual estimates of the population of Costa Rica (Centro Latino-Americano de Demografia, San Jose).

AVERAGE ANNUAL POPULATION: 1980–1983

Age	Male	Female
0	36998	35262
1–4	132757	127176
5–9	145889	140094
10–14	143930	138331
0–14	459574	440863

Commentary

The incidence rate for all diagnoses taken together is one of the highest in this volume, the rate

Contd. p. 126

Costa Rica

MALE

1980 - 1983

DIAGNOSTIC GROUP	NUMBER OF CASES					REL. FREQUENCY(%)			RATES PER MILLION						Cum	HV(%)
	0	1-4	5-9	10-14	All	Crude	Adj.	Group	0	1-4	5-9	10-14	Crude	Adj.		
TOTAL	18	103	83	78	282	100.0	100.0	100.0	121.6	194.0	142.2	135.5	153.4	154.7	2286	88.7
I. LEUKAEMIAS	6	41	37	30	114	40.4	40.4	100.0	40.5	77.2	63.4	52.1	62.0	62.6	927	90.4
Acute lymphocytic	4	33	29	20	86	30.5	30.4	75.4	27.0	62.1	49.7	34.7	46.8	47.5	698	89.5
Other lymphocytic	0	2			2	0.7	0.7	1.8		3.8			1.1	1.2	15	50.0
Acute non-lymphocytic	0	5	4	7	16	5.7	5.8	14.0		9.4	6.9	12.2	8.7	8.7	133	93.8
Chronic myeloid	1	1	0	1	3	1.1	1.0	2.6	6.8	1.9		1.7	1.6	1.6	23	100.0
Other and unspecified	1	0	4	2	7	2.5	2.5	6.1	6.8		6.9	3.5	3.8	3.7	58	100.0
II. LYMPHOMAS	2	31	22	15	70	24.8	24.6	100.0	13.5	58.4	37.7	26.1	38.1	38.8	566	91.4
Hodgkin's disease	0	5	11	10	26	9.2	9.5	37.1		9.4	18.8	17.4	14.1	14.0	219	96.2
Non-Hodgkin lymphoma	0	13	3	3	19	6.7	6.5	27.1		24.5	5.1	5.2	10.3	10.8	150	84.2
Burkitt's lymphoma	0	1	0	0	1	0.4	0.3	1.4		1.9			0.5	0.6	8	100.0
Unspecified lymphoma	0	7	7	1	15	5.3	5.2	21.4		13.2	12.0	1.7	8.2	8.5	121	93.3
Histiocytosis X	0	3	1	1	5	1.8	1.7	7.1		5.6	1.7	1.7	2.7	2.8	40	80.0
Other reticuloendothelial	2	2	0	0	4	1.4	1.3	5.7	13.5	3.8			2.2	2.2	29	100.0
III. BRAIN AND SPINAL	2	7	13	11	33	11.7	11.9	100.0	13.5	13.2	22.3	19.1	18.0	17.9	273	84.8
Ependymoma	1	0	2	0	3	1.1	1.1	9.1	6.8		3.4		1.6	1.6	24	100.0
Astrocytoma	1	2	3	2	8	2.8	2.8	24.2	6.8	3.8	5.1	3.5	4.4	4.4	65	100.0
Medulloblastoma	0	2	5	7	14	5.0	5.2	42.4		3.8	8.6	12.2	7.6	7.5	119	71.4
Other glioma	0	3	3	1	7	2.5	2.5	21.2		5.6	5.1	1.7	3.9	3.9	57	85.7
Other and unspecified *	0	0	0	1	1	0.4	0.4	3.0				1.7	0.5	0.5	9	100.0
IV. SYMPATHETIC N.S.	2	6	1	1	10	3.5	3.4	100.0	13.5	11.3	1.7	1.7	5.4	5.6	76	80.0
Neuroblastoma	1	6	1	1	9	3.2	3.1	90.0	6.8	11.3	1.7	1.7	4.9	5.1	69	77.8
Other	1	0	0	0	1	0.4	0.3	10.0	6.8				0.5	0.5	7	100.0
V. RETINOBLASTOMA	1	5	0	0	6	2.1	2.0	100.0	6.8	9.4			3.3	3.4	44	100.0
VI. KIDNEY	2	3	1	1	7	2.5	2.4	100.0	13.5	5.6	1.7	1.7	3.8	3.9	53	71.4
Wilms' tumour	2	2	1	1	6	2.1	2.1	85.7	13.5	3.8	1.7	1.7	3.3	3.3	46	66.7
Renal carcinoma	0	0	0	0	0											
Other and unspecified	0	1	0	0	1	0.4	0.3	14.3		1.9			0.5	0.6	8	100.0
VII. LIVER	0	0	1	4	5	1.8	1.9	100.0			1.7	6.9	2.7	2.6	43	60.0
Hepatoblastoma	0	0	1	0	1	0.4	0.4	20.0			1.7		0.5	0.6	9	100.0
Hepatic carcinoma	0	0	0	4	4	1.4	1.5	80.0				6.9	2.2	2.0	35	50.0
Other and unspecified	0	0	0	0	0											
VIII. BONE	0	0	2	4	6	2.1	2.3	100.0			3.4	6.9	3.3	3.1	52	83.3
Osteosarcoma	0	0	1	1	2	0.7	0.7	33.3			1.7	1.7	1.1	1.1	17	50.0
Chondrosarcoma	0	0	0	1	1	0.4	0.4	16.7				1.7	0.5	0.5	9	100.0
Ewing's sarcoma	0	0	0	2	2	0.7	0.8	33.3				3.5	1.1	1.0	17	100.0
Other and unspecified	0	0	1	0	1	0.4	0.4	16.7			1.7		0.5	0.6	9	100.0
IX. SOFT TISSUE SARCOMAS	1	5	3	2	11	3.9	3.8	100.0	6.8	9.4	5.1	3.5	6.0	6.1	87	90.9
Rhabdomyosarcoma	0	4	2	0	6	2.1	2.0	54.5		7.5	3.4		3.3	3.4	47	83.3
Fibrosarcoma	0	0	0	1	1	0.4	0.4	9.1				1.7	0.5	0.5	9	100.0
Other and unspecified	1	1	1	1	4	1.4	1.4	36.4	6.8	1.9	1.7	1.7	2.2	2.2	32	100.0
X. GONADAL & GERM CELL	1	4	1	0	6	2.1	2.0	100.0	6.8	7.5	1.7		3.3	3.4	45	83.3
Non-gonadal germ cell	0	1	1	0	2	0.7	0.7	33.3		1.9	1.7		1.1	1.1	16	100.0
Gonadal germ cell	1	3	0	0	4	1.4	1.3	66.7	6.8	5.6			2.2	2.3	29	75.0
Gonadal carcinoma	0	0	0	0	0											
Other and unspecified	0	0	0	0	0											
XI. EPITHELIAL NEOPLASMS	0	1	2	10	14	5.0	5.2	100.0		1.9	3.4	17.4	7.6	7.3	118	92.9
Adrenocortical carcinoma	0	0	0	1	1	0.4	0.4	7.1				1.7	0.5	0.6	9	100.0
Thyroid carcinoma	0	0	0	7	7	2.5	2.7	50.0				12.2	3.8	3.5	61	100.0
Nasopharyngeal carcinoma	0	0	1	0	1	0.4	0.3	7.1			1.7		0.5	0.6	9	100.0
Melanoma	0	1	1	3	5	1.8	1.8	35.7		1.9	1.7	5.2	2.7	2.6	41	80.0
Other carcinoma	1	0	0	0	1				6.8						8	100.0
XII. OTHER	0	0	0	0	0											
* Specified as malignant	0	0	0	1	1	0.4	0.4					1.7	0.5	0.5	9	100.0

* Specified as malignant

Costa Rica

1980 – 1983

FEMALE

DIAGNOSTIC GROUP	NUMBER OF CASES					REL. FREQUENCY(%)			RATES PER MILLION							HV(%)
	0	1-4	5-9	10-14	All	Crude	Adj.	Group	0	1-4	5-9	10-14	Crude	Adj.	Cum	
TOTAL	12	80	51	66	209	100.0	100.0	100.0	85.1	157.3	91.0	119.3	118.5	119.3	1766	85.6
I. LEUKAEMIAS	4	38	26	30	98	46.9	47.2	100.0	28.4	74.7	46.4	54.2	55.6	56.0	830	87.8
Acute lymphocytic	2	29	22	20	73	34.9	35.5	74.5	14.2	57.0	39.3	36.1	41.4	41.9	619	94.5
Other lymphocytic	0	1	0	0	1	0.5	0.4	1.0	–	2.0	–	–	0.6	0.6	8	100.0
Acute non-lymphocytic	1	5	2	8	16	7.7	7.4	16.3	7.1	9.8	3.6	14.5	9.1	8.9	137	87.5
Chronic myeloid	0	0	0	0	0	–	–	–	–	–	–	–	–	–	–	–
Other and unspecified	1	3	2	2	8	3.8	3.8	8.2	7.1	5.9	3.6	3.6	4.5	4.6	67	25.0
II. LYMPHOMAS	1	15	6	8	30	14.4	14.1	100.0	7.1	29.5	10.7	14.5	17.0	17.3	251	90.0
Hodgkin's disease	0	5	2	6	13	6.2	6.1	43.3	–	9.8	3.6	10.8	7.4	7.3	111	100.0
Non-Hodgkin lymphoma	1	6	2	1	10	4.8	4.7	33.3	7.1	11.8	3.6	1.8	5.7	5.9	81	80.0
Burkitt's lymphoma	0	0	1	0	1	0.5	0.6	3.3	–	–	1.8	–	0.6	0.6	9	100.0
Unspecified lymphoma	0	1	1	0	2	1.0	1.0	6.7	–	2.0	1.8	–	1.1	1.2	17	100.0
Histiocytosis X	0	2	0	0	2	1.0	0.9	6.7	–	3.9	–	–	1.1	1.1	16	50.0
Other reticuloendothelial	0	1	0	1	2	1.0	0.9	6.7	–	2.0	–	1.8	1.1	1.1	17	100.0
III. BRAIN AND SPINAL	2	2	7	7	18	8.6	9.0	100.0	14.2	3.9	12.5	12.7	10.2	10.0	156	72.2
Ependymoma	0	0	0	0	0	–	–	–	–	–	–	–	–	–	–	–
Astrocytoma	1	1	1	4	7	3.3	3.3	38.9	7.1	2.0	1.8	7.2	4.0	3.8	60	85.7
Medulloblastoma	0	1	0	0	1	0.5	0.5	5.6	–	2.0	–	–	0.6	0.5	9	100.0
Other glioma	1	1	6	2	10	4.8	5.3	55.6	7.1	2.0	10.7	3.6	5.7	5.7	87	60.0
Other and unspecified *	0	0	0	0	0	–	–	–	–	–	–	–	–	–	–	–
IV. SYMPATHETIC N.S.	1	5	1	0	7	3.3	3.2	100.0	7.1	9.8	1.8	–	4.0	4.2	55	85.7
Neuroblastoma	1	5	1	0	7	3.3	3.2	100.0	7.1	9.8	1.8	–	4.0	4.2	55	85.7
Other	0	0	0	0	0	–	–	–	–	–	–	–	–	–	–	–
V. RETINOBLASTOMA	3	3	1	0	7	3.3	3.2	100.0	21.3	5.9	1.8	–	4.0	4.0	54	85.7
VI. KIDNEY	1	6	3	2	12	5.7	5.7	100.0	7.1	11.8	5.4	3.6	6.8	7.0	99	75.0
Wilms' tumour	1	6	3	2	12	5.7	5.7	100.0	7.1	11.8	5.4	3.6	6.8	7.0	99	75.0
Renal carcinoma	0	0	0	0	0	–	–	–	–	–	–	–	–	–	–	–
Other and unspecified	0	0	0	0	0	–	–	–	–	–	–	–	–	–	–	–
VII. LIVER	0	2	1	0	3	1.4	1.5	100.0	–	3.9	1.8	–	1.7	1.8	25	66.7
Hepatoblastoma	0	2	0	0	2	1.0	0.9	66.7	–	3.9	–	–	1.1	1.1	16	100.0
Hepatic carcinoma	0	0	1	0	1	0.5	0.6	33.3	–	–	1.8	–	0.6	0.6	9	–
Other and unspecified	0	0	0	0	0	–	–	–	–	–	–	–	–	–	–	–
VIII. BONE	0	0	0	7	7	3.3	3.2	100.0	–	–	–	12.7	4.0	3.7	63	85.7
Osteosarcoma	0	0	0	4	4	1.9	1.8	57.1	–	–	–	7.2	2.3	2.1	36	75.0
Chondrosarcoma	0	0	0	0	0	–	–	–	–	–	–	–	–	–	–	–
Ewing's sarcoma	0	0	0	3	3	1.4	1.4	42.9	–	–	–	5.4	1.7	1.6	27	100.0
Other and unspecified	0	0	0	0	0	–	–	–	–	–	–	–	–	–	–	–
IX. SOFT TISSUE SARCOMAS	0	7	3	1	11	5.3	5.3	100.0	–	13.8	5.4	1.8	6.2	6.5	91	81.8
Rhabdomyosarcoma	0	6	1	1	8	3.8	3.7	72.7	–	11.8	1.8	1.8	4.5	4.8	65	100.0
Fibrosarcoma	0	0	0	0	0	–	–	–	–	–	–	–	–	–	–	–
Other and unspecified	0	1	2	0	3	1.4	1.6	27.3	–	2.0	3.6	–	1.7	1.8	26	33.3
X. GONADAL & GERM CELL	0	1	1	6	8	3.8	3.8	100.0	–	2.0	1.8	10.8	4.5	4.3	71	87.5
Non-gonadal germ cell	0	1	0	1	2	1.0	0.9	25.0	–	2.0	–	1.8	1.1	1.1	17	50.0
Gonadal germ cell	0	0	1	5	6	2.9	2.9	75.0	–	–	1.8	9.0	3.4	3.2	54	100.0
Gonadal carcinoma	0	0	0	0	0	–	–	–	–	–	–	–	–	–	–	–
Other and unspecified	0	0	0	0	0	–	–	–	–	–	–	–	–	–	–	–
XI. EPITHELIAL NEOPLASMS	0	1	2	5	8	3.8	3.9	100.0	–	2.0	3.6	9.0	4.5	4.4	71	100.0
Adrenocortical carcinoma	0	0	1	1	1	0.5	0.5	12.5	–	–	–	1.8	0.6	0.5	9	100.0
Thyroid carcinoma	0	1	0	4	5	2.4	2.3	62.5	–	2.0	–	7.2	2.8	2.7	44	100.0
Nasopharyngeal carcinoma	0	0	0	0	0	–	–	–	–	–	–	–	–	–	–	–
Melanoma	0	0	1	0	1	0.5	0.6	12.5	–	–	1.8	–	0.6	0.6	9	100.0
Other carcinoma	0	0	1	0	1	0.5	0.6	12.5	–	–	1.8	–	0.6	0.6	9	100.0
XII. OTHER	0	0	0	0	0	–	–	–	–	–	–	–	–	–	–	–
* Specified as malignant	0	0	0	0	0	–	–	–	–	–	–	–	–	–	–	–

for leukaemia being the highest by a considerable margin; this high rate is observed particularly for acute lymphocytic leukaemia. The rate for lymphoma was also high; for Hodgkin's disease, both the total frequency and the rates at younger ages were high. Rates for CNS tumours and neuroblastoma were low. The rate for nasopharyngeal carcinoma was high, though this was based on only seven cases, all in boys.

Reference

Salas, J. (1973) Lymphoreticular tumours in Costa Rica. *J. natl Cancer Inst., 50,* 1657-1661

CUBA

National Cancer Registry, 1970–1981

M. Caraballoso

The Cuban National Cancer Registry was established in 1964 by the Cuban Ministry of Public Health, on the initiative of the National Institute of Oncology, which recognized the urgent need for information on the numbers and characteristics of the neoplasms in the country. The Registry was designed to provide information for administrative health purposes and to facilitate investigative epidemiological studies.

All the population have easy access to health services, so that most of the cancer cases are diagnosed in hospitals; they are reported to the Registry when the medical records are summarized.

Reporting of cancer cases is compulsory. Cancer case data are abstracted on a form which is sent, through the Provincial Health Statistics Services, to the Registry Office. On receipt, these are reviewed and further information requested if the data are incomplete. Registry personnel visit all hospitals of the capital, Havana, which has one-fifth of the country's population, to verify that cases diagnosed in pathology and haematology departments have been reported. In each province there are oncologists who review the cancer diagnoses and reports in their hospitals. Death certificates on which cancer is mentioned are checked in the index, and are included as new cases when they have not been previously reported. Coded data are sent to the Computer Department of the National Cancer Institute for processing. A publication is produced every three years.

Since 1959, health care has been provided free of charge for the whole country. The National Health System has three levels: polyclinics which provide primary care, specialized hospitals, and institutes which have more highly specialized facilities and methods of investigation. There are 256 hospitals in the country, including 91 urban general and 52 rural general. The remainder are paediatric, obstetric, gynaecological, and other specialized hospitals. All the general, paediatric and obstetric urban hospitals and some of the others have a department of pathology. Paediatric oncology services are provided initially in paediatric hospitals; cases may also be referred to Institutes for Oncology and Haematology.

The Registry covers the entire Republic of Cuba, comprising the main island of Cuba and the myriad of adjacent small islands and keys, with a total area of 110 860 square kilometres. The climate is tropical. Temperatures oscillate between 28.5° C and 31° C average maximum and 19.5° C and 24° C average minimum. The mean rainfall is 1500 mm in the west and 1000 mm in the east. At the 1981 census the population was 9 724 000, of whom 30% were younger than 15 years of age. The population density was 88 inhabitants per square kilometre. Of the total population, 69% is classified as urban.

Ethnically, the Cuban population is made up of the following main groups: white (66%), black (12%), yellow (0.2%) and mixed (21.8%). Life expectancy has increased from 61.8 years in 1958 to 73.5 in 1980. Cuba has one of the highest death rates from cancer in the Americas; it is the second cause of death in the country, with a crude rate of 109.1 per 100 000 inhabitants in 1981.

Some 36% of the population is economically active: agriculture accounts for 22%; industry 19%; construction 9%; commerce 9%; transportation 6%; education and scientific research 8%; medicine 2%; and others 25%.

Population

The population at risk is based on data from the censuses of 1970 and 1981 (Direccion Central de Estadisticas, Junta Central de Planificacion; and Comite Estatal de Estadisticas, Censo de Poblacion y Viviendas, 1981, Republica de Cuba), together with an estimate for 1975 based on these two censuses and data on births, deaths and migration.

Contd. p. 130

Cuba   MALE   1970 – 1981

DIAGNOSTIC GROUP	NUMBER OF CASES					REL. FREQUENCY(%)			RATES PER MILLION						Cum	HV(%)
	0	1-4	5-9	10-14	All	Crude	Adj.	Group	0	1-4	5-9	10-14	Crude	Adj.		
TOTAL	67	699	725	516	2007	100.0	100.0	100.0	60.0	136.4	104.0	78.1	101.3	103.1	1516	80.5
I. LEUKAEMIAS	23	211	231	170	635	31.6	31.7	100.0	20.6	41.2	33.1	25.7	32.0	32.5	480	75.3
Acute lymphocytic	8	115	94	72	289	14.4	14.5	45.5	7.2	22.4	13.5	10.9	14.6	15.0	219	79.8
Other lymphocytic	1	12	23	11	47	2.3	2.3	7.4	0.9	2.3	3.3	1.7	2.3	2.3	35	83.3
Acute non-lymphocytic	3	13	22	27	65	3.2	3.3	10.2	2.7	2.5	3.2	4.1	3.3	3.2	49	63.3
Chronic myeloid	0	3	4	6	13	0.6	0.7	2.0	–	0.6	0.6	0.9	0.7	0.6	10	60.0
Other and unspecified	11	68	88	54	221	11.0	10.9	34.8	9.8	13.3	12.6	8.2	11.2	11.3	167	68.2
II. LYMPHOMAS	10	191	253	145	599	29.8	29.4	100.0	9.0	37.3	36.3	22.0	30.2	30.3	449	87.5
Hodgkin's disease	1	19	60	58	138	6.9	6.9	23.0	0.9	3.7	8.6	8.8	7.0	6.5	103	92.2
Non-Hodgkin lymphoma	5	151	159	67	382	19.0	18.6	63.8	4.5	29.5	22.8	10.1	19.3	19.8	287	85.4
Burkitt's lymphoma	0	2	3	2	7	0.3	0.4	1.2	–	0.4	0.4	0.3	0.4	0.3	5	100.0
Unspecified lymphoma	3	18	30	17	68	3.4	3.3	11.4	2.7	3.5	4.3	2.6	3.4	3.4	51	84.6
Histiocytosis X	0	0	0	0	0	–	–	–	–	–	–	–	–	–	–	–
Other reticuloendothelial	1	1	2	0	4	0.2	0.2	0.7	0.9	0.2	0.3	–	0.2	0.2	3	–
III. BRAIN AND SPINAL	4	59	105	80	248	12.4	12.3	100.0	3.6	11.5	15.1	12.1	12.5	12.2	186	68.0
Ependymoma	1	5	11	8	25	1.2	1.2	10.1	0.9	1.0	1.6	1.2	1.3	1.2	19	80.0
Astrocytoma	1	18	26	19	64	3.2	3.2	25.8	0.9	3.5	3.7	2.9	3.2	3.2	48	94.6
Medulloblastoma	2	16	30	17	65	3.2	3.2	26.2	1.8	3.1	4.3	2.6	3.3	3.2	49	88.6
Other glioma	0	12	18	19	49	2.4	2.5	19.8	–	2.3	2.6	2.9	2.5	2.4	37	29.2
Other and unspecified *	0	8	20	17	45	2.2	2.2	18.1	–	1.6	2.9	2.6	2.3	2.2	33	21.1
IV. SYMPATHETIC N.S.	10	62	25	12	109	5.4	5.5	100.0	9.0	12.1	3.6	1.8	5.5	6.1	84	77.4
Neuroblastoma	10	62	25	12	109	5.4	5.5	100.0	9.0	12.1	3.6	1.8	5.5	6.1	84	77.4
Other	0	0	0	0	0	–	–	–	–	–	–	–	–	–	–	–
V. RETINOBLASTOMA	6	50	4	2	62	3.1	3.2	100.0	5.4	9.8	0.6	0.3	3.1	3.7	49	74.5
VI. KIDNEY	4	52	35	4	95	4.7	4.6	100.0	3.6	10.1	5.0	0.6	4.8	5.2	72	91.4
Wilms' tumour	4	50	33	3	90	4.5	4.4	94.7	3.6	9.8	4.7	0.5	4.5	5.0	69	91.1
Renal carcinoma	0	0	1	1	2	0.1	0.1	2.1	–	–	0.1	0.2	0.1	0.1	1	100.0
Other and unspecified	0	2	1	0	3	0.1	0.1	3.2	–	0.4	0.1	–	0.2	0.2	2	100.0
VII. LIVER	1	4	4	4	13	0.6	0.7	100.0	0.9	0.8	0.6	0.6	0.7	0.7	10	66.7
Hepatoblastoma	0	0	0	0	0	–	–	–	–	–	–	–	–	–	–	–
Hepatic carcinoma	1	2	2	3	8	0.4	0.4	61.5	0.9	0.4	0.3	0.5	0.4	0.4	6	66.7
Other and unspecified	0	2	2	1	5	0.2	0.2	38.5	–	0.4	0.3	0.2	0.3	0.3	4	–
VIII. BONE	0	5	21	40	66	3.3	3.5	100.0	–	1.0	3.0	6.1	3.3	3.0	49	83.7
Osteosarcoma	0	1	9	24	34	1.7	1.8	51.5	–	0.2	1.3	3.6	1.7	1.5	25	76.2
Chondrosarcoma	0	0	0	1	1	0.1	0.1	1.5	–	–	–	–	0.1	–	1	100.0
Ewing's sarcoma	0	1	10	12	23	1.1	1.2	34.8	–	0.2	1.4	1.8	1.2	1.1	17	87.5
Other and unspecified	0	3	2	3	8	0.4	0.4	12.1	–	0.6	0.3	0.5	0.4	0.4	6	100.0
IX. SOFT TISSUE SARCOMAS	5	26	29	20	80	4.0	4.0	100.0	4.5	5.1	4.2	3.0	4.0	4.1	61	92.0
Rhabdomyosarcoma	3	15	10	7	35	1.7	1.8	43.8	2.7	2.9	1.4	1.1	1.8	1.9	27	89.5
Fibrosarcoma	0	1	2	4	7	0.4	0.4	8.8	–	0.2	0.3	0.6	0.4	0.3	5	100.0
Other and unspecified	2	10	17	9	38	1.9	1.9	47.5	1.8	2.0	2.4	1.4	1.9	1.9	29	92.3
X. GONADAL & GERM CELL	2	6	2	2	12	0.6	0.6	100.0	1.8	1.2	0.3	0.3	0.6	0.7	9	100.0
Non-gonadal germ cell	0	2	0	2	4	0.2	0.2	33.3	–	0.4	–	0.3	0.2	0.2	3	100.0
Gonadal germ cell	2	1	1	0	4	0.2	0.2	33.3	1.8	0.2	0.1	–	0.2	0.2	3	100.0
Gonadal carcinoma	0	2	0	0	2	0.1	0.1	16.7	–	0.4	–	–	0.1	0.1	2	100.0
Other and unspecified	0	1	1	0	2	0.1	0.1	16.7	–	0.2	0.1	–	0.1	0.1	2	100.0
XI. EPITHELIAL NEOPLASMS	2	12	11	24	49	2.4	2.6	100.0	1.8	2.3	1.6	3.6	2.5	2.4	37	74.2
Adrenocortical carcinoma	0	0	0	0	0	–	–	–	–	–	–	–	–	–	–	–
Thyroid carcinoma	0	0	4	6	10	0.5	0.5	20.4	–	–	0.6	0.9	0.5	0.4	7	50.0
Nasopharyngeal carcinoma	0	2	0	5	7	0.3	0.3	14.3	–	0.4	–	0.8	0.4	0.3	5	80.0
Melanoma	0	3	0	1	4	0.2	0.2	8.2	–	0.6	–	0.2	0.2	0.2	3	100.0
Other carcinoma	2	7	7	12	28	1.4	1.5	57.1	1.8	1.4	1.0	1.8	1.4	1.4	21	80.0
XII. OTHER	0	21	5	13	39	1.9	2.1	100.0	–	4.1	0.7	2.0	2.0	2.1	30	20.0
* Specified as malignant	0	8	16	14	38	1.9	1.9	100.0	–	1.6	2.3	2.1	1.9	1.8	28	21.4

Cuba   FEMALE

1970 – 1981

DIAGNOSTIC GROUP	NUMBER OF CASES					REL. FREQUENCY (%)			RATES PER MILLION						Cum	HV(%)
	0	1-4	5-9	10-14	All	Crude	Adj.	Group	0	1-4	5-9	10-14	Crude	Adj.		
TOTAL	49	486	520	416	1471	100.0	100.0	100.0	45.9	99.3	78.0	66.1	77.8	78.7	1164	81.1
I. LEUKAEMIAS	18	160	200	126	504	34.3	33.9	100.0	16.9	32.7	30.0	20.0	26.6	26.9	398	81.2
Acute lymphocytic	4	78	96	49	227	15.4	15.2	45.0	3.8	15.9	14.4	7.8	12.0	12.1	178	81.9
other lymphocytic	0	13	15	7	35	2.4	2.3	6.9	-	2.7	2.3	1.1	1.9	1.9	27	86.7
Acute non-lymphocytic	2	18	18	29	67	4.6	4.6	13.3	1.9	3.7	2.7	4.6	3.5	3.5	53	82.4
Chronic myeloid	1	2	2	5	10	0.7	0.7	2.0	0.9	0.4	0.3	0.8	0.5	0.5	8	80.0
Other and unspecified	11	49	69	36	165	11.2	11.1	32.7	10.3	10.0	10.4	5.7	8.7	8.9	131	72.2
II. LYMPHOMAS	4	101	90	66	261	17.7	17.8	100.0	3.8	20.6	13.5	10.5	13.8	14.1	206	87.8
Hodgkin's disease	0	4	25	31	60	4.1	4.0	23.0	-	0.8	3.7	4.9	3.2	2.9	47	91.7
Non-Hodgkin lymphoma	3	81	52	24	160	10.9	11.0	61.3	2.8	16.5	7.8	3.8	8.5	9.0	127	88.5
Burkitt's lymphoma	0	1	2	0	3	0.2	0.2	1.1	-	0.2	0.3	-	0.2	0.2	2	100.0
Unspecified lymphoma	0	14	11	11	37	2.5	2.5	14.2	-	2.9	1.7	1.7	2.0	2.0	29	71.4
Histiocytosis X	0	0	0	0	0	-	-	-	-	-	-	-	-	-	-	-
Other reticuloendothelial	0	1	0	0	1	0.1	0.1	0.4	-	0.2	-	-	0.1	0.1	1	100.0
III. BRAIN AND SPINAL	3	47	106	64	220	15.0	14.5	100.0	2.8	9.6	15.9	10.2	11.6	11.3	172	61.9
Ependymoma	1	5	5	2	13	0.9	0.9	5.9	0.9	1.0	0.8	0.3	0.7	0.7	10	100.0
Astrocytoma	1	11	27	28	67	4.6	4.5	30.5	0.9	2.0	4.1	4.5	3.5	3.4	52	83.8
Medulloblastoma	1	10	22	7	40	2.7	2.6	18.2	0.9	2.0	3.3	1.1	2.1	2.1	31	89.5
Other glioma	0	11	25	13	49	3.3	3.2	22.3	-	2.2	3.8	2.1	2.6	2.5	38	31.6
Other and unspecified	0	10	27	14	51	3.5	3.3	23.2	-	2.0	4.1	2.2	2.7	2.6	40	15.8
IV. SYMPATHETIC N.S.	5	42	18	7	72	4.9	5.1	100.0	4.7	8.6	2.7	1.1	3.8	4.2	58	83.3
Neuroblastoma	5	42	18	7	72	4.9	5.1	100.0	4.7	8.6	2.7	1.1	3.8	4.2	58	83.3
Other	0	0	0	0	0	-	-	-	-	-	-	-	-	-	-	-
V. RETINOBLASTOMA	6	42	9	1	58	3.9	4.2	100.0	5.6	8.6	1.4	0.2	3.1	3.6	47	81.8
VI. KIDNEY	4	47	26	9	86	5.8	6.0	100.0	3.8	9.6	3.9	1.4	4.5	4.9	69	86.4
Wilms' tumour	4	47	24	8	83	5.6	5.8	96.5	3.8	9.6	3.6	1.3	4.4	4.8	67	86.4
Renal carcinoma	0	0	0	0	0	-	-	-	-	-	-	-	-	-	-	-
Other and unspecified	0	0	2	1	3	0.2	0.2	3.5	-	-	0.3	0.2	0.2	0.1	2	-
VII. LIVER	0	5	2	3	10	0.7	0.7	100.0	-	1.0	0.3	0.5	0.5	0.6	8	100.0
Hepatoblastoma	0	0	0	0	0	-	-	-	-	-	-	-	-	-	-	-
Hepatic carcinoma	0	3	2	2	7	0.5	0.5	70.0	-	0.6	0.3	0.3	0.4	0.4	6	100.0
Other and unspecified	0	2	0	1	3	0.2	0.2	30.0	-	0.4	-	0.2	0.2	0.2	2	100.0
VIII. BONE	2	2	14	47	65	4.4	4.5	100.0	1.9	0.4	2.1	7.5	3.4	3.1	51	76.2
Osteosarcoma	2	0	6	24	32	2.2	2.2	49.2	1.9	-	0.9	3.8	1.7	1.5	25	75.0
Chondrosarcoma	0	0	0	3	3	0.2	0.2	4.6	-	-	-	0.5	0.1	0.1	2	100.0
Ewing's sarcoma	0	2	7	14	23	1.6	1.6	35.4	-	0.4	1.1	2.2	1.2	1.1	18	81.3
Other and unspecified	0	0	1	6	7	0.5	0.5	10.8	-	-	0.2	1.0	0.4	0.3	6	50.0
IX. SOFT TISSUE SARCOMAS	4	19	28	29	80	5.4	5.4	100.0	3.8	3.9	4.2	4.6	4.2	4.2	63	91.5
Rhabdomyosarcoma	0	9	16	14	39	2.7	2.6	48.8	-	1.8	2.4	2.2	2.1	2.0	30	91.3
Fibrosarcoma	0	1	0	5	6	0.4	0.4	7.5	-	0.2	-	0.8	0.3	0.3	5	100.0
Other and unspecified	4	9	12	10	35	2.4	2.4	43.8	3.8	1.8	1.8	1.6	1.9	1.9	28	89.5
X. GONADAL & GERM CELL	0	7	6	19	32	2.2	2.2	100.0	-	1.4	0.9	3.0	1.7	1.6	25	90.9
Non-gonadal germ cell	0	4	0	2	6	0.4	0.4	18.8	-	0.8	-	0.3	0.3	0.3	5	85.7
Gonadal germ cell	0	0	3	11	14	1.0	1.0	43.8	-	-	0.5	1.7	0.7	0.7	6	100.0
Gonadal carcinoma	0	2	1	4	7	0.5	0.5	21.9	-	0.4	0.2	0.6	0.4	0.4	6	100.0
Other and unspecified	0	1	2	2	5	0.3	0.3	15.6	-	0.2	0.3	0.3	0.3	0.3	4	100.0
XI. EPITHELIAL NEOPLASMS	1	6	8	36	51	3.5	3.6	100.0	0.9	1.2	1.2	5.7	2.7	2.5	40	89.7
Adrenocortical carcinoma	0	1	0	1	2	0.1	0.1	3.9	-	0.2	-	0.2	0.1	0.1	1	100.0
Thyroid carcinoma	0	0	0	22	22	1.5	1.6	43.1	-	-	-	3.5	1.2	1.0	17	85.0
Nasopharyngeal carcinoma	0	0	3	2	5	0.3	0.3	9.8	-	-	0.4	0.3	0.3	0.3	4	100.0
Melanoma	0	1	1	0	2	0.1	0.1	3.9	-	0.2	0.2	-	0.1	0.1	2	100.0
Other carcinoma	1	4	4	11	20	1.4	1.4	39.2	0.9	0.8	0.6	1.7	1.1	1.0	16	91.7
XII. OTHER	2	8	13	9	32	2.2	2.1	100.0	1.9	1.6	2.0	1.4	1.7	1.7	25	16.7
* Specified as malignant	0	10	26	13	49	3.3	3.2	100.0	-	2.0	3.9	2.1	2.6	2.5	38	15.8

* Specified as malignant

AVERAGE ANNUAL POPULATION: 1970–1981

Age	Male	Female
0	93083	88872
1–4	427147	407884
5–9	580890	555541
10–14	550228	524060
0–14	1651348	1576357

Commentary

A very high proportion of the cases were registered on the basis of information recorded on death certificates; the percentage of these 'death certificate only' (DCO) cases for each of the major diagnostic groups is given below.

Diagnostic group		Percentage DCO	
		Male	Female
Total		44.0	45.3
I	Leukaemias	64.1	65.1
II	Lymphomas	34.6	38.7
III	Brain and spinal neoplasms	33.9	38.6
IV	Sympathetic nervous system tumours	45.0	40.3
V	Retinoblastoma	17.7	13.8
VI	Kidney tumours	28.4	27.9
VII	Liver tumours	76.9	80.0
VIII	Bone tumours	30.3	27.7
IX	Soft-tissue sarcomas	27.5	30.0
X	Gonadal amd germ-cell neoplasms	16.7	28.1
XI	Epithelial neoplasms	26.5	15.7
XII	Other	79.5	75.0

The proportion of the DCO cases which had been diagnosed on the basis of histological evidence was unknown, although presumably some had been, since morphological type had been specified; for this reason the 'histologically verified' (HV) column of the main table has been calculated excluding DCO cases.

The total rate and those for leukaemia and for CNS tumours were lower than other American or European rates. Rates for lymphoma were high; this was mainly accounted for by lymphomas other than Hodgkin's disease or Burkitt's lymphoma. The incidence rates for this group are particularly high in the first ten years of life, and are even more striking at ages 1–4.

Reference

Alert, J. & Jimenez, J. (1980) Malignant tumours in Cuban children. Fourth triennial 1973-1975 of the National Cancer Registry. *Neoplasma, 27*, 739-744

JAMAICA

Kingston and St. Andrew, 1968-1981

B. Hanchard & S.E.H. Brooks

The Jamaica Cancer Registry was founded in 1958 in order to provide information on cancer incidence for research, teaching and health care planning. Registration was limited to the predominantly urban area of Kingston and St. Andrew, where the concentration of medical facilities would contribute to the completeness of registration. The Registry is currently headed by Professor S.E.H. Brooks and is attached to the Pathology Department of the University of the West Indies at Mona. The routine work of the Registry is carried out by two nurses.

Registration is active; Registry staff visit all wards of the two large general hospitals in the area at least weekly, interview all cancer patients or suspected cases, note relevant investigations and check permanent addresses to ensure that only those permanently resident in Kingston and St. Andrew are used for incidence and epidemiological studies. Other Government institutions, such as the Chest Hospital and Children's Hospital, are visited monthly, as are private nursing homes and hospitals. The X-ray departments of the hospitals record suspicious cases, and these lists are available for checking. Pathology records at the two large hospitals and those of pathologists in private practice are examined. Although notification cards are sent to private practitioners, few co-operate and visits from Registry staff are necessary to trace cases not attending the general hospitals; about 10% of cases were derived from private practitioners only.

Data from each patient are recorded on a separate card and filed by site and by year of diagnosis. Duplication is avoided by means of an alphabetical card file. No patient is registered twice, except when there is more than one primary malignancy, proven by histology. Data are used by many departments in the medical school for teaching and background in research projects, but personal information is kept strictly confidential.

The Registry covers the predominantly urban community of Kingston and St. Andrew with an estimated population of 586 930 in 1982. Kingston is a seaboard city, spreading over the coastal plain to the foothills of the Blue Mountains. Of adjacent St. Andrew, roughly half is less than 300 m above sea level, the remainder going up to over 1500 m. The total registration area is 490 square kilometres.

The Registry does not gather information on ethnic group or occupation. The population is 65% Black, 1% White, 2% East Indian, 1% Chinese and Asian and 30% mixed blood. The majority of the population belong to a Christian denomination. There are smaller groups of Rastafarians, Hindus and Moslems. Occupations in the registration area include light industry, commerce, government administration, service occupations, construction and other forms of manual labour. There are also a considerable number of unemployed.

Migration to the island from other areas is minimal. There is, however, considerable internal migration of younger people from the rural areas to Kingston in search of jobs.

Population

The average annual population at risk is derived from data from the censuses of 1970 and 1982 (Department of Statistics, Jamaica).

AVERAGE ANNUAL POPULATION: 1968-1981

Age	Male	Female
0-4	37940	37686
5-9	36728	37690
10-14	30477	32008
0-14	105145	107384

Commentary

Overall the incidence rate for childhood cancer was rather low. There was a relatively high

Contd p. 134

Jamaica   1968 – 1981   MALE

DIAGNOSTIC GROUP	NUMBER OF CASES					REL. FREQUENCY(%)			RATES PER MILLION					Cum	HV(%)
	0	1-4	5-9	10-14	All	Crude	Adj.	Group	0-4	5-9	10-14	Crude	Adj.		
TOTAL	4	50	36	38	128	100.0	100.0	100.0	101.7	70.0	89.1	87.0	87.8	1304	97.7
I. LEUKAEMIAS	1	15	8	11	35	27.3	27.2	100.0	30.1	15.6	25.8	23.8	24.2	357	100.0
Acute lymphocytic	0	10	4	4	19	14.8	14.6	54.3	20.7	7.8	9.4	12.9	13.2	189	100.0
Other lymphocytic	0	0	0	1	1	0.8	0.8	2.9	-	-	2.3	0.7	0.7	12	100.0
Acute non-lymphocytic	0	2	4	4	10	7.8	8.0	28.6	3.8	7.8	9.4	6.8	6.7	105	100.0
Chronic myeloid	0	0	0	1	1	0.8	0.8	2.9	-	-	2.3	0.7	0.7	12	100.0
Other and unspecified	1	3	0	1	4	3.1	3.0	11.4	5.6	-	2.3	2.7	2.9	40	100.0
II. LYMPHOMAS	0	4	11	9	24	18.8	19.2	100.0	7.5	21.4	21.1	16.3	15.9	250	100.0
Hodgkin's disease	0	1	5	2	8	6.3	6.5	33.3	1.9	9.7	4.7	5.4	5.2	81	100.0
Non-Hodgkin lymphoma	0	1	5	6	12	9.4	9.6	50.0	1.9	9.7	14.1	8.2	7.9	128	100.0
Burkitt's lymphoma	0	0	0	0	0	-	-	-	-	-	-	-	-	-	-
Unspecified lymphoma	0	1	1	1	3	2.3	2.4	12.5	1.9	1.9	2.3	2.0	2.0	31	100.0
Histiocytosis X	0	1	0	0	1	0.8	0.7	4.2	1.9	-	-	0.7	0.7	9	100.0
Other reticuloendothelial	0	0	0	0	0	-	-	-	-	-	-	-	-	-	-
III. BRAIN AND SPINAL	0	4	9	9	22	17.2	17.6	100.0	7.5	17.5	21.1	14.9	14.7	231	95.5
Ependymoma	0	1	1	2	4	3.1	3.2	18.2	1.9	1.9	4.7	2.7	2.7	43	100.0
Astrocytoma	0	1	5	5	11	8.6	8.9	50.0	1.9	9.7	11.7	7.5	7.3	117	100.0
Medulloblastoma	0	1	2	1	4	3.1	3.2	18.2	1.9	3.9	-	2.7	2.7	41	100.0
Other glioma	0	0	1	0	1	0.8	0.8	4.5	-	1.9	-	0.7	0.6	10	100.0
Other and unspecified *	0	1	0	1	2	1.6	1.5	9.1	1.9	-	2.3	1.4	1.4	21	50.0
IV. SYMPATHETIC N.S.	3	6	4	0	13	10.2	10.0	100.0	16.9	7.8	-	8.8	9.1	124	92.3
Neuroblastoma	3	5	4	0	12	9.4	9.3	92.3	15.1	7.8	-	8.2	8.3	114	91.7
Other	0	1	0	0	1	0.8	0.7	7.7	1.9	-	-	0.7	0.7	9	100.0
V. RETINOBLASTOMA	0	7	0	0	7	5.5	5.2	100.0	13.2	-	-	4.8	5.1	66	85.7
VI. KIDNEY	0	8	3	0	11	8.6	8.4	100.0	15.1	5.8	-	7.5	7.7	104	100.0
Wilms' tumour	0	8	3	0	11	8.6	8.4	100.0	15.1	5.8	-	7.5	7.7	104	100.0
Renal carcinoma	0	0	0	0	0	-	-	-	-	-	-	-	-	-	-
Other and unspecified	0	0	0	0	0	-	-	-	-	-	-	-	-	-	-
VII. LIVER	0	0	0	0	0	-	-	-	-	-	-	-	-	-	-
Hepatoblastoma	0	0	0	0	0	-	-	-	-	-	-	-	-	-	-
Hepatic carcinoma	0	0	0	0	0	-	-	-	-	-	-	-	-	-	-
Other and unspecified	0	0	0	0	0	-	-	-	-	-	-	-	-	-	-
VIII. BONE	0	0	1	5	6	4.7	4.8	100.0	-	1.9	11.7	4.1	4.0	68	100.0
Osteosarcoma	0	0	0	5	5	3.9	3.9	83.3	-	-	11.7	3.4	3.4	59	100.0
Chondrosarcoma	0	0	0	0	0	-	-	-	-	-	-	-	-	-	-
Ewing's sarcoma	0	0	1	0	1	0.8	0.8	16.7	-	1.9	-	0.7	0.6	10	100.0
Other and unspecified	0	0	0	0	0	-	-	-	-	-	-	-	-	-	-
IX. SOFT TISSUE SARCOMAS	0	6	0	2	8	6.3	6.0	100.0	11.3	-	4.7	5.4	5.7	80	100.0
Rhabdomyosarcoma	0	4	0	0	4	3.1	3.0	50.0	7.5	-	-	2.7	2.9	38	100.0
Fibrosarcoma	0	1	0	0	1	0.8	0.7	12.5	1.9	-	-	0.7	0.7	9	100.0
Other and unspecified	0	1	0	2	3	2.3	2.3	37.5	1.9	-	4.7	2.0	2.1	33	100.0
X. GONADAL & GERM CELL	0	0	0	0	0	-	-	-	-	-	-	-	-	-	-
Non-gonadal germ cell	0	0	0	0	0	-	-	-	-	-	-	-	-	-	-
Gonadal germ cell	0	0	0	0	0	-	-	-	-	-	-	-	-	-	-
Gonadal carcinoma	0	0	0	0	0	-	-	-	-	-	-	-	-	-	-
Other and unspecified	0	0	0	0	0	-	-	-	-	-	-	-	-	-	-
XI. EPITHELIAL NEOPLASMS	0	0	0	2	2	1.6	1.6	100.0	-	-	4.7	1.4	1.4	23	100.0
Adrenocortical carcinoma	0	0	0	0	0	-	-	-	-	-	-	-	-	-	-
Thyroid carcinoma	0	0	0	0	0	-	-	-	-	-	-	-	-	-	-
Nasopharyngeal carcinoma	0	0	0	1	1	0.8	0.8	50.0	-	-	2.3	0.7	0.7	12	100.0
Melanoma	0	0	0	0	0	-	-	-	-	-	-	-	-	-	-
Other carcinoma	0	0	0	1	1	0.8	0.8	50.0	-	-	2.3	0.7	0.7	12	100.0
XII. OTHER	0	1	0	0	1	0.8	0.7	100.0	1.9	-	-	0.7	0.7	9	100.0

* Specified as malignant

Jamaica   FEMALE

1968 – 1981

DIAGNOSTIC GROUP	NUMBER OF CASES					REL. FREQUENCY(%)			RATES PER MILLION						HV(%)
	0	1-4	5-9	10-14	All	Crude	Adj.	Group	0-4	5-9	10-14	Crude	Adj.	Cum	
TOTAL	7	38	32	27	104	100.0	100.0	100.0	85.3	60.6	60.3	69.2	70.1	1031	100.0
I. LEUKAEMIAS	2	13	9	6	30	28.8	28.4	100.0	28.4	17.1	13.4	20.0	20.4	294	100.0
Acute lymphocytic	2	11	7	4	24	23.1	22.6	80.0	24.6	13.3	8.9	16.0	16.4	234	100.0
Other lymphocytic	0	0	0	0	0	-	-	-	-	-	-	-	-	-	-
Acute non-lymphocytic	0	0	1	1	2	1.9	2.0	6.7	-	1.9	2.2	1.3	1.3	21	100.0
Chronic myeloid	0	0	1	0	1	1.0	1.1	3.3	-	1.9	-	0.7	0.6	11	100.0
Other and unspecified	0	2	1	0	3	2.9	2.7	10.0	3.8	1.9	-	2.0	2.1	28	100.0
II. LYMPHOMAS	1	3	3	3	10	9.6	9.7	100.0	7.6	5.7	6.7	6.7	6.7	100	100.0
Hodgkin's disease	0	1	0	1	2	1.9	2.0	20.0	1.9	-	2.2	1.3	1.4	21	100.0
Non-Hodgkin lymphoma	1	0	3	2	6	5.8	5.9	60.0	1.9	5.7	4.5	4.0	3.9	60	100.0
Burkitt's lymphoma	0	0	0	0	0	-	-	-	-	-	-	-	-	-	-
Unspecified lymphoma	0	0	0	1	1	1.0	0.9	10.0	-	-	-	0.7	0.7	9	100.0
Histiocytosis X	0	0	0	0	0	-	-	-	-	-	-	-	-	-	-
Other reticuloendothelial	0	1	0	0	1	1.0	0.9	10.0	1.9	-	-	0.7	0.7	9	100.0
III. BRAIN AND SPINAL	1	3	10	4	18	17.3	17.4	100.0	7.6	19.0	8.9	12.0	11.6	177	100.0
Ependymoma	0	0	0	0	0	-	-	-	-	-	-	-	-	-	-
Astrocytoma	1	2	7	3	13	12.5	12.6	72.2	5.7	13.3	6.7	8.6	8.4	128	100.0
Medulloblastoma	0	1	2	0	3	2.9	2.8	16.7	1.9	3.8	-	2.0	2.0	28	100.0
Other glioma	0	0	1	1	2	1.9	2.0	11.1	-	1.9	2.2	1.3	1.3	21	100.0
Other and unspecified *	0	0	0	0	0	-	-	-	-	-	-	-	-	-	-
IV. SYMPATHETIC N.S.	1	5	5	1	12	11.5	11.1	100.0	11.4	9.5	2.2	8.0	8.1	115	100.0
Neuroblastoma	1	5	5	1	12	11.5	11.1	100.0	11.4	9.5	2.2	8.0	8.1	115	100.0
Other	0	0	0	0	0	-	-	-	-	-	-	-	-	-	-
V. RETINOBLASTOMA	0	6	0	0	6	5.8	5.3	100.0	11.4	-	-	4.0	4.4	57	100.0
VI. KIDNEY	1	2	4	0	7	6.7	6.4	100.0	5.7	7.6	-	4.7	4.6	66	100.0
Wilms' tumour	1	2	4	0	7	6.7	6.4	100.0	5.7	7.6	-	4.7	4.6	66	100.0
Renal carcinoma	0	0	0	0	0	-	-	-	-	-	-	-	-	-	-
Other and unspecified	0	0	0	0	0	-	-	-	-	-	-	-	-	-	-
VII. LIVER	0	1	0	0	1	1.0	0.9	100.0	1.9	-	-	0.7	0.7	9	100.0
Hepatoblastoma	0	1	0	0	1	1.0	0.9	100.0	1.9	-	-	0.7	0.7	9	100.0
Hepatic carcinoma	0	0	0	0	0	-	-	-	-	-	-	-	-	-	-
Other and unspecified	0	0	0	0	0	-	-	-	-	-	-	-	-	-	-
VIII. BONE	0	1	1	2	4	3.8	4.0	100.0	1.9	1.9	4.5	2.7	2.6	41	100.0
Osteosarcoma	0	0	1	2	3	2.9	3.2	75.0	-	1.9	4.5	2.0	1.9	32	100.0
Chondrosarcoma	0	0	0	0	0	-	-	-	-	-	-	-	-	-	-
Ewing's sarcoma	0	0	0	0	0	-	-	-	-	-	-	-	-	-	-
Other and unspecified	0	1	0	0	1	1.0	0.9	25.0	1.9	-	-	0.7	0.7	9	100.0
IX. SOFT TISSUE SARCOMAS	0	3	0	2	5	4.8	4.9	100.0	5.7	-	4.5	3.3	3.5	51	100.0
Rhabdomyosarcoma	0	3	0	1	4	3.8	3.8	80.0	5.7	-	2.2	2.7	2.8	40	100.0
Fibrosarcoma	0	0	0	0	0	-	-	-	-	-	-	-	-	-	-
Other and unspecified	0	0	0	1	1	1.0	1.1	20.0	-	-	2.2	0.7	0.6	11	100.0
X. GONADAL & GERM CELL	1	1	0	4	6	5.8	6.2	100.0	3.8	-	8.9	4.0	4.1	64	100.0
Non-gonadal germ cell	1	1	0	2	4	3.8	4.0	66.7	3.8	-	4.5	2.7	2.8	41	100.0
Gonadal germ cell	0	0	0	1	1	1.0	1.1	16.7	-	-	2.2	0.7	0.6	11	100.0
Gonadal carcinoma	0	0	0	0	0	-	-	-	-	-	-	-	-	-	-
Other and unspecified	0	0	0	1	1	1.0	1.1	16.7	-	-	2.2	0.7	0.6	11	100.0
XI. EPITHELIAL NEOPLASMS	0	0	0	3	3	2.9	3.3	100.0	-	-	6.7	2.0	1.9	33	100.0
Adrenocortical carcinoma	0	0	0	0	0	-	-	-	-	-	-	-	-	-	-
Thyroid carcinoma	0	0	0	0	0	-	-	-	-	-	-	-	-	-	-
Nasopharyngeal carcinoma	0	0	0	1	1	1.0	1.1	33.3	-	-	2.2	0.7	0.6	11	100.0
Melanoma	0	0	0	0	0	-	-	-	-	-	-	-	-	-	-
Other carcinoma	0	0	0	2	2	1.9	2.2	66.7	-	-	4.5	1.3	1.3	22	100.0
XII. OTHER	0	0	0	2	2	1.9	2.2	100.0	-	-	4.5	1.3	1.3	22	100.0
* Specified as malignant	0	0	0	0	0	-	-	-	-	-	-	-	-	-	-

frequency of lymphomas (especially non-Hodgkin), neuroblastoma, retinoblastoma and osteosarcoma, with a correspondingly low frequency of leukaemia. Only one of the 13 cases of retinoblastoma was bilateral. Ewing's sarcoma was particularly rare.

Reference

Bras, G., Cole, H., Ashmeade-Dyer, J. & Watler, D.C. (1969) Report of 151 childhood malignancies observed in Jamaica. *J. natl Cancer Inst.*, *43*, 417-421

PUERTO RICO

Central Cancer Registry of Puerto Rico, 1973–1982

I. Martinez, R. Torres, L. Echevarria, N.E. Zea,
J.R. Marrero, N.E. Perez & M.M. Rivera

The Central Cancer Registry is a section of the Cancer Control Program of the Puerto Rico Department of Health. All cancer cases diagnosed in all hospitals, clinics and private offices of physicians in Puerto Rico are analysed and registered. In addition to the legally required reporting of cancer cases, the Registry makes a systematic search for unreported cases. In 90% of cancer cases first reported to the Central Cancer Registry the notification was based on a clinical abstract or a biopsy report.

Each record of the Central Cancer Registry consists of four basic documents: a clinical abstract completed by medical records clerks from the Registry or from the hospital, or by physicians in private cases; a carbon copy of the biopsy report from the pathologist; follow-up forms with the yearly information; and a photocopy of the death certificate from the Vital Statistics Office of the Department of Health. A large proportion of records also contain photocopies of those sections of the patient's hospital medical record which are important for substantiating the clinical abstract information.

Since 1976 ICD-O has been used for coding topographic and histological diagnosis; from 1970 to 1975 the *Manual of Tumor Nomenclature and Coding* of the American Cancer Society was used.

If more than one primary tumour is detected in the same person, each tumour is registered as a different case. Carcinoma of the skin has not been registered since 1976.

Regular epidemiological and clinical studies are planned using Registry data. An annual report is published.

There are four levels of medical care in Puerto Rico: (*a*) the primary level (health centres, etc.), where the cancer cases are usually suspected or detected and referred to (*b*) the secondary level (subregional), where the diagnosis is usually made and some tumours are also treated; many cases are referred to complete the diagnosis, stage or treatment to (*c*) the tertiary level (regional) or (*d*) the supratertiary level (oncological hospitals), where all facilities for cancer treatment are located. There is close liaison between the Central Cancer Registry and the medical care facilities in the island, including assistance with and supervision of their hospital tumour registries.

Puerto Rico is a rectangular-shaped island east of Hispaniola in the West Indies with an area of 8897 square kilometres. It is surrounded by the Atlantic Ocean to the north and the Caribbean Sea to the south. It is formed by a chain of mountains running from east to west. There is sunshine most of the year and the average temperature is 25° C (range 21 to 29° C). Trade winds make the climate agreeable, but also bring abundant rain (average annual rainfall 188 cm).

The population is 80% white and mixed blood, 20% black. Of the total population, 58% live in conurbations of more than 100 000; 98% are reported to be Catholics. Spanish and English are the official languages. The main economic activities are manufacturing, tourism, service industries and agriculture.

Population

Annual population estimates are available, based on the results of the censuses of 1970 and 1980 (US Bureau of the Census).

AVERAGE ANNUAL POPULATION: 1973–1982

Age	Male	Female
0–4	170761	165315
5–9	169685	164317
10–14	172530	166294
0–14	512976	495926

Contd p. 138

Puerto Rico   MALE   1973 - 1982

DIAGNOSTIC GROUP	NUMBER OF CASES 0	1-4	5-9	10-14	All	REL. FREQUENCY(%) Crude	Adj.	Group	RATES PER MILLION 0-4	5-9	10-14	Crude	Adj.	Cum	HV(%)
TOTAL	49	217	162	153	581	100.0	100.0	100.0	155.8	95.5	88.7	113.3	116.8	1700	97.7
I. LEUKAEMIAS	10	91	52	42	195	33.6	33.1	100.0	59.1	30.6	24.3	38.0	39.8	571	99.0
Acute lymphocytic	3	67	37	29	136	23.4	23.1	69.7	41.0	21.8	16.8	26.5	27.8	398	100.0
Other lymphocytic	0	0	2	0	2	0.3	0.4	1.0	-	1.2	-	0.4	0.4	6	100.0
Acute non-lymphocytic	6	12	8	8	34	5.9	5.8	17.4	10.5	4.7	4.6	6.6	6.9	99	100.0
Chronic myeloid	1	1	0	0	2	0.3	0.3	1.0	1.2	-	-	0.4	0.5	6	100.0
Other and unspecified	0	11	5	5	21	3.6	3.6	10.8	6.4	2.9	2.9	4.1	4.3	61	89.5
II. LYMPHOMAS	0	26	41	41	108	18.6	19.5	100.0	15.2	24.2	23.8	21.1	20.6	316	99.1
Hodgkin's disease	0	6	18	20	44	7.6	8.2	40.7	3.5	10.6	11.6	8.6	8.1	129	100.0
Non-Hodgkin lymphoma	0	9	10	12	31	5.3	5.6	28.7	5.3	5.9	7.0	6.0	6.0	91	100.0
Burkitt's lymphoma	0	3	5	2	10	1.7	1.8	9.3	1.8	2.9	1.2	1.9	2.0	29	100.0
Unspecified lymphoma	0	5	7	6	18	3.1	3.2	16.7	2.9	4.1	3.5	3.5	3.5	53	94.4
Histiocytosis X	0	0	0	0	0										
Other reticuloendothelial	0	3	1	1	5	0.9	0.8	4.6	1.8	0.6	0.6	1.0	1.0	15	100.0
III. BRAIN AND SPINAL	6	31	29	23	89	15.3	15.4	100.0	21.7	17.1	13.3	17.3	17.8	260	93.1
Ependymoma	2	8	2	0	12	2.1	1.9	13.5	5.9	1.2	-	2.3	2.6	35	100.0
Astrocytoma	3	16	16	15	50	8.6	8.8	56.2	11.1	9.4	8.7	9.7	9.9	146	98.0
Medulloblastoma	0	7	7	3	17	2.9	2.9	19.1	4.1	4.1	1.7	3.3	3.4	50	100.0
Other glioma	1	0	3	2	6	1.0	1.1	6.7	0.6	1.8	1.2	1.2	1.1	18	33.3
Other and unspecified *	0	0	1	3	4	0.7	0.8	4.5	-	0.6	1.7	0.8	0.7	12	50.0
IV. SYMPATHETIC N.S.	9	15	7	3	34	5.9	5.5	100.0	14.1	4.1	1.7	6.6	7.3	100	100.0
Neuroblastoma	9	15	7	2	33	5.7	5.3	97.1	14.1	4.1	1.2	6.4	7.1	97	100.0
Other	0	0	0	1	1	0.2	0.2	2.9	-	-	0.6	0.2	0.2	3	100.0
V. RETINOBLASTOMA	2	15	1	0	18	3.1	2.7	100.0	10.0	0.6	-	3.5	4.0	53	100.0
VI. KIDNEY	8	20	8	3	39	6.7	6.3	100.0	16.4	4.7	1.7	7.6	8.4	114	100.0
Wilms' tumour	8	20	7	3	38	6.5	6.1	97.4	16.4	4.1	1.7	7.4	8.2	111	100.0
Renal carcinoma	0	0	0	0	0										
Other and unspecified	0	0	1	0	1	0.2	0.2	2.6	-	0.6	-	0.2	0.2	3	100.0
VII. LIVER	4	1	2	1	8	1.4	1.3	100.0	2.9	1.2	0.6	1.6	1.7	23	75.0
Hepatoblastoma	3	1	1	0	5	0.9	0.8	62.5	2.3	0.6	-	1.0	1.1	15	100.0
Hepatic carcinoma	0	0	1	0	1	0.3	0.3	12.5	-	0.6	-	0.2	0.2		100.0
Other and unspecified	1	0	0	1	2	0.3	0.3	25.0	0.6	-	0.6	0.4	0.4	6	100.0
VIII. BONE	1	1	4	18	24	4.1	4.6	100.0	1.2	2.4	10.4	4.7	4.2	70	95.8
Osteosarcoma	0	0	2	9	11	1.9	2.1	45.8	-	1.2	5.2	2.1	1.9	32	100.0
Chondrosarcoma	0	0	0	2	2	0.3	0.4	8.3	-	-	1.2	0.4	0.3	3	100.0
Ewing's sarcoma	0	1	2	6	9	1.5	1.7	37.5	0.6	1.2	3.5	1.8	1.6	26	88.9
Other and unspecified	1	0	0	1	2	0.3	0.3	8.3	0.6	-	0.6	0.4	0.4	6	100.0
IX. SOFT TISSUE SARCOMAS	6	9	13	13	41	7.1	7.2	100.0	8.8	7.7	7.5	8.0	8.1	120	100.0
Rhabdomyosarcoma	2	6	6	5	19	3.3	3.3	46.3	4.7	3.5	2.9	3.7	3.8	56	100.0
Fibrosarcoma	0	1	3	2	6	1.0	1.1	14.6	0.6	1.8	1.2	1.2	1.1	18	100.0
Other and unspecified	4	2	4	6	16	2.8	2.8	39.0	3.5	2.4	3.5	3.1	3.1	47	100.0
X. GONADAL & GERM CELL	2	5	1	3	11	1.9	1.8	100.0	4.1	0.6	1.7	2.1	2.3	32	100.0
Non-gonadal germ cell	0	1	1	2	4	0.7	0.7	36.4	0.6	0.6	1.2	0.8	0.8	12	100.0
Gonadal germ cell	2	3	0	1	6	1.0	0.9	54.5	2.9	-	0.6	1.2	1.3	18	100.0
Gonadal carcinoma	0	1	0	0	1	0.2	0.2	9.1	0.6	-	-	0.2	0.2	3	100.0
Other and unspecified	0	0	0	0	0										
XI. EPITHELIAL NEOPLASMS	0	0	3	4	7	1.2	1.3	100.0	-	1.8	2.3	1.4	1.2	20	100.0
Adrenocortical carcinoma	0	0	0	0	0										
Thyroid carcinoma	0	0	1	2	3	0.5	0.6	42.9	-	0.6	1.2	0.6	0.5	9	100.0
Nasopharyngeal carcinoma	0	0	0	0	0										
Melanoma	0	0	0	2	2	0.3	0.4	28.6	-	-	1.2	0.4	0.4	6	100.0
Other carcinoma	0	0	2	0	2	0.3	0.4	28.6	-	1.2	-	0.4	0.3	6	100.0
XII. OTHER	1	3	1	2	7	1.2	1.2	100.0	2.3	0.6	1.2	1.4	1.4	20	83.3
* Specified as malignant	0	0	1	3	4	0.7	0.8	100.0	-	0.6	1.7	0.8	0.7	12	50.0

* Specified as malignant

Puerto Rico

1973 – 1982

FEMALE

DIAGNOSTIC GROUP	NUMBER OF CASES					REL. FREQUENCY(%)			RATES PER MILLION					Cum	HV(%)
	0	1-4	5-9	10-14	All	Crude	Adj.	Group	0-4	5-9	10-14	Crude	Adj.		
TOTAL	42	179	109	148	478	100.0	100.0	100.0	133.7	66.3	89.0	96.4	99.0	1445	97.4
I. LEUKAEMIAS	6	90	52	45	193	40.4	40.8	100.0	58.1	31.6	27.1	38.9	40.5	584	98.9
Acute lymphocytic	4	74	37	23	138	28.9	29.0	71.5	47.2	22.5	13.8	27.8	29.5	418	100.0
Other lymphocytic	0	3	0	1	4	0.8	0.8	2.1	1.8	0.6	–	0.8	0.9	12	100.0
Acute non-lymphocytic	0	7	11	14	32	6.7	7.1	16.6	4.2	6.7	8.4	6.5	6.2	97	100.0
Chronic myeloid	0	2	0	4	6	1.3	1.2	3.1	1.2	–	2.4	1.2	1.2	18	100.0
Other and unspecified	2	4	4	4	13	2.7	2.7	6.7	3.6	1.8	2.4	2.6	2.7	39	80.0
II. LYMPHOMAS	2	12	11	29	54	11.3	11.4	100.0	8.5	6.7	17.4	10.9	10.5	163	100.0
Hodgkin's disease	0	0	5	20	25	5.2	5.4	46.3	–	3.0	12.0	5.0	4.5	75	100.0
Non-Hodgkin lymphoma	0	6	4	6	16	3.3	3.4	29.6	3.6	2.4	3.6	3.2	3.2	48	100.0
Burkitt's lymphoma	0	1	1	1	3	0.6	0.7	5.6	0.6	0.6	0.6	0.6	0.6	9	100.0
Unspecified lymphoma	1	3	1	2	7	1.5	1.4	13.0	2.4	0.6	1.2	1.4	1.5	21	100.0
Histiocytosis X	1	0	0	0	1	0.2	0.2	1.9	0.6	–	–	0.2	0.2	3	100.0
Other reticuloendothelial	0	2	0	0	2	0.4	0.4	3.7	1.2	–	–	0.4	0.5	6	100.0
III. BRAIN AND SPINAL	5	22	19	20	66	13.8	14.2	100.0	16.3	11.6	12.0	13.3	13.5	200	87.7
Ependymoma	0	2	0	0	2	0.4	0.4	3.0	1.2	–	–	0.4	0.5	6	100.0
Astrocytoma	2	12	13	15	42	8.8	9.2	63.6	8.5	7.9	9.0	8.5	8.4	127	95.2
Medulloblastoma	1	2	4	4	11	2.3	2.5	16.7	1.8	2.4	2.4	2.2	2.2	33	100.0
Other glioma	0	4	1	1	6	1.3	1.2	9.1	2.4	0.6	0.6	1.2	1.3	18	40.0
Other and unspecified *	2	2	1	0	5	1.0	1.0	7.6	2.4	0.6	–	1.0	1.1	15	40.0
IV. SYMPATHETIC N.S.	6	18	1	0	25	5.2	4.6	100.0	14.5	0.6	–	5.0	5.8	76	100.0
Neuroblastoma	6	17	0	0	23	4.8	4.2	92.0	13.9	–	–	4.6	5.4	70	100.0
Other	0	1	1	0	2	0.4	0.5	8.0	0.6	0.6	–	0.4	0.4	6	100.0
V. RETINOBLASTOMA	6	12	0	0	18	3.8	3.3	100.0	10.9	–	–	3.6	4.2	54	100.0
VI. KIDNEY	5	13	8	2	28	5.9	5.9	100.0	10.9	4.9	1.2	5.6	6.1	85	100.0
Wilms' tumour	5	13	8	2	28	5.9	5.9	100.0	10.9	4.9	1.2	5.6	6.1	85	100.0
Renal carcinoma	0	0	0	0	0	–	–	–	–	–	–	–	–	–	–
Other and unspecified	0	0	0	0	0	–	–	–	–	–	–	–	–	–	–
VII. LIVER	2	2	0	0	4	0.8	0.7	100.0	2.4	–	–	0.8	0.9	12	100.0
Hepatoblastoma	2	1	0	0	3	0.6	0.5	75.0	1.8	–	–	0.6	0.7	9	100.0
Hepatic carcinoma	0	0	0	0	0	–	–	–	–	–	–	–	–	–	–
Other and unspecified	0	1	0	0	1	0.2	0.2	25.0	0.6	–	–	0.2	0.2	3	100.0
VIII. BONE	0	2	6	13	21	4.4	4.6	100.0	1.2	3.7	7.8	4.2	3.9	63	95.2
Osteosarcoma	0	1	3	7	11	2.3	2.4	52.4	0.6	1.8	4.2	2.2	2.0	33	100.0
Chondrosarcoma	0	0	1	1	2	0.4	0.5	9.5	–	0.6	0.6	0.4	0.4	6	100.0
Ewing's sarcoma	0	1	1	5	7	1.5	1.5	33.3	0.6	0.6	3.0	1.4	1.3	21	100.0
Other and unspecified	0	0	1	0	1	0.2	0.3	4.8	–	0.6	–	0.2	0.2	3	100.0
IX. SOFT TISSUE SARCOMAS	7	6	6	11	30	6.3	6.2	100.0	7.9	3.7	6.6	6.0	6.1	91	100.0
Rhabdomyosarcoma	3	5	4	6	18	3.8	3.8	60.0	4.8	2.4	3.6	3.6	3.7	54	100.0
Fibrosarcoma	0	0	1	2	3	0.6	0.7	10.0	–	0.6	1.2	0.6	0.5	9	100.0
Other and unspecified	4	1	1	3	9	1.9	1.8	30.0	3.0	0.6	1.8	1.8	1.9	27	100.0
X. GONADAL & GERM CELL	2	0	3	11	16	3.3	3.4	100.0	1.2	1.8	6.6	3.2	3.0	48	100.0
Non-gonadal germ cell	2	0	0	0	2	0.4	0.4	12.5	1.2	–	–	0.4	0.5	6	100.0
Gonadal germ cell	0	0	3	9	12	2.5	2.7	75.0	–	1.8	5.4	2.4	2.2	36	100.0
Gonadal carcinoma	0	0	0	0	0	–	–	–	–	–	–	–	–	–	–
Other and unspecified	0	0	0	2	2	0.4	0.4	12.5	–	–	1.2	0.4	0.3	6	100.0
XI. EPITHELIAL NEOPLASMS	0	1	2	17	20	4.2	4.2	100.0	0.6	1.2	10.2	4.0	3.6	60	100.0
Adrenocortical carcinoma	0	0	0	0	0	–	–	–	–	–	–	–	–	–	–
Thyroid carcinoma	0	0	1	6	7	1.5	1.5	35.0	–	0.6	3.6	1.4	1.2	21	100.0
Nasopharyngeal carcinoma	0	0	0	1	1	0.2	0.2	5.0	–	–	0.6	0.2	0.2	3	100.0
Melanoma	0	0	0	1	1	0.2	0.2	5.0	–	–	0.6	0.2	0.2	3	100.0
Other carcinoma	0	1	1	9	11	2.3	2.3	55.0	0.6	0.6	5.4	2.2	2.0	33	100.0
XII. OTHER	1	1	1	0	3	0.6	0.6	100.0	1.2	0.6	–	0.6	0.7	9	–
* Specified as malignant	2	2	1	0	5	1.0	1.0	100.0	2.4	0.6	–	1.0	1.1	15	40.0

Commentary

The overall incidence was lower than would be expected in populations containing a similar proportion of Whites and Blacks in the mainland United States. The difference was largely accounted for by low rates for acute lymphocytic leukaemia (in boys), neuroblastoma and brain tumours. The age-distribution for acute lymphocytic leukaemia showed the peak in the 1–4 age-group characteristic of western populations but the sex ratio was close to unity.

ASIA

BANGLADESH

Cancer Epidemiology Research Program, 1970–1981

M.A. Rahim

The Cancer Epidemiology Research Program (CERP) is a non-profit-making private organization. Its own tumour registry has been in operation since 1970. Sources of registration are the five radiotherapy departments of Bangladesh, where all oncological activities are carried out. Four of these are functioning under the Medical College Hospitals of Dacca (capital), Chittagong (sea port), Mymensingh and Rajshahi. The fifth is located in the district of Tangail and housed in a non-teaching private hospital, Kumudini Trust Hospital. Cancer patients from all the Medical College Hospitals (of which there are eight), specialized hospitals (seven), district hospitals and others are referred to these departments for radiotherapy and/or chemotherapy. Thus the Tumour Registry of CERP covers almost the whole country. However, because registration is done at the radiotherapy departments and reporting of cancer is not compulsory, incompleteness is unavoidable.

Autopsies are rarely performed, because of religious constraints. The pathology service is seriously short of resources so that biopsies of suspected tumours are rarely performed. This problem is exacerbated by the fact that 90% of cancer patients initially present with advanced disease. Birth and death registers are not properly maintained. Thus data from these sources could not be included. Technical difficulties preclude any attempt at follow-up. Age is estimated by the appearance of the patients, by use of historical events and physiological milestones.

Cancer patients receiving radiotherapy or chemotherapy are registered. Clinical data are recorded on uniform core-data forms. Optional data are recorded on a separate form and are used for special investigations. Completed forms are collected by the central cell of the CERP, situated at Dacca, where data are coded for site and histology. Anatomical sites are coded by ICD–8 (1970-1981), while histology, initially coded according to the *Manual of Tumor Nomenclature and Coding* of the American Cancer Society, has been recoded retrospectively according to ICD-O (1970-1981).

Indexes are used to identify individuals and specific anatomical sites. With the help of these indexes, each site is checked for valid code, age, sex, missing information and inclusion at more than one centre. Compilation and analysis is done manually and results are published in the *Bangladesh cancer reports*. Unpublished data are preserved for future use and further investigation.

Bangladesh formed the eastern wing of Pakistan until it became an independent state in 1971. It is a deltaic plain 144 000 square kilometres in area, located in the north-eastern region of the South Asian subcontinent. Mean annual temperatures vary between 14° C and 23° C. Annual rainfall varies from 125 cm in the west to 250 cm in the south-east and 500 cm in the submontane region of the Assam hills in the north.

The population is 90 million, of whom about 45% are aged under 15 (1981 census). The people are descended from several racial and subracial groups which entered the subcontinent over the past 5000 years. More than 85% of the population are Muslims, while the rest are Hindus, Christians, and Buddhists. There are 108 males per 100 females. The average population density is 591 per square kilometre. Bangladesh is primarily a rural country, with 87% of the population living in villages. The people are essentially peace-loving, poetic, lead a simple life and rarely travel more than 50 km from their homes. Rice is their staple food, which is eaten with curried fish, vegetables and pulses. Alcohol is prohibited by law and religion. Agriculture is the main occupation, employing 80% of the labour force.

The tables present the cases recorded as numbers and percentages. Incidence rates have not been calculated because of the low proportion of cases registered.

Contd. p. 142

Bangladesh, CERP　　　　1970 - 1981　　　　MALE

DIAGNOSTIC GROUP	NUMBER OF CASES					REL. FREQUENCY(%)			HV(%)
	0	1-4	5-9	10-14	All	Crude	Adj.	Group	
TOTAL	16	257	283	323	879	100.0	100.0	100.0	60.1
I. LEUKAEMIAS	0	13	27	33	73	8.3	7.8	100.0	100.0
Acute lymphocytic	0	9	8	4	21	2.4	2.5	28.8	100.0
Other lymphocytic	0	0	2	2	4	0.5	0.4	5.5	100.0
Acute non-lymphocytic	0	1	3	2	6	0.7	0.7	8.2	100.0
Chronic myeloid	0	0	1	15	16	1.8	1.5	21.9	100.0
Other and unspecified	0	3	13	10	26	3.0	2.7	35.6	100.0
II. LYMPHOMAS	0	13	67	90	170	19.3	17.4	100.0	92.9
Hodgkin's disease	0	6	36	29	71	8.1	7.4	41.8	91.5
Non-Hodgkin lymphoma	0	4	11	25	40	4.6	4.1	23.5	97.5
Burkitt's lymphoma	0	0	0	0	0	-	-	-	-
Unspecified lymphoma	0	3	20	35	58	6.6	5.8	34.1	91.4
Histiocytosis X	0	0	0	0	0	-	-	-	-
Other reticuloendothelial	0	0	0	1	1	0.1	0.1	0.6	100.0
III. BRAIN AND SPINAL	0	3	6	7	16	1.8	1.7	100.0	81.3
Ependymoma	0	0	0	0	0	-	-	-	-
Astrocytoma	0	2	2	3	7	0.8	0.8	43.8	100.0
Medulloblastoma	0	0	0	0	0	-	-	-	-
Other glioma	0	0	2	1	3	0.3	0.3	18.8	100.0
Other and unspecified *	0	1	2	3	6	0.7	0.6	37.5	50.0
IV. SYMPATHETIC N.S.	0	1	0	1	2	0.2	0.2	100.0	100.0
Neuroblastoma	0	1	0	1	2	0.2	0.2	100.0	100.0
Other	0	0	0	0	0	-	-	-	-
V. RETINOBLASTOMA	9	159	74	18	260	29.6	34.1	100.0	31.5
VI. KIDNEY	6	29	13	3	51	5.8	6.8	100.0	37.3
Wilms' tumour	5	29	13	3	50	5.7	6.6	98.0	38.0
Renal carcinoma	0	0	0	0	0	-	-	-	-
Other and unspecified	1	0	0	0	1	0.1	0.1	2.0	-
VII. LIVER	0	1	6	1	8	0.9	0.9	100.0	75.0
Hepatoblastoma	0	0	0	0	0	-	-	-	-
Hepatic carcinoma	0	1	4	1	6	0.7	0.7	75.0	100.0
Other and unspecified	0	2	0	0	2	0.2	0.2	25.0	-
VIII. BONE	0	6	30	61	97	11.0	9.7	100.0	40.2
Osteosarcoma	0	3	22	44	69	7.8	6.9	71.1	30.4
Chondrosarcoma	0	0	2	1	3	0.3	0.3	3.1	100.0
Ewing's sarcoma	0	1	4	8	13	1.5	1.3	13.4	61.5
Other and unspecified	0	2	2	8	12	1.4	1.2	12.4	58.3
IX. SOFT TISSUE SARCOMAS	1	8	18	27	54	6.1	5.7	100.0	75.9
Rhabdomyosarcoma	1	0	2	1	4	0.5	0.5	7.4	100.0
Fibrosarcoma	0	2	1	10	13	1.5	1.3	24.1	92.3
Other and unspecified	0	6	15	16	37	4.2	4.0	68.5	67.6
X. GONADAL & GERM CELL	0	3	4	4	11	1.3	1.2	100.0	90.9
Non-gonadal germ cell	0	0	0	0	0	-	-	-	-
Gonadal germ cell	0	3	4	3	10	1.1	1.1	90.9	100.0
Gonadal carcinoma	0	0	0	0	0	-	-	-	-
Other and unspecified	0	0	0	1	1	0.1	0.1	9.1	-
XI. EPITHELIAL NEOPLASMS	0	13	23	49	85	9.7	8.9	100.0	96.5
Adrenocortical carcinoma	0	0	0	0	0	-	-	-	-
Thyroid carcinoma	0	0	0	0	0	-	-	-	-
Nasopharyngeal carcinoma	0	0	5	23	28	3.2	2.7	32.9	100.0
Melanoma	0	1	1	1	3	0.3	0.3	3.5	33.3
Other carcinoma	0	12	17	25	54	6.1	5.9	63.5	98.1
XII. OTHER	0	8	15	29	52	5.9	5.5	100.0	5.8
* Specified as malignant	0	1	2	3	6	0.7	0.6	100.0	50.0

Bangladesh, CERP

1970 – 1981

FEMALE

DIAGNOSTIC GROUP	NUMBER OF CASES					REL. FREQUENCY(%)			HV(%)
	0	1-4	5-9	10-14	All	Crude	Adj.	Group	
TOTAL	8	134	121	151	414	100.0	100.0	100.0	58.5
I. LEUKAEMIAS	1	10	12	15	38	9.2	9.1	100.0	100.0
Acute lymphocytic	0	4	4	3	11	2.7	2.7	28.9	100.0
Other lymphocytic	0	1	0	1	2	0.5	0.5	5.3	100.0
Acute non-lymphocytic	0	2	2	2	6	1.4	1.5	15.8	100.0
Chronic myeloid	0	0	2	4	6	1.4	1.3	15.8	100.0
Other and unspecified	1	3	4	5	13	3.1	3.1	34.2	100.0
II. LYMPHOMAS	0	9	10	27	46	11.1	10.4	100.0	91.3
Hodgkin's disease	0	1	3	8	12	2.9	2.6	26.1	91.7
Non-Hodgkin lymphoma	0	2	2	7	11	2.7	2.4	23.9	100.0
Burkitt's lymphoma	0	0	0	0	0	-	-	-	-
Unspecified lymphoma	0	6	5	11	22	5.3	5.1	47.8	86.4
Histiocytosis X	0	0	0	0	0	-	-	-	-
Other reticuloendothelial	0	0	0	1	1	0.2	0.2	2.2	100.0
III. BRAIN AND SPINAL	0	1	2	2	5	1.2	1.2	100.0	80.0
Ependymoma	0	1	0	0	1	0.2	0.3	20.0	100.0
Astrocytoma	0	0	0	1	1	0.2	0.2	20.0	100.0
Medulloblastoma	0	0	0	0	0	-	-	-	-
Other glioma	0	0	1	0	1	0.2	0.2	20.0	100.0
Other and unspecified *	0	0	1	1	2	0.5	0.4	40.0	50.0
IV. SYMPATHETIC N.S.	0	0	1	1	2	0.5	0.4	100.0	100.0
Neuroblastoma	0	0	1	1	2	0.5	0.4	100.0	100.0
Other	0	0	0	0	0	-	-	-	-
V. RETINOBLASTOMA	3	81	44	5	133	32.1	35.6	100.0	36.1
VI. KIDNEY	0	6	9	3	18	4.3	4.5	100.0	33.3
Wilms' tumour	0	5	9	2	16	3.9	4.0	88.9	37.5
Renal carcinoma	0	0	0	0	0	-	-	-	-
Other and unspecified	0	1	0	1	2	0.5	0.5	11.1	-
VII. LIVER	0	3	7	5	15	3.6	3.6	100.0	93.3
Hepatoblastoma	0	1	0	0	1	0.2	0.2	6.7	100.0
Hepatic carcinoma	0	2	7	4	13	3.1	3.1	86.7	100.0
Other and unspecified	0	0	0	1	1	0.2	0.2	6.7	-
VIII. BONE	0	7	6	30	43	10.4	9.4	100.0	44.2
Osteosarcoma	0	4	6	22	32	7.7	7.0	74.4	28.1
Chondrosarcoma	0	0	0	0	0	-	-	-	-
Ewing's sarcoma	0	1	0	5	6	1.4	1.2	14.0	100.0
Other and unspecified	0	2	0	3	5	1.2	1.2	11.6	80.0
IX. SOFT TISSUE SARCOMAS	3	6	8	15	32	7.7	7.5	100.0	78.1
Rhabdomyosarcoma	1	1	0	3	5	1.2	1.1	15.6	100.0
Fibrosarcoma	0	2	1	0	3	0.7	0.8	9.4	100.0
Other and unspecified	2	3	7	12	24	5.8	5.6	75.0	70.8
X. GONADAL & GERM CELL	0	2	5	18	25	6.0	5.4	100.0	52.0
Non-gonadal germ cell	0	1	3	5	9	2.2	2.0	36.0	100.0
Gonadal germ cell	0	0	1	3	4	1.0	0.8	16.0	100.0
Gonadal carcinoma	0	1	1	10	12	2.9	2.5	48.0	-
Other and unspecified	0	0	0	0	0	-	-	-	-
XI. EPITHELIAL NEOPLASMS	0	3	10	18	31	7.5	6.9	100.0	96.8
Adrenocortical carcinoma	0	0	0	1	1	0.2	0.2	3.2	100.0
Thyroid carcinoma	0	0	1	2	3	0.7	0.6	9.7	100.0
Nasopharyngeal carcinoma	0	0	0	2	2	0.5	0.4	6.5	100.0
Melanoma	0	0	0	0	0	-	-	-	-
Other carcinoma	0	3	9	13	25	6.0	5.7	80.6	96.0
XII. OTHER	1	7	6	12	26	6.3	6.1	100.0	3.8
* Specified as malignant	0	0	1	1	2	0.5	0.4	100.0	50.0

Commentary

The most numerous diagnostic group was retino-blastoma, accounting for over 30% of all registrations. The laterality was given for all but one of the 393 cases of retinoblastoma; only 10 (2.6%) were bilateral, and all but one of these were diagnosed after 1976. Compared with European populations, there were high relative frequencies of lymphomas (both Hodgkin's disease and others), osteo-sarcoma, and carcinomas and unspecified tumours of the nasopharynx and oral cavity. Under 2% of registrations were for brain and spinal tumours, and under 0.5% for neuroblastoma. The ratio of male to female registrations overall was 2.12. As the ratio was almost as high (1.95) for retinoblastoma, for which the sex ratio is generally close to unity, the excess of boys could be partially attributable to less complete ascertainment among girls.

CHINA

Shanghai Cancer Registry, 1972–1979

Gao Yu-Tang & Jin Fan

Pursuant to the Regulation concerning the notification of cancer cases issued by the Shanghai Municipal Bureau of Public Health, the Shanghai Cancer Registry was established and started operating in 1963. It is a centralized population-based cancer registry, now affiliated to the Department of Epidemiology of the Shanghai Cancer Institute.

Under the above-mentioned Regulation, each medical facility in Shanghai is responsible for reporting all new cancer cases (including benign tumours of the central nervous system) after admission to hospital, whether as out-patients or in-patients. The notifications, completed by physicians or medical clerks of the medical facilities, are sent to the Cancer Registry. If an incorrect diagnosis has been made, the physician attending the cancer patient sends another notification card to correct the previous erroneous diagnosis. All new notification cards on cancer cases are collated with existing files to avoid duplicate registrations; these cases are searched for in the local Offices of Public Security to see whether the cancer patients are registered as residents of Shanghai urban area. New files are then established for these cases.

The Cancer Registry receives monthly notifications of all cancer deaths from the Section of Vital Statistics in each district of Shanghai. Several times every year Registry staff members visit the medical facilities responsible for reporting new cases to discuss with them problems related to improvement of the quality of reporting.

For the early years of the registry (1972–1979), no information on the precise histological diagnosis was recorded, but only the fact of a biopsy having being done. For the present study, therefore, a special search of medical and pathology records relating to cases diagnosed in this period was necessary. Unfortunately, a considerable proportion of records could not be found, as reflected in the high proportion of cases with general, rather than specific, diagnostic labels (e.g., leukaemia,

sarcoma), despite the relatively high percentages of histologically verified cancers.

Shanghai is situated in the middle part of China, on the east coast. Its altitude is about 4 m above sea level and it has an area of 6139 square kilometres (urban area about 223 square kilometres). Average annual temperature is about 15° C. It is the largest city in China, with about 11 million inhabitants. In 1980, the inhabitants in the urban area numbered 5 963 723. At the end of 1980 there were 15 037 physicians qualified in western medicine (2.52 per 1000 persons) in the urban area and 40 388 hospital beds (6.77 per 1000).

Population

Annual estimates of the population are available, based on the censuses of 1973 and 1979.

AVERAGE ANNUAL POPULATION: 1972–1979

Age	Male	Female
0	20457	19106
1–4	89511	83619
5–9	137695	129341
10–14	282187	264409
0–14	529850	496475

Commentary

The ratio of acute lymphocytic leukaemia (ALL) to acute non-lymphocytic leukaemia was 1.47:1. Peak incidence of ALL occurred in the 5–9-year age-group. Hodgkin's disease accounted for under 20% of lymphomas. No children with Burkitt's lymphoma were recorded.

Malignant kidney tumours were very rare, and half of those registered were in the 'other and unspecified' group.

Malignant liver tumours were relatively common, with a crude incidence rate similar to that for

Contd p. 146

China, Shanghai

1972 – 1979

MALE

DIAGNOSTIC GROUP	NUMBER OF CASES 0	1-4	5-9	10-14	All	REL. FREQUENCY(%) Crude	Adj.	Group	RATES PER MILLION 0	1-4	5-9	10-14	Crude	Adj.	Cum	HV(%)
TOTAL	27	84	127	225	463	100.0	100.0	100.0	165.0	117.3	115.3	99.7	109.2	115.2	1709	87.7
I. LEUKAEMIAS	6	30	62	86	184	39.7	39.1	100.0	36.7	41.9	56.3	38.1	43.4	45.0	676	100.0
Acute lymphocytic	2	13	30	39	84	18.1	17.7	45.7	12.2	18.2	27.2	17.3	19.8	20.4	307	100.0
Other lymphocytic	0	0	0	0	0											
Acute non-lymphocytic	0	9	21	27	57	12.3	11.8	31.0	–	12.6	19.1	12.0	13.4	13.5	205	100.0
Chronic myeloid	0	2	3	2	7	1.5	1.7	3.8	–	2.8	2.7	0.9	1.7	2.0	29	100.0
Other and unspecified	4	6	8	18	36	7.8	7.9	19.6	24.4	8.4	7.3	8.0	8.5	9.1	134	100.0
II. LYMPHOMAS	7	7	14	43	71	15.3	14.1	100.0	42.8	9.8	12.7	19.0	16.7	16.0	241	100.0
Hodgkin's disease	0	3	3	8	14	3.0	2.9	19.7	–	4.2	2.7	3.5	3.3	3.2	48	100.0
Non-Hodgkin lymphoma	1	2	9	24	36	7.8	6.4	50.7	6.1	2.8	8.2	10.6	8.5	7.1	111	100.0
Burkitt's lymphoma	0	0	0	0	0											
Unspecified lymphoma	2	1	1	4	8	1.7	1.9	11.3	12.2	1.4	0.9	1.8	1.9	2.2	31	100.0
Histiocytosis X	0	0	0	0	0											
Other reticuloendothelial	4	1	1	7	13	2.8	3.0	18.3	24.4	1.4	0.9	3.1	3.1	3.5	50	100.0
III. BRAIN AND SPINAL	1	11	35	33	80	17.3	17.0	100.0	6.1	15.4	31.8	14.6	18.9	19.7	300	61.3
Ependymoma	0	2	0	0	2	0.4	0.7	2.5	–	2.8	–	–	0.5	0.9	11	100.0
Astrocytoma	0	2	4	6	12	2.6	2.5	15.0	–	2.8	3.6	2.7	2.8	2.8	43	100.0
Medulloblastoma	0	1	5	0	6	1.3	1.5	7.5	–	1.4	4.5	–	1.4	1.9	28	100.0
Other glioma	0	0	3	2	5	1.1	1.0	6.3	–	–	2.7	0.9	1.2	1.1	18	100.0
Other and unspecified *	1	6	23	25	55	11.9	11.3	68.8	6.1	8.4	20.9	11.1	13.0	13.0	199	43.6
IV. SYMPATHETIC N.S.	2	8	3	2	15	3.2	4.6	100.0	12.2	11.2	2.7	0.9	3.5	5.5	75	100.0
Neuroblastoma	2	8	3	1	14	3.0	4.4	93.3	12.2	11.2	2.7	0.4	3.3	5.4	73	100.0
Other	0	0	0	1	1	0.2	0.1	6.7	–	–	–	0.4	0.2	0.1	2	100.0
V. RETINOBLASTOMA	2	4	1	0	7	1.5	2.4	100.0	12.2	5.6	0.9	–	1.7	3.0	39	100.0
VI. KIDNEY	2	4	2	0	8	1.7	2.6	100.0	12.2	5.6	1.8	–	1.9	3.3	44	100.0
Wilms' tumour	1	1	0	0	2	0.4	0.7	25.0	6.1	1.4	–	–	0.5	0.9	12	100.0
Renal carcinoma	0	0	1	0	1	0.2	0.2	12.5	–	–	0.9	–	0.2	0.3	5	100.0
Other and unspecified	1	3	1	0	5	1.1	1.7	62.5	6.1	4.2	0.9	–	1.2	2.1	27	100.0
VII. LIVER	3	3	1	16	23	5.0	4.5	100.0	18.3	4.2	0.9	7.1	5.4	5.1	75	17.4
Hepatoblastoma	1	1	0	0	2	0.4	0.7	8.7	6.1	1.4	–	–	0.5	0.9	12	100.0
Hepatic carcinoma	0	0	1	0	1	0.2	0.2	4.3	–	–	0.9	–	0.2	0.3	5	100.0
Other and unspecified	2	2	0	16	20	4.3	3.6	87.0	12.2	2.8	–	7.1	4.7	3.9	59	5.0
VIII. BONE	0	0	2	12	14	3.0	2.1	100.0	–	–	1.8	5.3	3.3	2.1	36	92.9
Osteosarcoma	0	0	2	7	9	1.9	1.4	64.3	–	–	1.8	3.1	2.1	1.5	25	100.0
Chondrosarcoma	0	0	0	0	0											
Ewing's sarcoma	0	0	0	2	2	0.4	0.3	14.3	–	–	–	0.9	0.5	0.3	4	100.0
Other and unspecified	0	0	0	3	3	0.6	0.4	21.4	–	–	–	1.3	0.7	0.4	7	66.7
IX. SOFT TISSUE SARCOMAS	1	3	1	8	13	2.8	2.7	100.0	6.1	4.2	0.9	3.5	3.1	3.1	45	100.0
Rhabdomyosarcoma	1	2	0	2	5	1.1	1.3	38.5	6.1	2.8	–	0.9	1.2	1.6	22	100.0
Fibrosarcoma	0	0	1	3	4	0.9	0.6	30.8	–	–	0.9	1.3	0.9	0.7	11	100.0
Other and unspecified	0	1	0	3	4	0.9	0.8	30.8	–	1.4	–	1.3	0.9	0.8	12	100.0
X. GONADAL & GERM CELL	1	8	0	2	11	2.4	3.5	100.0	6.1	11.2	–	0.9	2.6	4.2	55	100.0
Non-gonadal germ cell	0	5	0	1	6	1.3	1.9	54.5	–	7.0	–	0.4	1.4	2.3	30	100.0
Gonadal germ cell	1	3	0	0	4	0.9	1.4	36.4	6.1	4.2	–	–	0.9	1.8	23	100.0
Gonadal carcinoma	0	0	0	0	0											
Other and unspecified	0	0	0	1	1	0.2	0.1	9.1	–	–	–	0.4	0.2	0.1	2	100.0
XI. EPITHELIAL NEOPLASMS	0	1	1	7	9	1.9	1.5	100.0	–	1.4	0.9	3.1	2.1	1.6	26	100.0
Adrenocortical carcinoma	0	0	0	0	0											
Thyroid carcinoma	0	0	2	0	2	0.4	0.3	22.2	–	–	0.9	–	0.5	0.3	4	100.0
Nasopharyngeal carcinoma	0	0	0	0	0											
Melanoma	0	0	0	0	0											
Other carcinoma	0	1	1	5	7	1.5	1.3	77.8	–	1.4	0.9	2.2	1.7	1.4	21	100.0
XII. OTHER	2	5	5	16	28	6.0	5.8	100.0	12.2	7.0	4.5	7.1	6.6	6.6	98	78.6
* Specified as malignant	1	6	22	18	47	10.2	10.1	100.0	6.1	8.4	20.0	8.0	11.1	11.8	179	34.0

China, Shanghai

1972 - 1979

FEMALE

DIAGNOSTIC GROUP	NUMBER OF CASES 0	1-4	5-9	10-14	All	REL. FREQUENCY(%) Crude	Adj.	Group	RATES PER MILLION 0	1-4	5-9	10-14	Crude	Adj.	Cum	HV(%)
TOTAL	22	74	95	174	365	100.0	100.0	100.0	143.9	110.6	91.8	82.3	91.9	98.9	1457	86.6
I. LEUKAEMIAS	7	28	37	60	132	36.2	36.6	100.0	45.8	41.9	35.8	28.4	33.2	36.3	534	100.0
Acute lymphocytic	2	11	21	26	60	16.4	16.5	45.5	13.1	16.4	20.3	12.3	15.1	16.2	242	100.0
Other lymphocytic	0	2	0	0	2	0.5	0.8	1.5	-	3.0	-	-	0.5	0.9	12	100.0
Acute non-lymphocytic	1	8	11	21	41	11.2	10.8	31.1	6.5	12.0	10.6	9.9	10.3	10.5	157	100.0
Chronic myeloid	0	0	0	5	5	1.4	0.9	3.8	-	-	-	2.4	1.3	0.7	12	100.0
Other and unspecified	4	7	5	8	24	6.6	7.5	18.2	26.2	10.5	4.8	3.8	6.0	7.9	111	100.0
II. LYMPHOMAS	0	3	6	18	27	7.4	6.2	100.0	-	4.5	5.8	8.5	6.8	5.7	89	100.0
Hodgkin's disease	0	1	0	4	5	1.4	1.1	18.5	-	1.5	-	1.9	1.3	1.0	15	100.0
Non-Hodgkin lymphoma	0	0	6	7	13	3.6	3.1	48.1	-	-	5.8	3.3	3.3	2.8	46	100.0
Burkitt's lymphoma	0	0	0	0	0	-	-	-	-	-	-	-	-	-	-	-
Unspecified lymphoma	0	2	0	6	8	2.2	1.9	29.6	-	3.0	-	2.8	2.0	1.7	26	100.0
Histiocytosis X	0	0	0	0	0	-	-	-	-	-	-	-	-	-	-	-
Other reticuloendothelial	0	0	0	1	1	0.3	0.2	3.7	-	-	-	0.5	0.3	0.1	2	100.0
III. BRAIN AND SPINAL	2	13	32	23	70	19.2	20.3	100.0	13.1	19.4	30.9	10.9	17.6	20.2	300	52.9
Ependymoma	0	0	1	0	1	0.3	0.3	1.4	-	-	1.0	-	0.3	0.3	5	100.0
Astrocytoma	0	0	8	1	9	2.5	2.7	12.9	-	-	7.7	0.5	2.3	2.6	41	100.0
Medulloblastoma	0	0	4	2	6	1.6	1.6	8.6	-	-	3.9	0.9	1.5	1.4	24	100.0
Other glioma	2	0	2	4	8	2.2	1.7	11.4	13.1	-	1.9	1.9	2.0	1.4	24	100.0
Other and unspecified	0	13	17	16	46	12.6	14.0	65.7	-	19.4	16.4	7.6	11.6	14.3	206	28.3
IV. SYMPATHETIC N.S.	0	6	1	3	10	2.7	3.3	100.0	-	9.0	1.0	1.4	2.5	3.5	48	100.0
Neuroblastoma	0	6	1	3	10	2.7	3.3	100.0	-	9.0	1.0	1.4	2.5	3.5	48	100.0
Other	0	0	0	0	0	-	-	-	-	-	-	-	-	-	-	-
V. RETINOBLASTOMA	3	3	0	0	6	1.6	2.5	100.0	19.6	4.5	-	-	1.5	2.9	38	100.0
VI. KIDNEY	0	0	0	2	2	0.5	0.3	100.0	-	-	-	0.9	0.5	0.3	5	100.0
Wilms' tumour	0	0	0	2	2	0.5	0.3	100.0	-	-	-	0.9	0.5	0.3	5	100.0
Renal carcinoma	0	0	0	0	0	-	-	-	-	-	-	-	-	-	-	-
Other and unspecified	0	0	0	0	0	-	-	-	-	-	-	-	-	-	-	-
VII. LIVER	0	4	0	6	10	2.7	2.7	100.0	-	6.0	-	2.8	2.5	2.7	38	40.0
Hepatoblastoma	0	1	0	2	3	0.8	0.8	30.0	-	1.5	-	0.9	0.8	0.7	11	100.0
Hepatic carcinoma	0	0	0	1	1	0.3	0.2	10.0	-	-	-	0.5	0.3	0.1	2	100.0
Other and unspecified	0	3	0	3	6	1.6	1.8	60.0	-	4.5	-	1.4	1.5	1.8	25	-
VIII. BONE	0	0	8	20	28	7.7	6.0	100.0	-	-	7.7	9.5	7.0	5.2	86	92.9
Osteosarcoma	0	0	2	12	14	3.8	2.7	50.0	-	-	1.9	5.7	3.5	2.3	38	100.0
Chondrosarcoma	0	0	2	0	2	0.5	0.6	7.1	-	-	1.9	-	0.5	0.4	10	100.0
Ewing's sarcoma	0	0	0	3	3	0.8	0.5	10.7	-	-	-	1.4	0.8	0.6	7	100.0
Other and unspecified	0	0	4	5	9	2.5	2.1	32.1	-	-	3.9	2.4	2.3	1.9	31	77.8
IX. SOFT TISSUE SARCOMAS	3	6	5	7	21	5.8	6.5	100.0	19.6	9.0	4.8	3.3	5.3	6.8	96	100.0
Rhabdomyosarcoma	2	6	1	1	10	2.7	3.8	47.6	13.1	9.0	1.0	0.5	2.5	4.2	56	100.0
Fibrosarcoma	0	0	1	3	4	1.1	0.8	19.0	-	-	1.0	1.4	1.0	0.7	12	100.0
Other and unspecified	1	0	3	3	7	1.9	1.9	33.3	6.5	-	2.9	1.4	1.8	1.8	28	100.0
X. GONADAL & GERM CELL	3	4	3	11	21	5.8	5.8	100.0	19.6	6.0	2.9	5.2	5.3	5.8	84	100.0
Non-gonadal germ cell	2	4	0	1	7	1.9	2.7	33.3	13.1	6.0	-	0.5	1.8	3.0	39	100.0
Gonadal germ cell	0	0	1	6	7	1.9	1.4	33.3	-	-	1.0	2.8	1.8	1.1	19	100.0
Gonadal carcinoma	0	0	0	1	1	0.3	0.2	4.8	-	-	-	0.5	0.3	0.1	2	100.0
Other and unspecified	1	0	2	3	6	1.6	1.6	28.6	6.5	-	1.9	1.4	1.5	1.5	23	100.0
XI. EPITHELIAL NEOPLASMS	1	0	0	10	11	3.0	2.1	100.0	6.5	-	-	4.7	2.8	1.9	30	100.0
Adrenocortical carcinoma	1	0	0	2	3	0.8	0.5	27.3	6.5	-	-	0.9	0.8	0.4	7	100.0
Thyroid carcinoma	0	0	0	0	0	-	-	-	-	-	-	-	-	-	-	-
Nasopharyngeal carcinoma	0	0	0	2	2	0.5	0.3	18.2	-	-	-	0.9	0.5	0.3	5	100.0
Melanoma	0	0	0	0	0	-	-	-	-	-	-	-	-	-	-	-
Other carcinoma	0	0	0	6	6	1.6	1.3	54.5	-	-	-	2.8	1.5	1.2	18	100.0
XII. OTHER	3	7	3	14	27	7.4	7.5	100.0	19.6	10.5	2.9	6.6	6.8	7.6	109	70.4
* Specified as malignant	2	13	13	13	41	11.2	12.6	-	13.1	19.4	12.6	6.1	10.3	12.9	184	19.5

* Specified as malignant

neuroblastoma and Wilms' tumour combined. Only a quarter of the liver cancers were histologically verified, but as the great majority were in the 10–14 age-group they were presumably mostly carcinomas.

Ewing's sarcoma was rarely seen, as has been noted before in Chinese populations (Li *et al.*, 1980b).

The rates for non-gonadal germ-cell tumours in both sexes seem high.

References

Li, F.P., Jin, F. & Gao, Y.T. (1980a) Incidence of childhood leukaemia in Shanghai. *Int. J. Cancer, 25*, 701-703

Li, F.P., Tu, J.T., Liu, F.S. & Shiang, E.L. (1980b) Rarity of Ewing's sarcoma in China. *Lancet, i*, 1255

Tu, J. & Li, F.P. (1983) Incidence of childhood tumours in Shanghai, 1973-1977. *J. natl Cancer Inst., 70*, 589-592

Taipei: Central Cancer Registry, 1983–1984

K.Y. Chen & Ting Y. Kuan

The Central Cancer Registry was established in 1979. All hospitals throughout Taiwan with 50 or more beds were invited to participate in case reporting. In 1978, a meeting of hospital administrators was held, seeking to promote their participation and support, a workshop was conducted to train hospital tumour registrars, and a uniform notification form was designed to be used by all hospitals.

In 1983, one of the leading national teaching hospitals, the Veterans General Hospital (VGH), Taipei, was requested to conduct a technical project, 'Establishing the centralized cancer patient data system', financed by a grant from the Department of Health. A centralized database was created on the computer at VGH, and annual reports have been published since then. From 1983 the registry has been population-based. Benign neoplasms are not registered. Diagnoses are coded using ICD-O.

In 1984, hospital visits by project field investigators were initiated, and a questionnaire survey was undertaken to assess hospital compliance. The three largest independent pathology laboratories were added as new case-finding sources.

In 1985, a random abstract audit was undertaken by field investigators to assess the accuracy of data. Tumour registrar seminars were conducted in three regions to cover the whole area of Taiwan.

Currently, the sources of information are 113 hospital registries, and three independent laboratories. A pilot study was conducted to explore the possibility of case matching with death certificates. Cases are reported on a voluntary basis. A notification fee equivalent to US$ 0.5 is paid by the Bureau of Public Health for each case reported.

The island of Taiwan is located in the southeastern China Sea, with the Pacific Ocean on the east, and the Taiwan Strait on the west. The total land area is 36 000 square kilometres. Taiwan is 394 kilometres in length from north to south, and 144 kilometres in width from east to west at its widest point.

The mid-year population in 1984 was 18.9 million; the population density was 524 per square kilometre.

Population

The population at risk is available as annual estimates from official sources.

AVERAGE ANNUAL POPULATION: 1983–1984

Age	Male	Female
0	182220	170102
1–4	834770	784790
5–9	996629	940098
10–14	950923	899456
0–14	2964542	2794446

Commentary

The relative frequencies of the major diagnostic groups are similar to those observed in other east Asian registries. However, for nearly all groups the registration rates appear low. The data presented here are more recent than those from most other registries, and are from the first two years of operation as a population-based registry, and it is therefore plausible that the deficit is due to under-ascertainment rather than a generally abnormally low risk of childhood cancer. The main exceptions to this pattern of low incidence rate were liver tumours in males and testicular germ-cell tumours, which had correspondingly high relative frequencies. Among liver tumours, only half were of specified histological type and 64% of these were hepatic carcinoma; the age-distribution of unspecified liver tumours suggests that they were also

Contd p. 150

China, Taipei

1983 – 1984 MALE

DIAGNOSTIC GROUP	NUMBER OF CASES 0	1-4	5-9	10-14	All	REL. FREQUENCY(%) Crude	Adj.	Group	RATES PER MILLION 0	1-4	5-9	10-14	Crude	Adj.	Cum	HV(%)
TOTAL	51	185	135	138	509	100.0	100.0	100.0	139.9	110.8	67.7	72.6	85.8	88.1	1285	84.6
I. LEUKAEMIAS	10	68	49	47	174	34.2	34.3	100.0	27.4	40.7	24.6	24.7	29.3	29.8	437	100.0
Acute lymphocytic	6	58	35	23	122	24.0	23.6	70.1	16.5	34.7	17.6	12.1	20.6	21.2	304	100.0
Other lymphocytic	0	0	1	0	1	0.2	0.2	0.6			0.5		0.2		3	100.0
Acute non-lymphocytic	4	10	11	17	42	8.3	8.5	24.1	11.0	6.0	5.5	8.9	7.1	7.1	107	100.0
Chronic myeloid	0	0	1	2	6	1.2	1.3	3.4			0.5	2.6	1.0	0.9	16	100.0
Other and unspecified	0	0	1	2	3	0.6	0.7	1.7			0.5	1.1	0.5	0.5	8	100.0
II. LYMPHOMAS	0	19	19	16	54	10.6	10.9	100.0		11.4	9.5	8.4	9.1	9.0	135	100.0
Hodgkin's disease	0	1	2	2	5	1.0	1.0	9.3		0.6	1.0	1.1	0.8	0.8	13	100.0
Non-Hodgkin lymphoma	0	6	12	9	27	5.3	5.6	50.0		3.6	6.0	4.7	4.6	4.4	68	100.0
Burkitt's lymphoma	0	0	0	0	0											
Unspecified lymphoma	0	8	4	4	16	3.1	3.1	29.6		4.8	2.0	2.1	2.7	2.7	40	100.0
Histiocytosis X	0	2	0	0	2	0.4	0.4	3.7		1.2			0.3	0.4	5	100.0
Other reticuloendothelial	0	2	1	1	4	0.8	0.8	7.4		1.2	0.5	0.5	0.7	0.7	10	100.0
III. BRAIN AND SPINAL	4	18	23	20	65	12.8	13.2	100.0	11.0	10.8	11.5	10.5	11.0	11.0	164	78.5
Ependymoma	1	1	1	1	4	0.8	0.8	6.2	2.7	0.6	0.5	0.5	0.7	0.7	10	100.0
Astrocytoma	0	6	8	10	24	4.7	5.0	36.9		3.6	4.0	5.3	4.0	3.9	61	100.0
Medulloblastoma	1	6	8	4	19	3.7	3.8	29.2	2.7	3.6	4.0	2.1	3.2	3.2	48	100.0
Other glioma	1	0	1	0	2	0.4	0.4	3.1	2.7		0.5		0.3	0.4	5	100.0
Other and unspecified *	1	5	5	5	16	3.1	3.2	24.6	2.7	3.0	2.5	2.6	2.7	2.7	40	12.5
IV. SYMPATHETIC N.S.	5	15	2	2	24	4.7	4.3	100.0	13.7	9.0	1.0	1.1	4.0	4.5	60	100.0
Neuroblastoma	5	15	2	2	24	4.7	4.3	100.0	13.7	9.0	1.0	1.1	4.0	4.5	60	100.0
Other	0	0	0	0	0											
V. RETINOBLASTOMA	1	11	0	0	12	2.4	2.0	100.0	2.7	6.6			2.0	2.3	29	100.0
VI. KIDNEY	3	8	6	1	18	3.5	3.4	100.0	8.2	4.8	3.0	0.5	3.0	3.2	45	77.8
Wilms' tumour	2	6	2	1	11	2.2	2.0	61.1	5.5	3.6	1.0	0.5	1.9	2.0	28	100.0
Renal carcinoma	0	0	3	0	3	0.6	0.7	16.7			1.5		0.5		8	100.0
Other and unspecified	1	2	1	0	4	0.8	0.7	22.2	2.7	1.2	0.5		0.7	0.7	10	100.0
VII. LIVER	6	5	12	15	38	7.5	7.8	100.0	16.5	3.0	6.0	7.9	6.4	6.4	98	47.4
Hepatoblastoma	5	0	0	1	6	1.2	1.1	15.8	13.7			0.5	1.0	1.2	16	100.0
Hepatic carcinoma	0	0	6	6	12	2.4	2.6	31.6			3.0	3.2	2.0	1.9	31	100.0
Other and unspecified	1	5	6	8	20	3.9	4.1	52.6	2.7	3.0	3.0	4.2	3.4	3.3	51	
VIII. BONE	0	1	3	10	14	2.8	3.0	100.0		0.6	1.5	5.3	2.4	2.2	36	100.0
Osteosarcoma	0	1	2	9	12	2.4	2.6	85.7		0.6	1.0	4.7	2.0	1.9	31	100.0
Chondrosarcoma	0	0	0	0	0											
Ewing's sarcoma	0	0	1	1	2	0.4	0.4	14.3			0.5	0.5	0.3	0.3	5	100.0
Other and unspecified	0	0	0	0	0											
IX. SOFT TISSUE SARCOMAS	3	6	8	5	22	4.3	4.4	100.0	8.2	3.6	4.0	2.6	3.7	3.8	56	100.0
Rhabdomyosarcoma	1	4	2	2	9	1.8	1.7	40.9	2.7	2.4	1.0	1.1	1.5	1.6	23	100.0
Fibrosarcoma	1	1	2	1	5	1.0	1.0	22.7	2.7	0.6	1.0	0.5	0.8	0.9	13	100.0
Other and unspecified	1	1	4	2	8	1.6	1.7	36.4	2.7	0.6	2.0	1.1	1.3	1.4	20	100.0
X. GONADAL & GERM CELL	10	17	2	1	30	5.9	5.2	100.0	27.4	10.2	1.0	0.5	5.1	5.8	76	100.0
Non-gonadal germ cell	2	2	0	1	6	1.2	1.1	20.0	5.5	1.2		0.5	1.0	1.1	15	100.0
Gonadal germ cell	8	14	1	0	23	4.5	4.0	76.7	22.0	8.4	0.5		3.9	4.5	58	100.0
Gonadal carcinoma	0	1	0	0	1	0.2	0.2	3.3		0.6			0.2	0.2	2	100.0
Other and unspecified	0	0	0	0	0											
XI. EPITHELIAL NEOPLASMS	3	2	2	9	16	3.1	3.2	100.0	8.2	1.2	1.0	4.7	2.7	2.7	42	100.0
Adrenocortical carcinoma	0	1	0	1	2	0.4	0.4	12.5		0.6		0.5	0.3	0.3	5	100.0
Thyroid carcinoma	0	1	1	0	2	0.4	0.4	12.5		0.6	0.5		0.3	0.3	5	100.0
Nasopharyngeal carcinoma	0	0	0	3	3	0.6	0.7	18.8				1.6	0.5	0.5	8	100.0
Melanoma	0	0	0	0	0											
Other carcinoma	3	0	1	5	9	1.8	1.8	56.3	8.2		0.5	2.6	1.5	1.6	24	100.0
XII. OTHER	6	15	9	12	42	8.3	8.2	100.0	16.5	9.0	4.5	6.3	7.1	7.3	107	2.4
* Specified as malignant	1	5	5	5	16	3.1	3.2	100.0	2.7	3.0	2.5	2.6	2.7	2.7	40	12.5

China, Taipei

1983 - 1984

FEMALE

DIAGNOSTIC GROUP	NUMBER OF CASES 0	1-4	5-9	10-14	All	REL. FREQUENCY(%) Crude	Adj.	Group	RATES PER MILLION 0	1-4	5-9	10-14	Crude	Adj.	Cum	HV(%)
TOTAL	34	142	88	100	364	100.0	100.0	100.0	99.9	90.5	46.8	55.6	65.1	67.0	974	88.1
I. LEUKAEMIAS	10	61	35	26	132	36.3	35.9	100.0	29.4	38.9	18.6	14.5	23.6	24.5	350	100.0
Acute lymphocytic	8	41	24	14	87	23.9	23.5	65.9	23.5	26.1	12.8	7.8	15.6	16.3	231	100.0
Other lymphocytic	0	0	0	0	0	-	-	-	-	-	-	-	-	-	-	-
Acute non-lymphocytic	1	17	11	12	41	11.3	11.4	31.1	2.9	10.8	5.9	6.7	7.3	7.4	109	100.0
Chronic myeloid	0	1	0	0	1	0.3	0.2	0.8	-	0.6	-	-	0.2	0.2	3	100.0
Other and unspecified	1	2	0	0	3	0.8	0.7	2.3	2.9	1.3	-	-	0.5	0.6	8	100.0
II. LYMPHOMAS	4	18	8	16	46	12.6	12.5	100.0	11.8	11.5	4.3	8.9	8.2	8.4	123	100.0
Hodgkin's disease	0	0	1	0	1	0.3	0.3	2.2	-	-	0.5	-	0.2	0.2	3	100.0
Non-Hodgkin lymphoma	1	6	5	7	19	5.2	5.4	41.3	2.9	3.8	2.7	3.9	3.4	3.4	51	100.0
Burkitt's lymphoma	0	0	0	0	0	-	-	-	-	-	-	-	-	-	-	-
Unspecified lymphoma	2	7	2	6	17	4.7	4.7	37.0	5.9	4.5	1.1	3.3	3.0	3.0	45	100.0
Histiocytosis X	0	2	0	2	4	1.1	0.9	8.7	-	1.3	-	1.1	0.7	0.8	11	100.0
Other reticuloendothelial	1	3	0	1	5	1.4	1.2	10.9	2.9	1.9	-	0.6	0.9	1.0	13	100.0
III. BRAIN AND SPINAL	1	12	23	14	50	13.7	15.0	100.0	2.9	7.6	12.2	7.8	8.9	8.8	134	86.0
Ependymoma	0	1	0	0	1	0.3	0.2	2.0	-	0.6	-	-	0.2	0.2	3	100.0
Astrocytoma	1	7	9	7	24	6.6	7.0	48.0	2.9	4.5	4.8	3.9	4.3	4.3	64	100.0
Medulloblastoma	0	4	5	7	16	4.4	4.7	32.0	-	2.5	2.7	3.9	2.9	2.8	43	100.0
Other glioma	0	0	2	0	2	0.5	0.7	4.0	-	-	1.1	-	0.4	0.3	5	100.0
Other and unspecified *	0	0	7	0	7	1.9	2.4	14.0	-	-	3.7	-	1.3	1.2	19	-
IV. SYMPATHETIC N.S.	2	9	3	0	14	3.8	3.5	100.0	5.9	5.7	1.6	-	2.5	2.7	37	100.0
Neuroblastoma	2	9	3	0	14	3.8	3.5	100.0	5.9	5.7	1.6	-	2.5	2.7	37	100.0
Other	0	0	0	0	0	-	-	-	-	-	-	-	-	-	-	-
V. RETINOBLASTOMA	0	10	0	0	10	2.7	2.3	100.0	-	6.4	-	-	1.8	2.0	25	100.0
VI. KIDNEY	4	10	0	2	16	4.4	3.8	100.0	11.8	6.4	-	1.1	2.9	3.2	43	68.8
Wilms' tumour	3	4	0	1	8	2.2	1.9	50.0	8.8	2.5	-	0.6	1.4	1.6	22	100.0
Renal carcinoma	0	1	0	1	2	0.5	0.5	12.5	-	0.6	-	0.6	0.4	0.4	5	100.0
Other and unspecified	1	5	0	0	6	1.6	1.4	37.5	2.9	3.2	-	-	1.1	1.2	16	16.7
VII. LIVER	2	1	3	1	7	1.9	2.0	100.0	5.9	0.6	1.6	0.6	1.3	1.3	19	57.1
Hepatoblastoma	1	0	1	0	2	0.5	0.6	28.6	2.9	-	0.5	-	0.4	0.4	6	100.0
Hepatic carcinoma	1	0	1	0	2	0.5	0.6	28.6	2.9	-	0.5	-	0.4	0.4	6	100.0
Other and unspecified	0	1	1	1	3	0.8	0.9	42.9	-	0.6	0.5	0.6	0.5	0.5	8	100.0
VIII. BONE	0	0	2	8	10	2.7	3.1	100.0	-	-	1.1	4.4	1.8	1.6	28	100.0
Osteosarcoma	0	0	1	7	8	2.2	2.4	80.0	-	-	0.5	3.9	1.4	1.3	22	100.0
Chondrosarcoma	0	0	0	0	0	-	-	-	-	-	-	-	-	-	-	-
Ewing's sarcoma	0	0	1	1	2	0.5	0.6	20.0	-	-	0.5	0.6	0.4	0.3	5	100.0
Other and unspecified	0	0	0	0	0	-	-	-	-	-	-	-	-	-	-	-
IX. SOFT TISSUE SARCOMAS	2	2	3	6	13	3.6	3.7	100.0	5.9	1.3	1.6	3.3	2.3	2.3	36	100.0
Rhabdomyosarcoma	1	2	2	0	5	1.4	1.3	38.5	2.9	1.3	1.1	-	0.9	0.9	14	100.0
Fibrosarcoma	1	0	1	3	5	1.4	1.5	38.5	2.9	-	0.5	1.7	0.9	0.9	14	100.0
Other and unspecified	0	0	0	3	3	0.8	1.0	23.1	-	-	-	1.7	0.5	0.5	8	100.0
X. GONADAL & GERM CELL	5	5	3	7	20	5.5	5.4	100.0	14.7	3.2	1.6	3.9	3.6	3.8	55	100.0
Non-gonadal germ cell	5	3	1	1	10	2.7	2.5	50.0	14.7	1.9	0.5	0.6	1.8	2.1	28	100.0
Gonadal germ cell	0	1	1	3	5	1.4	1.5	25.0	-	0.6	0.5	1.7	0.9	0.9	14	100.0
Gonadal carcinoma	0	1	1	3	5	1.4	1.5	25.0	-	0.6	0.5	1.7	0.9	0.9	14	100.0
Other and unspecified	0	0	0	0	0	-	-	-	-	-	-	-	-	-	-	-
XI. EPITHELIAL NEOPLASMS	0	3	3	11	17	4.7	5.0	100.0	-	1.9	1.6	6.1	3.0	2.9	46	100.0
Adrenocortical carcinoma	0	1	0	0	1	0.3	0.2	5.9	-	0.6	-	-	0.2	0.2	3	100.0
Thyroid carcinoma	0	0	0	7	7	1.9	2.1	41.2	-	-	-	3.9	1.3	1.1	19	100.0
Nasopharyngeal carcinoma	0	0	0	2	2	0.5	0.6	11.8	-	-	-	1.1	0.4	0.3	6	100.0
Melanoma	0	0	0	0	0	-	-	-	-	-	-	-	-	-	-	-
Other carcinoma	0	2	3	2	7	1.9	2.1	41.2	-	1.3	1.6	1.1	1.3	1.2	19	100.0
XII. OTHER	4	11	5	9	29	8.0	7.8	100.0	11.8	7.0	2.7	5.0	5.2	5.4	78	-
* Specified as malignant	0	0	7	0	7	1.9	2.4	100.0	-	-	3.7	-	1.3	1.2	19	-

predominantly carcinomas. The incidence of retinoblastoma appeared to be rather low; however, if the
eight males and six females with unspecified eye
tumours had all in fact had retinoblastoma, this
would make the rates similar to those from the
other Chinese registries in the present volume.

HONG KONG

Hong Kong Cancer Registry, 1974-1979

H.C. Ho, K.K. Man, S.Y. Tsao & P.K. Chan

In 1963, a population-based Cancer Registry was established within the Medical and Health Department Institute of Radiology and Oncology of the Hong Kong Government; it became fully operational in 1965. Cancer notification is, however, still on a voluntary basis. Voluntary notification is never satisfactory, as most practising clinicians and pathologists, with their heavy commitments, are reluctant to fill in forms of any kind. They are, however, willing to co-operate in allowing registry clerks to extract data on clinical and histopathological diagnoses from their registers of cancer cases.

Because of staff limitations only modest objectives were feasible, namely: (1) to achieve as high a rate of registration of new cases as possible in order to obtain detailed incidence rates according to anatomical site and cells of origin and thus provide a basis for comparative geographical incidence studies; and (2) to provide, wherever possible, relevant data, e.g., sex, age, place of birth and origin, usual language or dialect spoken, place of residence, occupation, etc., for epidemiological studies.

The channels through which information is obtained are: (1) voluntary notification — simple notification forms distributed to hospitals and doctors in private practice; (2) the Medical and Health Department Institute of Radiology and Oncology based at Queen Elizabeth Hospital, which is the largest general hospital in Hong Kong, and Queen Mary Hospital, the teaching hospital of the University of Hong Kong. The Institute notifies approximately 4000 new cancer cases a year, and treats more than 90% of the patients referred for radiotherapy in Hong Kong. Most of the patients attend the Institute mainly for radiotherapy, but about 30% receive chemotherapy either alone or in combination with radiation; (3) one private hospital which provides radiotherapy; (4) Government and Government-subsidized hospitals — data from these are either collected by the Registry clerks or

supplied by the medical superintendents; (5) pathologists in private practice; (6) death certificates kept by the Government Deaths Registry — existing records can be up-dated with date of death, and cases for which data are derived from a death certificate only can be separately listed.

Notifications received are checked for duplication by a comprehensive cross-index system before they are registered. For the period included in the tables (1974-1979), the Registry did not systematically record histological diagnoses, so that for 40% of cases the basis of diagnosis was unknown, and an ICD-O code of 9990/3 was allocated. This accounts for the relatively large proportion of cases with general diagnostic labels (e.g., lymphoid leukaemia, brain tumours) appearing in the 'Other and unspecified' categories, despite an apparently high percentage of cases histologically verified. The Registry includes only malignant neoplasms; benign and unspecified tumours, even of the CNS, are excluded.

The total land area of Hong Kong is 1060 square kilometres. The population at the 1981 census was 5.1 million, of whom 25% were children. Of the total population, 98% were classified as Chinese, of whom 90.7% claimed the province of Guangdong as their place of origin. Hong Kong is one of the most densely populated places in the world with an overall population density of 4792 per square kilometre at the end of 1983.

Hong Kong has a low infant mortality rate (10.1 per 1000 live births in 1983), attributed to the provision of comprehensive family health care facilities as well as improvements in environmental and socioeconomic conditions. There is a Paediatric Tumor Study Group, whose members come from the medical staff of the University of Hong Kong and the Government Medical and Health Departments.

Contd p. 154

Hong Kong

1974 – 1979 MALE

DIAGNOSTIC GROUP	NUMBER OF CASES					REL. FREQUENCY(%)			RATES PER MILLION							HV (%)
	0	1-4	5-9	10-14	All	Crude	Adj.	Group	0	1-4	5-9	10-14	Crude	Adj.	Cum	
TOTAL	46	201	157	188	592	100.0	100.0	100.0	185.6	203.9	121.4	118.2	143.8	151.0	2199	96.6
I. LEUKAEMIAS	15	68	60	64	207	35.0	35.1	100.0	60.5	69.0	46.4	40.2	50.3	52.7	770	100.0
Acute lymphocytic	2	32	22	27	83	14.0	14.0	40.1	8.1	32.5	17.0	17.0	20.2	21.1	308	100.0
Other lymphocytic	2	13	14	11	40	6.8	6.9	19.3	8.1	13.2	10.8	6.9	9.7	10.2	150	100.0
Acute non-lymphocytic	0	3	4	1	8	1.4	1.4	3.9	–	3.0	3.1	0.6	1.9	2.1	31	100.0
Chronic myeloid	0	0	0	0	0	–	–	–	–	–	–	–	–	–	–	–
Other and unspecified	11	20	20	25	76	12.8	12.8	36.7	44.4	20.3	15.5	15.7	18.5	19.3	281	100.0
II. LYMPHOMAS	3	25	35	37	100	16.9	17.1	100.0	12.1	25.4	27.1	23.3	24.3	24.3	365	98.2
Hodgkin's disease	0	4	3	6	13	2.2	2.2	13.0	–	3.9	2.3	2.5	3.2	3.2	48	100.0
Non-Hodgkin lymphoma	2	10	15	19	46	7.8	7.8	46.0	8.1	10.1	11.6	11.9	11.2	11.0	166	100.0
Burkitt's lymphoma	0	0	2	2	4	0.7	0.7	4.0	–	–	0.8	1.3	1.0	0.9	14	100.0
Unspecified lymphoma	0	4	11	7	22	3.7	3.9	22.0	–	4.1	8.5	4.4	5.3	5.3	81	100.0
Histiocytosis X	1	7	3	3	14	2.4	2.3	14.0	–	7.1	2.3	2.5	3.4	3.7	53	92.9
Other reticuloendothelial	0	0	1	0	1	0.2	0.2	1.0	–	–	–	0.6	0.2	0.2	3	100.0
III. BRAIN AND SPINAL	0	22	20	18	60	10.1	10.3	100.0	–	22.3	15.5	11.3	14.6	15.2	223	78.1
Ependymoma	0	1	2	0	3	0.5	0.5	5.0	–	1.0	1.5	–	0.7	0.7	12	100.0
Astrocytoma	0	4	3	2	9	1.5	1.5	15.0	–	4.1	2.3	1.3	2.2	2.4	34	88.9
Medulloblastoma	0	1	5	4	10	1.7	1.8	16.7	–	1.0	3.9	2.5	2.4	2.3	36	100.0
Other glioma	0	1	1	2	4	0.7	0.7	6.7	–	1.0	0.8	1.0	1.0	0.9	14	100.0
Other and unspecified *	0	15	9	10	34	5.7	5.7	56.7	–	15.2	7.0	6.3	8.3	8.8	127	–
IV. SYMPATHETIC N.S.	5	11	3	2	21	3.5	3.5	100.0	20.2	11.2	2.3	1.3	5.1	6.1	83	95.2
Neuroblastoma	5	11	3	2	21	3.5	3.5	100.0	20.2	11.2	2.3	1.3	5.1	6.1	83	95.2
Other	0	0	0	0	0	–	–	–	–	–	–	–	–	–	–	–
V. RETINOBLASTOMA	1	13	0	0	14	2.4	2.3	100.0	4.0	13.2	–	–	3.4	4.4	57	85.7
VI. KIDNEY	6	14	3	1	24	4.1	4.0	100.0	24.2	14.2	2.3	0.6	5.8	7.2	96	95.8
Wilms' tumour	6	13	3	1	23	3.9	3.8	95.8	24.2	13.2	2.3	0.6	5.6	6.9	92	95.7
Renal carcinoma	0	1	0	0	1	0.2	0.2	4.2	–	1.0	–	–	0.2	0.3	4	100.0
Other and unspecified	0	0	0	0	0	–	–	–	–	–	–	–	–	–	–	–
VII. LIVER	3	3	9	9	24	4.1	4.1	100.0	12.1	3.0	7.0	5.7	5.8	5.8	87	100.0
Hepatoblastoma	3	0	0	0	3	0.5	0.5	12.5	12.1	–	–	–	0.7	0.7	12	100.0
Hepatic carcinoma	0	2	7	7	16	2.7	2.8	66.7	–	2.0	5.4	4.4	3.9	3.7	57	100.0
Other and unspecified	0	1	2	2	5	0.8	0.8	20.8	–	1.0	1.3	1.3	1.2	1.3	18	100.0
VIII. BONE	1	1	2	17	21	3.5	3.4	100.0	4.0	1.0	0.8	11.3	5.1	4.2	69	100.0
Osteosarcoma	0	0	0	8	8	1.4	1.3	38.1	–	–	–	5.0	1.9	1.5	25	100.0
Chondrosarcoma	0	0	0	2	2	0.3	0.3	9.5	–	–	–	1.3	0.5	0.4	6	100.0
Ewing's sarcoma	0	0	0	2	2	0.3	0.3	9.5	–	–	–	1.3	0.5	0.4	6	100.0
Other and unspecified	1	1	2	5	9	1.5	1.5	42.9	4.0	1.0	0.8	3.8	2.2	2.0	31	100.0
IX. SOFT TISSUE SARCOMAS	1	9	6	4	20	3.4	3.4	100.0	4.0	9.1	4.6	2.5	4.9	5.4	76	100.0
Rhabdomyosarcoma	1	4	3	0	8	1.4	1.4	40.0	4.0	4.1	2.3	–	1.9	2.3	32	100.0
Fibrosarcoma	0	4	3	4	11	1.9	1.9	55.0	–	4.1	2.3	2.5	2.7	2.7	40	100.0
Other and unspecified	0	1	0	0	1	0.2	0.2	5.0	–	1.0	–	–	0.2	0.3	4	100.0
X. GONADAL & GERM CELL	4	12	2	2	20	3.4	3.3	100.0	16.1	12.2	1.5	1.3	4.9	5.9	79	100.0
Non-gonadal germ cell	1	0	0	0	1	0.2	0.2	5.0	4.0	–	–	0.6	0.2	0.2	3	100.0
Gonadal germ cell	3	11	2	1	17	2.8	2.8	85.0	12.1	11.2	1.5	0.6	4.1	5.1	68	100.0
Gonadal carcinoma	0	1	0	0	1	0.2	0.2	5.0	–	1.0	–	–	0.2	0.2	4	100.0
Other and unspecified	0	0	0	1	1	0.2	0.2	5.0	–	–	–	0.6	0.2	0.3	4	100.0
XI. EPITHELIAL NEOPLASMS	1	3	7	16	27	4.6	4.6	100.0	4.0	3.0	6.2	9.4	6.6	6.0	94	100.0
Adrenocortical carcinoma	0	0	0	0	0	–	–	–	–	–	–	–	–	–	–	–
Thyroid carcinoma	0	0	1	2	3	0.5	0.5	11.1	–	–	1.5	1.3	0.7	0.5	9	100.0
Nasopharyngeal carcinoma	0	1	2	2	5	0.8	0.9	18.5	–	1.0	1.5	1.3	1.2	1.2	18	100.0
Melanoma	1	1	0	1	3	0.5	0.5	11.1	–	1.0	–	–	0.7	0.8	12	100.0
Other carcinoma	0	1	4	11	16	2.7	2.7	59.3	4.0	1.0	3.1	6.3	3.9	3.4	55	100.0
XII. OTHER	6	20	10	18	54	9.1	9.0	100.0	24.2	20.3	7.7	11.3	13.1	13.9	201	–
* Specified as malignant	0	15	9	10	34	5.7	5.7	100.0	–	15.2	7.0	6.3	8.3	8.8	127	–

* Specified as malignant

Hong Kong   1974 - 1979   FEMALE

DIAGNOSTIC GROUP	NUMBER OF CASES					REL. FREQUENCY(%)			RATES PER MILLION							HV(%)
	0	1-4	5-9	10-14	All	Crude	Adj.	Group	0	1-4	5-9	10-14	Crude	Adj.	Cum	
TOTAL	25	123	117	142	407	100.0	100.0	100.0	107.7	132.5	95.6	93.2	104.2	107.3	1582	93.4
I. LEUKAEMIAS	8	51	42	56	157	38.6	38.5	100.0	34.5	54.9	34.3	36.8	40.2	41.4	610	99.0
Acute lymphocytic	1	23	27	15	66	16.2	16.6	42.0	4.3	24.8	22.1	9.8	16.9	18.0	263	100.0
Other lymphocytic	2	7	10	10	29	7.1	7.1	18.5	8.6	7.5	8.2	6.6	7.4	7.5	112	100.0
Acute non-lymphocytic	2	7	0	9	18	4.4	4.3	11.5	8.6	7.5		5.9	4.6	4.7	68	100.0
Chronic myeloid	0	0	1	1	2	0.5	0.5	1.3			0.8	0.7	0.5	0.5	7	50.0
Other and unspecified	3	14	4	21	42	10.3	10.1	26.3	12.9	15.1	3.3	13.8	10.7	10.7	159	100.0
II. LYMPHOMAS	2	20	12	19	53	13.0	13.0	100.0	8.6	21.5	9.8	12.5	13.6	14.1	206	96.4
Hodgkin's disease	2	2	3	0	7	1.7	1.9	13.2	8.6	2.2	2.5		1.8	2.1	29	100.0
Non-Hodgkin lymphoma	0	9	6	13	28	6.9	6.7	52.8		9.7	4.9	8.5	7.2	7.1	106	100.0
Burkitt's lymphoma	0	2	1	2	5	1.2	1.2	9.4		2.2	0.8	1.3	1.3	1.3	19	100.0
Unspecified lymphoma	0	5	2	1	8	2.0	2.1	15.1		5.4	1.6	0.7	2.0	2.4	33	100.0
Histiocytosis X	0	2	0	2	4	1.0	1.0	7.5		2.2		1.3	1.0	1.0	15	75.0
Other reticuloendothelial	0	0	0	1	1	0.2	0.2	1.9				0.7	0.3	0.2	3	100.0
III. BRAIN AND SPINAL	1	10	25	9	45	11.1	11.3	100.0	4.3	10.8	20.4	5.9	11.5	12.0	179	66.7
Ependymoma	0	0	0	0	0											
Astrocytoma	0	2	6	2	10	2.5	2.5	22.2		2.2	4.9	1.3	2.6	2.6	40	100.0
Medulloblastoma	0	3	3	0	6	1.5	1.6	13.3		3.2	2.5		1.5	1.8	25	100.0
Other glioma	0	2	0	0	2	0.5	0.5	4.4		2.2			0.5	0.7	9	100.0
Other and unspecified *	1	3	16	7	27	6.6	6.7	60.0	4.3	3.2	13.1	4.6	6.9	6.9	106	
IV. SYMPATHETIC N.S.	3	5	3	2	13	3.2	3.4	100.0	12.9	5.4	2.5	1.3	3.3	3.8	53	92.3
Neuroblastoma	3	5	3	2	13	3.2	3.4	100.0	12.9	5.4	2.5	1.3	3.3	3.8	53	92.3
Other	0	0	0	0	0											
V. RETINOBLASTOMA	3	5	0	0	8	2.0	2.2	100.0	12.9	5.4			2.0	2.7	34	100.0
VI. KIDNEY	1	4	1	0	6	1.5	1.6	100.0	4.3	4.3	0.8		1.5	1.9	26	100.0
Wilms' tumour	1	4	1	0	6	1.5	1.6	100.0	4.3	4.3	0.8		1.5	1.9	26	100.0
Renal carcinoma	0	0	0	0	0											
Other and unspecified	0	0	0	0	0											
VII. LIVER	1	2	1	3	7	1.7	1.7	100.0	4.3	2.2	0.8	2.0	1.8	1.8	27	100.0
Hepatoblastoma	0	0	1	0	1	0.2	0.3	14.3			0.8		0.3	0.3	4	100.0
Hepatic carcinoma	0	0	0	2	2	0.5	0.4	28.6				1.3	0.5	0.4	7	100.0
Other and unspecified	1	2	0	1	4	1.0	1.0	57.1	4.3	2.2		0.7	1.0	1.2	16	
VIII. BONE	1	2	5	12	20	4.9	4.6	100.0	4.3	2.2	4.1	7.9	5.1	4.6	73	92.3
Osteosarcoma	0	0	2	8	10	2.5	2.2	50.0			1.6	5.3	2.6	2.1	35	90.0
Chondrosarcoma	0	0	0	0	0											
Ewing's sarcoma	0	0	2	0	2	0.5	0.5	10.0			1.6		0.5	0.5	8	100.0
Other and unspecified	1	2	1	4	8	2.0	1.9	40.0	4.3	2.2	0.8	2.6	2.0	2.0	30	100.0
IX. SOFT TISSUE SARCOMAS	2	4	10	5	21	5.2	5.2	100.0	8.6	4.3	8.2	3.3	5.4	5.6	83	100.0
Rhabdomyosarcoma	2	2	3	0	7	1.7	1.8	33.3	8.6	2.2	2.5		1.8	1.8	28	100.0
Fibrosarcoma	0	1	4	4	9	2.2	2.1	42.9		1.1	3.3	2.6	2.3	2.2	34	100.0
Other and unspecified	0	1	3	1	5	1.2	1.3	23.8		1.1	2.5	0.7	1.3	1.5	21	100.0
X. GONADAL & GERM CELL	0	2	2	6	10	2.5	2.3	100.0		2.2	1.6	3.9	2.6	2.3	36	100.0
Non-gonadal germ cell	0	0	0	0	0											
Gonadal germ cell	0	2	2	6	10	2.5	2.3	100.0		2.2	1.6	3.9	2.6	2.3	36	100.0
Gonadal carcinoma	0	0	0	0	0											
Other and unspecified	0	0	0	0	0											
XI. EPITHELIAL NEOPLASMS	0	2	3	15	20	4.9	4.5	100.0		2.2	2.5	9.8	5.1	4.3	70	94.1
Adrenocortical carcinoma	0	0	0	0	0											
Thyroid carcinoma	0	0	1	5	6	1.5	1.3	30.0			0.8	3.3	1.5	1.2	20	100.0
Nasopharyngeal carcinoma	0	0	0	3	3	0.7	0.6	15.0				2.0	0.8	0.6	10	100.0
Melanoma	0	1	1	4	6	1.5	1.4	30.0		1.1	0.8	2.6	1.5	1.4	22	66.7
Other carcinoma	0	1	1	3	5	1.2	1.2	25.0		1.1	0.8	2.0	1.3	1.2	18	100.0
XII. OTHER	3	16	13	15	47	11.5	11.6	100.0	12.9	17.2	10.6	9.8	12.0	12.6	184	
* Specified as malignant	1	3	16	7	27	6.6	6.7		4.3	3.2	13.1	4.6	6.9	6.9	106	

* Specified as malignant

Population

For the present volume, estimates of the child population were calculated by the Department of Census and Statistics, based on the 1971 census and taking account of births, deaths and migrations recorded by the Immigration Department.

AVERAGE ANNUAL POPULATION: 1974–1979

Age	Male	Female
0	41300	38700
1–4	164300	154700
5–9	215500	204000
10–14	265100	253900
0–14	686200	651300

Commentary

If it is assumed that the 'other lymphocytic' leukaemias are in fact entirely acute lymphocytic leukaemia (ALL), the incidence rate for childhood ALL appears to be similar to that in many Western populations but without any marked peak in younger children. Lymphomas were relatively common, with substantial numbers in the non-Hodgkin and unspecified categories, but Hodgkin's disease in childhood was comparatively rare. The rather low rate for brain and spinal tumours may be due to the fact that only tumours specified as malignant are registered. There was a high incidence of liver tumours, particularly in boys; these tumours were predominantly hepatic carcinomas. Osteosarcoma was more than four times as frequent as Ewing's sarcoma. There were unusually high rates of gonadal germ-cell tumours in both sexes, but these had the usual age-distribution, i.e., the highest incidence was in boys at age 0–4 and in girls at age 10–14. Nasopharyngeal carcinoma had the higher incidence typical of east Asian registries but still only accounted for 0.8% of all registrations. In the 'other and unspecified' category there was an unusually large number of lung tumours (10 males and three females; 1.3% of all registrations), but no lung carcinomas were registered in children.

INDIA

Bangalore Cancer Registry, 1982–1984

M.K. Bhargava, A. Nandakumar & K. Ramachandra Reddy

A population-based cancer registry was established in August 1981 at Kidwai Memorial Institute of Oncology, Bangalore, as part of the National Cancer Registry Project of the Indian Council of Medical Research. The Registry is one of six set up by the Council to provide an accurate and scientific foundation for studies on cancer epidemiology and control and other aspects of cancer research. The collection and regular compilation of data started in January 1982.

The main sources of patient information are teaching and other hospitals, nursing homes, and pathology and radiology departments. Social investigators, who form part of the staff of the Registry, collect information from these sources, including the pathology, radiology and medical records departments of the hospitals. The physicians concerned are consulted whenever necessary in order to clarify or complete patient information. Patients are interviewed by the social investigators, and a questionnaire is completed on their way of life and other matters. The co-operation of ward personnel and other senior and clerical staff in the hospitals, nursing homes and laboratories is reassuring. The completeness of coverage and therefore of registration is believed to be over 90%. However, data available from death certificates are far from satisfactory. Efforts to improve this by administrative reforms are under way. Registration is voluntary.

Kidwai Memorial Institute of Oncology is a referral hospital for cancer patients, and over 70% of residents of Bangalore diagnosed as having cancer are referred to the Institute; collection of detailed patient information is therefore relatively easy. Co-operation in the contribution of information by the various other institutions has been exemplary.

Bangalore, a conurbation, is the capital of the state of Karnataka in the south of India, occupying an area of 215 square kilometres, and is located at an altitude of 900 m above sea level. In the period 1971–1981, the population grew by 76%; it is the fastest growing city in the country.

Population

The estimate of the population at risk is based on the 1981 census, allowance being made for births and deaths (but not for migration).

AVERAGE ANNUAL POPULATION: 1982–1984

Age	Male	Female
0–4	198164	197311
5–9	207516	204881
10–14	172113	172381
0–14	577793	574573

Commentary

Overall incidence rates are low. Leukaemias and lymphomas were equally frequent in the series, each accounting for 23% of registrations. The relative frequencies of most other major diagnostic groups were broadly similar to those in European registries, though brain and spinal tumours appear to be under-represented.

India, Bangalore

1982 – 1984   MALE

DIAGNOSTIC GROUP	NUMBER OF CASES					REL. FREQUENCY(%)			RATES PER MILLION					Cum	HV(%)
	0	1-4	5-9	10-14	All	Crude	Adj.	Group	0-4	5-9	10-14	Crude	Adj.		
TOTAL	2	39	48	42	132¤	100.0	100.0	100.0	69.0	77.1	81.3	76.2	75.2	1137	98.5
I. LEUKAEMIAS	1	6	18	8	34¤	25.8	23.8	100.0	11.8	28.9	15.5	19.6	18.4	281	100.0
Acute lymphocytic	1	6	10	1	19¤	14.4	13.8	55.9	11.8	16.1	1.9	11.0	10.3	149	100.0
Other lymphocytic	0	0	1	3	4	3.0	2.8	11.8	–	1.6	5.8	2.3	2.2	37	100.0
Acute non-lymphocytic	0	0	4	3	7	5.3	4.6	20.6	–	6.4	5.8	4.0	3.8	61	100.0
Chronic myeloid	0	0	1	1	1	0.8	0.7	2.9	–	–	1.9	0.6	0.6	10	100.0
Other and unspecified	0	0	3	0	3	2.3	1.9	8.8	–	4.8	–	1.7	1.6	24	100.0
II. LYMPHOMAS	0	6	17	16	39	29.5	27.9	100.0	10.1	27.3	31.0	22.5	21.7	342	97.4
Hodgkin's disease	0	1	6	8	15	11.4	10.4	38.5	1.7	9.6	15.5	8.7	8.3	134	100.0
Non-Hodgkin lymphoma	0	4	6	5	15	11.4	11.2	38.5	6.7	9.6	9.7	8.7	8.5	130	100.0
Burkitt's lymphoma	0	1	1	0	2	1.5	1.6	5.1	1.7	1.6	–	1.2	1.2	16	100.0
Unspecified lymphoma	0	0	4	2	6	4.5	3.9	15.4	–	6.4	3.9	3.5	3.2	51	83.3
Histiocytosis X	0	0	0	0	0	–	–	–	–	–	–	–	–	–	–
Other reticuloendothelial	0	0	0	1	1	0.8	0.7	2.6	–	–	1.9	0.6	0.6	10	100.0
III. BRAIN AND SPINAL	0	3	6	3	12	9.1	8.8	100.0	5.0	9.6	5.8	6.9	6.7	102	100.0
Ependymoma	0	1	1	0	2	1.5	1.6	16.7	1.7	1.6	–	1.2	1.2	16	100.0
Astrocytoma	0	0	3	0	3	2.3	1.9	25.0	–	4.8	–	1.7	1.6	24	100.0
Medulloblastoma	0	2	1	1	4	3.0	3.3	33.3	3.4	1.6	1.9	2.3	2.4	35	100.0
Other glioma	0	0	1	2	3	2.3	2.1	25.0	–	1.6	3.9	1.7	1.6	27	100.0
Other and unspecified *	0	0	0	0	0	–	–	–	–	–	–	–	–	–	–
IV. SYMPATHETIC N.S.	0	7	2	2	11	8.3	9.5	100.0	11.8	3.2	3.9	6.3	6.7	94	100.0
Neuroblastoma	0	7	2	2	11	8.3	9.5	100.0	11.8	3.2	3.9	6.3	6.7	94	100.0
Other	0	0	0	0	0	–	–	–	–	–	–	–	–	–	–
V. RETINOBLASTOMA	0	4	1	0	5	3.8	4.5	100.0	6.7	1.6	–	2.9	3.1	42	100.0
VI. KIDNEY	1	7	0	2	10	7.6	9.2	100.0	13.5	–	3.9	5.8	6.3	87	100.0
Wilms' tumour	1	7	0	2	10	7.6	9.2	100.0	13.5	–	3.9	5.8	6.3	87	100.0
Renal carcinoma	0	0	0	0	0	–	–	–	–	–	–	–	–	–	–
Other and unspecified	0	0	0	0	0	–	–	–	–	–	–	–	–	–	–
VII. LIVER	0	1	1	0	2	1.5	1.6	100.0	1.7	1.6	–	1.2	1.2	16	100.0
Hepatoblastoma	0	1	0	0	1	–	–	–	–	–	–	–	–	–	–
Hepatic carcinoma	0	1	1	0	2	1.5	1.6	100.0	1.7	1.6	–	1.2	1.2	16	100.0
Other and unspecified	0	0	0	0	0	–	–	–	–	–	–	–	–	–	–
VIII. BONE	0	0	1	6	7	5.3	4.9	100.0	–	1.6	11.6	4.0	3.9	66	100.0
Osteosarcoma	0	0	1	3	4	3.0	2.8	57.1	–	1.6	5.8	2.3	2.2	37	100.0
Chondrosarcoma	0	0	0	1	1	0.8	0.7	14.3	–	–	1.9	0.6	0.6	10	100.0
Ewing's sarcoma	0	0	0	2	2	1.5	1.4	28.6	–	–	3.9	1.2	1.1	19	100.0
Other and unspecified	0	0	0	0	0	–	–	–	–	–	–	–	–	–	–
IX. SOFT TISSUE SARCOMAS	0	2	1	3	6	4.5	4.7	100.0	3.4	1.6	5.8	3.5	3.5	54	100.0
Rhabdomyosarcoma	0	2	1	2	5	3.8	4.0	83.3	3.4	1.6	3.9	2.9	2.9	44	100.0
Fibrosarcoma	0	0	0	0	0	–	–	–	–	–	–	–	–	–	–
Other and unspecified	0	0	0	1	1	0.8	0.7	16.7	–	–	1.9	0.6	0.6	10	100.0
X. GONADAL & GERM CELL	0	2	0	0	2	1.5	2.0	100.0	3.4	–	–	1.2	1.3	17	100.0
Non-gonadal germ cell	0	0	0	0	0	–	–	–	–	–	–	–	–	–	–
Gonadal germ cell	0	2	0	0	2	1.5	2.0	100.0	3.4	–	–	1.2	1.3	17	100.0
Gonadal carcinoma	0	0	0	0	0	–	–	–	–	–	–	–	–	–	–
Other and unspecified	0	0	0	0	0	–	–	–	–	–	–	–	–	–	–
XI. EPITHELIAL NEOPLASMS	0	0	0	2	2	1.5	1.4	100.0	–	–	3.9	1.2	1.1	19	100.0
Adrenocortical carcinoma	0	0	0	0	0	–	–	–	–	–	–	–	–	–	–
Thyroid carcinoma	0	0	0	1	1	0.8	0.7	50.0	–	–	1.9	0.6	0.7	10	100.0
Nasopharyngeal carcinoma	0	0	0	1	1	0.8	0.7	50.0	–	–	1.9	0.6	0.7	10	100.0
Melanoma	0	0	0	0	0	–	–	–	–	–	–	–	–	–	–
Other carcinoma	0	0	0	0	0	–	–	–	–	–	–	–	–	–	–
XII. OTHER	0	1	1	0	2	1.5	1.6	100.0	1.7	1.6	–	1.2	1.2	16	50.0
* Specified as malignant	0	0	0	0	0	–	–	–	–	–	–	–	–	–	–
¤ Includes age unknown															

India, Bangalore

1982 – 1984

FEMALE

DIAGNOSTIC GROUP	NUMBER OF CASES					REL. FREQUENCY(%)			RATES PER MILLION						
	0	1-4	5-9	10-14	All	Crude	Adj.	Group	0-4	5-9	10-14	Crude	Adj.	Cum	HV(%)
TOTAL	3	23	25	21	72	100.0	100.0	100.0	43.9	40.7	40.6	41.8	41.9	626	98.6
I. LEUKAEMIAS	1	3	6	2	12	16.7	16.2	100.0	6.8	9.8	3.9	7.0	6.9	102	100.0
Acute lymphocytic	0	2	5	0	7	9.7	9.1	58.3	3.4	8.1	-	4.1	3.9	58	100.0
Other lymphocytic	0	0	0	1	1	1.4	1.4	8.3	-	-	1.9	0.6	0.6	10	100.0
Acute non-lymphocytic	0	0	0	0	0	-	-	-	-	-	-	-	-	-	-
Chronic myeloid	0	0	0	1	1	1.4	1.4	8.3	-	1.6	1.9	0.6	0.6	10	100.0
Other and unspecified	1	1	1	0	3	4.2	4.3	25.0	3.4	1.6	-	1.7	1.8	25	100.0
II. LYMPHOMAS	0	1	4	2	7	9.7	9.2	100.0	1.7	6.5	3.9	4.1	3.9	60	100.0
Hodgkin's disease	0	0	1	1	2	2.8	2.6	28.6	-	1.6	1.9	1.2	1.1	18	100.0
Non-Hodgkin lymphoma	0	1	3	1	5	6.9	6.6	71.4	1.7	4.9	1.9	2.9	2.8	43	100.0
Burkitt's lymphoma	0	0	0	0	0	-	-	-	-	-	-	-	-	-	-
Unspecified lymphoma	0	0	0	0	0	-	-	-	-	-	-	-	-	-	-
Histiocytosis X	0	0	0	0	0	-	-	-	-	-	-	-	-	-	-
Other reticuloendothelial	0	0	0	0	0	-	-	-	-	-	-	-	-	-	-
III. BRAIN AND SPINAL	0	3	9	4	16	22.2	21.1	100.0	5.1	14.6	7.7	9.3	8.9	137	100.0
Ependymoma	0	0	1	0	1	1.4	1.2	6.3	-	1.6	-	0.6	0.5	8	100.0
Astrocytoma	0	2	4	1	7	9.7	9.3	43.8	3.4	6.5	1.9	4.1	4.0	59	100.0
Medulloblastoma	0	1	4	3	8	11.1	10.6	50.0	1.7	6.5	5.8	4.6	4.4	70	100.0
Other glioma	0	0	0	0	0	-	-	-	-	-	-	-	-	-	-
Other and unspecified *	0	0	0	0	0	-	-	-	-	-	-	-	-	-	-
IV. SYMPATHETIC N.S.	0	2	1	2	5	6.9	7.1	100.0	3.4	1.6	3.9	2.9	3.0	44	100.0
Neuroblastoma	0	2	1	2	5	6.9	7.1	100.0	3.4	1.6	3.9	2.9	3.0	44	100.0
Other	0	0	0	0	0	-	-	-	-	-	-	-	-	-	-
V. RETINOBLASTOMA	0	5	0	0	5	6.9	7.7	100.0	8.4	-	-	2.9	3.3	42	100.0
VI. KIDNEY	1	4	1	0	6	8.3	8.9	100.0	8.4	1.6	-	3.5	3.8	50	100.0
Wilms' tumour	1	4	1	0	6	8.3	8.9	100.0	8.4	1.6	-	3.5	3.8	50	100.0
Renal carcinoma	0	0	0	0	0	-	-	-	-	-	-	-	-	-	-
Other and unspecified	0	0	0	0	0	-	-	-	-	-	-	-	-	-	-
VII. LIVER	0	0	0	0	0	-	-	-	-	-	-	-	-	-	-
Hepatoblastoma	0	0	0	0	0	-	-	-	-	-	-	-	-	-	-
Hepatic carcinoma	0	0	0	0	0	-	-	-	-	-	-	-	-	-	-
Other and unspecified	0	0	0	0	0	-	-	-	-	-	-	-	-	-	-
VIII. BONE	0	0	0	0	0	-	-	-	-	-	-	-	-	-	-
Osteosarcoma	0	0	0	0	0	-	-	-	-	-	-	-	-	-	-
Chondrosarcoma	0	0	0	0	0	-	-	-	-	-	-	-	-	-	-
Ewing's sarcoma	0	0	0	0	0	-	-	-	-	-	-	-	-	-	-
Other and unspecified	0	0	0	0	0	-	-	-	-	-	-	-	-	-	-
IX. SOFT TISSUE SARCOMAS	1	2	1	2	6	8.3	8.7	100.0	5.1	1.6	3.9	3.5	3.6	53	100.0
Rhabdomyosarcoma	0	1	1	2	4	5.6	5.6	66.7	1.7	1.6	3.9	2.3	2.3	36	100.0
Fibrosarcoma	0	0	0	0	0	-	-	-	-	-	-	-	-	-	-
Other and unspecified	1	1	0	0	2	2.8	3.1	33.3	3.4	-	-	1.2	1.3	17	100.0
X. GONADAL & GERM CELL	0	2	2	1	5	6.9	6.9	100.0	3.4	3.3	1.9	2.9	2.9	43	100.0
Non-gonadal germ cell	0	2	1	0	3	4.2	4.3	60.0	3.4	1.6	-	1.7	1.8	25	100.0
Gonadal germ cell	0	0	1	0	1	1.4	1.4	20.0	-	1.6	-	0.6	0.6	10	100.0
Gonadal carcinoma	0	0	0	0	0	-	-	-	-	-	-	-	-	-	-
Other and unspecified	0	0	0	1	1	1.4	1.2	20.0	-	-	1.9	0.6	0.5	8	100.0
XI. EPITHELIAL NEOPLASMS	0	1	0	8	9	12.5	13.0	100.0	1.7	-	15.5	5.2	5.1	86	100.0
Adrenocortical carcinoma	0	0	0	0	0	-	-	-	-	-	-	-	-	-	-
Thyroid carcinoma	0	0	0	3	3	4.2	4.3	33.3	-	-	5.8	1.7	1.7	29	100.0
Nasopharyngeal carcinoma	0	0	0	2	2	2.8	2.9	22.2	-	-	3.9	1.2	1.1	19	100.0
Melanoma	0	0	0	1	1	1.4	1.4	11.1	-	-	1.9	0.6	0.6	10	100.0
Other carcinoma	0	1	0	2	3	4.2	4.4	33.3	1.7	-	3.9	1.7	1.8	28	100.0
XII. OTHER	0	0	1	0	1	1.4	1.2	100.0	-	1.6	-	0.6	0.5	8	-

* Specified as malignant
□ Includes age unknown

Bombay: The Bombay Cancer Registry, 1970–1979

D.J. Jussawalla & B.B. Yeole

The Bombay Cancer Registry was established in June 1963 as a unit of the Indian Cancer Society at Bombay, with the aim of obtaining reliable morbidity data on cancer from a precisely defined urban population (Greater Bombay). The actual compilation of data could only begin in 1964. Until then, no continuing survey had been undertaken anywhere in India. Initially, the project started in collaboration with, and received financial support up to 1975 from, the Biometry Branch of the National Cancer Institute in Bethesda, USA. During 1976–1980 the project received financial support from the Department of Science and Technology, Government of India, New Delhi, from the Indian Council of Medical Research, New Delhi, and from the Indian Cancer Society.

Information is obtained on all cancer patients registered in 102 private and public hospitals in Bombay and under the care of 315 specialists practising in the city (115 surgeons/physicians, 40 pathologists, 35 radiologists and 125 gynaecologists). The majority of hospitals in Bombay are maintained by the Municipal Corporation and State Government, which are responsible for the organization of public health and medical services in the city. The major source of data is the Tata Memorial Centre (q.v.), which is a postgraduate university teaching centre for cancer research. The city has four medical colleges. The diagnosis and treatment of cancer is centralized in certain hospitals in Bombay. Facilities for cobalt-60 therapy are available in three hospitals in the city while orthovoltage deep X-ray therapy is available in ten. There are no special facilities for paediatric oncology.

General medical practitioners are not contacted individually, as at one stage or another almost all cancer patients are referred to specialists. Staff members of the Registry visit the wards of all cooperating hospitals at least once a week to interview persons suspected of having cancer, as well as each cancer patient. All files maintained by the various departments of these hospitals are also crosschecked individually. With the exception of the Tata Memorial Hospital for Cancer at Bombay, hospital out-patient records are not included in the survey because of a paucity of clinical details and lack of information on residential status. Supplementary information is gleaned from the death records maintained by the Bombay Municipal Corporation. Every cancer death not traceable to an entry in the files is labelled as an unmatched death and is so registered for the corresponding year. No patient is followed up directly by the Registry staff. A total of 19 270 hospital beds are covered in the survey.

The Registry includes all malignant neoplasms and a few specific types of non-malignant tumours, but the policy is that benign and unspecified CNS tumours are not registered.

The Registry covers the resident population of Greater Bombay, a densely populated metropolis (approximately 13 670 inhabitants per square kilometre) on the west coast of India, occupying an area of 603 square kilometres. Greater Bombay is, in fact, an island, joined to the mainland by bridges, and has a warm, humid climate.

The 1981 census enumerated a population of 8.24 million, of whom approximately 69% are Hindus, 14% Moslems, 6% Christians (mostly Hindu converts), 5% Neo-Buddhists, 4% Jains, 1% Parsis (Zoroastrians), 0.7% Sikhs and 0.1% others. In 1981, approximately 50% of the workforce were employed in industry; Greater Bombay is the industrial heart of India. Immigration to Bombay continues unabated and the population now includes sizeable numbers of people from every state in the Union.

Population

The population at risk is based on annual estimates prepared by the Bombay Cancer Registry, using data from the censuses of 1961 and 1971, and information on migration patterns.

Contd p. 162

India, Bombay Cancer Registry   1970 - 1979   MALE

DIAGNOSTIC GROUP	NUMBER OF CASES					REL. FREQUENCY(%)			RATES PER MILLION					Cum	HV(%)
	0	1-4	5-9	10-14	All	Crude	Adj.	Group	0-4	5-9	10-14	Crude	Adj.		
TOTAL	56	306	285	315	962	100.0	100.0	100.0	94.7	75.4	87.2	85.8	86.3	1287	69.8
I. LEUKAEMIAS	14	100	101	79	294	30.6	30.8	100.0	29.8	26.7	21.9	26.2	26.5	392	66.3
Acute lymphocytic	6	55	46	39	146	15.2	15.3	49.7	16.0	12.2	10.8	13.0	13.2	195	79.5
Other lymphocytic	2	5	6	4	17	1.8	1.8	5.8	1.8	1.6	1.1	1.5	1.5	23	70.6
Acute non-lymphocytic	2	10	17	11	40	4.2	4.2	13.6	3.1	4.5	3.0	3.6	3.6	53	75.0
Chronic myeloid	0	3	6	3	12	1.2	1.2	4.1	0.8	1.6	0.8	1.1	1.1	16	91.7
Other and unspecified	4	27	26	22	79	8.2	8.3	26.9	8.1	6.9	6.1	7.0	7.1	105	32.9
II. LYMPHOMAS	3	34	75	92	204	21.2	20.7	100.0	9.7	19.8	25.5	18.2	17.5	275	78.3
Hodgkin's disease	1	5	37	40	83	8.6	8.4	40.7	1.6	9.8	11.1	7.4	7.0	112	85.5
Non-Hodgkin lymphoma	1	23	25	33	82	8.5	8.4	40.2	6.3	6.6	9.1	7.3	7.2	110	69.5
Burkitt's lymphoma	0	1	0	1	2	0.2	0.2	1.0	0.3	-	0.3	0.2	0.2	3	-
Unspecified lymphoma	1	4	11	18	34	3.5	3.4	16.7	1.3	2.9	5.0	3.0	2.9	46	85.3
Histiocytosis X	0	1	0	0	1	0.1	0.1	0.5	0.3	-	-	0.1	0.1	1	100.0
Other reticuloendothelial	0	0	2	0	2	0.2	0.2	1.0	-	0.5	-	0.2	0.2	3	50.0
III. BRAIN AND SPINAL	1	17	40	40	98	10.2	10.0	100.0	4.7	10.6	11.1	8.7	8.5	132	66.0
Ependymoma	0	3	2	0	5	0.5	0.5	5.1	0.8	0.5	-	0.4	0.5	7	80.0
Astrocytoma	1	3	13	15	32	3.3	3.2	32.7	1.0	3.4	4.2	2.9	2.7	43	100.0
Medulloblastoma	0	2	6	12	20	2.1	2.0	20.4	0.5	1.6	3.3	1.8	1.7	27	90.0
Other glioma	0	4	3	3	10	1.0	1.0	10.2	0.5	0.8	0.8	0.9	0.9	13	60.0
Other and unspecified *	0	5	16	10	31	3.2	3.2	31.6	1.3	4.2	2.8	2.8	2.7	42	13.3
IV. SYMPATHETIC N.S.	6	16	15	4	41	4.3	4.4	100.0	5.8	4.0	1.1	3.7	3.8	54	85.4
Neuroblastoma	6	16	15	4	41	4.3	4.4	100.0	5.8	4.0	1.1	3.7	3.8	54	85.4
Other	0	0	0	0	0	-	-	-	-	-	-	-	-	-	-
V. RETINOBLASTOMA	7	46	9	1	63	6.5	6.9	100.0	13.9	2.4	0.3	5.6	6.2	83	54.0
VI. KIDNEY	7	29	7	4	47	4.9	5.1	100.0	9.4	1.9	1.1	4.2	4.6	62	61.7
Wilms' tumour	3	24	7	4	38	4.0	4.1	80.9	7.1	1.9	1.1	3.4	3.7	50	71.1
Renal carcinoma	0	1	0	0	1	0.1	0.1	2.1	0.3	-	-	0.1	0.1	1	100.0
Other and unspecified	4	4	0	0	8	0.8	0.9	17.0	2.1	-	-	0.7	0.8	10	12.5
VII. LIVER	8	11	3	3	25	2.6	2.7	100.0	5.0	0.8	0.8	2.2	2.4	33	68.0
Hepatoblastoma	6	8	2	0	16	1.7	1.8	64.0	3.7	0.5	-	1.4	1.6	21	81.3
Hepatic carcinoma	2	0	1	3	6	0.6	0.6	24.0	0.5	0.3	0.8	0.5	0.5	8	66.7
Other and unspecified	0	3	0	0	3	0.3	0.3	12.0	0.8	-	-	0.3	0.3	4	-
VIII. BONE	0	4	12	43	59	6.1	5.8	100.0	1.0	3.2	11.9	5.3	4.9	81	81.4
Osteosarcoma	0	2	4	14	20	2.1	2.0	33.9	0.5	1.1	3.9	1.8	1.7	27	85.0
Chondrosarcoma	0	0	0	0	0	-	-	-	-	-	-	-	-	-	-
Ewing's sarcoma	0	1	7	20	28	2.9	2.8	47.5	0.3	1.9	5.5	2.5	2.3	38	100.0
Other and unspecified	0	1	1	9	11	1.1	1.1	18.6	0.3	0.3	2.5	1.0	0.9	15	27.3
IX. SOFT TISSUE SARCOMAS	4	19	8	16	47	4.9	4.9	100.0	6.0	2.1	4.4	4.2	4.3	63	89.4
Rhabdomyosarcoma	2	11	4	3	20	2.1	2.1	42.6	3.4	1.1	0.8	1.8	1.9	26	90.0
Fibrosarcoma	0	4	3	9	16	1.7	1.6	34.0	1.0	0.8	2.5	1.4	1.4	22	93.8
Other and unspecified	2	4	1	4	11	1.1	1.1	23.4	1.6	0.3	1.1	1.0	1.0	15	81.8
X. GONADAL & GERM CELL	3	12	1	5	21	2.2	2.2	100.0	3.9	0.3	1.4	1.9	2.0	28	81.0
Non-gonadal germ cell	2	3	0	0	5	0.5	0.6	23.8	1.3	-	-	0.4	0.5	7	100.0
Gonadal germ cell	1	6	0	5	12	1.2	1.2	57.1	1.8	-	1.4	1.1	1.1	16	91.7
Gonadal carcinoma	0	0	1	0	1	0.1	0.1	4.8	-	0.3	-	0.1	0.1	1	100.0
Other and unspecified	0	3	0	0	3	0.3	0.3	14.3	0.5	-	-	0.3	0.3	4	-
XI. EPITHELIAL NEOPLASMS	1	1	7	18	27	2.8	2.7	100.0	0.5	1.9	5.0	2.4	2.2	37	92.6
Adrenocortical carcinoma	0	0	0	0	0	-	-	-	-	-	-	-	-	-	-
Thyroid carcinoma	0	0	1	3	4	0.4	0.4	14.8	-	0.3	0.8	0.4	0.3	5	100.0
Nasopharyngeal carcinoma	0	0	1	5	6	0.6	0.6	22.2	-	0.3	1.4	0.5	0.5	8	100.0
Melanoma	0	0	0	2	2	0.2	0.5	7.4	-	-	0.6	0.2	0.2	3	100.0
Other carcinoma	1	1	5	8	15	1.6	1.2	55.6	0.5	1.3	2.2	1.3	1.3	20	86.7
XII. OTHER	2	17	7	10	36	3.7	3.8	100.0	5.0	1.9	2.8	3.2	3.3	48	13.9
* Specified as malignant	0	5	13	8	26	2.7	2.7	100.0	1.3	3.4	2.2	2.3	2.3	35	4.0

India, Bombay Cancer Registry   1970 - 1979   FEMALE

DIAGNOSTIC GROUP	NUMBER OF CASES					REL. FREQUENCY(%)			RATES PER MILLION						HV(%)
	0	1-4	5-9	10-14	All	Crude	Adj.	Group	0-4	5-9	10-14	Crude	Adj.	Cum	
TOTAL	25	198	162	181	566	100.0	100.0	100.0	61.8	44.8	55.5	54.0	54.5	810	73.1
I. LEUKAEMIAS	5	69	64	61	199	35.2	35.2	100.0	20.5	17.7	18.7	19.0	19.1	285	67.3
Acute lymphocytic	0	31	34	25	90	15.9	16.0	45.2	8.6	9.4	7.7	8.6	8.6	128	77.8
Other lymphocytic	0	4	3	3	10	1.8	1.8	5.0	1.1	0.8	0.9	1.0	1.0	14	70.0
Acute non-lymphocytic	1	10	9	12	32	5.7	5.6	16.1	3.0	2.5	3.7	3.1	3.1	46	75.0
Chronic myeloid	0	1	6	4	11	1.9	2.0	5.5	0.3	1.7	1.2	1.0	1.0	16	81.8
Other and unspecified	4	23	12	17	56	9.9	9.9	28.1	7.5	3.3	5.2	5.3	5.5	80	42.9
II. LYMPHOMAS	0	15	22	14	51	9.0	9.1	100.0	4.2	6.1	4.3	4.9	4.8	73	74.5
Hodgkin's disease	0	2	7	4	13	2.3	2.3	25.5	0.6	1.9	1.2	1.2	1.2	19	84.6
Non-Hodgkin lymphoma	0	5	9	5	19	3.4	3.4	37.3	1.4	2.5	1.5	1.8	1.8	27	78.9
Burkitt's lymphoma	0	2	4	0	6	1.1	1.1	11.8	0.6	1.1	-	0.6	0.6	8	83.3
Unspecified lymphoma	0	6	2	5	13	2.3	2.3	25.5	1.7	0.6	1.5	1.2	1.3	19	53.8
Histiocytosis X	0	0	0	0	0	-	-	-	-	-	-	-	-	-	-
Other reticuloendothelial	0	0	0	0	0	-	-	-	-	-	-	-	-	-	-
III. BRAIN AND SPINAL	0	9	33	34	76	13.4	13.4	100.0	2.5	9.1	10.4	7.2	6.9	110	71.1
Ependymoma	0	0	3	3	6	1.1	1.1	7.9	-	0.8	0.9	0.6	0.5	9	100.0
Astrocytoma	0	3	17	15	35	6.2	6.2	46.1	0.8	4.7	4.6	3.3	3.2	51	91.4
Medulloblastoma	0	2	4	9	15	2.7	2.6	19.7	0.6	1.1	2.8	1.4	1.4	22	80.0
Other glioma	0	2	2	0	4	0.7	0.7	5.3	0.6	0.6	-	0.4	0.4	6	50.0
Other and unspecified *	0	2	7	7	16	2.8	2.8	21.1	0.6	1.9	2.1	1.5	1.5	23	12.5
IV. SYMPATHETIC N.S.	4	17	2	1	24	4.2	4.3	100.0	5.8	0.6	0.3	2.3	2.5	33	91.7
Neuroblastoma	4	16	2	1	23	4.1	4.1	95.8	5.5	0.6	0.3	2.2	2.4	32	91.3
Other	0	1	0	0	1	0.2	0.2	4.2	0.3	-	-	0.1	0.1	1	100.0
V. RETINOBLASTOMA	1	33	5	1	40	7.1	7.2	100.0	9.4	1.4	0.3	3.8	4.2	56	70.0
VI. KIDNEY	7	26	5	3	41	7.2	7.3	100.0	9.1	1.4	0.9	3.9	4.3	57	90.2
Wilms' tumour	6	25	5	1	37	6.5	6.7	90.2	8.6	1.4	0.3	3.5	3.9	51	91.9
Renal carcinoma	0	1	0	2	3	0.5	0.5	7.3	0.3	-	0.6	0.3	0.3	4	66.7
Other and unspecified	1	0	0	0	1	0.2	0.2	2.4	0.3	-	-	0.1	0.1	1	100.0
VII. LIVER	2	2	2	2	8	1.4	1.4	100.0	1.1	0.6	0.6	0.8	0.8	11	62.5
Hepatoblastoma	2	0	2	0	4	0.7	0.7	50.0	0.6	0.6	-	0.4	0.4	6	100.0
Hepatic carcinoma	0	1	0	0	1	0.2	0.2	12.5	0.3	-	-	0.1	0.1	1	100.0
Other and unspecified	0	1	0	2	3	0.5	0.5	37.5	0.3	-	0.6	0.3	0.3	4	-
VIII. BONE	0	2	14	32	48	8.5	8.3	100.0	0.6	3.9	9.8	4.6	4.3	71	77.1
Osteosarcoma	0	0	4	14	18	3.2	3.1	37.5	-	1.1	4.3	1.7	1.6	27	77.8
Chondrosarcoma	0	1	0	0	1	0.2	0.2	2.1	0.3	-	-	0.1	0.1	1	100.0
Ewing's sarcoma	0	1	6	15	22	3.9	3.8	45.8	0.3	1.7	4.6	2.1	2.0	33	95.5
Other and unspecified	0	0	4	3	7	1.2	1.2	14.6	-	1.1	0.9	0.7	0.6	10	14.3
IX. SOFT TISSUE SARCOMAS	2	10	7	6	25	4.4	4.4	100.0	3.3	1.9	1.8	2.4	2.4	36	92.0
Rhabdomyosarcoma	2	6	4	3	15	2.7	2.7	60.0	2.2	1.1	0.9	1.4	1.5	21	93.3
Fibrosarcoma	0	2	1	3	6	1.1	1.0	24.0	0.6	0.3	0.9	0.6	0.6	9	83.3
Other and unspecified	0	2	2	0	4	0.7	0.7	16.0	0.6	0.6	-	0.4	0.4	6	100.0
X. GONADAL & GERM CELL	2	4	2	10	18	3.2	3.1	100.0	1.7	0.6	3.1	1.7	1.7	26	88.9
Non-gonadal germ cell	1	2	0	1	4	0.7	0.7	22.2	0.8	-	0.3	0.4	0.4	6	100.0
Gonadal germ cell	1	2	1	7	11	1.9	1.9	61.1	0.8	0.3	2.1	1.0	1.0	16	100.0
Gonadal carcinoma	0	0	1	0	1	0.4	0.4	5.6	-	0.3	-	0.1	0.1	1	100.0
Other and unspecified	0	0	1	1	2	0.4	0.4	11.1	-	0.3	0.3	0.2	0.2	3	-
XI. EPITHELIAL NEOPLASMS	0	2	2	8	12	2.1	2.1	100.0	0.6	0.6	2.5	1.1	1.1	18	100.0
Adrenocortical carcinoma	0	0	0	0	0	0.2	0.2	8.3	-	-	0.3	0.1	0.1	2	100.0
Thyroid carcinoma	0	0	0	1	1	0.2	0.2	8.3	-	-	0.3	0.1	0.1	2	100.0
Nasopharyngeal carcinoma	0	0	0	1	1	-	-	-	-	-	-	-	-	-	-
Melanoma	0	0	0	0	0	-	-	-	-	-	-	-	-	-	-
Other carcinoma	2	2	2	6	10	1.8	1.7	83.3	0.6	0.6	1.8	1.0	0.9	15	100.0
XII. OTHER	2	9	4	9	24	4.2	4.2	100.0	3.0	1.1	2.8	2.3	2.3	35	33.3
* Specified as malignant	0	2	6	6	14	2.5	2.5	100.0	0.6	1.7	1.8	1.3	1.3	20	-

AVERAGE ANNUAL POPULATION: 1970–1979

Age	Male	Female
0–4	382383	360896
5–9	377850	361373
10–14	361154	326273
0–14	1121387	1048542

Commentary

Since many of the records in the registry refer to children who were patients at the Tata Memorial Hospital, Bombay, they will also have been included in the tables for that centre (see page 163).

The overall incidence rate is among the lowest for any population-based registry included in the present volume. There was a very high sex ratio for all diagnoses combined (M/F = 1.58).

Lymphomas, both Hodgkin's disease and non-Hodgkin lymphoma, were relatively frequent. Registration rates for brain and spinal tumours were low, possibly because, with rare exception, only those specified as malignant are registered. The rates for neuroblastoma and Wilms' tumour were low, while those for retinoblastoma, which was the commonest embryonal tumour, were comparatively high. Only 15% (15/103) of retinoblastomas were reported to be bilateral. Males, but not females, had a high rate of malignant liver tumours, most of which were hepatoblastoma.

Reference

Jussawalla, D.J., Yeole, B.B. & Natekar, N.V. (1975) Cancer in children in Greater Bombay, (1964-1972): comparative study. *Indian J. Cancer*, *12*, 135-143

Bombay: Cancer Registry of the Tata Memorial Hospital, 1970–1979

P.B. Desai

The Tata Memorial Centre — the pioneer cancer hospital and research centre in India — was established in 1941 for the diagnosis and treatment of cancer and to conduct research on basic aspects of the disease. The Centre consists of two units, viz. Tata Memorial Hospital and the Cancer Research Institute, and is under the administrative control of the Government of India's Department of Atomic Energy. The Tata Memorial Hospital is a well-equipped comprehensive care cancer hospital consisting of the Departments of Surgery, Pathology, Biochemistry, Cytology, Anaesthesiology, Radio-diagnosis, Radiotherapy, Internal Medicine, Blood Bank, Chemotherapy, Medical Records and Statistics, Social Service, Rehabilitation and Administration. The Hospital has a total staff of 1794, consisting of 274 medical and scientific, 380 technical, 99 administrative and 1041 auxiliary staff.

Patients come for treatment from all parts of India and also from the neighbouring countries of the Middle East, East Africa and South-east Asia. The majority of the patients come from the neighbouring states, particularly Gujarat and Maharashtra.

The Department of Medical Records and Statistics has functioned as a hospital tumour registry ever since the inception of the Hospital. All medical records of patients are maintained in this Department. Patients attending Tata Memorial Hospital are registered only once, their medical records being updated as and when they attend the Hospital. The medical record is used both for in-patient and out-patient activities. All procedures carried out on a particular patient, such as radiotherapy, chemotherapy, and surgery, are included in the same medical record. Each medical record contains information on the patient's demographic status, e.g., age, sex, mother tongue, duration of stay in Bombay, occupation, socioeconomic status, complete address, and medical information.

Hospital medical records are extensively used for clinical research, and form part of the educational material for students registered for MD and MS courses. The population-based Bombay Cancer Registry of the Indian Cancer Society has functioned since 1963, and Tata Memorial Hospital records are used for identifying cancer cases occurring in the city of Greater Bombay. About 60% of the material collected by the Bombay Cancer Registry is from the Tata Memorial Hospital medical records.

Commentary

Since many of the children were residents of Greater Bombay, they will also have been included in the tables for the Bombay Cancer Registry (see page 159).

The commonest diagnostic groups were leukaemia (25% of all cases) and lymphomas (20%). Over half the lymphomas were Hodgkin's disease. The most common embryonal tumour was retinoblastoma, accounting for 11% of all cases and more than all other embryonal tumours combined. Laterality was not recorded for retinoblastoma. Brain and spinal tumours were relatively infrequent. Among boys, especially in the 10–14 age-range, there was a large number of nasopharyngeal carcinomas but this tumour was much less common in girls. Over half of the 'other carcinoma' group were in the oral cavity, etc.

By comparison with the population-based Bombay Cancer Registry, there were relatively high frequencies of retinoblastoma, bone and soft-tissue sarcomas and nasopharyngeal carcinoma. There are several possible explanations for this: patients with these tumours (or at least those resident outside Greater Bombay) may be more likely to be treated at the Tata Memorial Hospital, or these diagnostic groups may account for a larger proportion of the total incidence of childhood cancer outside Bombay.

India, Tata Hospital, Bombay   1970 – 1979   MALE

DIAGNOSTIC GROUP	NUMBER OF CASES					REL. FREQUENCY(%)			HV(%)
	0	1-4	5-9	10-14	All	Crude	Adj.	Group	
TOTAL	50	434	519	610	1614¤	100.0	100.0	100.0	80.9
I. LEUKAEMIAS	9	98	155	152	414	25.7	25.3	100.0	100.0
Acute lymphocytic	4	74	111	85	274	17.0	17.0	66.2	100.0
Other lymphocytic	0	1	1	5	7	0.4	0.4	1.7	100.0
Acute non-lymphocytic	4	8	20	37	69	4.3	4.0	16.7	100.0
Chronic myeloid	0	2	8	6	16	1.0	0.9	3.9	100.0
Other and unspecified	1	13	15	19	48	3.0	3.0	11.6	100.0
II. LYMPHOMAS	0	38	168	180	386	23.9	21.7	100.0	83.7
Hodgkin's disease	0	17	104	101	222	13.8	12.4	57.5	86.5
Non-Hodgkin lymphoma	0	9	30	35	74	4.6	4.2	19.2	85.1
Burkitt's lymphoma	0	0	2	0	2	0.1	0.1	0.5	100.0
Unspecified lymphoma	0	12	31	44	87	5.4	4.9	22.5	74.7
Histiocytosis X	0	0	0	0	0	–	–	–	–
Other reticuloendothelial	0	0	1	0	1	0.1	0.1	0.3	100.0
III. BRAIN AND SPINAL	2	12	44	40	99¤	6.1	5.7	100.0	51.5
Ependymoma	0	3	1	0	4	0.2	0.3	4.0	75.0
Astrocytoma	0	1	13	22	36	2.2	1.9	36.4	66.7
Medulloblastoma	1	3	12	8	25¤	1.5	1.4	25.3	88.0
Other glioma	0	3	6	6	15	0.9	0.9	15.2	6.7
Other and unspecified *	1	2	12	4	19	1.2	1.1	19.2	5.3
IV. SYMPATHETIC N.S.	7	28	30	9	74	4.6	5.1	100.0	74.3
Neuroblastoma	7	28	30	9	74	4.6	5.1	100.0	74.3
Other	0	0	0	0	0	–	–	–	–
V. RETINOBLASTOMA	16	126	20	2	164	10.2	13.0	100.0	61.0
VI. KIDNEY	3	44	18	5	70	4.3	5.2	100.0	75.7
Wilms' tumour	3	43	18	5	69	4.3	5.1	98.6	75.4
Renal carcinoma	0	0	0	0	0	–	–	–	–
Other and unspecified	0	1	0	0	1	0.1	0.1	1.4	100.0
VII. LIVER	0	2	2	4	8	0.5	0.5	100.0	87.5
Hepatoblastoma	0	2	0	0	2	0.1	0.2	25.0	100.0
Hepatic carcinoma	0	0	2	4	6	0.4	0.3	75.0	83.3
Other and unspecified	0	0	0	0	0	–	–	–	–
VIII. BONE	1	8	37	113	159	9.9	8.4	100.0	78.0
Osteosarcoma	1	1	7	54	62	3.8	3.1	39.0	74.2
Chondrosarcoma	0	0	0	0	0	–	–	–	–
Ewing's sarcoma	1	5	22	43	71	4.4	3.9	44.7	85.9
Other and unspecified	0	2	8	16	26	1.6	1.4	16.4	65.4
IX. SOFT TISSUE SARCOMAS	11	44	24	39	118	7.3	7.9	100.0	80.5
Rhabdomyosarcoma	8	33	17	10	68	4.2	4.9	57.6	85.3
Fibrosarcoma	2	4	3	16	25	1.5	1.5	21.2	96.0
Other and unspecified	1	7	4	13	25	1.5	1.5	21.2	52.0
X. GONADAL & GERM CELL	0	18	1	6	25	1.5	1.8	100.0	80.0
Non-gonadal germ cell	0	3	1	1	5	0.3	0.4	20.0	100.0
Gonadal germ cell	0	9	0	3	12	0.7	0.9	48.0	91.7
Gonadal carcinoma	0	4	0	2	6	0.4	0.4	24.0	66.7
Other and unspecified	0	2	0	0	2	0.1	0.2	8.0	–
XI. EPITHELIAL NEOPLASMS	0	6	12	51	69	4.3	3.7	100.0	66.7
Adrenocortical carcinoma	0	0	0	0	0	–	–	–	–
Thyroid carcinoma	0	0	3	9	12	0.7	0.6	17.4	75.0
Nasopharyngeal carcinoma	0	1	4	26	31	1.9	1.6	44.9	67.7
Melanoma	0	0	0	0	0	–	–	–	–
Other carcinoma	0	5	5	16	26	1.6	1.5	37.7	61.5
XII. OTHER	1	10	8	9	28	1.7	1.8	100.0	60.7
* Specified as malignant	1	2	12	4	19	1.2	1.1	100.0	5.3

¤ Includes age unknown

India, Tata Hospital, Bombay

1970 - 1979

FEMALE

DIAGNOSTIC GROUP	NUMBER OF CASES					REL. FREQUENCY(%)			HV(%)
	0	1-4	5-9	10-14	All	Crude	Adj.	Group	
TOTAL	26	260	212	254	752	100.0	100.0	100.0	77.3
I. LEUKAEMIAS	3	56	69	53	181	24.1	24.3	100.0	100.0
Acute lymphocytic	1	42	44	32	119	15.8	16.0	65.7	100.0
Other lymphocytic	0	1	1	0	2	0.3	0.3	1.1	100.0
Acute non-lymphocytic	1	6	10	9	26	3.5	3.5	14.4	100.0
Chronic myeloid	0	1	9	4	14	1.9	1.9	7.7	100.0
Other and unspecified	1	6	5	8	20	2.7	2.6	11.0	100.0
II. LYMPHOMAS	1	18	40	36	95	12.6	12.6	100.0	74.7
Hodgkin's disease	0	3	19	17	39	5.2	5.1	41.1	79.5
Non-Hodgkin lymphoma	1	7	7	8	23	3.1	3.1	24.2	73.9
Burkitt's lymphoma	0	1	1	0	2	0.3	0.3	2.1	100.0
Unspecified lymphoma	0	7	13	11	31	4.1	4.1	32.6	67.7
Histiocytosis X	0	0	0	0	0	-	-	-	-
Other reticuloendothelial	0	0	0	0	0	-	-	-	-
III. BRAIN AND SPINAL	1	7	27	32	67	8.9	8.7	100.0	50.7
Ependymoma	0	0	0	3	3	0.4	0.4	4.5	100.0
Astrocytoma	0	2	11	12	25	3.3	3.3	37.3	72.0
Medulloblastoma	0	2	6	5	13	1.7	1.7	19.4	76.9
Other glioma	0	2	4	4	10	1.3	1.3	14.9	30.0
Other and unspecified *	1	1	5	9	16	2.1	2.1	23.9	-
IV. SYMPATHETIC N.S.	7	26	12	5	50	6.6	6.9	100.0	74.0
Neuroblastoma	7	26	12	5	50	6.6	6.9	100.0	74.0
Other	0	0	0	0	0	-	-	-	-
V. RETINOBLASTOMA	5	74	13	1	93	12.4	13.0	100.0	63.4
VI. KIDNEY	3	41	8	0	52	6.9	7.3	100.0	75.0
Wilms' tumour	3	41	8	0	52	6.9	7.3	100.0	75.0
Renal carcinoma	0	0	0	0	0	-	-	-	-
Other and unspecified	0	0	0	0	0	-	-	-	-
VII. LIVER	1	2	1	0	4	0.5	0.6	100.0	100.0
Hepatoblastoma	1	2	1	0	4	0.5	0.6	100.0	100.0
Hepatic carcinoma	0	0	0	0	0	-	-	-	-
Other and unspecified	0	0	0	0	0	-	-	-	-
VIII. BONE	0	1	20	65	86	11.4	10.6	100.0	76.7
Osteosarcoma	0	0	6	25	31	4.1	3.8	36.0	87.1
Chondrosarcoma	0	0	0	0	0	-	-	-	-
Ewing's sarcoma	0	1	12	28	41	5.5	5.1	47.7	85.4
Other and unspecified	0	0	2	12	14	1.9	1.7	16.3	28.6
IX. SOFT TISSUE SARCOMAS	5	24	10	20	59	7.8	7.8	100.0	72.9
Rhabdomyosarcoma	4	19	7	5	35	4.7	4.8	59.3	80.0
Fibrosarcoma	0	2	1	6	9	1.2	1.1	15.3	66.7
Other and unspecified	1	3	2	9	15	2.0	1.9	25.4	60.0
X. GONADAL & GERM CELL	0	3	6	17	26	3.5	3.3	100.0	84.6
Non-gonadal germ cell	0	1	1	0	2	0.3	0.3	7.7	100.0
Gonadal germ cell	0	1	3	14	18	2.4	2.2	69.2	88.9
Gonadal carcinoma	0	1	0	1	2	0.3	0.3	7.7	100.0
Other and unspecified	0	0	2	2	4	0.5	0.5	15.4	50.0
XI. EPITHELIAL NEOPLASMS	0	2	4	17	23	3.1	2.9	100.0	69.6
Adrenocortical carcinoma	0	0	0	0	0	-	-	-	-
Thyroid carcinoma	0	0	1	3	4	0.5	0.5	17.4	75.0
Nasopharyngeal carcinoma	0	0	0	5	5	0.7	0.6	21.7	60.0
Melanoma	0	0	1	0	1	0.1	0.1	4.3	100.0
Other carcinoma	0	2	2	9	13	1.7	1.6	56.5	69.2
XII. OTHER	0	6	2	8	16	2.1	2.1	100.0	56.3
	1	1	5	9	16	2.1	2.1	100.0	-

* Specified as malignant
¤ Includes age unknown

INDONESIA

Yogyakarta Pathology Registry, 1973–1983

Soeripto & E. Soetristi

The registry was established in 1973. Until that time there was no cancer registry in the region, and there was a need for cancer data for comparative studies in Indonesia.

The sources of data are the Department of Pathology in the Medical Faculty of Gadjah Mada University, the pathology laboratory of Waskitha, and the pathology laboratory of Bethesda Hospital. Reporting of cases is voluntary.

Data are collected at the University Department of Pathology. Some hospital-based surveys were done in 1981 and 1982. An intensive population-based survey was done during 1983–1985 in one district with a population of about 26 500 in the special region of Yogyakarta. During the period of this survey, a trial was undertaken of ways to motivate health centres to participate in cancer registration. The results were due to be presented in mid-1985. Death certificates are not used for registration and autopsy is rare.

The data are used for comparative studies of trends in cancer in the departments of pathology and hospitals in the area.

There are five government hospitals, one military hospital and three private hospitals. One of the government hospitals is a referral and teaching hospital. This hospital and the three private ones are in Yogyakarta town; the others are located elsewhere in the province. Overall there are 0.15 doctors and 8–9 hospital beds per 1000 population.

The registry covers the Province of Yogyakarta, which has an area of 3021 square kilometres and consists of four counties (rural areas) and one town (Yogyakarta town). The total population, as given by the Statistical Bureau of Yogyakarta Province in 1981, is 2 750 128, of whom about 35% were children aged 0–14. The four counties of Kulon Progo, Bantul, Gunung Kidul and Sleman together contain 86% of the population of the Province and take up 99% of the area. The average population density is 787 persons per square kilometre in the four rural counties, 12 250 per square kilometre in Yogyakarta town and 910 per square kilometre overall. The great majority of the population (92%) are Moslem, with 5% Roman Catholic, 2% other Christians and under 1% each Hindus and Buddhists. Ethnically, the people are predominantly Malays, with a small number of Chinese in Yogyakarta town and the capitals of the counties. The main occupation is farming. A small number of people work in animal husbandry and a few as fishermen.

The tables present registered cases as numbers and percentages. Incidence rates have not been calculated because of the selective nature of the series.

Commentary

Leukaemias are not included in the registry, and there was only a single recorded case of a brain tumour. The most numerous diagnostic group was the lymphomas, accounting for 27% of all registrations; of these, about three-quarters were of non-Hodgkin type and a further 10% unspecified or Burkitt's lymphomas. The next most frequent diagnosis was retinoblastoma, with 19% of the total and more than twice the number of cases for all other embryonal tumours combined. There were no cases of Ewing's sarcoma.

Indonesia, Yogyakarta Path. Dept. 1973 - 1983 MALE

DIAGNOSTIC GROUP	NUMBER OF CASES					REL. FREQUENCY(%)			HV(%)
	0	1-4	5-9	10-14	All	Crude	Adj.	Group	
TOTAL	8	43	23	39	113	100.0	100.0	100.0	100.0
I. LEUKAEMIAS	0	0	0	0	0	-	-	-	-
Acute lymphocytic	0	0	0	0	0	-	-	-	-
Other lymphocytic	0	0	0	0	0	-	-	-	-
Acute non-lymphocytic	0	0	0	0	0	-	-	-	-
Chronic myeloid	0	0	0	0	0	-	-	-	-
Other and unspecified	0	0	0	0	0	-	-	-	-
II. LYMPHOMAS	4	4	10	17	35	31.0	32.4	100.0	100.0
Hodgkin's disease	0	1	1	6	8	7.1	6.7	22.9	100.0
Non-Hodgkin lymphoma	4	2	9	10	25	22.1	24.2	71.4	100.0
Burkitt's lymphoma	0	0	0	0	0	-	-	-	100.0
Unspecified lymphoma	0	1	0	1	2	1.8	1.6	5.7	-
Histiocytosis X	0	0	0	0	0	-	-	-	100.0
Other reticuloendothelial	0	0	0	0	0	-	-	-	-
III. BRAIN AND SPINAL	0	0	0	0	0	-	-	-	-
Ependymoma	0	0	0	0	0	-	-	-	-
Astrocytoma	0	0	0	0	0	-	-	-	-
Medulloblastoma	0	0	0	0	0	-	-	-	-
Other glioma	0	0	0	0	0	-	-	-	-
Other and unspecified *	0	0	0	0	0	-	-	-	-
IV. SYMPATHETIC N.S.	3	2	0	0	5	4.4	3.9	100.0	100.0
Neuroblastoma	3	2	0	0	5	4.4	3.9	100.0	100.0
Other	0	0	0	0	0	-	-	-	-
V. RETINOBLASTOMA	0	20	1	0	21	18.6	17.0	100.0	100.0
VI. KIDNEY	0	4	0	0	4	3.5	3.1	100.0	100.0
Wilms' tumour	0	4	0	0	4	3.5	3.1	100.0	100.0
Renal carcinoma	0	0	0	0	0	-	-	-	100.0
Other and unspecified	0	0	0	0	0	-	-	-	-
VII. LIVER	0	0	1	1	2	1.8	2.1	100.0	100.0
Hepatoblastoma	0	0	0	0	0	-	-	-	-
Hepatic carcinoma	0	0	1	1	2	1.8	2.1	100.0	100.0
Other and unspecified	0	0	0	0	0	-	-	-	-
VIII. BONE	0	0	2	5	7	6.2	5.4	100.0	100.0
Osteosarcoma	0	0	2	3	5	4.4	3.8	71.4	100.0
Chondrosarcoma	0	0	0	2	2	1.8	1.5	28.6	100.0
Ewing's sarcoma	0	0	0	0	0	-	-	-	-
Other and unspecified	0	0	0	0	0	-	-	-	-
IX. SOFT TISSUE SARCOMAS	0	1	6	6	13	11.5	10.6	100.0	100.0
Rhabdomyosarcoma	0	0	5	5	10	8.8	7.7	76.9	100.0
Fibrosarcoma	0	1	0	0	1	0.9	0.8	7.7	100.0
Other and unspecified	0	0	1	1	2	1.8	2.1	15.4	100.0
X. GONADAL & GERM CELL	1	2	1	7	11	9.7	8.6	100.0	100.0
Non-gonadal germ cell	1	2	0	0	3	2.7	2.3	27.3	100.0
Gonadal germ cell	0	0	1	7	8	7.1	6.3	72.7	100.0
Gonadal carcinoma	0	0	0	0	0	-	-	-	-
Other and unspecified	0	0	0	0	0	-	-	-	-
XI. EPITHELIAL NEOPLASMS	0	10	2	3	15	13.3	16.9	100.0	100.0
Adrenocortical carcinoma	0	0	0	0	0	-	-	-	-
Thyroid carcinoma	0	0	0	0	0	-	-	-	-
Nasopharyngeal carcinoma	0	0	0	1	1	0.9	0.8	6.7	100.0
Melanoma	0	2	0	0	2	1.8	2.6	13.3	100.0
Other carcinoma	0	8	2	2	12	10.6	13.5	80.0	100.0
XII. OTHER	0	0	0	0	0	-	-	-	-

* Specified as malignant

FEMALE

Indonesia, Yogyakarta Path. Dept.

1973 - 1983

DIAGNOSTIC GROUP	NUMBER OF CASES					REL. FREQUENCY(%)			HV(%)
	0	1-4	5-9	10-14	All	Crude	Adj.	Group	
TOTAL	6	31	23	42	102	100.0	100.0	100.0	100.0
I. LEUKAEMIAS	0	0	0	0	0	–	–	–	–
Acute lymphocytic	0	0	0	0	0	–	–	–	–
Other lymphocytic	0	0	0	0	0	–	–	–	–
Acute non-lymphocytic	0	0	0	0	0	–	–	–	–
Chronic myeloid	0	0	0	0	0	–	–	–	–
Other and unspecified	0	0	0	0	0	–	–	–	–
II. LYMPHOMAS	2	6	8	8	24	23.5	24.8	100.0	100.0
Hodgkin's disease	0	0	0	1	1	1.0	0.7	4.2	100.0
Non-Hodgkin lymphoma	2	4	7	6	19	18.6	19.9	79.2	100.0
Burkitt's lymphoma	0	1	0	0	1	1.0	1.1	4.2	100.0
Unspecified lymphoma	0	1	1	1	3	2.9	3.1	12.5	100.0
Histiocytosis X	0	0	0	0	0	–	–	–	–
Other reticuloendothelial	0	0	0	0	0	–	–	–	–
III. BRAIN AND SPINAL	0	1	0	0	1	1.0	1.1	100.0	100.0
Ependymoma	0	0	0	0	0	–	–	–	–
Astrocytoma	0	0	0	0	0	–	–	–	–
Medulloblastoma	0	1	0	0	1	1.0	1.1	100.0	100.0
Other glioma	0	0	0	0	0	–	–	–	–
Other and unspecified *	0	0	0	0	0	–	–	–	–
IV. SYMPATHETIC N.S.	0	2	2	0	4	3.9	4.8	100.0	100.0
Neuroblastoma	0	2	2	0	4	3.9	4.8	100.0	100.0
Other	0	0	0	0	0	–	–	–	–
V. RETINOBLASTOMA	1	15	4	0	20	19.6	22.5	100.0	100.0
VI. KIDNEY	0	4	1	1	6	5.9	6.3	100.0	100.0
Wilms' tumour	0	4	1	0	5	4.9	5.6	83.3	100.0
Renal carcinoma	0	0	0	1	1	1.0	0.7	16.7	100.0
Other and unspecified	0	0	0	0	0	–	–	–	–
VII. LIVER	0	0	0	2	2	2.0	1.4	100.0	100.0
Hepatoblastoma	0	0	0	0	0	–	–	–	–
Hepatic carcinoma	0	0	0	2	2	2.0	1.4	100.0	100.0
Other and unspecified	0	0	0	0	0	–	–	–	–
VIII. BONE	0	0	1	5	6	5.9	4.9	100.0	100.0
Osteosarcoma	0	0	0	4	4	3.9	2.9	66.7	100.0
Chondrosarcoma	0	0	0	1	1	1.0	0.7	16.7	100.0
Ewing's sarcoma	0	0	0	0	0	–	–	–	–
Other and unspecified	0	0	1	0	1	1.0	1.3	16.7	100.0
IX. SOFT TISSUE SARCOMAS	3	3	3	7	16	15.7	15.4	100.0	100.0
Rhabdomyosarcoma	3	2	2	5	12	11.8	11.6	75.0	100.0
Fibrosarcoma	0	0	0	1	1	1.0	0.7	6.3	100.0
Other and unspecified	0	1	1	1	3	2.9	3.1	18.8	100.0
X. GONADAL & GERM CELL	0	0	3	6	9	8.8	8.2	100.0	100.0
Non-gonadal germ cell	0	0	1	0	1	1.0	1.3	11.1	100.0
Gonadal germ cell	0	0	1	5	6	5.9	4.9	66.7	100.0
Gonadal carcinoma	0	0	1	1	2	2.0	2.0	22.2	100.0
Other and unspecified	0	0	0	0	0	–	–	–	–
XI. EPITHELIAL NEOPLASMS	0	0	1	13	14	13.7	10.6	100.0	100.0
Adrenocortical carcinoma	0	0	0	0	0	–	–	–	–
Thyroid carcinoma	0	0	0	0	0	–	–	–	–
Nasopharyngeal carcinoma	0	0	0	4	4	3.9	2.9	28.6	100.0
Melanoma	0	0	0	0	0	–	–	–	–
Other carcinoma	0	0	1	9	10	9.8	7.7	71.4	100.0
XII. OTHER	0	0	0	0	0	–	–	–	–
* Specified as malignant	0	0	0	0	0	–	–	–	–

IRAQ

Baghdad Cancer Registry, 1976-1984

A. Al-Fouadi

The Baghdad Cancer Registry was started in 1975. It is located in the Central Public Health Laboratory, which provides pathology services to a number of government hospitals. Data collection involves regular visits to the medical statistics departments of some of the main hospitals in the city, including the Medical City Teaching Hospital of the College of Medicine, University of Baghdad, from which about 50% of the registrations come. The remainder derive from several other general and specialist hospitals, including the Children's Hospital and the Hospital for Radiotherapy and Nuclear Medicine, which notifies cases directly to the Registry on a special form. Other data are derived from pathology reports, including those from private laboratories, which provide reports on cases of cancer diagnosed in private hospitals and clinics. A few hospitals in Baghdad are not covered by the Registry; however, most of their cases of childhood cancer are referred to the specialized teaching or other hospitals which do report to it.

Death certificates are not used as a source of information. A very high proportion of the cases registered in children (98.8%) have microscopic verification of tumour type, which implies that pathology departments, rather than hospital clinical records, are the major data source for the Register.

Although registrations are derived from most potential sources of cancer patients in the city, it is not possible to distinguish residents of Baghdad from cases of cancer referred from elsewhere in Iraq. Thus, it is not possible to calculate rates of incidence, which, in any case, would have represented estimates of minimum incidence. Data from the Registry, including an analysis of childhood cancer cases, were published recently (Al-Fouadi & Parkin, 1984).

Commentary

Leukaemia and lymphoma each accounted for 30% of the cases registered in boys and for 27% and 22%, respectively, of those in girls. The ratio of acute lymphocytic to acute non-lymphocytic leukaemia was about 4:1, a ratio similar to those found in European and North American registries. Approximately 30% of the lymphomas were specified to be of Burkitt's type, a very high figure for a registry outside Africa. Retinoblastoma, nasopharyngeal carcinoma and germ-cell tumours also appear to be frequent. Of the miscellaneous carcinomas, 15 were skin cancers, and five were in the bladder (of which three were squamous-cell).

Reference

Al-Fouadi, A. & Parkin, D.M. (1984) Cancer in Iraq: seven years' data from the Baghdad tumour registry. *Int. J. Cancer, 34*, 207-213

Iraq, Baghdad   1976 – 1984   MALE

DIAGNOSTIC GROUP	NUMBER OF CASES					REL. FREQUENCY(%)			HV(%)
	0	1-4	5-9	10-14	All	Crude	Adj.	Group	
TOTAL	49	451	552	542	1594	100.0	100.0	100.0	98.7
I. LEUKAEMIAS	14	126	171	172	483	30.3	30.0	100.0	97.9
Acute lymphocytic	5	97	124	127	353	22.1	21.9	73.1	100.0
Other lymphocytic	0	0	1	0	1	0.1	0.1	0.2	100.0
Acute non-lymphocytic	3	15	32	27	77	4.8	4.7	15.9	100.0
Chronic myeloid	1	1	0	2	4	0.3	0.3	0.8	100.0
Other and unspecified	5	13	14	16	48	3.0	3.1	9.9	79.2
II. LYMPHOMAS	2	126	206	151	485	30.4	29.8	100.0	100.0
Hodgkin's disease	0	28	67	62	157	9.8	9.3	32.4	100.0
Non-Hodgkin lymphoma	0	36	62	42	140	8.8	8.6	28.9	100.0
Burkitt's lymphoma	0	56	58	28	142	8.9	9.2	29.3	100.0
Unspecified lymphoma	1	6	18	19	44	2.8	2.6	9.1	100.0
Histiocytosis X	1	0	1	0	2	0.1	0.1	0.4	100.0
Other reticuloendothelial	0	0	0	0	0	-	-	-	-
III. BRAIN AND SPINAL	1	17	70	53	141	8.8	8.2	100.0	98.6
Ependymoma	0	3	6	4	13	0.8	0.8	9.2	100.0
Astrocytoma	1	10	26	33	70	4.4	4.1	49.6	100.0
Medulloblastoma	0	3	25	6	34	2.1	1.9	24.1	100.0
Other glioma	0	1	8	4	13	0.7	0.7	9.2	100.0
Other and unspecified *	0	0	5	6	11	0.7	0.6	7.8	81.8
IV. SYMPATHETIC N.S.	7	49	8	3	67	4.2	5.1	100.0	98.5
Neuroblastoma	7	49	7	3	66	4.1	5.0	98.5	98.5
Other	0	0	1	0	1	0.1	0.1	1.5	100.0
V. RETINOBLASTOMA	7	41	13	3	64	4.0	4.7	100.0	100.0
VI. KIDNEY	8	30	14	3	55	3.5	4.0	100.0	100.0
Wilms' tumour	8	30	14	3	55	3.5	4.0	100.0	100.0
Renal carcinoma	0	0	0	0	0	-	-	-	-
Other and unspecified	0	0	0	0	0	-	-	-	-
VII. LIVER	1	1	1	1	4	0.3	0.3	100.0	100.0
Hepatoblastoma	1	0	0	0	1	0.1	0.1	25.0	100.0
Hepatic carcinoma	0	1	1	1	3	0.2	0.2	75.0	100.0
Other and unspecified	0	0	0	0	0	-	-	-	-
VIII. BONE	0	3	17	72	92	5.8	5.1	100.0	100.0
Osteosarcoma	0	1	7	36	44	2.8	2.5	47.8	100.0
Chondrosarcoma	0	0	1	6	7	0.4	0.4	7.6	100.0
Ewing's sarcoma	0	2	8	29	39	2.4	2.2	42.4	100.0
Other and unspecified	0	0	1	1	2	0.1	0.1	2.2	100.0
IX. SOFT TISSUE SARCOMAS	3	24	24	27	78	4.9	5.0	100.0	100.0
Rhabdomyosarcoma	0	16	10	3	29	1.8	2.0	37.2	100.0
Fibrosarcoma	1	3	8	13	25	1.6	1.5	32.1	100.0
Other and unspecified	2	5	6	11	24	1.5	1.5	30.8	100.0
X. GONADAL & GERM CELL	5	17	9	11	42	2.6	2.9	100.0	100.0
Non-gonadal germ cell	4	9	3	7	23	1.4	1.6	54.8	100.0
Gonadal germ cell	1	8	5	3	17	1.1	1.2	40.5	100.0
Gonadal carcinoma	0	0	0	1	1	0.1	0.1	2.4	100.0
Other and unspecified	0	0	1	0	1	0.1	0.1	2.4	100.0
XI. EPITHELIAL NEOPLASMS	0	12	13	38	63	4.0	3.8	100.0	100.0
Adrenocortical carcinoma	0	0	0	0	0	-	-	-	-
Thyroid carcinoma	0	0	0	3	3	0.2	0.2	4.8	100.0
Nasopharyngeal carcinoma	0	0	2	8	10	0.6	0.6	15.9	100.0
Melanoma	0	0	2	1	3	0.2	0.2	4.8	100.0
Other carcinoma	0	12	9	26	47	2.9	2.9	74.6	100.0
XII. OTHER	1	5	6	8	20	1.3	1.2	100.0	60.0
	0	0	4	4	8	0.5	0.4	100.0	75.0

* Specified as malignant
□ Includes age unknown

Iraq, Baghdad

1976 - 1984

FEMALE

DIAGNOSTIC GROUP	NUMBER OF CASES					REL. FREQUENCY(%)			HV(%)
	0	1-4	5-9	10-14	All	Crude	Adj.	Group	
TOTAL	27	250	252	286	816¤	100.0	100.0	100.0	98.9
I. LEUKAEMIAS	2	62	73	83	220	27.0	26.6	100.0	98.6
Acute lymphocytic	2	52	53	46	153	18.8	18.9	69.5	100.0
Other lymphocytic	0	0	0	0	0	-	-	-	-
Acute non-lymphocytic	0	3	11	28	42	5.1	4.7	19.1	100.0
Chronic myeloid	0	0	2	1	3	0.4	0.3	1.4	100.0
Other and unspecified	0	7	7	8	22	2.7	2.7	10.0	86.4
II. LYMPHOMAS	0	56	67	58	181	22.2	22.1	100.0	100.0
Hodgkin's disease	0	5	22	25	52	6.4	6.0	28.7	100.0
Non-Hodgkin lymphoma	0	8	15	14	37	4.5	4.4	20.4	100.0
Burkitt's lymphoma	0	36	23	5	64	7.8	8.5	35.4	100.0
Unspecified lymphoma	0	6	7	13	26	3.2	3.1	14.4	100.0
Histiocytosis X	0	0	0	0	0	-	-	-	-
Other reticuloendothelial	0	1	0	1	2	0.2	0.2	1.1	100.0
III. BRAIN AND SPINAL	1	15	36	32	84	10.3	10.0	100.0	98.8
Ependymoma	0	1	4	1	6	0.7	0.7	7.1	100.0
Astrocytoma	1	6	19	20	46	5.6	5.4	54.8	100.0
Medulloblastoma	0	4	9	8	21	2.6	2.5	25.0	100.0
Other glioma	0	1	2	1	4	0.5	0.5	4.8	100.0
Other and unspecified *	0	3	2	2	7	0.9	0.9	8.3	85.7
IV. SYMPATHETIC N.S.	5	22	12	10	49	6.0	6.4	100.0	100.0
Neuroblastoma	5	22	12	10	49	6.0	6.4	100.0	100.0
Other	0	0	0	0	0	-	-	-	-
V. RETINOBLASTOMA	3	35	8	0	47¤	5.8	6.4	100.0	100.0
VI. KIDNEY	7	30	7	4	48	5.9	6.6	100.0	100.0
Wilms' tumour	6	29	7	3	45	5.5	6.2	93.8	100.0
Renal carcinoma	1	1	0	1	3	0.4	0.4	6.3	100.0
Other and unspecified	0	0	0	0	0	-	-	-	-
VII. LIVER	2	2	0	1	5	0.6	0.7	100.0	100.0
Hepatoblastoma	0	1	0	0	1	0.1	0.1	20.0	100.0
Hepatic carcinoma	2	1	0	1	4	0.5	0.5	80.0	100.0
Other and unspecified	0	0	0	0	0	-	-	-	-
VIII. BONE	1	1	11	35	48	5.9	5.3	100.0	100.0
Osteosarcoma	0	0	4	20	24	2.9	2.6	50.0	100.0
Chondrosarcoma	0	0	0	2	2	0.2	0.2	4.2	100.0
Ewing's sarcoma	0	1	6	9	16	2.0	1.8	33.3	100.0
Other and unspecified	1	0	1	4	6	0.7	0.7	12.5	100.0
IX. SOFT TISSUE SARCOMAS	2	11	17	11	41	5.0	5.1	100.0	100.0
Rhabdomyosarcoma	1	8	9	3	21	2.6	2.7	51.2	100.0
Fibrosarcoma	1	0	6	2	9	1.1	1.1	22.0	100.0
Other and unspecified	0	3	2	6	11	1.3	1.3	26.8	100.0
X. GONADAL & GERM CELL	4	13	7	21	45	5.5	5.5	100.0	100.0
Non-gonadal germ cell	4	11	3	3	21	2.6	2.8	46.7	100.0
Gonadal germ cell	0	2	3	17	22	2.7	2.4	48.9	100.0
Gonadal carcinoma	0	0	1	1	2	0.2	0.2	4.4	100.0
Other and unspecified	0	0	0	0	0	-	-	-	-
XI. EPITHELIAL NEOPLASMS	0	1	10	28	39	4.8	4.3	100.0	100.0
Adrenocortical carcinoma	0	0	0	0	0	-	-	-	-
Thyroid carcinoma	0	0	2	6	8	1.0	0.9	20.5	100.0
Nasopharyngeal carcinoma	0	0	0	4	4	0.5	0.4	10.3	100.0
Melanoma	0	0	0	4	4	0.5	0.4	10.3	100.0
Other carcinoma	0	1	8	14	23	2.8	2.6	59.0	100.0
XII. OTHER	0	2	4	3	9	1.1	1.1	100.0	37.5
	0	3	2	2	7	0.9	0.9	100.0	85.7

* Specified as malignant
¤ Includes age unknown

ISRAEL

Israel Cancer Registry, 1970-1979

L. Katz & R. Steinitz

The Israel Cancer Registry (ICR) was set up in January 1960 by the Ministry of Health to undertake incidence and mortality studies in various population groups, as a tool for planning and evaluation of services and as an aid to research workers. Since 1973, it has been linked by contract to the SEER Program of the National Cancer Institute of the National Institutes of Health of the United States. Registration aims at complete coverage of incidence in the whole of Israel. Non-resident cancer patients coming to the attention of the Israeli medical services, such as tourists and a large number of inhabitants of the Israel Administered Territories, are also registered. Special codes differentiate these from the resident population.

Until 1982, reporting was partly compulsory (to medical record personnel pursuant to an administrative order) and partly voluntary (e.g., from pathology institutes). In 1982, an amendment to the Public Health Ordinance made all reporting compulsory, thus forestalling objections to reporting for reasons of confidentiality.

Rather than rely on special notification forms, the ICR utilizes existing records as far as possible. Copies of pathology reports, hospital case summaries (first and subsequent) and death certificates are the main sources of information, supplemented by notifications from oncological centres and chest clinics, and the monthly diagnostic list of deaths obtained from the Central Bureau of Statistics. This multiple-source intake increases completeness of coverage and quality of information, but a constant look-out for possible duplicate registrations is necessary.

Data are processed manually in batches, coded and entered on disks containing the 'active file' (cases not known to be dead by a certain cut-off date) with the help of a minicomputer. The master file is kept on magnetic tape and a mainframe computer used for periodic updating and the production of case listings.

Medical information is checked and coded by the physicians on the Registry staff, the code being a modification of ICD-O. The Registry includes benign and unspecified tumours of the CNS and some other non-malignant tumours, but registration of squamous-cell and basal-cell cancers of the skin was discontinued from 1967.

For computing incidence rates, particular care is taken to verify residency status in order to exclude non-residents and immigrants diagnosed prior to immigration. Cancer cases in inhabitants of the occupied territories are reported by Israeli hospitals only, and reporting is therefore incomplete.

Over 90% of Israel's population is covered by prepaid medical insurance. Most hospitals are publicly owned and are accessible to the insured. Standards of medical practice are high and medical records are adequate. In 1982 there were 2.92 general hospital beds per 1000 population. The best estimate for the number of physicians is 11 394 in 1980. There are facilities for paediatric oncology in the major oncology centres.

The population of Israel comprises approximately 3 373 000 Jews and 690 000 non-Jews (mainly Moslem and Christian Arabs). The Jewish population consists of those born in the country and of immigrants from about 70 countries.

The total area covered is 20 700 square kilometres, and the altitude varies from 397 m below to 1208 m above sea level.

An account of childhood cancer incidence in Israel during 1961-1965 was published by Virag and Modan (1969) and incidence rates for leukaemia and non-Hodgkin lymphoma have been estimated for the Jewish and Arab populations from a clinical survey covering the years 1976-1981 (Ramot *et al.*, 1984). The present volume gives incidence separately for Jews and non-Jews.

Contd p. 180

Israel, Jews

1970 - 1979

MALE

DIAGNOSTIC GROUP	NUMBER OF CASES 0	1-4	5-9	10-14	All	REL. FREQUENCY(%) Crude	Adj.	Group	RATES PER MILLION 0	1-4	5-9	10-14	Crude	Adj.	Cum	HV(%)
TOTAL	75	247	197	145	664	100.0	100.0	100.0	214.5	185.1	134.4	108.7	148.1	148.8	2170	93.7
I. LEUKAEMIAS	14	73	48	32	167	25.2	24.7	100.0	40.0	54.7	32.8	24.0	37.2	37.6	543	99.4
Acute lymphocytic	3	43	32	16	94	14.2	13.9	56.3	8.6	32.2	21.8	12.0	21.0	21.2	307	98.9
Other lymphocytic	0	1	1	0	2	0.3	0.3	1.2	–	–	0.7	–	0.4	0.5	6	100.0
Acute non-lymphocytic	7	15	10	12	44	6.6	6.7	26.3	20.0	11.2	6.8	9.0	9.8	9.8	144	100.0
Chronic myeloid	0	0	2	1	3	0.5	0.5	1.8	–	–	–	0.7	0.7	0.7	10	100.0
Other and unspecified	4	12	5	3	24	3.6	3.4	14.4	11.4	9.0	3.4	2.2	5.4	5.4	76	100.0
II. LYMPHOMAS	8	54	61	38	161	24.2	24.9	100.0	22.9	40.5	41.6	28.5	35.9	36.0	535	96.3
Hodgkin's disease	0	9	17	13	39	5.9	6.4	24.2	–	6.7	11.6	9.7	8.7	8.7	134	97.4
Non-Hodgkin lymphoma	1	27	35	12	75	11.3	11.3	46.6	2.9	20.2	23.9	9.0	16.7	16.8	248	100.0
Burkitt's lymphoma	1	13	5	6	25	3.8	3.7	15.5	2.9	9.7	3.4	4.5	5.6	5.6	81	100.0
Unspecified lymphoma	5	2	3	6	16	2.4	2.6	9.9	14.3	1.5	2.0	4.5	3.6	3.5	53	68.8
Histiocytosis X	0	2	1	0	3	0.5	0.4	1.9	–	1.5	–	–	0.7	0.7	10	100.0
Other reticuloendothelial	1	1	0	1	3	0.5	0.4	1.9	2.9	0.7	0.7	0.7	0.7	0.7	9	100.0
III. BRAIN AND SPINAL	8	38	41	25	112	16.9	17.1	100.0	22.9	28.5	28.0	18.7	25.0	25.1	370	75.9
Ependymoma	2	4	3	2	11	1.7	1.6	9.8	5.7	3.0	2.0	1.5	2.5	2.5	35	100.0
Astrocytoma	1	12	12	9	34	5.1	5.3	30.4	2.9	9.0	8.2	6.7	7.6	7.6	113	97.1
Medulloblastoma	2	11	9	4	26	3.9	3.8	23.2	5.7	8.2	6.1	3.0	5.8	5.8	84	96.2
Other glioma	0	2	2	4	8	1.2	1.4	7.1	–	1.5	1.4	3.0	1.8	1.8	28	100.0
Other and unspecified *	3	9	15	6	33	5.0	5.0	29.5	8.6	6.7	10.2	4.5	7.4	7.4	109	24.2
IV. SYMPATHETIC N.S.	22	28	11	5	66	9.9	8.9	100.0	62.9	21.0	7.5	3.7	14.7	14.9	203	100.0
Neuroblastoma	22	27	11	5	65	9.8	8.8	98.5	62.9	20.2	7.5	3.7	14.5	14.6	200	100.0
Other					1	0.2	0.1	1.5	–	0.7	–	–	0.2	0.2	3	100.0
V. RETINOBLASTOMA	2	9	1	0	12	1.8	1.5	100.0	5.7	6.7	0.7	–	2.7	2.8	36	75.0
VI. KIDNEY	6	17	3	1	27	4.1	3.5	100.0	17.2	12.7	2.0	0.7	6.0	6.2	82	100.0
Wilms' tumour	6	17	3	1	27	4.1	3.5	100.0	17.2	12.7	2.0	0.7	6.0	6.2	82	100.0
Renal carcinoma	0	0	0	0	0	–	–	–	–	–	–	–	–	–	–	–
Other and unspecified	0	0	0	0	0	–	–	–	–	–	–	–	–	–	–	–
VII. LIVER	1	1	0	1	3	0.5	0.5	100.0	2.9	0.7	–	0.7	0.7	0.7	10	–
Hepatoblastoma	1	1	0	0	2	0.3	0.2	66.7	2.9	0.7	–	–	0.4	0.5	6	100.0
Hepatic carcinoma	0	0	0	1	1	0.2	0.2	33.3	–	–	–	0.7	0.2	0.2	4	100.0
Other and unspecified	0	0	0	0	0	–	–	–	–	–	–	–	–	–	–	–
VIII. BONE	2	1	11	15	29	4.4	5.2	100.0	5.7	0.7	7.5	11.2	6.5	6.4	102	96.6
Osteosarcoma	0	0	5	10	15	2.3	2.8	51.7	–	–	3.4	7.5	3.3	3.3	55	100.0
Chondrosarcoma	0	0	0	0	0	–	–	–	–	–	–	–	–	–	–	–
Ewing's sarcoma	0	1	6	3	10	1.5	1.7	34.5	–	0.7	4.1	2.2	2.2	2.2	35	100.0
Other and unspecified	2	0	0	2	4	0.6	0.7	13.8	5.7	–	–	1.5	0.9	0.9	13	75.0
IX. SOFT TISSUE SARCOMAS	3	13	16	13	45	6.8	7.1	100.0	8.6	9.7	10.9	9.7	10.0	10.0	151	100.0
Rhabdomyosarcoma	3	8	6	5	20	3.0	3.1	44.4	8.6	6.0	4.1	3.7	4.5	4.5	66	100.0
Fibrosarcoma	2	1	1	1	5	0.8	0.7	11.1	5.7	0.7	0.7	0.7	1.1	1.1	16	100.0
Other and unspecified	0	4	9	7	20	3.0	3.3	44.4	–	3.0	6.1	5.2	4.5	4.4	69	100.0
X. GONADAL & GERM CELL	5	7	2	1	15	2.3	2.0	100.0	14.3	5.2	1.4	0.7	3.3	3.4	46	93.3
Non-gonadal germ cell	1	0	0	1	2	0.3	0.3	13.3	2.9	–	–	0.7	0.4	0.4	7	100.0
Gonadal germ cell	3	7	2	0	12	1.8	1.5	80.0	8.6	5.2	1.4	–	2.7	2.7	36	100.0
Gonadal carcinoma	0	0	0	0	0	–	–	–	–	–	–	–	–	–	–	–
Other and unspecified	1	0	0	0	1	0.2	0.1	6.7	2.9	–	–	–	0.2	0.2	3	–
XI. EPITHELIAL NEOPLASMS	2	3	3	12	20	3.0	3.6	100.0	5.7	2.2	2.0	9.0	4.5	4.4	70	100.0
Adrenocortical carcinoma	0	0	0	0	0	–	–	–	–	–	–	–	–	–	–	–
Thyroid carcinoma	0	0	1	2	3	0.5	0.6	15.0	–	–	0.7	1.5	0.7	0.7	11	100.0
Nasopharyngeal carcinoma	0	0	0	3	3	0.5	0.6	15.0	–	–	–	2.2	0.7	0.7	11	100.0
Melanoma	2	2	2	4	8	1.2	1.3	40.0	5.7	1.5	–	3.0	1.8	1.8	27	100.0
Other carcinoma	0	1	2	3	6	0.9	1.0	30.0	–	0.7	1.4	2.2	1.3	1.3	21	100.0
XII. OTHER	2	3	0	2	7	1.1	1.0	100.0	5.7	2.2	–	1.5	1.6	1.6	22	57.1
* Specified as malignant	1	4	10	2	17	2.6	2.6		2.9	3.0	6.8	1.5	3.8	3.8	56	29.4

Israel, Jews

1970 - 1979

FEMALE

DIAGNOSTIC GROUP	NUMBER OF CASES					REL. FREQUENCY(%)			RATES PER MILLION							HV(%)
	0	1-4	5-9	10-14	All	Crude	Adj.	Group	0	1-4	5-9	10-14	Crude	Adj.	Cum	
TOTAL	61	194	125	123	503	100.0	100.0	100.0	184.0	153.1	89.8	97.2	118.2	118.9	1732	91.3
I. LEUKAEMIAS	11	55	26	24	116	23.1	22.4	100.0	33.2	43.4	18.7	19.0	27.3	27.5	395	99.1
Acute lymphocytic	5	47	16	16	84	16.7	15.9	72.4	15.1	37.1	11.5	12.6	19.7	20.0	284	98.8
Other lymphocytic	-	-	-	-	0	-	-	-	-	-	-	-	-	-	-	-
Acute non-lymphocytic	2	2	5	5	14	2.8	3.0	12.1	6.0	1.6	3.6	3.9	3.3	3.3	50	100.0
Chronic myeloid	-	2	3	0	5	1.0	1.0	4.3	-	1.6	2.2	-	1.2	1.2	17	100.0
Other and unspecified	4	4	2	3	13	2.6	2.5	11.2	12.1	3.2	1.4	2.4	3.1	3.1	44	100.0
II. LYMPHOMAS	3	35	16	24	78	15.5	15.7	100.0	9.1	27.6	11.5	19.0	18.3	18.5	272	98.7
Hodgkin's disease	1	3	6	16	26	5.2	6.0	33.3	3.0	2.4	4.3	12.6	6.1	6.0	97	96.2
Non-Hodgkin lymphoma	-	14	7	4	25	5.0	4.9	32.1	-	11.1	5.0	3.2	5.9	6.0	85	100.0
Burkitt's lymphoma	-	8	0	3	11	2.2	2.0	14.1	-	6.3	-	2.4	2.6	2.1	37	100.0
Unspecified lymphoma	1	5	2	1	9	1.8	1.7	11.5	3.0	3.9	1.4	0.8	2.1	2.1	30	100.0
Histiocytosis X	-	2	-	-	2	0.4	0.3	2.6	-	1.6	-	-	0.5	0.5	6	100.0
Other reticuloendothelial	1	3	1	-	5	1.0	0.9	6.4	3.0	2.4	0.7	-	1.2	1.2	16	100.0
III. BRAIN AND SPINAL	3	32	40	21	96	19.1	20.2	100.0	9.1	25.3	28.7	16.6	22.6	22.6	337	68.8
Ependymoma	1	4	1	1	7	1.4	1.3	7.3	3.0	3.2	0.7	0.8	1.6	1.7	23	100.0
Astrocytoma	1	9	17	9	36	7.2	7.8	37.5	3.0	7.1	12.2	7.1	8.5	8.4	128	83.3
Medulloblastoma	-	10	10	3	23	4.6	4.7	24.0	-	7.9	7.2	2.4	5.4	5.5	79	100.0
Other glioma	-	-	1	1	2	0.4	0.5	2.1	-	-	0.7	0.8	0.5	0.5	8	100.0
Other and unspecified *	1	9	11	7	28	5.6	5.9	29.2	3.0	7.1	7.9	5.5	6.6	6.6	99	14.3
IV. SYMPATHETIC N.S.	19	18	6	2	45	8.9	7.7	100.0	57.3	14.2	4.3	1.6	10.6	10.7	144	100.0
Neuroblastoma	19	17	6	2	44	8.7	7.6	97.8	57.3	13.4	4.3	1.6	10.3	10.4	140	100.0
Other	-	1	-	-	1	0.2	0.2	2.2	-	0.8	-	-	0.2	0.2	3	100.0
V. RETINOBLASTOMA	5	9	-	-	14	2.8	2.8	100.0	15.1	7.1	-	-	3.3	3.4	44	100.0
VI. KIDNEY	7	17	9	2	35	7.0	6.4	100.0	21.1	13.4	6.5	1.6	8.2	8.3	115	97.1
Wilms' tumour	7	17	7	-	31	6.2	5.4	88.6	21.1	13.4	5.0	-	7.3	7.4	100	96.8
Renal carcinoma	-	-	-	-	0	-	-	-	-	-	-	-	-	-	-	-
Other and unspecified	-	-	2	2	4	0.8	1.0	11.4	-	-	1.4	1.6	0.9	0.9	15	100.0
VII. LIVER	1	1	1	-	3	0.6	0.6	100.0	3.0	0.8	0.7	-	0.7	0.7	10	66.7
Hepatoblastoma	1	1	-	-	2	0.4	0.4	66.7	3.0	0.8	-	-	0.5	0.5	7	100.0
Hepatic carcinoma	-	-	1	-	1	0.2	0.2	33.3	-	-	0.7	-	0.2	0.2	3	100.0
Other and unspecified	-	-	-	-	0	-	-	-	-	-	-	-	-	-	-	-
VIII. BONE	1	4	8	12	25	5.0	5.6	100.0	3.0	3.2	5.7	9.5	5.9	5.8	92	96.0
Osteosarcoma	-	1	5	5	11	2.2	2.5	44.0	-	0.8	3.6	3.9	2.6	2.6	40	100.0
Chondrosarcoma	-	-	-	2	2	0.4	0.4	8.0	-	-	-	1.6	0.5	0.5	7	100.0
Ewing's sarcoma	-	-	3	5	8	1.6	1.9	32.0	-	-	2.2	3.9	1.9	1.8	31	75.0
Other and unspecified	1	3	-	-	4	0.8	0.8	16.0	3.0	2.4	-	-	0.9	0.9	14	100.0
IX. SOFT TISSUE SARCOMAS	4	12	10	8	34	6.8	6.9	100.0	12.1	9.5	7.2	6.3	8.0	8.0	117	97.1
Rhabdomyosarcoma	2	7	1	1	11	2.2	2.1	32.4	6.0	5.5	0.7	0.8	2.6	2.6	37	100.0
Fibrosarcoma	1	3	6	5	15	3.0	3.1	44.1	3.0	2.4	4.3	3.9	3.5	3.5	52	93.3
Other and unspecified	1	2	3	2	8	1.6	1.7	23.5	3.0	1.6	2.2	1.6	1.9	1.9	28	100.0
X. GONADAL & GERM CELL	2	4	3	8	17	3.4	3.6	100.0	6.0	3.2	2.2	6.3	4.0	4.0	61	88.2
Non-gonadal germ cell	2	4	-	1	7	1.4	1.2	41.2	6.0	3.2	-	0.8	1.6	1.7	23	85.7
Gonadal germ cell	-	-	2	6	8	1.6	1.9	47.1	-	-	1.4	4.7	1.9	1.8	31	93.3
Gonadal carcinoma	-	-	1	-	1	0.2	0.2	5.9	-	-	0.7	-	0.2	0.2	4	100.0
Other and unspecified	-	-	-	1	1	0.2	0.2	5.9	-	-	-	0.8	0.2	0.2	4	-
XI. EPITHELIAL NEOPLASMS	1	6	5	18	30	6.0	6.7	100.0	3.0	4.7	3.6	14.2	7.0	7.0	111	100.0
Adrenocortical carcinoma	-	1	-	-	1	0.2	0.2	3.3	-	0.8	-	-	0.2	0.2	3	100.0
Thyroid carcinoma	-	-	-	8	8	1.6	2.0	26.7	-	-	-	6.3	1.9	1.9	32	100.0
Nasopharyngeal carcinoma	-	-	-	2	2	0.4	0.5	6.7	-	-	-	1.6	0.5	0.5	8	100.0
Melanoma	1	4	1	2	8	1.6	1.6	26.7	3.0	3.2	0.7	1.6	1.9	1.9	28	100.0
Other carcinoma	-	1	4	6	11	2.2	2.5	36.7	-	0.8	2.9	4.7	2.6	2.6	40	100.0
XII. OTHER	4	1	1	4	10	2.0	2.0	100.0	12.1	0.8	0.7	3.2	2.3	2.3	35	40.0
* Specified as malignant	-	5	2	5	12	2.4	2.5	-	-	3.9	1.4	3.9	2.8	2.8	43	25.0

ISRAEL

Israel, non Jews

1970 - 1979   MALE

	NUMBER OF CASES					REL. FREQUENCY(%)			RATES PER MILLION							HV(%)
DIAGNOSTIC GROUP	0	1-4	5-9	10-14	All	Crude	Adj.	Group	0	1-4	5-9	10-14	Crude	Adj.	Cum	
TOTAL	15	77	38	32	162	100.0	100.0	100.0	135.3	188.1	85.4	85.5	120.9	121.1	1742	90.7
I. LEUKAEMIAS	2	23	13	7	45	27.8	27.7	100.0	18.0	56.2	29.2	18.7	33.6	33.7	482	100.0
Acute lymphocytic	0	12	8	3	23	14.2	14.3	51.1	-	29.3	18.0	8.0	17.2	17.2	247	100.0
Other lymphocytic	1	0	0	1	2	1.2	1.4	4.4	9.0	-	-	2.7	1.5	1.5	22	100.0
Acute non-lymphocytic	0	6	3	2	11	6.8	6.9	24.4	-	14.7	6.7	5.3	8.2	8.3	119	100.0
Chronic myeloid	0	1	0	0	1	0.6	0.4	2.2	-	2.4	-	-	0.7	0.8	10	100.0
Other and unspecified	1	4	2	1	8	4.9	4.7	17.8	9.0	9.8	4.5	2.7	6.0	6.0	84	100.0
II. LYMPHOMAS	3	29	18	7	57	35.2	34.7	100.0	27.1	70.8	40.5	18.7	42.6	42.5	606	94.7
Hodgkin's disease	1	5	6	3	15	9.3	10.2	26.3	9.0	12.2	13.5	8.0	11.2	11.2	165	100.0
Non-Hodgkin lymphoma	0	10	9	4	23	14.2	15.2	40.4	-	24.4	20.2	10.7	17.2	17.2	252	100.0
Burkitt's lymphoma	0	10	2	0	12	7.4	5.9	21.1	-	24.4	4.5	-	9.0	9.0	120	100.0
Unspecified lymphoma	2	4	0	0	6	3.7	2.6	10.5	18.0	9.8	-	-	4.5	4.4	57	50.0
Histiocytosis X	0	0	0	0	0	-	-	-	-	-	-	-	-	-	-	-
Other reticuloendothelial	0	0	1	0	1	0.6	0.8	1.8	-	-	2.2	-	0.7	0.7	11	100.0
III. BRAIN AND SPINAL	1	4	5	10	20	12.3	15.5	100.0	9.0	9.8	11.2	26.7	14.9	15.1	238	60.0
Ependymoma	0	1	0	2	3	1.9	2.7	15.0	-	2.4	-	5.3	2.2	2.3	36	100.0
Astrocytoma	0	0	1	2	3	1.9	2.7	15.0	-	-	2.2	5.3	2.2	2.3	38	100.0
Medulloblastoma	0	1	3	2	6	3.7	4.7	30.0	-	2.4	6.7	5.3	4.5	4.5	70	100.0
Other glioma	0	0	0	0	0	-	-	-	-	-	-	-	-	-	-	-
Other and unspecified *	1	2	1	4	8	4.9	5.8	40.0	9.0	4.9	2.2	10.7	6.0	6.0	93	-
IV. SYMPATHETIC N.S.	3	10	0	0	13	8.0	5.7	100.0	27.1	24.4	-	-	9.7	9.7	125	100.0
Neuroblastoma	3	10	0	0	13	8.0	5.7	100.0	27.1	24.4	-	-	9.7	9.7	125	100.0
Other	0	0	0	0	0	-	-	-	-	-	-	-	-	-	-	-
V. RETINOBLASTOMA	2	2	1	0	5	3.1	2.5	100.0	18.0	4.9	2.2	-	3.7	3.6	49	100.0
VI. KIDNEY	1	5	0	0	6	3.7	2.6	100.0	9.0	12.2	-	-	4.5	4.5	58	83.3
Wilms' tumour	1	5	0	0	6	3.7	2.6	100.0	9.0	12.2	-	-	4.5	4.5	58	83.3
Renal carcinoma	0	0	0	0	0	-	-	-	-	-	-	-	-	-	-	-
Other and unspecified	0	0	0	0	0	-	-	-	-	-	-	-	-	-	-	-
VII. LIVER	0	0	0	0	0	-	-	-	-	-	-	-	-	-	-	-
Hepatoblastoma	0	0	0	0	0	-	-	-	-	-	-	-	-	-	-	-
Hepatic carcinoma	0	0	0	0	0	-	-	-	-	-	-	-	-	-	-	-
Other and unspecified	0	0	0	0	0	-	-	-	-	-	-	-	-	-	-	-
VIII. BONE	1	0	0	2	3	1.9	2.3	100.0	9.0	-	-	5.3	2.2	2.2	36	100.0
Osteosarcoma	0	0	0	2	2	1.2	1.9	66.7	-	-	-	5.3	1.5	1.6	27	100.0
Chondrosarcoma	0	0	0	0	0	-	-	-	-	-	-	-	-	-	-	-
Ewing's sarcoma	0	0	0	0	0	-	-	-	-	-	-	-	-	-	-	-
Other and unspecified	1	0	0	0	1	0.6	0.4	33.3	9.0	-	-	-	0.7	0.7	9	100.0
IX. SOFT TISSUE SARCOMAS	0	3	0	2	5	3.1	3.2	100.0	-	7.3	-	5.3	3.7	3.8	56	100.0
Rhabdomyosarcoma	0	0	0	1	1	0.6	0.9	20.0	-	-	-	2.7	0.7	0.9	13	100.0
Fibrosarcoma	0	1	0	0	1	0.6	0.8	20.0	-	2.4	-	-	0.7	0.8	10	100.0
Other and unspecified	0	2	0	1	3	1.9	1.8	60.0	-	4.9	-	2.7	2.2	2.3	33	100.0
X. GONADAL & GERM CELL	1	1	0	0	2	1.2	0.9	100.0	9.0	2.4	-	-	1.5	1.5	19	50.0
Non-gonadal germ cell	1	0	0	0	1	0.6	0.4	50.0	9.0	-	-	-	0.7	0.7	9	100.0
Gonadal germ cell	0	1	0	0	1	0.6	0.4	50.0	-	2.4	-	-	0.7	0.8	10	-
Gonadal carcinoma	0	0	0	0	0	-	-	-	-	-	-	-	-	-	-	-
Other and unspecified	0	0	0	0	0	-	-	-	-	-	-	-	-	-	-	-
XI. EPITHELIAL NEOPLASMS	0	0	0	4	4	2.5	3.8	100.0	-	-	-	10.7	3.0	3.1	53	100.0
Adrenocortical carcinoma	0	0	0	0	0	-	-	-	-	-	-	-	-	-	-	-
Thyroid carcinoma	0	0	0	3	3	1.9	2.8	75.0	-	-	-	8.0	2.2	2.3	40	100.0
Nasopharyngeal carcinoma	0	0	0	1	1	0.6	0.9	25.0	-	-	-	2.7	0.7	0.8	13	100.0
Melanoma	0	0	0	0	0	-	-	-	-	-	-	-	-	-	-	-
Other carcinoma	0	0	0	0	0	-	-	-	-	-	-	-	-	-	-	-
XII. OTHER	1	0	1	0	2	1.2	1.2	100.0	9.0	-	2.2	-	1.5	1.4	20	-

* Specified as malignant

Israel, non Jews

1970 - 1979 FEMALE

DIAGNOSTIC GROUP	NUMBER OF CASES					REL. FREQUENCY(%)			RATES PER MILLION						Cum	HV(%)
	0	1-4	5-9	10-14	All	Crude	Adj.	Group	0	1-4	5-9	10-14	Crude	Adj.		
TOTAL	20	38	18	22	98	100.0	100.0	100.0	189.4	100.4	43.3	63.5	78.6	78.2	1125	87.4
I. LEUKAEMIAS	4	9	7	2	22	22.4	23.4	100.0	37.9	23.8	16.8	5.8	17.7	17.4	246	95.2
Acute lymphocytic	2	7	3	2	14	14.3	13.9	63.6	18.9	18.5	7.2	5.8	11.2	11.2	158	100.0
Other lymphocytic	1	0	0	0	1	1.0	0.7	4.5	9.5	-	-	-	0.8	0.7	9	-
Acute non-lymphocytic	1	0	1	0	2	2.0	2.4	9.1	9.5	-	2.4	-	1.6	1.5	21	100.0
Chronic myeloid	0	1	0	0	1	1.0	0.7	4.5	-	2.6	-	-	0.8	0.8	11	100.0
Other and unspecified	0	1	3	0	4	4.1	5.7	18.2	-	2.6	7.2	-	3.2	3.1	47	75.0
II. LYMPHOMAS	1	7	2	6	16	16.3	17.0	100.0	9.5	18.5	4.8	17.3	12.8	13.0	194	100.0
Hodgkin's disease	0	2	1	4	7	7.1	8.5	43.8	-	5.3	2.4	11.6	5.6	5.8	91	100.0
Non-Hodgkin lymphoma	0	1	0	2	3	3.1	3.4	18.8	-	2.6	-	5.8	2.4	2.5	39	100.0
Burkitt's lymphoma	1	4	0	0	5	5.1	3.4	31.3	9.5	10.6	-	-	4.0	4.0	52	100.0
Unspecified lymphoma	0	0	1	0	1	1.0	1.7	6.3	-	-	2.4	-	0.8	0.8	12	100.0
Histiocytosis X	0	0	0	0	0	-	-	-	-	-	-	-	-	-	-	-
Other reticuloendothelial	0	0	0	0	0	-	-	-	-	-	-	-	-	-	-	-
III. BRAIN AND SPINAL	4	7	5	7	23	23.5	25.5	100.0	37.9	18.5	12.0	20.2	18.5	18.4	273	72.7
Ependymoma	1	2	0	1	4	4.1	3.4	17.4	9.5	5.3	-	2.9	3.2	3.2	45	100.0
Astrocytoma	0	2	4	1	7	7.1	9.4	30.4	-	5.3	9.6	2.9	5.6	5.6	84	100.0
Medulloblastoma	0	1	1	1	3	3.1	3.7	13.0	-	2.6	2.4	2.9	2.4	2.4	37	100.0
Other glioma	0	0	0	1	1	1.0	1.4	4.3	-	-	-	2.9	0.8	0.8	14	100.0
Other and unspecified *	3	2	0	3	8	8.2	7.5	34.8	28.4	5.3	-	8.7	6.4	6.4	93	14.3
IV. SYMPATHETIC N.S.	4	3	1	1	9	9.2	7.9	100.0	37.9	7.9	2.4	2.9	7.2	7.0	96	100.0
Neuroblastoma	4	3	1	1	9	9.2	7.9	100.0	37.9	7.9	2.4	2.9	7.2	7.0	96	100.0
Other	0	0	0	0	0	-	-	-	-	-	-	-	-	-	-	-
V. RETINOBLASTOMA	1	3	0	0	4	4.1	2.8	100.0	9.5	7.9	-	-	3.2	3.2	41	100.0
VI. KIDNEY	3	2	0	1	6	6.1	4.8	100.0	28.4	5.3	-	2.9	4.8	4.7	64	83.3
Wilms' tumour	3	2	0	1	6	6.1	4.8	100.0	28.4	5.3	-	2.9	4.8	4.7	64	83.3
Renal carcinoma	0	0	0	0	0	-	-	-	-	-	-	-	-	-	-	-
Other and unspecified	0	0	0	0	0	-	-	-	-	-	-	-	-	-	-	-
VII. LIVER	0	0	0	0	0	-	-	-	-	-	-	-	-	-	-	-
Hepatoblastoma	0	0	0	0	0	-	-	-	-	-	-	-	-	-	-	-
Hepatic carcinoma	0	0	0	0	0	-	-	-	-	-	-	-	-	-	-	-
Other and unspecified	0	0	0	0	0	-	-	-	-	-	-	-	-	-	-	-
VIII. BONE	1	2	1	3	7	7.1	7.8	100.0	9.5	5.3	2.4	8.7	5.6	5.7	86	71.4
Osteosarcoma	0	1	1	1	3	3.1	3.7	42.9	-	2.6	2.4	2.9	2.4	2.4	37	100.0
Chondrosarcoma	0	0	0	0	0	-	-	-	-	-	-	-	-	-	-	-
Ewing's sarcoma	0	1	0	1	2	2.0	2.1	28.6	-	2.6	-	2.9	1.6	1.7	25	100.0
Other and unspecified	1	0	0	1	2	2.0	2.1	28.6	9.5	-	-	2.9	1.6	1.6	24	-
IX. SOFT TISSUE SARCOMAS	0	4	1	1	6	6.1	5.8	100.0	-	10.6	2.4	2.9	4.8	4.9	69	100.0
Rhabdomyosarcoma	0	3	0	0	3	3.1	2.1	50.0	-	7.9	-	-	2.4	2.5	32	100.0
Fibrosarcoma	0	0	0	0	0	-	-	-	-	-	-	-	-	-	-	-
Other and unspecified	0	1	1	1	3	3.1	3.7	50.0	-	2.6	2.4	2.9	2.4	2.4	37	100.0
X. GONADAL & GERM CELL	0	1	0	0	1	1.0	0.7	100.0	-	2.6	-	-	0.8	0.8	11	100.0
Non-gonadal germ cell	0	1	0	0	1	1.0	0.7	100.0	-	2.6	-	-	0.8	0.8	11	100.0
Gonadal germ cell	0	0	0	0	0	-	-	-	-	-	-	-	-	-	-	-
Gonadal carcinoma	0	0	0	0	0	-	-	-	-	-	-	-	-	-	-	-
Other and unspecified	0	0	0	0	0	-	-	-	-	-	-	-	-	-	-	-
XI. EPITHELIAL NEOPLASMS	0	0	0	1	1	1.0	1.4	100.0	-	-	-	2.9	0.8	0.8	14	100.0
Adrenocortical carcinoma	0	0	0	0	0	-	-	-	-	-	-	-	-	-	-	-
Thyroid carcinoma	0	0	0	0	0	-	-	-	-	-	-	-	-	-	-	-
Nasopharyngeal carcinoma	0	0	0	0	0	-	-	-	-	-	-	-	-	-	-	-
Melanoma	0	0	0	0	0	-	-	-	-	-	-	-	-	-	-	-
Other carcinoma	0	0	0	1	1	1.0	1.4	100.0	-	-	-	2.9	0.8	0.8	14	100.0
XII. OTHER	2	0	1	0	3	3.1	3.0	100.0	18.9	-	2.4	-	2.4	2.2	31	33.3
* Specified as malignant	1	0	0	2	3	3.1	3.4	100.0	9.5	-	-	5.8	2.4	2.4	38	-

Population

The average population at risk for Jewish and non-Jewish residents has been calculated from annual estimates provided by the Population, Demography and Health Division of the Central Bureau of Statistics.

AVERAGE ANNUAL POPULATION: 1970–1979

Age	Male	Female
Jews		
0	34962	33143
1–4	133443	126684
5–9	146540	139147
10–14	133445	126590
0–14	448390	425564
Non-Jews		
0	11084	10562
1–4	40932	37864
5–9	44491	41558
10–14	37437	34619
0–14	133944	124603

Commentary

The ratios of the total incidence rates for Jews and non-Jews are 1.23:1 for males and 1.52:1 for females. The rates for lymphomas and retinoblastoma among Jews and non-Jews are similar, but for all other major diagnostic groups the rate is higher for Jews. Apart from liver tumours, of which no cases were registered among non-Jews, the greatest difference was in gonadal and germ-cell tumours, which were three times as common in Jews as in non-Jews.

The overall incidence rates presented here are broadly similar to those given by Virag and Modan for 1961–1965 for children aged under 10, but show a drop of about a third for those aged 10–14. This decline in incidence rates in the oldest age-group is concentrated among the leukaemias and brain/spinal tumours. There was also a less marked reduction in the incidence of leukaemia in the 5–9 age-group. In consequence, the rates of leukaemia during 1970–1979 exhibit the peak in the 1–4 age-group commonly observed in Western populations and reported in Israeli Jews in 1976–1981 (Ramot *et al.*, 1984) but not in the earlier series from 1961 to 1965. The emergence of this peak thus seems to be due to a reduction in incidence in older children rather than an increase in the younger age-groups. The peak is present for both Jews and non-Jews.

References

Ramot, B., Ben-Bassat, J., Brecher, A., Zaizov, R. & Modan, M. (1984) The epidemiology of childhood acute lymphoblastic leukaemia and non-Hodgkin's lymphoma in Israel between 1976 and 1981. *Leukaemia Res., 8*, 691-699

Virag, I. & Modan, B. (1969) Epidemiological aspects of neoplastic diseases in Israeli immigrant population: II, malignant neoplasms in childhood. *Cancer, 23*, 137-141

JAPAN

Kanagawa Cancer Registry, 1975–1979

R. Inoue

The Kanagawa Cancer Registry began operation as a population-based cancer registry in January 1970. It was initially a project of the Cancer Epidemiology Study Group (Ministry of Health), organized to study the size and nature of the cancer burden in the area. It is now operated by the local government, with the full support of the Kanagawa Medical Association and the Centre for Adult Diseases of Kanagawa.

The sources of information are hospitals, outpatient clinics and death certificates. Although registration is not compulsory, a check on the various sources is made to ensure that reporting is carried out.

The cases diagnosed as cancer in all medical facilities in the Prefecture are notified to the Kanagawa Medical Association. This material is then sent to the Centre for Adult Diseases of Kanagawa, where the data are coded, processed by computer and analysed.

There are well-established communications networks between the Kanagawa Medical Association and the health departments, and all death certificates are reported to the health centres. Death certificates are received from the health centres and these are also processed by computer.

Cross-checking for duplication and correction of errors is done on a master tape which is based on the patient data and on death certificates. Benign and unspecified brain tumours are not included in the registry. All diagnostic coding is done using ICD-O.

The data are used to study cancer incidence in Kanagawa, the epidemio logical patterns and characteristics of the disease, the current status of cancer detection, diagnosis and treatment, and prognosis of cancer patients.

In Kanagawa Prefecture, there are 10 medical college hospitals, one centre (adult disease centre), 314 hospitals, 4114 clinics, 39 health centres, and one paediatric hospital with a department of oncology.

The registration area comprises the whole of Kanagawa Prefecture, which is located approximately in the centre of Japan. Kanagawa Prefecture adjoins Metropolitan Tokyo. Extending 77 kilometres from east to west, and approximately 60 kilometres from north to south, it covers an area of 2390 square kilometres. The Keihin industrial zone in the south-east includes Kawasaki city and Yokohama city.

The population was 6.9 million at the 1980 national census, giving a population density of 2889 per square kilometre; 99.5% of the population are Japanese.

The main occupational groups at the census were: craftsmen, production workers and labourers (33.1%), clerical and related workers (20.5%), sales workers (14.4%), professional and technical workers (10.4%), and farmers, lumbermen and fishermen (2.1%).

Of the total population, 95% was classified as urban and 5% as rural.

Population

The population used is that of the 1975 census, provided by the Japanese Bureau of Statistics.

AVERAGE ANNUAL POPULATION: 1975–1979

Age	Male	Female
0	61400	58537
1–4	266540	252703
5–9	283699	268930
10–14	226064	214148
0–14	837703	794318

Commentary

By comparison with Western registries, there were relatively high incidence rates for acute non-lymphocytic leukaemia and correspondingly low rates for

Contd. p. 184

Japan, Kanagawa　　　　　　　　　　1975 – 1979　　　　　　　　　　MALE

DIAGNOSTIC GROUP	NUMBER OF CASES 0	1-4	5-9	10-14	All	REL. FREQUENCY(%) Crude	Adj.	Group	RATES PER MILLION 0	1-4	5-9	10-14	Crude	Adj.	Cum	HV(%)
TOTAL	51	168	121	73	413	100.0	100.0	100.0	166.1	126.1	85.3	64.6	98.6	98.2	1420	89.0
I. LEUKAEMIAS	13	74	48	32	167	40.4	40.9	100.0	42.3	55.5	33.8	28.3	39.9	39.6	575	97.4
Acute lymphocytic	2	41	21	11	75	18.2	17.6	44.9	6.5	30.8	14.8	9.7	17.9	17.6	252	94.7
Other lymphocytic	0	0	0	0	0	-	-	-	-	-	-	-	-	-	-	-
Acute non-lymphocytic	5	17	21	7	50	12.1	12.1	29.9	16.3	12.8	14.8	6.2	11.9	11.8	172	100.0
Chronic myeloid	1	3	1	4	9	2.2	2.6	5.4	3.3	2.3	0.7	3.5	2.1	2.0	33	100.0
Other and unspecified	5	13	5	10	33	8.0	8.6	19.8	16.3	9.8	3.5	8.8	7.9	8.0	117	100.0
II. LYMPHOMAS	2	6	14	8	30	7.3	8.2	100.0	6.5	4.5	9.9	7.1	7.2	7.1	109	100.0
Hodgkin's disease	0	0	3	0	3	0.7	0.7	10.0	-	-	2.1	-	0.7	0.7	11	100.0
Non-Hodgkin lymphoma	0	1	4	1	6	1.5	1.6	20.0	-	0.8	2.8	0.9	1.4	1.4	22	100.0
Burkitt's lymphoma	0	0	0	2	2	0.5	0.8	6.7	-	-	-	1.8	0.5	0.5	9	100.0
Unspecified lymphoma	0	4	5	3	12	2.9	3.2	40.0	-	3.0	3.5	2.7	2.9	2.8	43	100.0
Histiocytosis X	1	0	0	0	1	0.2	0.2	3.3	3.3	-	-	-	0.2	0.3	-	-
Other reticuloendothelial	1	1	2	2	6	1.5	1.7	20.0	3.3	0.8	1.4	1.8	1.4	1.5	22	100.0
III. BRAIN AND SPINAL	9	25	27	16	77	18.6	19.5	100.0	29.3	18.8	19.0	14.2	18.4	18.3	270	73.8
Ependymoma	0	1	1	1	3	0.7	0.9	3.9	-	0.8	1.4	0.9	0.7	0.7	10	100.0
Astrocytoma	2	4	6	6	18	4.4	5.0	23.4	6.5	3.0	4.2	5.3	4.3	4.3	66	100.0
Medulloblastoma	0	6	6	1	13	3.1	3.0	16.9	-	4.5	4.2	0.9	3.1	3.0	44	100.0
Other glioma	0	2	2	0	4	1.0	1.0	5.2	-	1.5	1.4	-	1.0	0.9	14	100.0
Other and unspecified *	7	12	12	8	39	9.4	9.7	50.6	22.8	9.0	8.5	7.1	9.4	9.3	137	37.0
IV. SYMPATHETIC N.S.	7	20	5	1	33	8.0	6.6	100.0	22.8	15.0	3.5	0.9	7.9	7.8	105	81.8
Neuroblastoma	7	20	5	1	33	8.0	6.6	100.0	22.8	15.0	3.5	0.9	7.9	7.8	105	81.8
Other	0	0	0	0	0	-	-	-	-	-	-	-	-	-	-	-
V. RETINOBLASTOMA	6	6	1	0	13	3.1	2.4	100.0	19.5	4.5	0.7	-	3.1	3.1	41	100.0
VI. KIDNEY	3	9	3	0	15	3.6	2.9	100.0	9.8	6.8	2.1	-	3.6	3.5	47	90.0
Wilms' tumour	1	6	2	0	9	2.2	1.8	60.0	3.3	4.5	1.4	-	2.2	2.1	28	100.0
Renal carcinoma	0	0	0	0	0	-	-	-	-	-	-	-	-	-	-	100.0
Other and unspecified	2	3	1	0	6	1.5	1.2	40.0	6.5	2.3	0.7	-	1.4	1.4	19	100.0
VII. LIVER	2	8	3	2	15	3.6	3.4	100.0	6.5	6.0	2.1	1.8	3.6	3.4	50	64.3
Hepatoblastoma	0	7	0	0	7	1.7	1.3	46.7	-	5.3	-	-	1.7	1.3	21	100.0
Hepatic carcinoma	0	0	1	0	1	0.2	0.2	6.7	-	-	0.7	-	0.2	0.2	4	100.0
Other and unspecified	2	1	2	2	7	1.7	1.9	46.7	6.5	0.8	1.4	1.8	1.7	1.7	25	16.7
VIII. BONE	0	1	6	4	11	2.7	3.3	100.0	-	0.8	4.2	3.5	2.6	2.6	42	85.7
Osteosarcoma	0	0	0	4	4	1.0	1.2	36.4	-	-	-	3.5	1.0	0.9	15	100.0
Chondrosarcoma	0	0	1	0	1	0.2	0.2	9.1	-	-	0.7	-	0.2	0.2	4	100.0
Ewing's sarcoma	0	0	1	0	1	0.2	0.2	9.1	-	-	0.7	-	0.2	0.2	4	100.0
Other and unspecified	0	1	4	0	5	1.2	1.7	45.5	-	0.8	2.7	-	1.2	1.2	20	100.0
IX. SOFT TISSUE SARCOMAS	2	5	4	4	15	3.6	3.9	100.0	6.5	3.8	2.8	3.5	3.6	3.6	53	100.0
Rhabdomyosarcoma	2	4	3	0	9	2.2	1.8	60.0	6.5	3.0	2.1	-	2.1	2.1	29	100.0
Fibrosarcoma	0	1	0	1	2	0.5	0.6	13.3	-	0.8	-	0.9	0.5	0.5	7	100.0
Other and unspecified	0	0	1	3	4	1.0	1.5	26.7	-	-	0.7	2.7	1.0	1.0	17	100.0
X. GONADAL & GERM CELL	3	9	4	4	20	4.8	4.8	100.0	9.8	6.8	2.8	3.5	4.8	4.8	69	100.0
Non-gonadal germ cell	1	3	4	4	12	2.9	3.4	60.0	3.3	2.3	2.8	3.5	2.9	2.9	44	100.0
Gonadal germ cell	2	6	0	0	8	1.9	1.5	40.0	6.5	4.5	-	-	1.9	1.9	25	100.0
Gonadal carcinoma	0	0	0	0	0	-	-	-	-	-	-	-	-	-	-	-
Other and unspecified	0	0	0	0	0	-	-	-	-	-	-	-	-	-	-	-
XI. EPITHELIAL NEOPLASMS	0	0	3	1	4	1.0	1.2	100.0	-	-	2.1	0.9	1.0	0.9	15	100.0
Adrenocortical carcinoma	0	0	0	0	0	-	-	-	-	-	-	-	-	-	-	-
Thyroid carcinoma	0	0	0	0	0	-	-	-	-	-	-	-	-	-	-	-
Nasopharyngeal carcinoma	0	0	0	0	0	-	-	-	-	-	-	-	-	-	-	-
Melanoma	0	0	1	0	1	0.2	0.2	25.0	-	-	0.7	-	0.2	0.2	4	100.0
Other carcinoma	0	0	2	1	3	0.7	0.9	75.0	-	-	1.4	0.9	0.7	0.7	11	100.0
XII. OTHER	4	5	3	1	13	3.1	2.8	100.0	13.0	3.8	2.1	0.9	3.1	3.1	43	40.0
* Specified as malignant	7	10	12	8	37	9.0	9.4	100.0	22.8	7.5	8.5	7.1	8.8	8.9	131	32.0

* Specified as malignant

Japan, Kanagawa

1975 - 1979 FEMALE

DIAGNOSTIC GROUP	NUMBER OF CASES					REL. FREQUENCY(%)			RATES PER MILLION						Cum	HV(%)
	0	1-4	5-9	10-14	All	Crude	Adj.	Group	0	1-4	5-9	10-14	Crude	Adj.		
TOTAL	45	137	90	66	338	100.0	100.0	100.0	153.7	108.4	66.9	61.6	85.1	85.0	1230	87.0
I. LEUKAEMIAS	18	67	42	21	148	43.8	42.2	100.0	61.5	53.0	31.2	19.6	37.3	37.0	528	89.2
Acute lymphocytic	6	36	20	5	67	19.8	18.2	45.3	20.5	28.5	14.9	4.7	16.9	16.6	232	82.1
Other lymphocytic	0	1	0	0	1	0.3	0.2	0.7	-	0.8	-	-	0.3	0.2	3	100.0
Acute non-lymphocytic	3	16	9	12	40	11.8	12.6	27.0	10.2	12.7	6.7	11.2	10.1	10.1	150	97.1
Chronic myeloid	0	1	2	1	4	1.2	1.3	2.7	-	0.8	1.5	0.9	1.0	1.0	15	75.0
Other and unspecified	9	13	11	3	36	10.7	9.9	24.3	30.7	10.3	8.2	2.8	9.1	9.0	127	100.0
II. LYMPHOMAS	5	5	8	6	24	7.1	7.6	100.0	17.1	4.0	5.9	5.6	6.0	6.1	91	86.4
Hodgkin's disease	0	0	1	1	2	0.6	0.8	8.3	-	-	0.7	0.9	0.5	0.5	8	50.0
Non-Hodgkin lymphoma	0	3	2	3	8	2.4	2.7	33.3	-	2.4	1.5	2.8	2.0	2.0	31	100.0
Burkitt's lymphoma	0	0	0	0	0	-	-	-	-	-	-	-	-	-	-	-
Unspecified lymphoma	0	0	3	1	4	1.2	1.5	16.7	-	-	2.2	0.9	1.0	1.0	16	100.0
Histiocytosis X	4	0	1	0	5	1.5	1.2	20.8	13.7	-	0.7	-	1.3	1.3	17	50.0
Other reticuloendothelial	1	2	1	1	5	1.5	1.4	20.8	3.4	1.6	0.7	0.9	1.3	1.3	18	100.0
III. BRAIN AND SPINAL	4	22	22	16	64	18.9	20.3	100.0	13.7	17.4	16.4	14.9	16.1	16.1	240	79.2
Ependymoma	0	3	3	0	3	0.9	0.7	4.7	-	2.4	-	-	0.8	0.7	9	100.0
Astrocytoma	0	6	8	5	19	5.6	6.3	29.7	-	4.7	5.9	4.7	4.8	4.7	72	100.0
Medulloblastoma	0	6	3	3	12	3.6	3.7	18.8	-	4.7	2.2	2.8	3.0	3.0	44	100.0
Other glioma	1	0	2	4	7	2.1	2.7	10.9	3.4	-	1.5	3.7	1.8	1.8	30	71.4
Other and unspecified *	3	7	9	4	23	6.8	7.0	35.9	10.2	5.5	6.7	3.7	5.8	5.8	85	25.0
IV. SYMPATHETIC N.S.	4	18	1	2	25	7.4	6.1	100.0	13.7	14.2	0.7	1.9	6.3	6.3	84	96.0
Neuroblastoma	4	17	1	2	24	7.1	5.9	96.0	13.7	13.5	0.7	1.9	6.0	6.0	81	95.8
Other	0	1	0	0	1	0.3	0.2	4.0	-	0.8	-	-	0.3	0.2	3	100.0
V. RETINOBLASTOMA	6	3	0	0	9	2.7	2.0	100.0	20.5	2.4	-	-	2.3	2.3	30	100.0
VI. KIDNEY	0	7	1	0	8	2.4	1.9	100.0	-	5.5	0.7	-	2.0	2.0	26	100.0
Wilms' tumour	0	4	1	0	5	1.5	1.2	62.5	-	3.2	0.7	-	1.3	1.2	16	100.0
Renal carcinoma	0	0	0	0	0	-	-	-	-	-	-	-	-	-	-	-
Other and unspecified	0	3	0	0	3	0.9	0.7	37.5	-	2.4	-	-	0.8	0.8	9	100.0
VII. LIVER	3	2	0	0	5	1.5	1.1	100.0	10.2	1.6	-	-	1.3	1.3	17	100.0
Hepatoblastoma	2	1	0	0	3	0.9	0.7	60.0	6.8	0.8	-	-	0.8	0.8	10	100.0
Hepatic carcinoma	0	0	0	0	1	0.3	0.2	20.0	-	-	-	-	0.3	0.2	3	100.0
Other and unspecified	1	0	0	0	1	0.3	0.2	20.0	3.4	0.8	-	-	0.3	0.3	3	-
VIII. BONE	0	0	4	4	8	2.4	3.2	100.0	-	-	3.0	3.7	2.0	2.0	34	100.0
Osteosarcoma	0	0	1	2	3	0.9	1.2	37.5	-	-	0.7	1.9	0.8	0.8	13	100.0
Chondrosarcoma	0	0	1	0	1	0.3	0.3	12.5	-	-	0.7	-	0.3	0.2	4	100.0
Ewing's sarcoma	0	0	1	1	1	0.3	0.5	12.5	-	-	0.7	0.9	0.3	0.3	5	100.0
Other and unspecified	0	0	2	1	3	0.9	1.1	37.5	-	-	1.5	0.9	0.8	0.8	12	100.0
IX. SOFT TISSUE SARCOMAS	2	4	4	6	16	4.7	5.4	100.0	6.8	3.2	3.0	5.6	4.0	4.1	62	93.8
Rhabdomyosarcoma	1	0	3	4	8	2.4	3.0	50.0	3.4	-	2.2	3.7	2.0	2.1	33	87.5
Fibrosarcoma	0	0	1	0	1	0.3	0.3	6.3	-	-	0.7	-	0.3	0.2	4	100.0
Other and unspecified	1	4	0	2	7	2.1	2.0	43.8	3.4	3.2	-	1.9	1.8	1.8	25	100.0
X. GONADAL & GERM CELL	0	5	5	6	16	4.7	5.5	100.0	-	4.0	3.7	5.6	4.0	4.1	62	66.7
Non-gonadal germ cell	0	3	0	0	6	1.8	2.0	37.5	-	2.4	-	-	1.5	1.5	24	83.3
Gonadal germ cell	0	1	3	3	6	1.5	1.7	31.3	-	0.8	2.2	2.8	1.3	1.2	19	80.0
Gonadal carcinoma	0	0	1	1	1	0.3	0.3	6.3	-	-	0.7	0.9	0.3	0.2	4	100.0
Other and unspecified	0	1	1	2	4	1.2	1.5	25.0	-	0.8	0.7	1.9	1.0	1.0	16	-
XI. EPITHELIAL NEOPLASMS	0	2	0	3	5	1.5	1.8	100.0	-	1.6	-	2.8	1.3	1.3	20	100.0
Adrenocortical carcinoma	0	1	0	0	0	0.3	0.2	20.0	-	0.8	-	-	0.3	0.2	3	100.0
Thyroid carcinoma	0	0	0	0	0	-	-	-	-	-	-	-	-	-	-	-
Nasopharyngeal carcinoma	0	0	0	1	1	0.3	0.5	20.0	-	-	-	0.9	0.3	0.3	5	100.0
Melanoma	0	1	0	0	1	0.3	0.2	20.0	-	0.8	-	-	0.3	0.2	3	100.0
Other carcinoma	0	0	0	2	2	0.6	0.9	40.0	-	-	-	1.9	0.5	0.5	9	100.0
XII. OTHER	3	2	3	2	10	3.0	3.0	100.0	10.2	1.6	2.2	1.9	2.5	2.5	37	-
* Specified as malignant	3	7	9	4	23	6.8	7.0	100.0	10.2	5.5	6.7	3.7	5.8	5.8	85	25.0

acute lymphocytic leukaemia; these findings are similar to those for the other two Japanese registries reported here. Hodgkin's disease was extremely rare, and there were also relatively low rates for kidney tumours and bone and soft-tissue sarcomas. Among males only, liver tumours and nongonadal germ-cell tumours appeared to be relatively common, but these observations are based on small numbers of cases.

Miyagi Prefecture Cancer Registry, 1971–1979

Y. Okuno & A. Takano

The Miyagi Prefectural Cancer Registry (formerly Miyagi Cancer Registry) covers the entire Prefecture, and was initiated in 1951 by the late Professor Mitsuo Segi at the Department of Public Health, Tohoku University School of Medicine in Sendai. The Registry is now located in the Miyagi Cancer Society. Miyagi Prefecture makes grants to the Registry, and the Miyagi Cancer Society also supports it financially. The work of the Registry is entirely the responsibility of the Registry Committee, which consists of representatives of the Miyagi Medical Association, Tohoku University School of Medicine, public and private medical institutions, Miyagi Prefecture and the Miyagi Cancer Society.

The sources of information are clinics and hospitals (in-patients and out-patients); radiology and pathology departments; autopsy records; mass-screening records; and death certificates. Since reporting by clinics and hospitals is voluntary, information on all cancer cases has been actively sought from the beginning. However, it was not until 1974 that this active method of information collection was emphasized. Except for the cases reported from clinics and a few hospitals, all the rest are collected by abstracting the relevant details from the medical records of hospitals, pathology and autopsy records, etc. About 80% of the yearly incidence reports are collected by this active method of seeking information. The records of the past four years show an average of 1.5 reports on each patient, exclusive of death certificates. Although there is a delay between diagnosis and registration, this active information collection increases completeness of registration.

All the death certificates of Miyagi Prefecture are collated with the registered cases. Those which have not been registered are assigned an estimated incident year according to the 'duration of illness', and are registered as cases of that estimated year. The percentage registered from death certificates was 13.8% of all cases diagnosed during 1981.

Few patients from Miyagi go to other prefectures for treatment; however, the number is increasing slightly. Therefore, regular visits by Registry staff to hospitals in other prefectures are becoming necessary. Completeness of coverage has been gradually improving; this may be partly due to the improvement of medical record administration.

Data are held both manually and on computer (up to 1977 on magnetic tape and on disks since then). The computer has been used since 1972, but the present system was introduced in 1981. Our own data base system which uses a small-scale computer is effective for information retrieval. Data are entered and updated by VDU directly. Multiple neoplasms for the same person are counted separately.

Miyagi Prefecture is situated in the north of Honshu, and is flanked on the east by the Pacific Ocean. Sendai, the prefectural seat of Miyagi Prefecture, is situated about 350 kilometres north of Tokyo. The yearly mean temperature in Sendai is 12.3° C, and the annual rainfall about 1200 mm. The altitude of the Prefecture varies from sea level to 1841 m. The total area is 7291 square kilometres.

In general, the Japanese are, with very few exceptions, of a single religion, race and language, and there are very few immigrants in Japan. There are only 4000 foreigners in the Prefecture's total population of 2 million.

Population

The average annual population has been calculated from data from the censuses of 1970, 1975 and 1980, provided by the Japanese Bureau of Statistics.

AVERAGE ANNUAL POPULATION: 1971-1979

Age	Male	Female
0	16250	15399
1–4	65168	61984
5–9	77869	74137
10–14	77629	74176
0–14	236916	225696

Commentary

Over 40% of registrations were for leukaemia. Of these, 66/160 (41%) were acute lymphocytic and 45/160 (28%) were acute non-lymphocytic; 42 (26%) were of 'other and unspecified' cell type. Hodgkin's disease was very rare (only one case out of 374). The incidence rate for liver tumours, of which only one case out of 13 was hepatoblastoma, was similar to that for kidney tumours.

Japan, Miyagi

1971 - 1979   MALE

DIAGNOSTIC GROUP	__ NUMBER OF CASES __ 0	1-4	5-9	10-14	All	REL. FREQ. Crude	Adj.	Group	RATES PER MILLION 0	1-4	5-9	10-14	Crude	Adj.	Cum	HV(%)
TOTAL	35	76	45	48	204	100.0	100.0	100.0	239.3	129.6	64.2	68.7	95.7	99.3	1422	65.2
I. LEUKAEMIAS	11	32	21	19	83	40.7	41.4	100.0	75.2	54.6	30.0	27.2	38.9	40.3	579	44.3
Acute lymphocytic	0	20	11	4	35	17.2	17.0	42.2	-	34.1	15.7	5.7	16.4	17.3	243	39.4
Other lymphocytic	0	0	0	2	2	1.0		2.4	-	-	-	2.9	0.9	0.8	14	100.0
Acute non-lymphocytic	3	6	6	10	25	12.3	13.5	30.1	20.5	10.2	8.6	14.3	11.7	11.7	176	52.4
Chronic myeloid	0	1	1	1	3	1.5	1.7	3.6	-	1.7	1.4	1.4	1.4	1.4	21	100.0
Other and unspecified	8	5	3	2	18	8.8	7.9	21.7	54.7	8.5	4.3	2.9	8.4	9.1	125	25.0
II. LYMPHOMAS	0	1	3	7	11	5.4	6.7	100.0	-	1.7	4.3	10.0	5.2	4.8	78	77.8
Hodgkin's disease	0	0	0	1	1	0.5	0.6	9.1	-	-	-	1.4	0.5	0.4	7	100.0
Non-Hodgkin lymphoma	0	0	3	1	4	2.0	2.6	36.4	-	-	4.3	1.4	1.9	1.8	29	75.0
Burkitt's lymphoma	0	0	0	1	1	0.5	0.6	9.1	-	-	-	1.4	0.5	0.4	7	100.0
Unspecified lymphoma	0	1	0	4	5	2.5	2.9	45.5	-	1.7	-	5.7	2.3	2.2	35	66.7
Histiocytosis X	0	0	0	0	0	-	-	-	-	-	-	-	-	-	-	-
Other reticuloendothelial	0	0	0	0	0	-	-	-	-	-	-	-	-	-	-	-
III. BRAIN AND SPINAL	1	7	5	5	18	8.8	9.3	100.0	6.8	11.9	7.1	7.2	8.4	8.6	126	61.1
Ependymoma	0	1	0	0	1	0.5	0.4	5.6	-	1.7	-	-	0.5	0.5	7	100.0
Astrocytoma	0	1	2	2	5	2.5	2.5	27.8	-	1.7	2.9	2.9	2.3	2.3	35	100.0
Medulloblastoma	1	1	1	1	4	2.0	2.0	22.2	6.8	1.7	1.4	1.4	1.9	1.9	28	100.0
Other glioma	0	0	0	0	0	-	-	-	-	-	-	-	-	-	-	-
Other and unspecified *	0	4	2	2	8	3.9	4.0	44.4	-	6.8	2.9	2.9	3.8	3.9	56	12.5
IV. SYMPATHETIC N.S.	5	8	0	1	14	6.9	5.3	100.0	34.2	13.6	-	1.4	6.6	7.3	96	100.0
Neuroblastoma	5	8	0	1	14	6.9	5.3	100.0	34.2	13.6	-	1.4	6.6	7.3	96	100.0
Other	0	0	0	0	0	-	-	-	-	-	-	-	-	-	-	-
V. RETINOBLASTOMA	5	5	0	0	10	4.9	3.6	100.0	34.2	8.5	-	-	4.7	5.3	68	100.0
VI. KIDNEY	1	7	2	0	10	4.9	4.2	100.0	6.8	11.9	2.9	-	4.7	5.1	69	70.0
Wilms' tumour	1	6	0	0	7	3.4	2.5	70.0	6.8	10.2	-	-	3.3	3.7	48	100.0
Renal carcinoma	0	0	0	0	0	-	-	-	-	-	-	-	-	-	-	-
Other and unspecified	0	1	2	0	3	1.5	1.7	30.0	-	1.7	2.9	-	1.4	1.4	21	-
VII. LIVER	3	3	2	2	10	4.9	4.7	100.0	20.5	5.1	2.9	2.9	4.7	4.9	70	87.5
Hepatoblastoma	0	1	0	0	1	0.5	0.4	10.0	-	1.7	-	-	0.5	0.5	7	100.0
Hepatic carcinoma	1	2	2	1	6	2.9	3.0	60.0	6.8	3.4	2.9	1.4	2.8	2.9	42	100.0
Other and unspecified	2	0	0	1	3	1.5	1.3	30.0	13.7	-	-	1.4	1.4	1.5	21	-
VIII. BONE	1	0	2	4	7	3.4	4.2	100.0	6.8	-	2.9	5.7	3.3	3.1	50	57.1
Osteosarcoma	0	0	1	2	3	1.5	1.9	42.9	-	-	1.4	2.9	1.4	1.3	21	100.0
Chondrosarcoma	0	0	0	0	0	-	-	-	-	-	-	-	-	-	-	-
Ewing's sarcoma	0	0	0	1	1	0.5	0.6	14.3	-	-	-	1.4	0.5	0.4	7	100.0
Other and unspecified	1	0	1	1	3	1.5	1.7	42.9	6.8	-	1.4	1.4	1.4	1.4	21	-
IX. SOFT TISSUE SARCOMAS	4	4	2	5	15	7.4	7.3	100.0	27.3	6.8	2.9	7.2	7.0	7.2	105	100.0
Rhabdomyosarcoma	1	4	1	1	7	3.4	3.1	46.7	6.8	6.8	1.4	1.4	3.3	3.1	48	100.0
Fibrosarcoma	0	0	0	1	1	0.5	0.6	6.7	-	-	-	1.4	0.5	0.4	7	100.0
Other and unspecified	3	0	1	3	7	3.4	3.6	46.7	20.5	-	1.4	4.3	3.3	3.3	49	100.0
X. GONADAL & GERM CELL	2	8	1	2	13	6.4	5.5	100.0	13.7	13.6	1.4	2.9	6.1	6.6	90	83.3
Non-gonadal germ cell	1	1	0	1	3	1.5	1.6	23.1	6.8	1.7	-	1.4	1.4	1.7	21	66.7
Gonadal germ cell	1	7	0	0	8	3.9	2.9	61.5	6.8	11.9	-	-	3.8	4.2	55	100.0
Gonadal carcinoma	0	0	0	0	0	-	-	-	-	-	-	-	-	-	-	-
Other and unspecified	0	0	1	1	2	1.0		15.4	-	-	1.4	1.4	0.9	1.0	14	-
XI. EPITHELIAL NEOPLASMS	1	0	2	2	5	2.5	2.9	100.0	6.8	-	2.9	2.9	2.3	2.3	35	80.0
Adrenocortical carcinoma	0	0	0	0	0	-	-	-	-	-	-	-	-	-	-	-
Thyroid carcinoma	0	0	0	0	0	-	-	-	-	-	-	-	-	-	-	-
Nasopharyngeal carcinoma	0	0	0	0	0	-	-	-	-	-	-	-	-	-	-	-
Melanoma	1	0	1	0	2	1.0	1.0	40.0	6.8	-	1.4	-	0.9	1.0	14	50.0
Other carcinoma	0	0	1	2	3	1.5	1.9	60.0	-	-	1.4	2.9	1.4	1.3	21	100.0
XII. OTHER	1	1	5	1	8	3.9	4.7	100.0	6.8	1.7	7.1	1.4	3.8	3.8	56	14.3
* Specified as malignant	0	4	2	1	7	3.4	3.4	100.0	-	6.8	2.9	1.4	3.3	3.4	49	14.3

Japan, Miyagi

1971 – 1979

FEMALE

DIAGNOSTIC GROUP	NUMBER OF CASES 0	1-4	5-9	10-14	All	REL. FREQUENCY(%) Crude	Adj.	Group	RATES PER MILLION 0	1-4	5-9	10-14	Crude	Adj.	Cum	HV(%)
TOTAL	18	58	44	50	170	100.0	100.0	100.0	129.9	104.0	65.9	74.9	83.7	85.3	1250	69.9
I. LEUKAEMIAS	7	26	24	20	77	45.3	45.7	100.0	50.5	46.6	36.0	30.0	37.9	38.6	567	56.9
Acute lymphocytic	1	11	12	7	31	18.2	18.7	40.3	7.2	19.7	18.0	10.5	15.3	15.5	228	70.0
Other lymphocytic	0	0	0	1	1	0.6	0.6	1.3	-	-	-	1.5	0.5	0.4	7	100.0
Acute non-lymphocytic	2	7	6	5	20	11.8	11.8	26.0	14.4	12.5	9.0	7.5	9.8	10.1	147	58.8
Chronic myeloid	0	0	1	0	1	0.6	0.6	1.3	-	-	1.5	-	0.5	0.4	7	100.0
Other and unspecified	4	8	5	7	24	14.1	14.0	31.2	28.9	14.3	9.0	9.0	11.8	12.2	176	25.0
II. LYMPHOMAS	1	1	3	0	5	2.9	3.1	100.0	7.2	1.8	4.5	-	2.5	2.6	37	60.0
Hodgkin's disease	0	0	0	0	0	-	-	-	-	-	-	-	-	-	-	-
Non-Hodgkin lymphoma	0	0	0	0	0	-	-	-	-	-	-	-	-	-	-	-
Burkitt's lymphoma	0	0	0	0	0	-	-	-	-	-	-	-	-	-	-	-
Unspecified lymphoma	0	1	2	0	3	1.8	1.9	60.0	-	1.8	3.0	-	1.5	1.5	22	33.3
Histiocytosis X	1	0	0	0	1	0.6	0.5	20.0	7.2	-	-	-	0.5	0.6	7	100.0
Other reticuloendothelial	0	0	1	0	1	0.6	0.7	20.0	-	-	1.5	-	0.5	0.5	7	100.0
III. BRAIN AND SPINAL	3	9	5	3	20	11.8	11.5	100.0	21.6	16.1	7.5	4.5	9.8	10.4	146	82.4
Ependymoma	0	1	0	0	1	0.6	0.5	5.0	-	1.8	-	-	0.5	0.6	7	100.0
Astrocytoma	0	2	3	2	7	4.1	4.3	35.0	-	3.6	4.5	3.0	3.4	3.4	52	100.0
Medulloblastoma	1	2	2	1	6	3.5	3.5	30.0	7.2	3.6	3.0	1.5	3.0	3.1	44	100.0
Other glioma	0	0	0	0	0	-	-	-	-	-	-	-	-	-	-	-
Other and unspecified *	2	4	0	0	6	3.5	3.2	30.0	14.4	7.2	-	-	3.0	3.3	43	-
IV. SYMPATHETIC N.S.	1	9	1	2	13	7.6	7.1	100.0	7.2	16.1	1.5	3.0	6.4	6.9	94	84.6
Neuroblastoma	1	9	1	2	13	7.6	7.1	100.0	7.2	16.1	1.5	3.0	6.4	6.9	94	84.6
Other	0	0	0	0	0	-	-	-	-	-	-	-	-	-	-	-
V. RETINOBLASTOMA	2	4	0	0	6	3.5	3.2	100.0	14.4	7.2	-	-	3.0	3.3	43	100.0
VI. KIDNEY	0	4	2	0	6	3.5	3.5	100.0	-	7.2	3.0	-	3.0	3.2	44	83.3
Wilms' tumour	0	4	0	0	4	2.4	2.1	66.7	-	7.2	-	-	2.0	2.2	29	100.0
Renal carcinoma	0	0	1	0	1	0.6	0.7	16.7	-	-	1.5	-	0.5	0.5	7	100.0
Other and unspecified	0	0	1	0	1	0.6	0.7	16.7	-	-	1.5	-	0.5	0.5	7	-
VII. LIVER	1	1	0	1	3	1.8	1.7	100.0	7.2	1.8	-	1.5	1.5	1.5	22	66.7
Hepatoblastoma	0	0	0	0	0	-	-	-	-	-	-	-	-	-	-	-
Hepatic carcinoma	1	0	0	1	2	1.2	1.1	66.7	7.2	-	-	1.5	1.0	1.0	15	100.0
Other and unspecified	0	1	0	0	1	0.6	0.5	33.3	-	1.8	-	-	0.5	0.6	7	-
VIII. BONE	1	0	3	7	11	6.5	6.8	100.0	7.2	-	4.5	10.5	5.4	5.1	82	72.7
Osteosarcoma	0	0	1	5	6	3.5	3.7	54.5	-	-	1.5	7.5	3.0	2.7	45	100.0
Chondrosarcoma	0	0	0	0	0	-	-	-	-	-	-	-	-	-	-	-
Ewing's sarcoma	0	0	1	1	2	1.2	1.3	18.2	-	-	1.5	1.5	1.0	0.9	15	100.0
Other and unspecified	1	0	1	1	3	1.8	1.8	27.3	7.2	-	1.5	1.5	1.5	1.5	22	-
IX. SOFT TISSUE SARCOMAS	1	1	2	2	6	3.5	3.6	100.0	7.2	1.8	3.0	3.0	3.0	3.0	44	100.0
Rhabdomyosarcoma	0	1	2	0	3	1.8	1.9	50.0	-	1.8	3.0	-	1.5	1.9	22	100.0
Fibrosarcoma	1	0	0	0	1	0.6	0.5	16.7	7.2	-	-	-	0.5	0.5	7	100.0
Other and unspecified	0	0	0	2	2	1.2	1.2	33.3	-	-	-	3.0	1.0	0.6	15	100.0
X. GONADAL & GERM CELL	0	1	3	9	13	7.6	8.0	100.0	-	1.8	4.5	13.5	6.4	5.9	97	75.0
Non-gonadal germ cell	0	1	0	1	2	1.2	1.1	15.4	-	1.8	-	1.5	1.0	1.0	15	100.0
Gonadal germ cell	0	0	2	4	6	3.5	3.8	46.2	-	-	3.0	6.0	3.0	3.8	45	100.0
Gonadal carcinoma	0	0	0	1	1	0.6	0.6	7.7	-	-	-	1.5	0.5	0.4	7	100.0
Other and unspecified	0	0	1	3	4	2.4	2.5	30.8	-	-	1.5	4.5	2.0	1.8	30	100.0
XI. EPITHELIAL NEOPLASMS	0	0	1	5	6	3.5	3.7	100.0	-	-	1.5	7.5	3.0	2.7	45	100.0
Adrenocortical carcinoma	0	0	0	0	0	-	-	-	-	-	-	-	-	-	-	-
Thyroid carcinoma	0	0	1	3	4	2.4	2.5	66.7	-	-	1.5	4.5	2.0	1.8	30	100.0
Nasopharyngeal carcinoma	0	0	0	0	0	-	-	-	-	-	-	-	-	-	-	-
Melanoma	0	0	0	0	0	-	-	-	-	-	-	-	-	-	-	-
Other carcinoma	0	0	0	2	2	1.2	1.2	33.3	-	-	-	3.0	1.0	0.9	15	100.0
XII. OTHER	1	2	0	1	4	2.4	2.2	100.0	7.2	3.6	-	1.5	2.0	2.1	29	-
* Specified as malignant	2	4	0	0	6	3.5	3.2	100.0	14.4	7.2	-	-	3.0	3.3	43	-

Osaka Cancer Registry, 1971–1980

I. Fujimoto & A. Hanai

In 1962 the Osaka Prefectural Government, the Osaka Medical Association (OMA) and the Centre for Adult Diseases (CAD), Osaka, decided to start prefecture-wide cancer registration on a voluntary basis in order to obtain information about the nature and extent of the cancer problem in Osaka and to assist in planning cancer control programmes.

The OMA requests physicians and hospital doctors to prepare reports on cases of cancer that they diagnose and send them to the OMA. The Osaka Prefectural Health Department is responsible for the budgetary support of registration.

The Registry operates within the Department of Field Research, CAD. Every month, it receives a batch of cancer reports from the OMA and collects the cancer death certificates from the health centres. Cancer reports and cancer death cards are checked for consistency, then coded, punched and stored on the computer file. All information is cross-checked for inconsistencies.

Registration procedures are computerized. Collation is carried out by computer, using six items (date of birth, name, sex, area, detailed address, site of cancer). A list of possible duplicates is printed out by computer and checked by hand by the Registry staff against the original cards. Multiple primary cancers in the same patient are counted separately. The registry includes all malignant neoplasms, and benign and unspecified brain and spinal tumours. Since 1979, histiocytosis X has also been registered. Diagnostic coding is by ICD-9 (site) and ICD-O (morphology).

Two kinds of statistical output have been routinely prepared, the first being patient (tumour)-oriented and the other hospital-oriented. Physicians or hospital doctors may request and obtain information on the cases that they reported. The Registry data are also used for epidemiological studies and for preparing and evaluating cancer control programmes.

It is estimated from the various indices obtained from Registry data that the number of registered cases currently corresponds to 85–94% of all cancer cases in Osaka.

Osaka Prefecture is located in the south of Honshu. It is the second smallest prefecture but its population density is the highest of all prefectures in Japan. In the past 20 years the population has increased from 6.0 to 8.5 million; 98% of the population is Japanese, 1.9% being Korean and 0.1% Chinese and other.

In the Prefecture, the city of Osaka is surrounded by 30 satellite cities, 13 towns and one village. Of the workers, 33% are engaged in industry, 27% in commerce, 16% in personal services, etc., and 1% in agriculture.

Population

The population at risk has been calculated from the data from the 1970, 1975 and 1980 censuses (Japanese Bureau of Statistics).

AVERAGE ANNUAL POPULATION: 1971–1980

Age	Male	Female
0	73842	69918
1–4	307092	291068
5–9	363524	344573
10–14	305055	289818
0–14	1049513	995377

Commentary

As with the other Japanese registries, a relatively high proportion of leukaemias were acute non-lymphocytic and correspondingly fewer were acute lymphocytic; the ratio of acute lymphocytic leukaemia to acute non-lymphocytic leukaemia was 2.1:1, compared with the ratios of over 4:1 commonly observed in Western children. Hodgkin's disease was very rare. Among embryonal tumours, Wilms' tumour had a relatively low incidence and retinoblastoma a relatively high one. Laterality was recorded for 75 (74%) of retinoblastomas; of these, 75% were unilateral and 25% bilateral. Liver tumours were also relatively common, and 86% of those whose histological type was known were hepatoblastoma. Over a third of liver tumours were of unknown histology but their age distribution was similar to that for those known to be hepatoblastoma and they were therefore probably also mostly hepatoblastoma. Ewing's sarcoma was rare. There were high rates for germ-cell tumours of both gonadal and non-gonadal sites, especially in boys.

Japan, Osaka

1971 - 1980

MALE

DIAGNOSTIC GROUP	NUMBER OF CASES 0	1-4	5-9	10-14	All	REL. FREQUENCY(%) Crude	Adj.	Group	RATES PER MILLION 0	1-4	5-9	10-14	Crude	Adj.	Cum	HV(%)
TOTAL	207	524	333	241	1305	100.0	100.0	100.0	280.3	170.6	91.6	79.0	124.3	127.0	1816	83.5
I. LEUKAEMIAS	39	187	140	65	431	33.0	33.1	100.0	52.8	60.9	38.5	21.3	41.1	41.6	595	90.7
Acute lymphocytic	12	119	71	32	234	17.9	17.5	54.3	16.3	38.8	19.5	10.5	22.3	22.6	321	93.5
Other lymphocytic	1	0	1	0	2	0.2	0.1	0.5	1.4	–	0.3	–	0.2	0.2	3	50.0
Acute non-lymphocytic	13	37	42	21	113	8.7	9.1	26.2	17.6	12.0	11.6	6.9	10.8	10.8	158	96.4
Chronic myeloid	2	6	7	4	19	1.5	1.6	4.4	2.7	2.0	1.9	1.3	1.8	1.8	27	100.0
Other and unspecified	11	25	19	8	63	4.8	4.7	14.6	14.9	8.1	5.2	2.6	6.1	6.1	87	66.1
II. LYMPHOMAS	12	45	30	37	124	9.5	10.4	100.0	16.3	14.7	8.3	12.1	11.8	12.0	177	89.9
Hodgkin's disease	0	1	1	7	9	0.7	1.0	7.3	–	0.3	0.3	2.3	0.9	0.9	14	100.0
Non-Hodgkin lymphoma	6	21	14	17	58	4.4	4.9	46.8	8.1	6.8	3.9	5.6	5.5	5.6	83	98.2
Burkitt's lymphoma	0	2	1	0	3	0.2	0.2	2.4	–	0.7	0.3	–	0.3	0.2	4	100.0
Unspecified lymphoma	4	14	12	11	41	3.1	3.4	33.1	5.4	4.6	3.3	3.6	3.9	3.9	58	76.9
Histiocytosis X	1	0	0	0	1	0.1	0.1	0.8	1.4	–	–	–	0.1	0.1	1	100.0
Other reticuloendothelial	1	7	2	2	12	0.9	0.9	9.7	1.4	2.3	0.6	0.7	1.1	1.2	17	100.0
III. BRAIN AND SPINAL	31	80	93	77	281	21.5	24.0	100.0	42.0	26.1	25.6	25.2	26.8	26.9	400	60.1
Ependymoma	3	6	4	3	16	1.2	1.2	5.7	4.1	2.0	1.1	1.0	1.5	1.6	22	100.0
Astrocytoma	0	6	11	9	26	2.0	2.4	9.3	–	2.0	3.0	2.9	2.5	2.4	38	100.0
Medulloblastoma	1	14	10	5	30	2.3	2.3	10.7	1.4	4.6	2.8	1.6	2.9	2.9	42	100.0
Other glioma	0	4	8	3	15	1.1	1.3	5.3	–	1.3	2.2	1.0	1.4	1.4	21	100.0
Other and unspecified *	27	50	60	57	194	14.9	16.7	69.0	36.6	16.3	16.5	18.7	18.5	18.6	278	40.3
IV. SYMPATHETIC N.S.	20	62	15	4	101	7.7	6.3	100.0	27.1	20.2	4.1	1.3	9.6	10.1	135	100.0
Neuroblastoma	20	62	15	4	101	7.7	6.3	100.0	27.1	20.2	4.1	1.3	9.6	10.1	135	100.0
Other	0	0	0	0	0	–	–	–	–	–	–	–	–	–	–	–
V. RETINOBLASTOMA	16	39	1	0	56	4.3	3.1	100.0	21.7	12.7	0.3	–	5.3	5.7	74	100.0
VI. KIDNEY	28	21	5	1	55	4.2	3.3	100.0	37.9	6.8	1.4	0.3	5.2	5.6	74	92.3
Wilms' tumour	24	18	4	1	47	3.6	2.8	85.5	32.5	5.9	1.1	0.3	4.5	4.8	63	100.0
Renal carcinoma	0	0	0	0	0	–	–	–	–	–	–	–	–	–	–	–
Other and unspecified	4	3	1	0	8	0.6	0.5	14.5	5.4	1.0	0.3	–	0.8	0.8	11	20.0
VII. LIVER	9	15	5	4	33	2.5	2.3	100.0	12.2	4.9	1.4	1.3	3.1	3.3	45	72.7
Hepatoblastoma	4	11	4	1	20	1.5	1.3	60.6	5.4	3.6	1.1	0.3	1.9	2.0	27	100.0
Hepatic carcinoma	0	1	1	1	3	0.2	0.2	9.1	–	0.3	0.3	0.3	0.3	0.3	5	100.0
Other and unspecified	5	3	0	2	10	0.8	0.7	30.3	6.8	1.0	–	0.7	1.0	1.0	14	10.0
VIII. BONE	2	6	9	22	39	3.0	4.0	100.0	2.7	2.0	2.5	7.2	3.7	3.7	59	87.2
Osteosarcoma	0	3	6	15	24	1.8	2.6	61.5	–	1.0	1.7	4.9	2.3	2.3	37	100.0
Chondrosarcoma	1	0	0	0	1	0.1	0.1	2.6	1.4	–	–	0.3	0.1	0.1	1	100.0
Ewing's sarcoma	0	0	3	2	5	0.4	0.5	12.8	–	–	0.8	0.7	0.5	0.5	7	100.0
Other and unspecified	1	3	0	5	9	0.7	0.8	23.1	1.4	1.0	–	1.6	0.9	0.9	13	44.4
IX. SOFT TISSUE SARCOMAS	11	16	14	8	49	3.8	3.7	100.0	14.9	5.2	3.9	2.6	4.7	4.8	68	100.0
Rhabdomyosarcoma	4	10	8	3	25	1.9	1.9	51.0	5.4	3.3	2.2	1.0	2.4	2.4	34	100.0
Fibrosarcoma	3	0	1	2	6	0.5	0.5	12.2	4.1	–	0.3	0.7	0.6	0.6	9	100.0
Other and unspecified	4	6	5	3	18	1.4	1.4	36.7	5.4	2.0	1.4	1.0	1.7	1.8	25	100.0
X. GONADAL & GERM CELL	26	37	8	11	82	6.3	5.5	100.0	35.2	12.0	2.2	3.6	7.8	8.2	112	90.2
Non-gonadal germ cell	1	7	7	10	25	1.9	2.3	30.5	1.4	2.3	1.9	3.3	2.4	2.4	36	100.0
Gonadal germ cell	17	24	0	1	42	3.2	2.4	51.2	23.0	7.8	–	0.3	4.0	4.3	56	100.0
Gonadal carcinoma	2	1	0	0	3	0.2	0.2	3.7	2.7	0.3	–	–	0.3	0.3	4	100.0
Other and unspecified	6	5	1	0	12	0.9	0.7	14.6	8.1	1.6	0.3	–	1.1	1.2	16	33.3
XI. EPITHELIAL NEOPLASMS	2	4	4	6	16	1.2	1.4	100.0	2.7	1.3	1.1	2.0	1.5	1.5	23	100.0
Adrenocortical carcinoma	0	0	0	0	0	–	–	–	–	–	–	–	–	–	–	–
Thyroid carcinoma	0	0	0	1	2	0.2	0.2	12.5	–	–	–	0.3	0.2	0.2	3	100.0
Nasopharyngeal carcinoma	0	0	0	1	1	0.1	0.1	6.3	–	–	–	0.3	0.1	0.1	4	100.0
Melanoma	0	2	0	1	3	0.2	0.2	18.8	–	0.7	–	0.3	0.2	0.3	4	100.0
Other carcinoma	2	0	4	3	10	0.8	0.9	62.5	2.7	–	1.1	1.0	0.8	1.0	14	100.0
XII. OTHER	11	12	9	6	38	2.9	2.8	100.0	14.9	3.9	2.5	2.0	3.6	3.7	53	22.9
* Specified as malignant	26	40	46	42	154	11.8	13.0	100.0	35.2	13.0	12.7	13.8	14.7	14.8	219	22.8

Japan, Osaka

1971 - 1980

FEMALE

DIAGNOSTIC GROUP	NUMBER OF CASES					REL. FREQUENCY(%)			RATES PER MILLION							HV(%)
	0	1-4	5-9	10-14	All	Crude	Adj.	Group	0	1-4	5-9	10-14	Crude	Adj.	Cum	
TOTAL	155	350	265	213	983	100.0	100.0	100.0	221.7	120.2	76.9	73.5	98.8	100.5	1455	82.3
I. LEUKAEMIAS	32	143	105	65	345	35.1	34.9	100.0	45.8	49.1	30.5	22.4	34.7	35.1	507	87.8
Acute lymphocytic	11	87	66	26	190	19.3	18.9	55.1	15.7	29.9	19.2	9.0	19.1	19.3	276	94.5
Other lymphocytic	0	2	0	1	3	0.3	-	0.9	-	0.7	-	0.3	0.3	0.3	4	100.0
Acute non-lymphocytic	6	30	28	21	85	8.6	9.0	24.6	8.6	10.3	8.1	7.2	8.5	8.6	127	92.9
Chronic myeloid	1	0	3	6	10	1.0	1.3	2.9	1.4	-	0.9	2.1	1.0	1.0	16	80.0
Other and unspecified	14	24	8	11	57	5.8	5.5	16.5	20.0	8.2	2.3	3.8	5.7	6.0	84	58.2
II. LYMPHOMAS	7	16	26	18	67	6.8	7.3	100.0	10.0	5.5	7.5	6.2	6.7	6.7	101	92.1
Hodgkin's disease	0	1	4	1	6	0.6	0.7	9.0	-	0.3	1.2	0.3	0.6	0.6	9	66.7
Non-Hodgkin lymphoma	1	6	13	10	30	3.1	3.4	44.8	1.4	2.1	3.8	3.5	3.0	3.0	46	96.7
Burkitt's lymphoma	0	3	0	0	3	0.3	0.4	4.5	-	1.0	-	-	0.3	0.3	5	100.0
Unspecified lymphoma	4	5	7	3	19	1.9	1.9	28.4	5.7	1.7	2.0	1.0	1.9	1.9	28	88.2
Histiocytosis X	0	0	0	0	0	-	-	-	-	-	-	-	-	-	-	-
Other reticuloendothelial	2	1	2	4	9	0.9	0.8	13.4	2.9	0.3	0.6	1.4	0.9	0.9	13	100.0
III. BRAIN AND SPINAL	22	63	74	51	210	21.4	22.3	100.0	31.5	21.6	21.5	17.6	21.1	21.2	313	60.1
Ependymoma	1	9	5	2	17	1.7	1.6	8.1	1.4	3.1	1.5	0.7	1.7	1.7	25	100.0
Astrocytoma	3	10	11	10	34	3.5	3.7	16.2	4.3	3.4	3.2	3.5	3.4	3.4	51	100.0
Medulloblastoma	1	6	4	5	16	1.6	1.9	7.6	1.4	2.1	1.2	1.7	1.6	1.6	25	100.0
Other glioma	0	3	6	4	13	1.3	1.3	6.2	-	1.0	1.7	1.4	1.3	1.3	19	100.0
Other and unspecified *	17	35	48	30	130	13.2	13.8	61.9	24.3	12.0	13.9	10.4	13.1	13.1	194	33.1
IV. SYMPATHETIC N.S.	19	43	11	2	75	7.6	6.4	100.0	27.2	14.8	3.2	0.7	7.5	7.9	106	100.0
Neuroblastoma	19	43	11	2	75	7.6	6.4	100.0	27.2	14.8	3.2	0.7	7.5	7.9	106	100.0
Other	0	0	0	0	0	-	-	-	-	-	-	-	-	-	-	-
V. RETINOBLASTOMA	13	29	3	0	45	4.6	3.7	100.0	18.6	10.0	0.9	-	4.5	4.8	63	100.0
VI. KIDNEY	9	17	4	2	32	3.3	2.8	100.0	12.9	5.8	1.2	0.7	3.2	3.4	45	93.8
Wilms' tumour	8	17	3	1	29	3.0	2.5	90.6	11.4	5.8	0.9	0.3	2.9	3.1	41	100.0
Renal carcinoma	0	0	0	0	0	-	-	-	-	-	-	-	-	-	-	-
Other and unspecified	1	0	1	1	3	0.3	0.3	9.4	1.4	-	0.3	0.3	0.3	0.3	5	33.3
VII. LIVER	14	8	3	2	27	2.7	2.4	100.0	20.0	2.7	0.9	0.7	2.7	2.9	39	63.0
Hepatoblastoma	5	6	1	0	12	1.2	1.0	44.4	7.2	2.1	0.3	-	1.2	1.3	17	100.0
Hepatic carcinoma	1	0	0	1	2	0.2	0.2	7.4	1.4	-	-	0.3	0.2	0.2	3	100.0
Other and unspecified	8	2	2	1	13	1.3	1.2	48.1	11.4	0.7	0.6	0.3	1.3	1.4	19	23.1
VIII. BONE	1	2	9	27	39	4.0	5.1	100.0	1.4	0.7	2.6	9.3	3.9	3.9	64	87.2
Osteosarcoma	0	0	3	16	19	1.9	2.6	48.7	-	-	0.9	5.5	1.9	1.9	32	100.0
Chondrosarcoma	0	0	0	0	0	-	-	-	-	-	-	-	-	-	-	-
Ewing's sarcoma	1	2	2	2	7	0.7	0.8	17.9	1.4	0.7	0.6	0.7	0.7	0.7	11	100.0
Other and unspecified	0	0	4	9	13	1.3	1.7	33.3	-	-	1.2	3.1	1.3	1.3	21	61.5
IX. SOFT TISSUE SARCOMAS	17	8	12	10	47	4.8	4.7	100.0	24.3	2.7	3.5	3.5	4.7	4.9	70	100.0
Rhabdomyosarcoma	7	2	6	3	18	1.8	1.8	38.3	10.0	0.7	1.7	1.0	1.8	1.9	27	100.0
Fibrosarcoma	2	1	1	5	9	0.9	1.0	19.1	2.9	0.3	0.3	1.7	0.9	0.9	14	100.0
Other and unspecified	8	5	5	2	20	2.0	1.9	42.6	11.4	1.7	1.5	0.7	2.0	2.1	29	100.0
X. GONADAL & GERM CELL	10	5	10	20	45	4.6	5.1	100.0	14.3	1.7	2.9	6.9	4.5	4.6	70	95.6
Non-gonadal germ cell	9	3	3	0	15	1.5	1.4	33.3	12.9	1.0	0.9	-	1.5	1.6	22	100.0
Gonadal germ cell	0	1	5	18	24	2.4	3.0	53.3	-	0.3	1.5	6.2	2.4	2.4	38	100.0
Gonadal carcinoma	0	0	0	1	1	0.1	0.1	2.2	-	-	-	0.3	0.1	0.1	2	100.0
Other and unspecified	1	1	2	1	5	0.5	0.6	11.1	1.4	0.3	0.6	0.3	0.5	0.5	8	60.0
XI. EPITHELIAL NEOPLASMS	0	5	3	9	17	1.7	2.0	100.0	-	1.7	0.9	3.1	1.7	1.7	27	100.0
Adrenocortical carcinoma	0	0	0	0	0	-	-	-	-	-	-	-	-	-	-	-
Thyroid carcinoma	0	0	0	1	1	0.1	0.1	5.9	-	-	-	0.3	0.1	0.1	2	100.0
Nasopharyngeal carcinoma	0	0	0	0	0	-	-	-	-	-	-	-	-	-	-	-
Melanoma	0	2	1	2	5	0.5	0.6	29.4	-	0.7	0.3	0.7	0.5	0.5	8	100.0
Other carcinoma	0	3	2	6	11	1.1	1.3	64.7	-	1.0	0.6	2.1	1.1	1.1	17	100.0
XII. OTHER	11	11	5	7	34	3.5	3.3	100.0	15.7	3.8	1.5	2.4	3.4	3.6	50	19.4
* Specified as malignant	16	28	41	26	111	11.3	11.8	100.0	22.9	9.6	11.9	9.0	11.2	11.2	166	20.2

KUWAIT

Kuwait Cancer Registry, 1974–1982

Y. T. Omar

In 1971, the Radiotherapy Department of Al-Sabah hospital set up a departmental cancer registry. This covered only minimal data, which included age, sex, site and histology. However, it was soon realized that, to assist in the planning of a cancer control programme for the country, a population-based cancer registry was required. The creation of such a registry was possible since at that time there were only six hospitals and one pathology department in Kuwait, and there was a large network of clinics in various districts which referred suspected cancer cases to hospital. Health facilities are accessible and free of charge to the whole of the population of Kuwait. Registration was also facilitated by the small size of the country and the good road system. By 1981, the total bed capacity of the Ministry of Health hospitals was 5756 (4.1 per 1000 inhabitants) and the number of medical practitioners was 2580 (1.8 per 1000 inhabitants). There are special facilities for surgical and medical paediatric oncology.

The data collected by the Registry were expanded to include patient identification, clinical data, tumour, node, metastasis (TNM) classification, modality of treatments and their chronology, and follow-up data. The data for the five-year period 1974–1978 were extremely helpful in the planning of the extension of oncological services in Kuwait and led to the development of a comprehensive cancer control centre in 1982, the Registry becoming a separate department of this centre. A further range of data items corresponding to those recommended by WHO for hospital-based cancer registries was added in 1979, bringing the total number to 98. The Registry includes all neoplasms not specified as benign. Since 1979, diagnoses have been coded using ICD-O.

Notification of cancer is compulsory under a Ministerial Decree. The sources of information available to the Registry are: medical records of the various hospitals in Kuwait, including the Cancer Centre, all reports from pathology departments mentioning cancer, and mortality data from the Vital and Health Statistics Division of the Ministry of Health.

The data are used to: estimate cancer mortality and incidence rates; monitor trends in incidence in relation to geographical area and demographic characteristics of the population; determine the survival of cancer patients; monitor trends in survival in relation to site, extent of disease, type of therapy, demographic and other prognostic parameters; and conduct special epidemiological studies of etiology.

Cases notified from death certificates not previously recorded and for which no verification of the cause of death was available are not included in the data presented here. However, it was decided that from 1983 onwards such cases should be included in incidence figures, as this group accounted for nearly 13.7% of cases registered.

The State of Kuwait is situated in the north-western corner of the Arabian Gulf. The climate is of the dry, hot, desert type, the principal characteristics of which are the great extremes of temperature, little and variable rainfall, and frequent dust storms.

Kuwait is an oil-producing country with an area of 17 820 square kilometres. It is generally flat, with the exception of a few rocky hills ranging from 180 to 300 m above sea-level.

A national population census has been carried out every five years since 1960. According to the 1980 census, the total population was 1.4 million, of whom Kuwaiti nationals constituted 41.7%, the rest being immigrants, mainly Arab and Asian in origin.

Population

The population at risk is based on the census populations of 1975 and 1980, for both Kuwaiti nationals and non-Kuwaiti residents.

Contd. p. 198

Kuwait, Kuwaiti　　　　　　1974 - 1982　　　　　　MALE

DIAGNOSTIC GROUP	NUMBER OF CASES					REL. FREQUENCY(%)			RATES PER MILLION						HV(%)
	0	1-4	5-9	10-14	All	Crude	Adj.	Group	0-4	5-9	10-14	Crude	Adj.	Cum	
TOTAL	2	27	25	24	78	100.0	100.0	100.0	70.9	71.6	85.8	75.2	75.4	1141	97.4
I. LEUKAEMIAS	0	6	0	6	12	15.4	15.8	100.0	14.7	-	21.4	11.6	11.9	181	100.0
Acute lymphocytic	0	6	0	5	11	14.1	14.5	91.7	14.7	-	17.9	10.6	10.9	163	100.0
Other lymphocytic	0	0	0	0	0	-	-	-	-	-	-	-	-	-	-
Acute non-lymphocytic	0	0	0	1	1	1.3	1.3	8.3	-	-	3.6	1.0	1.0	18	100.0
Chronic myeloid	0	0	0	0	0	-	-	-	-	-	-	-	-	-	-
Other and unspecified	0	0	0	0	0	-	-	-	-	-	-	-	-	-	-
II. LYMPHOMAS	0	6	18	10	34	43.6	42.4	100.0	14.7	51.5	35.7	32.8	32.7	510	100.0
Hodgkin's disease	0	2	6	6	14	17.9	17.5	41.2	4.9	17.2	21.4	13.5	13.7	218	100.0
Non-Hodgkin lymphoma	0	2	11	3	16	20.5	19.7	47.1	4.9	31.5	10.7	15.4	15.2	236	100.0
Burkitt's lymphoma	0	1	0	0	1	1.3	1.4	2.9	2.4	-	-	1.3	0.9	12	100.0
Unspecified lymphoma	0	0	1	1	2	2.6	2.5	5.9	-	2.9	3.6	1.9	2.0	32	100.0
Histiocytosis X	0	1	0	0	1	1.3	1.4	2.9	2.4	-	-	1.0	0.9	12	100.0
Other reticuloendothelial	0	0	0	0	0	-	-	-	-	-	-	-	-	-	-
III. BRAIN AND SPINAL	0	3	2	0	5	6.4	6.5	100.0	7.3	5.7	-	4.8	4.7	65	80.0
Ependymoma	0	2	0	0	2	2.6	2.8	40.0	4.9	-	-	1.9	1.9	24	100.0
Astrocytoma	0	0	0	0	1	1.3	1.2	20.0	-	2.9	-	1.0	0.9	14	100.0
Medulloblastoma	0	0	0	0	0	-	-	-	-	-	-	-	-	-	-
Other glioma	0	0	1	0	1	1.3	1.2	20.0	-	2.9	-	1.0	0.9	14	100.0
Other and unspecified *	0	1	0	0	1	1.3	1.4	20.0	2.4	-	-	1.0	0.9	12	-
IV. SYMPATHETIC N.S.	1	4	0	1	6	7.7	8.1	100.0	12.2	-	3.6	5.8	5.8	79	83.3
Neuroblastoma	1	4	0	1	6	7.7	8.1	100.0	12.2	-	3.6	5.8	5.8	79	83.3
Other	0	0	0	0	0	-	-	-	-	-	-	-	-	-	-
V. RETINOBLASTOMA	1	1	0	0	2	2.6	2.8	100.0	4.9	-	-	1.9	1.9	24	100.0
VI. KIDNEY	0	3	1	1	5	6.4	6.6	100.0	7.3	2.9	3.6	4.8	4.8	69	100.0
Wilms' tumour	0	2	1	0	3	3.8	4.0	60.0	4.9	2.9	-	2.9	2.8	39	100.0
Renal carcinoma	0	0	0	1	1	1.3	1.3	20.0	-	-	3.6	1.0	1.0	18	100.0
Other and unspecified	0	1	0	0	1	1.3	1.4	20.0	2.4	-	-	1.0	0.9	12	100.0
VII. LIVER	0	0	0	0	0	-	-	-	-	-	-	-	-	-	-
Hepatoblastoma	0	0	0	0	0	-	-	-	-	-	-	-	-	-	-
Hepatic carcinoma	0	0	0	0	0	-	-	-	-	-	-	-	-	-	-
Other and unspecified	0	0	0	0	0	-	-	-	-	-	-	-	-	-	-
VIII. BONE	0	0	2	3	5	6.4	6.2	100.0	-	5.7	10.7	4.8	5.0	82	100.0
Osteosarcoma	0	0	0	3	3	3.8	3.8	60.0	-	-	10.7	2.9	3.1	54	100.0
Chondrosarcoma	0	0	0	0	0	-	-	-	-	-	-	-	-	-	-
Ewing's sarcoma	0	0	1	0	1	1.3	1.2	20.0	-	2.9	-	1.0	0.9	14	100.0
Other and unspecified	0	0	1	0	1	1.3	1.2	20.0	-	2.9	-	1.0	0.9	14	100.0
IX. SOFT TISSUE SARCOMAS	0	2	2	1	5	6.4	6.4	100.0	4.9	5.7	3.6	4.8	4.8	71	100.0
Rhabdomyosarcoma	0	2	1	1	4	5.1	5.2	80.0	4.9	2.9	3.6	3.9	3.9	57	100.0
Fibrosarcoma	0	0	0	0	0	-	-	-	-	-	-	-	-	-	-
Other and unspecified	0	0	1	0	1	1.3	1.2	20.0	-	2.9	-	1.0	0.9	14	100.0
X. GONADAL & GERM CELL	0	1	0	0	1	1.3	1.4	100.0	2.4	-	-	1.0	0.9	12	100.0
Non-gonadal germ cell	0	1	0	0	1	1.3	1.4	100.0	2.4	-	-	1.0	0.9	12	100.0
Gonadal germ cell	0	0	0	0	0	-	-	-	-	-	-	-	-	-	-
Gonadal carcinoma	0	0	0	0	0	1.3	1.4	100.0	2.4	-	-	1.0	0.9	12	100.0
Other and unspecified	0	0	0	0	0	-	-	-	-	-	-	-	-	-	-
XI. EPITHELIAL NEOPLASMS	0	1	0	2	3	3.8	3.9	100.0	2.4	-	7.1	2.9	3.0	48	100.0
Adrenocortical carcinoma	0	0	0	0	0	-	-	-	-	-	-	-	-	-	-
Thyroid carcinoma	0	0	0	0	0	-	-	-	-	-	-	-	-	-	-
Nasopharyngeal carcinoma	0	0	0	1	1	1.3	1.3	33.3	-	-	3.6	1.0	1.0	18	100.0
Melanoma	0	0	0	0	0	-	-	-	-	-	-	-	-	-	-
Other carcinoma	0	1	0	1	2	2.6	2.6	66.7	2.4	-	3.6	1.9	2.0	30	100.0
XII. OTHER	0	0	0	0	0	-	-	-	-	-	-	-	-	-	-
* Specified as malignant	0	1	0	0	1	1.3	1.4	100.0	2.4	-	-	1.0	0.9	12	-

Kuwait, Kuwaiti

1974 - 1982

FEMALE

DIAGNOSTIC GROUP	NUMBER OF CASES					REL. FREQUENCY(%)			RATES PER MILLION					Cum	HV(%)
	0	1-4	5-9	10-14	All	Crude	Adj.	Group	0-4	5-9	10-14	Crude	Adj.		
TOTAL	5	24	18	17	64	100.0	100.0	100.0	73.0	52.3	62.1	63.1	63.2	937	96.9
I. LEUKAEMIAS	2	5	2	5	14	21.9	21.8	100.0	17.6	5.8	18.3	13.8	14.0	209	100.0
Acute lymphocytic	2	5	2	4	13	20.3	20.0	92.9	17.6	5.8	14.6	12.8	12.9	190	100.0
Other lymphocytic	0	0	0	0	0	-	-	-	-	-	-	-	-	-	-
Acute non-lymphocytic	0	0	0	1	1	1.6	1.8	7.1	-	-	3.7	1.0	1.1	18	100.0
Chronic myeloid	0	0	0	0	0	-	-	-	-	-	-	-	-	-	-
Other and unspecified	0	0	0	0	0	-	-	-	-	-	-	-	-	-	-
II. LYMPHOMAS	0	6	9	4	19	29.7	30.3	100.0	15.1	26.1	14.6	18.7	18.5	279	94.7
Hodgkin's disease	0	1	3	3	7	10.9	11.7	36.8	2.5	8.7	11.0	6.9	7.0	111	100.0
Non-Hodgkin lymphoma	0	2	2	1	5	7.8	7.9	26.3	5.0	5.8	3.7	4.9	4.9	73	80.0
Burkitt's lymphoma	0	3	3	0	6	9.4	9.1	31.6	7.6	8.7	-	5.9	5.7	81	100.0
Unspecified lymphoma	0	0	0	0	0	-	-	-	-	-	-	-	-	-	-
Histiocytosis X	0	0	0	0	0	-	-	-	-	-	-	-	-	-	-
Other reticuloendothelial	0	0	1	0	1	1.6	1.7	5.3	-	2.9	-	1.0	0.9	15	100.0
III. BRAIN AND SPINAL	0	0	2	3	5	7.8	8.6	100.0	-	5.8	11.0	4.9	5.1	84	80.0
Ependymoma	0	0	0	1	1	1.6	1.8	20.0	-	-	3.7	1.0	1.1	18	100.0
Astrocytoma	0	0	1	2	3	4.7	5.2	60.0	-	2.9	7.3	3.0	3.1	51	100.0
Medulloblastoma	0	0	0	0	0	-	-	-	-	-	-	-	-	-	-
Other glioma	0	0	0	0	0	-	-	-	-	-	-	-	-	-	-
Other and unspecified *	0	0	1	0	1	1.6	1.7	20.0	-	2.9	-	1.0	0.9	15	-
IV. SYMPATHETIC N.S.	1	2	1	1	5	7.8	7.6	100.0	7.6	2.9	3.7	4.9	4.9	71	100.0
Neuroblastoma	1	2	1	1	5	7.8	7.6	100.0	7.6	2.9	3.7	4.9	4.9	71	100.0
Other	0	0	0	0	0	-	-	-	-	-	-	-	-	-	-
V. RETINOBLASTOMA	0	3	0	0	3	4.7	4.1	100.0	7.6	-	-	3.0	2.9	38	100.0
VI. KIDNEY	0	6	0	0	6	9.4	8.3	100.0	15.1	-	-	5.9	5.8	76	100.0
Wilms' tumour	0	5	0	0	5	7.8	6.9	83.3	12.6	-	-	4.9	4.9	63	100.0
Renal carcinoma	0	0	0	0	0	-	-	-	-	-	-	-	-	-	-
Other and unspecified	0	1	0	0	1	1.6	1.4	16.7	2.5	-	-	1.0	1.0	13	100.0
VII. LIVER	1	0	0	0	1	1.6	1.4	100.0	2.5	-	-	1.0	1.0	13	100.0
Hepatoblastoma	1	0	0	0	1	1.6	1.4	100.0	2.5	-	-	1.0	1.0	13	100.0
Hepatic carcinoma	0	0	0	0	0	-	-	-	-	-	-	-	-	-	-
Other and unspecified	0	0	0	0	0	-	-	-	-	-	-	-	-	-	-
VIII. BONE	1	1	1	3	6	9.4	9.7	100.0	5.0	2.9	11.0	5.9	6.1	95	100.0
Osteosarcoma	0	0	0	2	2	3.1	3.5	33.3	-	-	7.3	2.0	2.1	37	100.0
Chondrosarcoma	0	0	0	0	0	-	-	-	-	-	-	-	-	-	-
Ewing's sarcoma	0	1	1	1	3	4.7	4.8	50.0	2.5	2.9	3.7	3.0	3.0	45	100.0
Other and unspecified	1	0	0	0	1	1.6	1.4	16.7	2.5	-	-	1.0	1.0	13	100.0
IX. SOFT TISSUE SARCOMAS	0	1	1	1	3	4.7	4.8	100.0	2.5	2.9	3.7	3.0	3.0	45	100.0
Rhabdomyosarcoma	0	1	0	1	2	3.1	3.1	66.7	2.5	-	3.7	2.0	2.0	31	100.0
Fibrosarcoma	0	0	0	0	0	-	-	-	-	-	-	-	-	-	-
Other and unspecified	0	0	1	0	1	1.6	1.7	33.3	-	2.9	-	1.0	0.9	15	100.0
X. GONADAL & GERM CELL	0	0	0	0	0	-	-	-	-	-	-	-	-	-	-
Non-gonadal germ cell	0	0	0	0	0	-	-	-	-	-	-	-	-	-	-
Gonadal germ cell	0	0	0	0	0	-	-	-	-	-	-	-	-	-	-
Gonadal carcinoma	0	0	0	0	0	-	-	-	-	-	-	-	-	-	-
Other and unspecified	0	0	0	0	0	-	-	-	-	-	-	-	-	-	-
XI. EPITHELIAL NEOPLASMS	0	0	2	0	2	3.1	3.3	100.0	-	5.8	-	2.0	1.9	29	100.0
Adrenocortical carcinoma	0	0	0	0	0	-	-	-	-	-	-	-	-	-	-
Thyroid carcinoma	0	0	0	0	0	-	-	-	-	-	-	-	-	-	-
Nasopharyngeal carcinoma	0	0	0	0	0	-	-	-	-	-	-	-	-	-	-
Melanoma	0	0	0	0	0	-	-	-	-	-	-	-	-	-	-
Other carcinoma	0	0	2	0	2	3.1	3.3	100.0	-	5.8	-	2.0	1.9	29	100.0
XII. OTHER	0	0	0	0	0	-	-	-	-	-	-	-	-	-	-
* Specified as malignant	0	0	1	0	1	1.6	1.7	100.0	-	2.9	-	1.0	0.9	15	-

Kuwait, non Kuwaiti

1974 – 1982 MALE

DIAGNOSTIC GROUP	NUMBER OF CASES 0	1-4	5-9	10-14	All	REL. FREQUENCY(%) Crude	Adj.	Group	RATES PER MILLION 0-4	5-9	10-14	Crude	Adj.	Cum	HV(%)
TOTAL	6	67	45	23	141	100.0	100.0	100.0	187.0	134.3	94.1	145.4	143.0	2077	57.1
I. LEUKAEMIAS	0	19	15	3	37	26.2	24.3	100.0	48.7	44.8	12.3	38.1	36.8	529	81.1
Acute lymphocytic	0	19	14	3	36	25.5	23.7	97.3	48.7	41.8	12.3	37.1	35.9	514	80.6
Other lymphocytic	0	0	0	0	0	-	-	-	-	-	-	-	-	-	-
Acute non-lymphocytic	0	0	1	0	1	0.7	0.7	2.7	-	3.0	-	1.0	1.0	15	100.0
Chronic myeloid	0	0	0	0	0	-	-	-	-	-	-	-	-	-	-
Other and unspecified	0	0	0	0	0	-	-	-	-	-	-	-	-	-	-
II. LYMPHOMAS	0	17	15	6	38	27.0	27.1	100.0	43.6	44.8	24.5	39.2	38.4	564	56.8
Hodgkin's disease	0	3	7	2	12	8.5	8.9	31.6	7.7	20.9	8.2	12.4	12.1	184	63.6
Non-Hodgkin lymphoma	0	6	5	3	14	9.9	10.5	36.8	15.4	14.9	12.3	14.4	14.3	213	35.7
Burkitt's lymphoma	0	2	2	0	4	2.8	2.4	10.5	5.1	6.0	-	4.1	3.9	55	100.0
Unspecified lymphoma	0	0	0	1	1	0.7	1.3	2.6	-	-	4.1	1.0	1.2	20	-
Histiocytosis X	0	5	0	0	5	3.5	2.7	13.2	12.8	-	-	5.2	5.0	64	80.0
Other reticuloendothelial	0	1	1	0	2	1.4	1.2	5.3	2.6	3.0	-	2.1	2.0	28	50.0
III. BRAIN AND SPINAL	1	4	6	2	13	9.2	9.3	100.0	12.8	17.9	8.2	13.4	13.1	194	38.5
Ependymoma	0	1	1	0	2	1.4	1.2	15.4	2.6	3.0	-	2.1	2.0	28	50.0
Astrocytoma	1	1	1	1	4	2.8	3.1	30.8	5.1	3.0	4.1	4.1	4.1	61	75.0
Medulloblastoma	0	1	1	0	2	1.4	1.2	15.4	2.6	3.0	-	2.1	2.0	28	50.0
Other glioma	0	1	0	0	1	0.7	0.5	7.7	2.6	-	-	1.0	1.0	13	-
Other and unspecified *	0	0	3	1	4	2.8	3.3	30.8	-	9.0	4.1	4.1	4.1	65	-
IV. SYMPATHETIC N.S.	0	4	2	1	7	5.0	4.8	100.0	10.2	6.0	4.1	7.2	7.1	102	71.4
Neuroblastoma	0	4	2	1	7	5.0	4.8	100.0	10.2	6.0	4.1	7.2	7.1	102	71.4
Other	0	0	0	0	0	-	-	-	-	-	-	-	-	-	-
V. RETINOBLASTOMA	1	4	1	0	6	4.3	3.4	100.0	12.8	3.0	-	6.2	5.9	79	16.7
VI. KIDNEY	1	4	3	0	8	5.7	4.7	100.0	12.8	9.0	-	8.2	7.8	109	62.5
Wilms' tumour	1	4	2	0	7	5.0	4.1	87.5	12.8	6.0	-	7.2	6.9	94	57.1
Renal carcinoma	0	0	0	0	0	-	-	-	-	-	-	-	-	-	-
Other and unspecified	0	0	1	0	1	0.7	0.7	12.5	-	3.0	-	1.0	1.0	15	100.0
VII. LIVER	2	0	0	0	2	1.4	1.1	100.0	5.1	-	-	2.1	2.0	26	-
Hepatoblastoma	2	0	0	0	2	1.4	1.1	100.0	5.1	-	-	2.1	2.0	26	-
Hepatic carcinoma	0	0	0	0	0	-	-	-	-	-	-	-	-	-	-
Other and unspecified	0	0	0	0	0	-	-	-	-	-	-	-	-	-	-
VIII. BONE	0	2	1	7	10	7.1	10.9	100.0	5.1	3.0	28.6	10.3	11.3	184	50.0
Osteosarcoma	0	0	1	1	2	1.4	2.0	20.0	-	3.0	4.1	2.1	2.2	35	-
Chondrosarcoma	0	0	0	1	1	0.7	1.3	10.0	-	-	4.1	1.0	1.2	20	100.0
Ewing's sarcoma	0	2	0	5	7	5.0	7.6	70.0	5.1	-	20.5	7.2	7.9	128	57.1
Other and unspecified	0	0	0	0	0	-	-	-	-	-	-	-	-	-	-
IX. SOFT TISSUE SARCOMAS	1	6	0	1	8	5.7	5.1	100.0	17.9	-	4.1	8.2	8.1	110	62.5
Rhabdomyosarcoma	1	3	0	0	4	2.8	2.2	50.0	10.2	-	-	4.1	4.0	51	50.0
Fibrosarcoma	0	1	0	0	1	0.7	0.5	12.5	2.6	-	-	1.0	1.0	13	100.0
Other and unspecified	0	2	0	1	3	2.1	2.4	37.5	5.1	-	4.1	3.1	3.2	46	66.7
X. GONADAL & GERM CELL	0	2	2	0	4	2.8	2.4	100.0	5.1	6.0	-	4.1	3.9	55	25.0
Non-gonadal germ cell	0	1	0	0	1	0.7	0.5	25.0	2.6	-	-	1.0	1.0	13	100.0
Gonadal germ cell	0	1	1	0	2	1.4	1.2	50.0	2.6	3.0	-	2.1	2.0	28	-
Gonadal carcinoma	0	0	0	0	0	-	-	-	-	-	-	-	-	-	-
Other and unspecified	0	0	1	0	1	0.7	0.7	25.0	-	3.0	-	1.0	1.0	15	-
XI. EPITHELIAL NEOPLASMS	0	1	0	2	3	2.1	3.2	100.0	2.6	-	8.2	3.1	3.4	54	33.3
Adrenocortical carcinoma	0	0	0	0	0	-	-	-	-	-	-	-	-	-	-
Thyroid carcinoma	0	0	0	1	1	0.7	1.3	33.3	-	-	4.1	1.0	1.2	20	100.0
Nasopharyngeal carcinoma	0	0	0	1	1	0.7	1.3	33.3	-	-	4.1	1.0	1.2	20	-
Melanoma	0	0	0	0	0	-	-	-	-	-	-	-	-	-	-
Other carcinoma	0	1	0	0	1	0.7	0.5	33.3	2.6	-	-	1.0	1.0	13	-
XII. OTHER	0	4	0	1	5	3.5	3.5	100.0	10.2	-	4.1	5.2	5.2	72	20.0
* Specified as malignant	0	0	3	0	3	2.1	2.0	100.0	-	9.0	-	3.1	2.9	45	-

Kuwait, non Kuwaiti

1974 - 1982

FEMALE

DIAGNOSTIC GROUP	NUMBER OF CASES					REL. FREQUENCY(%)			RATES PER MILLION						HV(%)
	0	1-4	5-9	10-14	All	Crude	Adj.	Group	0-4	5-9	10-14	Crude	Adj.	Cum	
TOTAL	12	37	37	11	97	100.0	100.0	100.0	130.4	115.6	47.5	104.6	101.6	1468	62.5
I. LEUKAEMIAS	1	14	12	4	31	32.0	32.9	100.0	39.9	37.5	17.3	33.4	32.6	473	93.5
Acute lymphocytic	1	14	10	3	28	28.9	28.5	90.3	39.9	31.2	13.0	30.2	29.3	421	92.9
Other lymphocytic	0	0	0	0	0	-	-	-	-	-	-	-	-	-	-
Acute non-lymphocytic	0	0	1	1	2	2.1	3.5	6.5	-	3.1	4.3	2.2	2.3	37	100.0
Chronic myeloid	0	0	1	0	1	1.0	0.8	3.2	-	3.1	-	1.1	1.1	16	100.0
Other and unspecified	0	0	0	0	0	-	-	-	-	-	-	-	-	-	-
II. LYMPHOMAS	0	7	10	4	21	21.6	24.7	100.0	18.6	31.2	17.3	22.6	22.3	336	40.0
Hodgkin's disease	0	1	5	1	7	7.2	7.6	33.3	2.7	15.6	4.3	7.5	7.3	113	42.9
Non-Hodgkin lymphoma	0	5	3	3	11	11.3	14.7	52.4	13.3	9.4	13.0	11.9	11.9	178	30.0
Burkitt's lymphoma	0	0	0	0	0	-	-	-	-	-	-	-	-	-	-
Unspecified lymphoma	0	1	0	0	1	1.0	0.8	4.8	2.7	-	-	1.1	1.0	13	-
Histiocytosis X	0	0	2	0	2	2.1	1.6	9.5	-	6.2	-	2.2	2.0	31	100.0
Other reticuloendothelial	0	0	0	0	0	-	-	-	-	-	-	-	-	-	-
III. BRAIN AND SPINAL	2	0	7	1	10	10.3	10.0	100.0	5.3	21.9	4.3	10.8	10.4	158	50.0
Ependymoma	0	0	0	1	1	1.0	2.7	10.0	-	-	4.3	1.1	1.3	22	100.0
Astrocytoma	1	0	3	0	4	4.1	3.2	40.0	2.7	9.4	-	4.3	4.1	60	50.0
Medulloblastoma	1	0	2	0	3	3.1	2.4	30.0	2.7	6.2	-	3.2	3.0	45	33.3
Other glioma	0	0	1	0	1	1.0	0.8	10.0	-	3.1	-	1.1	1.0	16	100.0
Other and unspecified *	0	0	1	0	1	1.0	0.8	10.0	-	3.1	-	1.1	1.0	16	-
IV. SYMPATHETIC N.S.	6	6	1	0	13	13.4	10.6	100.0	31.9	3.1	-	14.0	13.4	175	53.8
Neuroblastoma	6	6	1	0	13	13.4	10.6	100.0	31.9	3.1	-	14.0	13.4	175	53.8
Other	0	0	0	0	0	-	-	-	-	-	-	-	-	-	-
V. RETINOBLASTOMA	0	2	0	0	2	2.1	1.6	100.0	5.3	-	-	2.2	2.1	27	50.0
VI. KIDNEY	0	4	1	0	5	5.2	4.1	100.0	10.6	3.1	-	5.4	5.1	69	40.0
Wilms' tumour	0	4	1	0	5	5.2	4.1	100.0	10.6	3.1	-	5.4	5.1	69	40.0
Renal carcinoma	0	0	0	0	0	-	-	-	-	-	-	-	-	-	-
Other and unspecified	0	0	0	0	0	-	-	-	-	-	-	-	-	-	-
VII. LIVER	2	1	0	0	3	3.1	2.4	100.0	8.0	-	-	3.2	3.1	40	66.7
Hepatoblastoma	1	1	0	0	2	2.1	1.6	66.7	5.3	-	-	2.2	2.1	27	50.0
Hepatic carcinoma	1	0	0	0	1	1.0	0.8	33.3	2.7	-	-	1.1	1.0	13	100.0
Other and unspecified	0	0	0	0	0	-	-	-	-	-	-	-	-	-	-
VIII. BONE	0	0	3	0	3	3.1	2.4	100.0	-	9.4	-	3.2	3.0	47	100.0
Osteosarcoma	0	0	1	0	1	1.0	0.8	33.3	-	3.1	-	1.1	1.0	16	100.0
Chondrosarcoma	0	0	0	0	0	-	-	-	-	-	-	-	-	-	-
Ewing's sarcoma	0	0	2	0	2	2.1	1.6	66.7	-	6.2	-	2.2	2.0	31	100.0
Other and unspecified	0	0	0	0	0	-	-	-	-	-	-	-	-	-	-
IX. SOFT TISSUE SARCOMAS	0	0	0	0	0	-	-	-	-	-	-	-	-	-	-
Rhabdomyosarcoma	0	0	0	0	0	-	-	-	-	-	-	-	-	-	-
Fibrosarcoma	0	0	0	0	0	-	-	-	-	-	-	-	-	-	-
Other and unspecified	0	0	0	0	0	-	-	-	-	-	-	-	-	-	-
X. GONADAL & GERM CELL	0	1	1	1	3	3.1	4.4	100.0	2.7	3.1	4.3	3.2	3.3	51	66.7
Non-gonadal germ cell	0	1	1	0	2	2.1	1.6	66.7	2.7	3.1	-	2.2	2.0	29	100.0
Gonadal germ cell	0	0	0	1	1	1.0	2.7	33.3	-	-	4.3	1.1	1.3	22	-
Gonadal carcinoma	0	0	0	0	0	-	-	-	-	-	-	-	-	-	-
Other and unspecified	0	0	0	0	0	-	-	-	-	-	-	-	-	-	-
XI. EPITHELIAL NEOPLASMS	0	1	2	0	3	3.1	2.4	100.0	2.7	6.2	-	3.2	3.0	45	33.3
Adrenocortical carcinoma	0	0	0	0	0	-	-	-	-	-	-	-	-	-	-
Thyroid carcinoma	0	0	1	0	1	1.0	0.8	33.3	-	3.1	-	1.1	1.0	16	100.0
Nasopharyngeal carcinoma	0	0	1	0	1	1.0	0.8	33.3	-	3.1	-	1.1	1.0	16	-
Melanoma	0	0	0	0	0	-	-	-	-	-	-	-	-	-	-
Other carcinoma	0	1	0	0	1	1.0	0.8	33.3	2.7	-	-	1.1	1.0	13	-
XII. OTHER	1	1	0	1	3	3.1	4.4	100.0	5.3	-	4.3	3.2	3.3	48	33.3
* Specified as malignant	0	0	1	0	1	1.0	0.8	100.0	-	3.1	-	1.1	1.0	16	-

AVERAGE ANNUAL POPULATION: 1974–1982

Age	Male	Female
Kuwaiti		
0–4	45416	44133
5–9	38813	38251
10–14	31094	30397
0–14	115323	112781
Non-Kuwaiti		
0–4	43366	41745
5–9	37241	35570
10–14	27162	25723
0–14	107769	103038

Commentary

The predominant diagnostic group was the lymphomas, accounting for 30% of all cases. Incidence rates were very high both for Hodgkin's disease and for other lymphomas. Leukaemia was somewhat less common than in Western populations, but over 90% of leukaemias were acute lymphocytic leukaemia. Only 8.7% of registrations were for brain and spinal tumours, in part due to the fact that only two non-malignant tumours are included. Overall, the incidence rate for non-Kuwaitis was 1.8 times that for Kuwaitis. The ratio of rates for non-Kuwaitis to Kuwaitis for individual major diagnostic groups ranged from 2.7:1 for leukaemias to 1.1:1 for soft-tissue sarcomas. Hodgkin's disease was slightly more common in Kuwaitis than in non-Kuwaitis.

PAKISTAN

Jinnah Post-graduate Medical Centre: 1979–1983

N.A. Jafarey & S.H.M. Zaidi

Jinnah Post-graduate Medical Centre (JPMC) is a major government hospital, offering free treatment and providing the only radiotherapy service in Karachi. It acts as a referral centre for a large number of hospitals and clinics, and contains a 200-bed children's hospital. It provides the only specialized oncological service for Karachi and the southern part of Sind Province.

A cancer registry, which receives information primarily from the Department of Radiotherapy, and the Department of Pathology, was established in the hospital in 1968. The information abstracted from the hospital records includes name, father's name, present and permanent address, sex, age, year of birth, mother tongue, duration of symptoms, diagnostic criteria, histopathological diagnosis and final diagnosis. The great majority of cases come from the District of Karachi (population in 1981: 5.44 million), with some from neighbouring parts of the Provinces of Sind and Baluchistan.

Although JPMC is the only hospital in the city providing special cancer facilities, not all cases diagnosed as cancer in other hospitals and laboratories are sent to the Centre and thus included in the registry.

The data from JPMC were included in a multicentre study in Pakistan, funded by the Pakistan Medical Research Council, and comprising since 1977, five different centres.

Previous results concerning childhood cancer cases seen in JPMC have been published by the present investigators for the periods 1968–1973 (Zaidi & Jafarey, 1977), and 1974–1978 (Khan *et al.*, 1983).

The tables show the numbers and frequencies of cases registered in the five-year period 1979–1983.

Commentary

Hodgkin's disease was particularly frequent, accounting for 15% of all registrations. Just over 10% of registrations were for retinoblastoma, which was twice as frequent as Wilms' tumour. There were no cases of neuroblastoma. There were 59 cases (18% of the total) in the 'other' group, almost entirely histologically unverified. These included eight boys and four girls with eye tumours.

References

Khan, A.B., Mc Keen, E.A. & Zaidi, S.H.M. (1983) Childhood cancer in Pakistan, with special reference to retinoblastoma. *J. Pakistan med. Assoc.*, *33*, 66-70

Zaidi, S.H.M. & Jafarey, N.A. (1977) Childhood tumours in Karachi. *J. Pakistan med. Assoc.*, *27*, 346-348

Pakistan, JPMC　　　　　　1979 - 1983　　　　　　MALE

DIAGNOSTIC GROUP	NUMBER OF CASES					REL. FREQUENCY(%)			HV(%)
	0	1-4	5-9	10-14	All	Crude	Adj.	Group	
TOTAL	8	62	66	72	212□	100.0	100.0	100.0	73.1
I. LEUKAEMIAS	0	5	8	5	18	8.5	8.6	100.0	94.4
Acute lymphocytic	0	4	6	3	13	6.1	6.3	72.2	100.0
Other lymphocytic	0	0	0	1	1	0.5	0.6	5.6	100.0
Acute non-lymphocytic	0	0	1	0	1	0.5	0.4	5.6	100.0
Chronic myeloid	0	0	0	0	0	-	-	-	-
Other and unspecified	0	0	2	1	3	1.4	1.3	16.7	66.7
II. LYMPHOMAS	2	10	21	25	59□	27.8	26.8	100.0	100.0
Hodgkin's disease	0	6	16	18	40	18.9	18.2	67.8	100.0
Non-Hodgkin lymphoma	1	4	4	4	13	6.1	6.3	22.0	100.0
Burkitt's lymphoma	0	0	0	0	1□	0.5	0.5	1.7	100.0
Unspecified lymphoma	1	0	1	2	4	1.9	1.9	6.8	100.0
Histiocytosis X	0	0	0	0	0	-	-	-	-
Other reticuloendothelial	0	0	0	1	1	0.5	0.4	1.7	100.0
III. BRAIN AND SPINAL	1	4	8	4	17	8.0	8.2	100.0	52.9
Ependymoma	0	0	0	0	0	-	-	-	-
Astrocytoma	0	0	3	3	6	2.8	2.6	35.3	100.0
Medulloblastoma	0	1	1	1	3	1.4	1.4	17.6	100.0
Other glioma	0	0	0	0	0	-	-	-	-
Other and unspecified *	1	3	4	0	8	3.8	4.1	47.1	-
IV. SYMPATHETIC N.S.	0	0	0	0	0	-	-	-	-
Neuroblastoma	0	0	0	0	0	-	-	-	-
Other	0	0	0	0	0	-	-	-	-
V. RETINOBLASTOMA	0	16	3	0	19	9.0	10.5	100.0	100.0
VI. KIDNEY	4	7	1	0	12	5.7	6.7	100.0	83.3
Wilms' tumour	3	6	1	0	10	4.7	5.6	83.3	100.0
Renal carcinoma	0	0	0	0	0	-	-	-	-
Other and unspecified	1	1	0	0	2	0.9	1.1	16.7	-
VII. LIVER	1	0	2	0	3	1.4	1.4	100.0	100.0
Hepatoblastoma	1	0	0	0	1	0.5	0.6	33.3	100.0
Hepatic carcinoma	0	0	2	0	2	0.9	0.8	66.7	100.0
Other and unspecified	0	0	0	0	0	-	-	-	-
VIII. BONE	0	1	4	11	17□	8.0	7.0	100.0	70.6
Osteosarcoma	0	0	0	3	3	1.4	1.3	17.6	100.0
Chondrosarcoma	0	0	0	1	1	0.5	0.4	5.9	100.0
Ewing's sarcoma	0	1	2	3	6	2.8	2.7	35.3	100.0
Other and unspecified	0	0	2	4	7□	3.3	2.6	41.2	28.6
IX. SOFT TISSUE SARCOMAS	0	2	4	3	9	4.2	4.2	100.0	100.0
Rhabdomyosarcoma	0	1	1	0	2	0.9	1.0	22.2	100.0
Fibrosarcoma	0	1	0	1	2	0.9	1.0	22.2	100.0
Other and unspecified	0	0	3	2	5	2.4	2.2	55.6	100.0
X. GONADAL & GERM CELL	0	4	1	0	7□	3.3	2.7	100.0	71.4
Non-gonadal germ cell	0	4	0	0	4□	1.9	1.7	57.1	100.0
Gonadal germ cell	0	0	0	0	0	-	-	-	-
Gonadal carcinoma	0	0	0	0	0	-	-	-	-
Other and unspecified	0	0	1	0	3□	1.4	1.0	42.9	33.3
XI. EPITHELIAL NEOPLASMS	0	2	3	6	11	5.2	5.0	100.0	100.0
Adrenocortical carcinoma	0	0	0	0	0	-	-	-	-
Thyroid carcinoma	0	0	1	0	1	0.5	0.5	9.1	100.0
Nasopharyngeal carcinoma	0	0	0	2	2	0.9	0.8	18.2	100.0
Melanoma	0	2	1	0	3	1.4	1.6	27.3	100.0
Other carcinoma	0	0	1	4	5	2.4	2.1	45.5	100.0
XII. OTHER	0	11	13	16	40	18.9	18.9	100.0	2.5
* Specified as malignant	1	3	4	0	8	3.8	4.1	100.0	-

□ Includes age unknown

Pakistan, JPMC FEMALE

1979 - 1983

DIAGNOSTIC GROUP	NUMBER OF CASES					REL. FREQUENCY(%)			HV(%)
	0	1-4	5-9	10-14	All	Crude	Adj.	Group	
TOTAL	3	33	44	39	119	100.0	100.0	100.0	71.4
I. LEUKAEMIAS	0	2	4	4	10	8.4	8.0	100.0	100.0
Acute lymphocytic	0	1	2	3	6	5.0	4.8	60.0	100.0
Other lymphocytic	0	0	0	0	0	–	–	–	–
Acute non-lymphocytic	0	1	1	1	3	2.5	2.6	30.0	100.0
Chronic myeloid	0	0	0	0	0	–	–	–	–
Other and unspecified	0	0	1	0	1	0.8	0.7	10.0	100.0
II. LYMPHOMAS	0	2	6	5	13	10.9	10.2	100.0	100.0
Hodgkin's disease	0	2	4	3	9	7.6	7.3	69.2	100.0
Non-Hodgkin lymphoma	0	0	2	0	2	1.7	1.5	15.4	100.0
Burkitt's lymphoma	0	0	0	0	0	–	–	–	–
Unspecified lymphoma	0	0	1	0	1	0.8	0.7	7.7	100.0
Histiocytosis X	0	0	0	0	0	–	–	–	–
Other reticuloendothelial	0	0	1	0	1	0.8	0.7	7.7	100.0
III. BRAIN AND SPINAL	0	1	10	4	15	12.6	11.0	100.0	53.3
Ependymoma	0	0	0	0	0	–	–	–	–
Astrocytoma	0	0	6	1	7	5.9	4.9	46.7	100.0
Medulloblastoma	0	0	1	0	1	0.8	0.7	6.7	100.0
Other glioma	0	0	0	0	0	–	–	–	–
Other and unspecified *	0	1	3	3	7	5.9	5.5	46.7	100.0
IV. SYMPATHETIC N.S.	0	0	1	0	1	0.8	0.7	100.0	100.0
Neuroblastoma	0	0	0	0	0	–	–	–	–
Other	0	0	1	0	1	0.8	0.7	100.0	100.0
V. RETINOBLASTOMA	0	12	2	1	15	12.6	15.5	100.0	100.0
VI. KIDNEY	0	3	2	0	5	4.2	4.7	100.0	80.0
Wilms' tumour	0	1	1	0	2	1.7	1.8	40.0	100.0
Renal carcinoma	0	2	0	0	2	1.7	2.2	40.0	100.0
Other and unspecified	0	0	1	0	1	0.8	0.7	20.0	–
VII. LIVER	0	1	0	0	1	0.8	1.1	100.0	100.0
Hepatoblastoma	0	0	0	0	0	–	–	–	–
Hepatic carcinoma	0	1	0	0	1	0.8	1.1	100.0	100.0
Other and unspecified	0	0	0	0	0	–	–	–	–
VIII. BONE	0	1	8	9	18	15.1	13.5	100.0	61.1
Osteosarcoma	0	1	0	2	3	2.5	2.6	16.7	100.0
Chondrosarcoma	0	0	1	0	1	0.8	0.8	5.6	100.0
Ewing's sarcoma	0	0	2	1	3	2.5	2.1	16.7	100.0
Other and unspecified	0	0	5	6	11	9.2	7.9	61.1	36.4
IX. SOFT TISSUE SARCOMAS	1	0	3	3	7	5.9	5.5	100.0	100.0
Rhabdomyosarcoma	0	0	0	0	0	–	–	–	–
Fibrosarcoma	0	0	1	1	2	1.7	1.5	28.6	100.0
Other and unspecified	1	0	2	2	5	4.2	4.0	71.4	100.0
X. GONADAL & GERM CELL	1	3	0	5	9	7.6	8.3	100.0	100.0
Non-gonadal germ cell	1	2	0	0	3	2.5	3.3	33.3	100.0
Gonadal germ cell	0	1	0	4	5	4.2	4.2	55.6	100.0
Gonadal carcinoma	0	0	0	0	0	–	–	–	–
Other and unspecified	0	0	0	1	1	0.8	0.8	11.1	100.0
XI. EPITHELIAL NEOPLASMS	0	0	2	4	6	5.0	4.4	100.0	100.0
Adrenocortical carcinoma	0	0	0	1	1	0.8	0.8	16.7	100.0
Thyroid carcinoma	0	0	0	0	0	–	–	–	–
Nasopharyngeal carcinoma	0	0	0	0	0	–	–	–	–
Melanoma	0	0	0	0	0	–	–	–	–
Other carcinoma	0	0	2	3	5	4.2	3.7	83.3	100.0
XII. OTHER	1	8	6	4	19	16.0	17.2	100.0	–
* Specified as malignant	0	1	3	3	7	5.9	5.5	100.0	–

□ Includes age unknown

PHILIPPINES

Metro Manila and Rizal Province, 1980–1982

T. Maramba (Central Tumor Registry of the Philippines),
A.V. Laudico & D. Esteban (Rizal Medical Center Cancer Registry)

Two population-based registries are located in the urban area of Metro Manila: the Central Tumor Registry of the Philippines (CTRP), which covers the population of the four cities (Manila, Caloocan, Pasay and Quezon City) at the centre of the area, and the Rizal Medical Center Cancer Registry (RMCCR), which covers the original province of Rizal with its 26 municipalities (see Fig. 3). At present, 12 of the municipalities of Rizal, together with the four cities and Valenzuela, a former municipality of Bulacan province, form the National Capital Region or metropolitan Manila (Valenzuela is not covered by either registry).

The CTRP was established in 1967 as a joint project of the Department of Health of the national Government and the Philippine Cancer Society. It was started as a hospital-based registry, passively collecting data from 25 hospitals, 24 in Metro Manila and one in the Visayan region. The aims of the registry were to:

— provide data on the survival of patients with cancer at different sites and in relation to treatment methods;

— classify by cancer site the patients treated annually;

— provide data on the methods of treatment used over time;

— describe the stage at diagnosis and monitor changes over time;

— provide data for planning cancer facilities and services.

The sources of data were the medical records (for both in-patients and out-patients), radiotherapy records and pathology files of the 25 hospitals covered, and, from 1975 to 1977, death certificates from the local civil registries. After a review of the operation of the CTRP in 1983, it was decided to convert the registry to a population-based one, as described below.

The RMCCR, a population-based registry, was founded in July 1974 as one of the projects of the Community Cancer Control Programme of Rizal. It covers the original province of Rizal with its 26 municipalities, encompassing a land area of 1860 square kilometres. The catchment area was maintained by the Registry in spite of the division of the province in 1975 (12 municipalities were incorporated into metropolitan Manila).

Initially, data collection was passive and reports were received from government and private hospitals and physicians in Metro Manila and Rizal. A high degree of under-reporting was noted. In 1980, active data collection was started retrospectively for the years 1977–1979, covering 61 primary, secondary and tertiary hospitals in the area. Cancer registry clerks were trained to abstract data on cancer patients resident in Rizal, both from hospital records and from death certificates. In 1983, the CTRP adopted the same method of data collection and the two registries worked together in a joint effort to cover 72 hospitals and 30 local civil registries. The CTRP registry clerks visited 47 hospitals, while the RMCCR clerks visited 25 hospitals. Each group gathered data for both registries for the years 1980–1982. Regular meetings were held to solve any problems and to exchange data between the registries. Death certificate abstracts were also gathered, the CTRP covering the four cities and the RMCCR the 26 municipalities.

Data sources include: medical records (out-patients and in-patients); pathology and haematology records; radiology, radiotherapy and chemotherapy records; nuclear medicine and ultrasonography reports; and hospital tumour registries and death certificates.

Hospital abstracts are checked for duplication and are subsequently cross-matched with the alpha-

Contd p. 206

Philippines, Metro Manila & Rizal   1980 - 1982   MALE

DIAGNOSTIC GROUP	\	NUMBER OF CASES				REL. FREQUENCY(%)			RATES PER MILLION						Cum	HV(%)
	0	1-4	5-9	10-14	All	Crude	Adj.	Group	0	1-4	5-9	10-14	Crude	Adj.		
TOTAL	17	114	92	96	319	100.0	100.0	100.0	51.0	110.3	87.8	100.6	94.7	95.6	1434	96.6
I. LEUKAEMIAS	11	60	58	41	170	53.3	53.4	100.0	33.0	58.0	55.3	43.0	50.4	50.8	757	99.0
Acute lymphocytic	3	34	25	20	82	25.7	25.7	48.2	9.0	32.9	23.8	21.0	24.3	24.7	365	100.0
Other lymphocytic	0	1	3	0	4	1.3	1.3	2.4	-	1.0	2.9	-	1.2	1.2	18	100.0
Acute non-lymphocytic	1	2	8	5	16	5.0	5.1	9.4	3.0	1.9	7.6	5.2	4.7	4.8	75	100.0
Chronic myeloid	0	0	1	3	4	1.3	1.3	2.4	-	-	1.0	3.1	1.2	1.2	20	100.0
Other and unspecified	7	23	21	13	64	20.1	20.1	37.6	21.0	22.3	20.0	13.6	19.0	18.9	278	94.7
II. LYMPHOMAS	1	10	12	11	34	10.7	10.7	100.0	3.0	9.7	11.4	11.5	10.1	10.3	157	100.0
Hodgkin's disease	0	0	4	2	6	1.9	1.9	17.6	-	-	2.9	3.1	1.8	1.8	30	100.0
Non-Hodgkin lymphoma	0	3	4	5	12	3.8	3.8	35.3	-	2.9	3.8	5.2	3.6	3.7	57	100.0
Burkitt's lymphoma	0	1	0	0	1	0.3	0.3	2.9	-	1.0	-	-	0.3	0.3	4	100.0
Unspecified lymphoma	1	6	5	3	15	4.7	4.7	44.1	3.0	5.8	4.8	3.1	4.5	4.5	66	100.0
Histiocytosis X	0	0	0	0	0	-	-	-	-	-	-	-	-	-	-	-
Other reticuloendothelial	0	0	0	0	0	-	-	-	-	-	-	-	-	-	-	-
III. BRAIN AND SPINAL	0	3	11	17	31	9.7	9.8	100.0	-	2.9	10.5	17.8	9.2	9.5	153	91.7
Ependymoma	0	0	0	0	0	-	-	-	-	-	-	-	-	-	-	-
Astrocytoma	0	1	3	4	8	2.5	2.5	25.8	-	1.0	2.9	4.2	2.4	2.4	39	100.0
Medulloblastoma	0	2	2	5	9	2.8	2.8	29.0	-	1.9	1.9	5.2	2.7	2.7	43	100.0
Other glioma	0	0	1	3	4	1.3	1.3	12.9	-	-	1.0	3.1	1.2	1.2	20	100.0
Other and unspecified *	0	0	5	5	10	3.1	3.2	32.3	-	-	4.8	5.2	3.0	3.1	50	50.0
IV. SYMPATHETIC N.S.	1	1	0	0	2	0.6	0.6	100.0	3.0	1.0	-	-	0.6	0.5	7	100.0
Neuroblastoma	1	1	0	0	2	0.6	0.6	100.0	3.0	1.0	-	-	0.6	0.5	7	100.0
Other	0	0	0	0	0	-	-	-	-	-	-	-	-	-	-	-
V. RETINOBLASTOMA	1	11	2	0	14	4.4	4.3	100.0	3.0	10.6	1.9	-	4.2	4.1	55	100.0
VI. KIDNEY	0	8	0	2	10	3.1	3.1	100.0	-	7.7	-	2.1	3.0	3.0	41	100.0
Wilms' tumour	0	6	0	0	6	1.9	1.8	60.0	-	5.8	-	-	1.8	1.8	23	100.0
Renal carcinoma	0	0	0	1	2	0.6	0.6	20.0	-	1.0	-	1.0	0.6	0.6	9	100.0
Other and unspecified	0	1	0	1	2	0.6	0.6	20.0	-	1.0	-	1.0	0.6	0.6	9	100.0
VII. LIVER	1	2	1	1	5	1.6	1.6	100.0	3.0	1.9	1.0	1.0	1.5	1.4	21	66.7
Hepatoblastoma	0	1	1	0	2	0.6	0.6	40.0	-	1.0	1.0	-	0.6	0.6	9	100.0
Hepatic carcinoma	0	0	0	0	0	-	-	-	-	-	-	-	-	-	-	-
Other and unspecified	1	1	0	1	3	0.9	0.9	60.0	3.0	1.0	-	1.0	0.9	0.8	12	100.0
VIII. BONE	0	2	1	8	11	3.4	3.4	100.0	-	1.9	1.0	8.4	3.3	3.3	54	85.7
Osteosarcoma	0	0	0	4	4	1.3	1.3	36.4	-	-	-	4.2	1.2	1.2	21	100.0
Chondrosarcoma	0	0	0	1	1	0.3	0.3	9.1	-	-	-	1.0	0.3	0.3	5	100.0
Ewing's sarcoma	0	1	0	1	2	0.6	0.6	18.2	-	1.0	-	1.0	0.6	0.6	9	100.0
Other and unspecified	0	1	1	2	4	1.3	1.3	36.4	-	1.0	1.0	2.1	1.2	1.2	19	100.0
IX. SOFT TISSUE SARCOMAS	0	7	1	3	11	3.4	3.4	100.0	-	6.8	1.0	3.1	3.3	3.3	48	100.0
Rhabdomyosarcoma	0	4	1	1	6	1.9	1.9	54.5	-	3.9	1.0	1.0	1.8	1.8	25	100.0
Fibrosarcoma	0	1	0	0	1	0.3	0.3	9.1	-	1.0	-	-	0.3	0.3	4	100.0
Other and unspecified	0	2	0	2	4	1.3	1.2	36.4	-	1.9	-	2.1	1.2	1.2	18	100.0
X. GONADAL & GERM CELL	1	5	0	1	7	2.2	2.1	100.0	3.0	4.8	-	1.0	2.1	2.0	28	100.0
Non-gonadal germ cell	1	1	0	1	3	0.9	0.9	42.9	3.0	1.0	-	1.0	0.9	0.8	12	100.0
Gonadal germ cell	0	4	0	0	4	1.3	1.2	57.1	-	3.9	-	-	1.3	1.2	15	100.0
Gonadal carcinoma	0	0	0	0	0	-	-	-	-	-	-	-	-	-	-	-
Other and unspecified	0	0	0	0	0	-	-	-	-	-	-	-	-	-	-	-
XI. EPITHELIAL NEOPLASMS	0	0	0	7	7	2.2	2.2	100.0	-	-	-	7.3	2.1	2.1	37	100.0
Adrenocortical carcinoma	0	0	0	0	0	-	-	-	-	-	-	-	-	-	-	-
Thyroid carcinoma	0	0	0	1	1	0.3	0.3	14.3	-	-	-	1.0	0.3	0.3	5	100.0
Nasopharyngeal carcinoma	0	0	0	2	2	0.6	0.6	28.6	-	-	-	2.1	0.6	0.6	10	100.0
Melanoma	0	0	0	0	0	-	-	-	-	-	-	-	-	-	-	-
Other carcinoma	0	0	0	4	4	1.3	1.3	57.1	-	-	-	4.2	1.2	1.2	21	100.0
XII. OTHER	1	5	6	5	17	5.3	5.4	100.0	3.0	4.8	5.7	5.2	5.0	5.1	77	33.3
* Specified as malignant	0	0	3	3	6	1.9	1.9	100.0	-	-	2.9	3.1	1.8	1.8	30	50.0

Philippines, Metro Manila & Rizal   1980 - 1982   FEMALE

DIAGNOSTIC GROUP	N 0	N 1-4	N 5-9	N 10-14	N All	RF Crude	RF Adj	RF Group	Rate 0	Rate 1-4	Rate 5-9	Rate 10-14	Rate Crude	Rate Adj	Cum	HV(%)
TOTAL	14	99	66	81	260	100.0	100.0	100.0	44.2	102.5	66.4	83.9	80.2	80.9	1206	93.4
I. LEUKAEMIAS	6	42	39	30	117	45.0	45.8	100.0	19.0	43.5	39.3	31.1	36.1	36.6	544	96.0
Acute lymphocytic	1	21	18	11	51	19.6	20.0	43.6	3.2	21.7	18.1	11.4	15.7	16.1	238	100.0
Other lymphocytic	1	1	0	1	3	1.2	1.1	2.6	3.2	1.0	-	1.0	0.9	0.9	12	100.0
Acute non-lymphocytic	0	7	3	3	13	5.0	5.0	11.1	-	7.2	3.0	3.1	4.0	4.1	60	91.7
Chronic myeloid	0	0	3	2	5	1.9	2.1	4.3	-	-	3.0	2.1	1.5	1.6	25	100.0
Other and unspecified	4	13	15	13	45	17.3	17.7	38.5	12.6	13.5	15.1	13.5	13.9	13.9	209	83.3
II. LYMPHOMAS	0	2	2	4	8	3.1	3.1	100.0	-	2.1	2.0	4.1	2.5	2.5	39	100.0
Hodgkin's disease	0	0	0	0	0	-	-	-	-	-	-	-	-	-	-	-
Non-Hodgkin lymphoma	0	1	0	2	3	1.2	1.1	37.5	-	1.0	-	2.1	0.9	0.9	14	100.0
Burkitt's lymphoma	0	0	0	0	0	-	-	-	-	-	-	-	-	-	-	-
Unspecified lymphoma	0	1	2	2	5	1.9	2.0	62.5	-	1.0	2.0	2.1	1.5	1.6	25	100.0
Histiocytosis X	0	0	0	0	0	-	-	-	-	-	-	-	-	-	-	-
Other reticuloendothelial	0	0	0	0	0	-	-	-	-	-	-	-	-	-	-	-
III. BRAIN AND SPINAL	0	2	10	9	21	8.1	8.6	100.0	-	2.1	10.1	9.3	6.5	6.6	105	76.9
Ependymoma	0	0	0	0	0	-	-	-	-	-	-	-	-	-	-	-
Astrocytoma	0	0	4	4	8	3.1	3.3	38.1	-	-	4.0	4.1	2.5	2.5	41	100.0
Medulloblastoma	0	1	0	1	2	0.8	0.7	9.5	-	1.0	-	1.0	0.6	0.6	9	100.0
Other glioma	0	0	0	0	0	-	-	-	-	-	-	-	-	-	-	-
Other and unspecified *	0	1	6	4	11	4.2	4.6	52.4	-	1.0	6.0	4.1	3.4	3.5	55	-
IV. SYMPATHETIC N.S.	2	2	1	0	5	1.9	1.9	100.0	6.3	2.1	1.0	-	1.5	1.5	20	100.0
Neuroblastoma	2	2	1	0	5	1.9	1.9	100.0	6.3	2.1	1.0	-	1.5	1.5	20	100.0
Other	0	0	0	0	0	-	-	-	-	-	-	-	-	-	-	-
V. RETINOBLASTOMA	1	18	2	0	21	8.1	7.6	100.0	3.2	18.6	2.0	-	6.5	6.7	88	100.0
VI. KIDNEY	1	14	2	1	18	6.9	6.6	100.0	3.2	14.5	2.0	1.0	5.6	5.7	76	81.3
Wilms' tumour	1	9	2	0	12	4.6	4.4	66.7	3.2	9.3	2.0	-	3.7	3.8	50	100.0
Renal carcinoma	0	0	0	1	1	0.4	0.4	5.6	-	-	-	1.0	0.3	0.3	5	100.0
Other and unspecified	0	5	0	0	5	1.9	1.8	27.8	-	5.2	-	-	1.5	1.6	21	-
VII. LIVER	0	0	2	0	2	0.8	0.9	100.0	-	-	2.0	-	0.6	0.6	10	-
Hepatoblastoma	0	0	0	0	0	-	-	-	-	-	-	-	-	-	-	-
Hepatic carcinoma	0	0	0	0	0	-	-	-	-	-	-	-	-	-	-	-
Other and unspecified	0	0	2	0	2	0.8	0.9	100.0	-	-	2.0	-	0.6	0.6	10	-
VIII. BONE	0	1	1	18	20	7.7	7.5	100.0	-	1.0	1.0	18.6	6.2	6.1	102	100.0
Osteosarcoma	0	0	1	9	10	3.8	3.8	50.0	-	-	1.0	9.3	3.1	3.0	52	100.0
Chondrosarcoma	0	0	0	1	1	0.4	0.4	5.0	-	-	-	1.0	0.3	0.3	5	100.0
Ewing's sarcoma	0	0	0	1	1	0.4	0.4	5.0	-	-	-	1.0	0.3	0.3	5	100.0
Other and unspecified	0	1	0	7	8	3.1	2.9	40.0	-	1.0	-	7.2	2.5	2.4	40	100.0
IX. SOFT TISSUE SARCOMAS	1	6	4	3	14	5.4	5.4	100.0	3.2	6.2	4.0	3.1	4.3	4.4	64	100.0
Rhabdomyosarcoma	1	6	2	0	9	3.5	3.4	64.3	3.2	6.2	2.0	-	2.8	2.8	38	100.0
Fibrosarcoma	0	0	0	3	3	1.2	1.1	21.4	-	-	-	3.1	0.9	0.9	16	100.0
Other and unspecified	0	0	2	0	2	0.8	0.9	14.3	-	-	2.0	-	0.6	0.6	10	100.0
X. GONADAL & GERM CELL	0	6	1	7	14	5.4	5.2	100.0	-	6.2	1.0	7.2	4.3	4.4	66	100.0
Non-gonadal germ cell	0	6	0	0	6	2.3	2.1	42.9	-	6.2	-	-	1.9	1.9	25	10.0
Gonadal germ cell	0	0	0	4	4	1.5	1.5	28.6	-	-	-	4.1	1.2	1.2	21	100.0
Gonadal carcinoma	0	0	1	2	3	1.2	1.2	21.4	-	-	1.0	2.1	0.9	0.9	15	100.0
Other and unspecified	0	0	0	1	1	0.4	0.4	7.1	-	-	-	1.0	0.3	0.3	5	-
XI. EPITHELIAL NEOPLASMS	0	0	1	4	5	1.9	1.9	100.0	-	-	1.0	4.1	1.5	1.5	26	100.0
Adrenocortical carcinoma	0	0	0	0	0	-	-	-	-	-	-	-	-	-	-	-
Thyroid carcinoma	0	0	0	1	1	0.4	0.4	20.0	-	-	-	1.0	0.3	0.3	5	100.0
Nasopharyngeal carcinoma	0	0	1	1	2	0.8	0.8	40.0	-	-	1.0	1.0	0.6	0.6	10	100.0
Melanoma	0	0	0	0	0	-	-	-	-	-	-	-	-	-	-	-
Other carcinoma	0	0	0	2	2	0.8	0.7	40.0	-	-	-	2.1	0.6	0.6	10	100.0
XII. OTHER	3	6	1	5	15	5.8	5.5	100.0	9.5	6.2	1.0	5.2	4.6	4.5	65	25.0
* Specified as malignant	0	0	4	3	7	2.7	2.9	-	-	-	4.0	3.1	2.2	2.2	36	-

* Specified as malignant

Figure 3. Surroundings of Manila Bay showing areas covered by the Rizal Medical Centre Cancer Registry and by the Central Tumour Registry of the Philippines

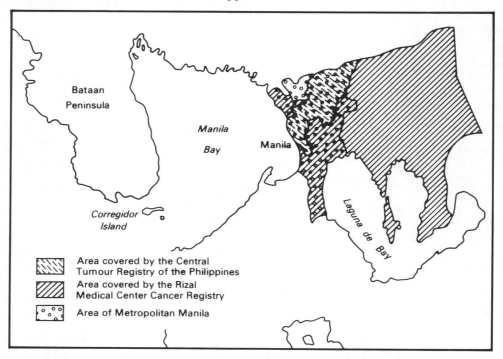

betical index file and the site index file before they are registered. Abstracts are filed numerically by year. A site accession register is maintained by both registries; the CTRP also has a tumour accession register.

Death certificates are matched with the hospital cases. If not previously registered, follow-back of cases is done with hospitals or with the physicians who signed the death certificate. Cases which cannot be traced are included under 'death certificates only' (DCO). The present percentage of DCO is 25–30%, and both registries are endeavouring to reduce this by a more intensive follow-back of DCOs.

The population of the four cities covered by the CTRP was 3.6 million in 1980, and for the 26 municipalities of the Rizal registry 2.7 million. Of the combined total, 35% were aged under 15 years. The total area covered by the two registries is 2134 square kilometres. The majority of this area is urbanized; only 4.4% of the population lives in areas designated as rural.

Population

The population at risk is taken from the census of 1980 (1980 Census of Population and Housing, National Census and Statistics Office, Manila).

AVERAGE ANNUAL POPULATION: 1980–1982

Age	Male	Female
0	111169	105510
1–4	344532	322046
5–9	349413	331112
10–14	318171	321948
0–14	1123285	1080616

Commentary

The largest diagnostic group was the leukaemias with almost half of all cases; although the majority are acute lymphocytic (the ratio of acute lymphocytic to acute non-lymphocytic leukaemia was 4.6:1), some 38% of the total were of 'other and unspecified' cell type. By contrast, lymphomas appear to be uncommon, the incidence in females being amongst the lowest recorded; this rarity applies particularly to Hodgkin's disease, for which only six cases, all in boys, were registered. Neuroblastoma is also very rare; the incidence rate for this tumour is the lowest of all the series in this volume. Ewing's sarcoma was hardly ever seen (three cases). The nasopharynx was the commonest site for carcinomas.

SINGAPORE

Singapore Cancer Registry, 1968–1982

H.P. Lee & K. Shanmugaratnam

Comprehensive population-based cancer registration began in January 1968. The Registry was established primarily to obtain information on cancer epidemiology.

Sources of data are: (*a*) cancer notifications from all sections of the medical profession; (*b*) pathology records; (*c*) hospital records; and (*d*) death certificates. Cancer notification is voluntary. All doctors in Singapore are provided with notification forms for which postage is prepaid. The Registry ensures that notifications are as complete as possible by checking all pathology reports and death certificates issued in Singapore as well as records of all Government hospitals. Cancer cases picked up from these sources are checked against registered cases and reminders are sent to doctors in charge of cases that have not been notified to the Registry. Cancer cases not notified by doctors (approximately 10%) are registered by the Registry staff on the basis of information derived from the sources mentioned above. Cancer registrations are reasonably comprehensive since all cases diagnosed histologically and all cases with mention of cancer in hospital discharge forms and death certificates are included. The registry includes all malignant neoplasms, and benign and unspecified CNS tumours.

There is no personal contact between patients and the Registry. Information on diagnosis and survival is obtained through hospital, pathology and death records.

The cancer notification forms and a register of cases are maintained on a current chronological basis. All relevant information is coded on to abstract cards and subsequently on to magnetic tapes. The Registry maintains two strip index panels of all cases, one filed alphabetically by name and the other by the patient's National Registration Identity Card Number. Duplication of cases is avoided by checking all new cases against these panels.

In 1980, there were 1976 registered medical practitioners (one medical practitioner per 1222 population), of whom 1121 were in private practice and 855 in the full-time service of the Ministry of Health and National University of Singapore. A total of 9579 hospital beds (3.97 hospital beds per 1000 population) were available — 8078 in 13 Government and institutional hospitals and 1501 in 13 private hospitals. Certification of death is virtually complete in Singapore. In 1980, 88.3% of all deaths were certified by qualified medical practitioners or the coroner and 11.7% by inspecting officers. The latter would certify a case as cancer only on the basis of a previous hospital diagnosis.

Registration covers the whole of the Republic of Singapore, comprising the main island of Singapore and several offshore islands with an area of 584 square kilometres. The island lies at the southern tip of the Malayan peninsula, with which it is connected by a road and rail causeway. On the southern part of the island are the port and city of Singapore. The island is rather flat, the highest point being a central granite hill 166 m high. The maximum temperature is around 31° C and the minimum 24° C. The island generally has rainfall throughout the year (total annual rainfall approximately 2400 mm), but is particularly wet during the monsoon season from November to January.

The population of Singapore in the 1980 census was 2 413 945. The population density was 4133 persons per square kilometre. The largest ethnic group are the Chinese (77% of the total population). They are for the most part derived from the south-eastern Chinese provinces of Fukien and Kwangtung. The principal linguistic or dialect groups are Hokkien (43.1%), Teochew (22.0%) and Cantonese (16.5%). Foreign-born migrants comprised 19.7% of the total Chinese population, and 7.1% of those aged under 30. The second largest

Contd p. 212

Singapore, Chinese

MALE

1968 - 1982

DIAGNOSTIC GROUP	NUMBER OF CASES					REL. FREQUENCY (%)			RATES PER MILLION						HV(%)
	0	1-4	5-9	10-14	All	Crude	Adj.	Group	0-4	5-9	10-14	Crude	Adj.	Cum	
TOTAL	31	134	117	138	420	100.0	100.0	100.0	134.9	81.5	92.0	101.0	105.2	1542	87.6
I. LEUKAEMIAS	8	62	56	41	167	39.8	40.2	100.0	57.2	39.0	27.3	40.2	42.7	618	91.6
Acute lymphocytic	2	43	32	21	98	23.3	23.7	58.7	36.8	22.3	14.0	23.6	25.5	365	92.9
Other lymphocytic	0	2	0	2	4	1.0	0.9	2.4	1.6	-	1.3	1.0	1.0	15	100.0
Acute non-lymphocytic	2	7	11	7	27	6.4	6.5	16.2	7.4	7.7	4.7	6.5	6.7	98	92.6
Chronic myeloid	1	3	4	9	17	4.0	4.0	10.2	3.3	2.8	6.0	4.1	3.9	60	94.1
Other and unspecified	3	7	9	2	21	5.0	5.2	12.6	8.2	6.3	1.3	5.0	5.6	79	81.0
II. LYMPHOMAS	4	9	22	23	58	13.8	13.8	100.0	10.6	15.3	15.3	13.9	13.5	206	91.4
Hodgkin's disease	1	8	0	2	11	2.6	2.7	19.0	0.8	5.6	1.3	2.6	2.5	39	100.0
Non-Hodgkin lymphoma	1	5	11	14	31	7.4	7.3	53.4	4.9	7.7	9.3	7.5	7.1	109	87.1
Burkitt's lymphoma	0	1	1	1	3	0.7	0.7	5.2	0.8	0.7	0.7	0.7	0.7	11	100.0
Unspecified lymphoma	2	1	2	5	10	2.4	2.3	17.2	2.5	1.4	3.3	2.4	2.4	36	90.0
Histiocytosis X	0	0	0	0	0	-	-	-	-	-	-	-	-	-	-
Other reticuloendothelial	1	1	0	1	3	0.7	0.7	5.2	1.6	-	0.7	0.7	0.8	12	100.0
III. BRAIN AND SPINAL	1	8	20	19	48	11.4	11.4	100.0	7.4	13.9	12.7	11.5	11.0	170	72.9
Ependymoma	1	0	1	0	2	0.5	0.5	4.2	0.8	-	0.7	0.5	0.5	7	100.0
Astrocytoma	0	3	4	6	13	3.1	3.1	27.1	2.5	2.8	4.0	3.1	3.0	46	100.0
Medulloblastoma	0	3	9	3	15	3.6	3.7	31.3	2.5	6.3	2.0	3.6	3.6	54	100.0
Other glioma	0	0	0	1	1	0.2	0.2	2.1	-	-	0.7	0.2	0.3	3	100.0
Other and unspecified *	0	2	7	8	17	4.0	4.0	35.4	1.6	4.9	5.3	4.1	3.8	59	23.5
IV. SYMPATHETIC N.S.	6	14	3	0	23	5.5	5.6	100.0	16.3	2.1	-	5.5	7.0	92	100.0
Neuroblastoma	6	14	3	0	23	5.5	5.6	100.0	16.3	2.1	-	5.5	7.0	92	100.0
Other	0	0	0	0	0	-	-	-	-	-	-	-	-	-	-
V. RETINOBLASTOMA	1	6	1	0	8	1.9	2.0	100.0	5.7	0.7	-	1.9	2.4	32	100.0
VI. KIDNEY	3	9	2	0	14	3.3	3.4	100.0	9.8	1.4	-	3.4	4.2	56	92.9
Wilms' tumour	3	8	1	0	12	2.9	2.9	85.7	9.0	0.7	-	2.9	3.7	48	100.0
Renal carcinoma	0	0	1	0	1	0.2	0.2	4.8	0.8	-	-	0.2	0.3	4	100.0
Other and unspecified	0	0	0	1	1	0.2	0.3	7.1	-	0.7	-	0.2	0.2	4	-
VII. LIVER	6	4	0	1	11	2.6	2.6	100.0	8.2	-	0.7	2.6	3.4	44	54.5
Hepatoblastoma	3	2	0	0	5	1.2	1.2	45.5	4.1	-	-	1.2	1.6	20	100.0
Hepatic carcinoma	0	0	0	1	1	0.2	0.2	9.1	-	-	0.7	0.2	0.2	3	100.0
Other and unspecified	3	2	0	0	5	1.2	1.2	45.5	4.1	-	-	1.2	1.6	20	-
VIII. BONE	0	0	3	18	21	5.0	4.7	100.0	-	2.1	12.0	5.0	4.2	70	90.5
Osteosarcoma	0	0	1	11	12	2.9	2.6	57.1	-	0.7	7.3	2.9	2.4	40	100.0
Chondrosarcoma	0	0	0	1	1	0.2	0.2	4.8	-	-	0.7	0.2	0.2	3	100.0
Ewing's sarcoma	0	0	0	3	3	0.7	0.7	14.3	-	-	2.0	0.7	0.6	10	100.0
Other and unspecified	0	0	2	3	5	1.2	1.2	23.8	-	1.4	2.0	1.2	1.0	17	60.0
IX. SOFT TISSUE SARCOMAS	1	6	4	8	19	4.5	4.5	100.0	5.7	2.8	5.3	4.6	4.7	69	100.0
Rhabdomyosarcoma	0	4	2	4	10	2.4	2.4	52.6	3.3	1.4	2.7	2.4	2.5	37	100.0
Fibrosarcoma	0	1	1	2	4	1.0	0.9	21.1	0.8	0.7	1.3	1.0	0.9	14	100.0
Other and unspecified	1	1	1	2	5	1.2	1.2	26.3	1.6	0.7	1.3	1.2	1.2	18	100.0
X. GONADAL & GERM CELL	1	9	1	2	13	3.1	3.1	100.0	8.2	0.7	1.3	3.1	3.8	51	100.0
Non-gonadal germ cell	0	1	1	1	3	0.7	0.7	23.1	0.8	0.7	0.7	0.7	0.7	11	100.0
Gonadal germ cell	1	5	0	1	7	1.7	1.7	53.8	4.9	-	0.7	1.7	2.1	28	100.0
Gonadal carcinoma	0	3	0	0	3	0.7	0.7	23.1	2.5	-	-	0.7	0.9	12	100.0
Other and unspecified	0	0	0	0	0	-	-	-	-	-	-	-	-	-	-
XI. EPITHELIAL NEOPLASMS	0	1	2	21	24	5.7	5.3	100.0	0.8	1.4	14.0	5.8	4.8	81	100.0
Adrenocortical carcinoma	0	0	0	0	0	-	-	-	-	-	-	-	-	-	-
Thyroid carcinoma	0	0	0	3	3	0.7	0.7	12.5	-	-	2.0	0.7	0.6	10	100.0
Nasopharyngeal carcinoma	0	0	0	7	7	1.7	1.5	29.2	-	-	4.7	1.7	1.4	23	100.0
Melanoma	0	0	1	0	1	0.2	0.2	4.2	-	-	0.7	0.2	0.2	3	100.0
Other carcinoma	0	1	2	10	13	3.1	2.9	54.2	0.8	1.4	6.7	3.1	2.7	44	100.0
XII. OTHER	0	6	3	5	14	3.3	3.3	100.0	4.9	2.1	3.3	3.4	3.5	52	14.3
* Specified as malignant	0	2	7	6	15	3.6	3.6	100.0	1.6	4.9	4.0	3.6	3.4	53	13.3

Singapore, Chinese

1968 – 1982

FEMALE

DIAGNOSTIC GROUP	NUMBER OF CASES					REL. FREQUENCY(%)			RATES PER MILLION					Cum	HV(%)
	0	1-4	5-9	10-14	All	Crude	Adj.	Group	0-4	5-9	10-14	Crude	Adj.		
TOTAL	21	117	89	99	326	100.0	100.0	100.0	121.7	66.2	70.0	83.7	88.8	1289	87.1
I. LEUKAEMIAS	5	52	33	25	115	35.3	35.2	100.0	50.3	24.5	17.7	29.5	32.5	462	92.2
Acute lymphocytic	2	35	20	15	72	22.1	22.0	62.6	32.6	14.9	10.6	18.5	20.5	291	93.1
Other lymphocytic	0	1	0	0	1	0.3	0.3	0.9	0.9	-	-	0.3	0.3	4	100.0
Acute non-lymphocytic	1	9	5	9	24	7.4	7.3	20.9	8.8	3.7	6.4	6.2	6.5	94	91.7
Chronic myeloid	1	2	3	1	7	2.1	2.2	6.1	2.6	2.2	0.7	1.8	1.9	28	100.0
Other and unspecified	1	5	5	0	11	3.4	3.4	9.6	5.3	3.7	-	2.8	3.2	45	81.8
II. LYMPHOMAS	2	9	10	9	30	9.2	9.3	100.0	9.7	7.4	6.4	7.7	8.0	117	83.3
Hodgkin's disease	0	2	1	0	3	0.9	1.0	10.0	1.8	0.7	-	0.8	0.7	11	100.0
Non-Hodgkin lymphoma	1	7	5	7	20	6.1	6.1	66.7	7.1	3.7	4.9	5.1	5.4	79	85.0
Burkitt's lymphoma	0	0	1	0	1	0.3	0.3	3.3	-	0.7	-	0.3	0.2	4	100.0
Unspecified lymphoma	0	0	1	2	3	0.9	0.9	10.0	-	0.7	1.4	0.8	0.9	13	100.0
Histiocytosis X	1	0	0	0	1	0.3	0.3	3.3	0.9	-	-	0.3	0.3	4	-
Other reticuloendothelial	0	0	2	0	2	0.6	0.7	6.7	-	1.5	-	0.5	0.5	7	50.0
III. BRAIN AND SPINAL	2	8	23	17	50	15.3	15.8	100.0	8.8	17.1	12.0	12.8	12.4	190	68.0
Ependymoma	1	1	2	0	4	1.2	1.3	8.0	1.8	1.5	-	1.0	1.2	16	100.0
Astrocytoma	0	5	6	7	18	5.5	5.6	36.0	4.4	4.5	4.9	4.6	4.6	69	100.0
Medulloblastoma	1	1	2	3	7	2.1	2.2	14.0	1.8	1.5	2.1	1.8	1.8	27	100.0
Other glioma	0	0	1	1	2	0.6	0.6	4.0	-	0.7	0.7	0.5	0.4	7	100.0
Other and unspecified *	0	1	12	6	19	5.8	6.2	38.0	0.9	8.9	4.2	4.9	4.5	70	15.8
IV. SYMPATHETIC N.S.	2	6	5	1	14	4.3	4.3	100.0	7.1	3.7	0.7	3.6	4.1	57	100.0
Neuroblastoma	2	6	4	1	13	4.0	4.0	92.9	7.1	3.0	0.7	3.3	3.9	54	100.0
Other	0	0	1	0	1	0.3	0.3	7.1	-	0.7	-	0.3	0.2	4	100.0
V. RETINOBLASTOMA	1	16	0	0	17	5.2	4.9	100.0	15.0	-	-	4.4	5.8	75	100.0
VI. KIDNEY	2	7	1	0	10	3.1	2.9	100.0	7.9	0.7	-	2.6	3.3	43	90.0
Wilms' tumour	2	7	0	0	9	2.8	2.6	90.0	7.9	-	-	2.3	3.1	40	100.0
Renal carcinoma	0	0	0	0	0	-	-	-	-	-	-	-	-	-	-
Other and unspecified	0	0	1	0	1	0.3	0.3	10.0	-	0.7	-	0.3	0.2	4	-
VII. LIVER	3	3	0	0	6	1.8	1.7	100.0	5.3	-	-	1.5	2.0	26	100.0
Hepatoblastoma	3	1	0	0	4	1.2	1.2	66.7	3.5	-	-	1.0	1.4	18	100.0
Hepatic carcinoma	0	2	0	0	2	0.6	0.6	33.3	1.8	-	-	0.5	0.7	9	100.0
Other and unspecified	0	0	0	0	0	-	-	-	-	-	-	-	-	-	-
VIII. BONE	1	2	5	13	21	6.4	6.5	100.0	2.6	3.7	9.2	5.4	4.9	78	95.2
Osteosarcoma	0	0	4	12	16	4.9	5.0	76.2	-	3.0	8.5	4.1	3.4	57	100.0
Chondrosarcoma	0	0	0	0	0	-	-	-	-	-	-	-	-	-	-
Ewing's sarcoma	0	1	0	0	1	0.3	0.3	4.8	0.9	-	-	0.3	0.3	4	100.0
Other and unspecified	1	1	1	1	4	1.2	1.2	19.0	1.8	0.7	0.7	1.0	1.1	16	75.0
IX. SOFT TISSUE SARCOMAS	1	5	8	4	18	5.5	5.6	100.0	5.3	6.0	2.8	4.6	4.8	70	100.0
Rhabdomyosarcoma	0	5	4	0	9	2.8	2.8	50.0	4.4	3.0	-	2.3	2.7	37	100.0
Fibrosarcoma	0	0	2	2	4	1.2	1.3	22.2	-	1.5	1.4	1.0	0.9	15	100.0
Other and unspecified	1	0	2	2	5	1.5	1.6	27.8	0.9	1.5	1.4	1.3	1.2	19	100.0
X. GONADAL & GERM CELL	0	3	2	12	17	5.2	5.2	100.0	2.6	1.5	8.5	4.4	4.0	63	100.0
Non-gonadal germ cell	0	3	0	0	3	0.9	0.9	17.6	2.6	-	-	0.8	1.0	13	100.0
Gonadal germ cell	0	0	2	8	10	3.1	3.1	58.8	-	1.5	5.7	2.6	2.1	36	100.0
Gonadal carcinoma	0	0	0	2	2	0.6	0.6	11.8	-	-	1.4	0.5	0.4	7	100.0
Other and unspecified	0	0	0	2	2	0.6	0.6	11.8	-	-	1.4	0.5	0.4	7	100.0
XI. EPITHELIAL NEOPLASMS	0	1	1	15	17	5.2	5.2	100.0	0.9	0.7	10.6	4.4	3.7	61	100.0
Adrenocortical carcinoma	0	0	0	0	0	-	-	-	-	-	-	-	-	-	-
Thyroid carcinoma	0	0	0	8	8	2.5	2.4	47.1	-	-	5.7	2.1	1.6	28	100.0
Nasopharyngeal carcinoma	0	0	0	2	2	0.6	0.6	11.8	-	-	1.4	0.5	0.4	7	100.0
Melanoma	0	0	0	0	0	-	-	-	-	-	-	-	-	-	-
Other carcinoma	0	1	1	5	7	2.1	2.1	41.2	0.9	0.7	3.5	1.8	1.6	26	100.0
XII. OTHER	2	5	1	3	11	3.4	3.3	100.0	6.2	0.7	2.1	2.8	3.2	45	9.1
* Specified as malignant	0	1	10	5	16	4.9	5.2	100.0	0.9	7.4	3.5	4.1	3.8	59	-

Singapore, Malay

1968 – 1982   MALE

DIAGNOSTIC GROUP	NUMBER OF CASES 0	1-4	5-9	10-14	All	REL. FREQUENCY(%) Crude	Adj.	Group	RATES PER MILLION 0-4	5-9	10-14	Crude	Adj.	Cum	HV(%)
TOTAL	5	24	25	26	80	100.0	100.0	100.0	105.2	76.9	80.7	86.7	89.0	1314	78.8
I. LEUKAEMIAS	2	13	20	9	44	55.0	55.0	100.0	54.4	61.5	27.9	47.7	49.0	719	84.1
Acute lymphocytic	1	8	12	5	26	32.5	32.6	59.1	32.6	36.9	15.5	28.2	29.1	425	92.3
Other lymphocytic	0	0	0	0	0	-	-	-	-	-	-	-	-	-	-
Acute non-lymphocytic	0	3	5	1	9	11.3	11.3	20.5	10.9	15.4	3.1	9.8	10.1	147	77.8
Chronic myeloid	0	0	2	2	4	5.0	4.7	9.1	-	6.2	6.2	4.3	3.8	62	100.0
Other and unspecified	1	2	1	1	5	6.3	6.5	11.4	10.9	3.1	3.1	5.4	6.1	85	40.0
II. LYMPHOMAS	0	3	2	5	10	12.5	12.3	100.0	10.9	6.2	15.5	10.8	10.7	163	90.0
Hodgkin's disease	0	1	0	1	2	2.5	2.5	20.0	3.6	-	3.1	2.2	2.3	34	100.0
Non-Hodgkin lymphoma	0	1	2	4	7	8.8	8.4	70.0	3.6	6.2	12.4	7.6	7.0	111	85.7
Burkitt's lymphoma	0	0	0	0	0	-	-	-	-	-	-	-	-	-	-
Unspecified lymphoma	0	0	0	0	0	-	-	-	-	-	-	-	-	-	-
Histiocytosis X	0	0	0	0	0	-	-	-	-	-	-	-	-	-	-
Other reticuloendothelial	0	1	0	0	1	1.3	1.4	10.0	3.6	-	-	1.1	1.4	18	100.0
III. BRAIN AND SPINAL	0	2	0	5	7	8.8	8.5	100.0	7.3	-	15.5	7.6	7.3	114	28.6
Ependymoma	0	0	0	0	0	-	-	-	-	-	-	-	-	-	-
Astrocytoma	0	0	0	2	2	2.5	2.3	28.6	-	-	6.2	2.2	1.8	31	100.0
Medulloblastoma	0	0	0	0	0	-	-	-	-	-	-	-	-	-	-
Other glioma	0	0	0	0	0	-	-	-	-	-	-	-	-	-	-
Other and unspecified *	0	2	0	3	5	6.3	6.2	71.4	7.3	-	9.3	5.4	5.5	83	-
IV. SYMPATHETIC N.S.	0	0	1	0	1	1.3	1.2	100.0	-	3.1	-	1.1	1.0	15	100.0
Neuroblastoma	0	0	1	0	1	1.3	1.2	100.0	-	3.1	-	1.1	1.0	15	100.0
Other	0	0	0	0	0	-	-	-	-	-	-	-	-	-	-
V. RETINOBLASTOMA	0	2	0	0	2	2.5	2.8	100.0	7.3	-	-	2.2	2.8	36	100.0
VI. KIDNEY	0	1	0	2	3	3.8	3.9	100.0	7.3	-	3.1	3.3	3.7	52	100.0
Wilms' tumour	0	1	0	1	2	2.5	2.8	66.7	7.3	-	3.1	2.2	2.8	36	100.0
Renal carcinoma	0	0	0	1	1	1.3	1.2	33.3	-	-	3.1	1.1	0.9	16	100.0
Other and unspecified	0	0	0	0	0	-	-	-	-	-	-	-	-	-	-
VII. LIVER	0	0	0	0	0	-	-	-	-	-	-	-	-	-	-
Hepatoblastoma	0	0	0	0	0	-	-	-	-	-	-	-	-	-	-
Hepatic carcinoma	0	0	0	0	0	-	-	-	-	-	-	-	-	-	-
Other and unspecified	0	0	0	0	0	-	-	-	-	-	-	-	-	-	-
VIII. BONE	0	1	0	3	4	5.0	4.8	100.0	3.6	-	9.3	4.3	4.1	65	75.0
Osteosarcoma	0	0	0	2	2	2.5	2.3	50.0	-	-	6.2	2.2	1.8	31	100.0
Chondrosarcoma	0	0	0	0	0	-	-	-	-	-	-	-	-	-	-
Ewing's sarcoma	0	1	0	0	1	1.3	1.4	25.0	3.6	-	-	1.1	1.4	18	100.0
Other and unspecified	0	0	0	1	1	1.3	1.2	25.0	-	-	3.1	1.1	0.9	16	100.0
IX. SOFT TISSUE SARCOMAS	0	0	0	1	1	1.3	1.2	100.0	-	-	3.1	1.1	0.9	16	100.0
Rhabdomyosarcoma	0	0	0	1	1	1.3	1.2	100.0	-	-	3.1	1.1	0.9	16	100.0
Fibrosarcoma	0	0	0	0	0	-	-	-	-	-	-	-	-	-	-
Other and unspecified	0	0	0	0	0	-	-	-	-	-	-	-	-	-	-
X. GONADAL & GERM CELL	0	2	0	0	2	2.5	2.8	100.0	7.3	-	-	2.2	2.8	36	50.0
Non-gonadal germ cell	0	1	0	0	1	1.3	1.4	50.0	3.6	-	-	1.1	1.4	18	100.0
Gonadal germ cell	0	0	0	0	0	-	-	-	-	-	-	-	-	-	-
Gonadal carcinoma	0	0	0	0	0	-	-	-	-	-	-	-	-	-	-
Other and unspecified	0	1	0	0	1	1.3	1.4	50.0	3.6	-	-	1.1	1.4	18	-
XI. EPITHELIAL NEOPLASMS	0	0	1	2	3	3.8	3.5	100.0	-	3.1	6.2	3.3	2.8	46	100.0
Adrenocortical carcinoma	0	0	0	0	0	-	-	-	-	-	-	-	-	-	-
Thyroid carcinoma	0	0	0	0	0	-	-	-	-	-	-	-	-	-	-
Nasopharyngeal carcinoma	0	0	1	1	2	2.5	2.4	66.7	-	3.1	3.1	2.2	1.9	31	100.0
Melanoma	0	0	0	1	1	1.3	1.2	33.3	-	-	3.1	1.1	0.9	16	100.0
Other carcinoma	0	0	0	0	0	-	-	-	-	-	-	-	-	-	-
XII. OTHER	2	0	1	0	3	3.8	4.0	100.0	7.3	3.1	-	3.3	3.8	52	33.3
* Specified as malignant	0	2	0	3	5	6.3	6.2	-	7.3	-	9.3	5.4	5.5	83	-

* Specified as malignant

Singapore, Malay

1968 - 1982

FEMALE

DIAGNOSTIC GROUP	NUMBER OF CASES 0	1-4	5-9	10-14	All	REL. FREQUENCY(%) Crude	Adj.	Group	RATES PER MILLION 0-4	5-9	10-14	Crude	Adj.	Cum	HV(%)
TOTAL	5	18	21	21	65	100.0	100.0	100.0	86.9	67.4	66.5	72.9	74.7	1104	80.0
I. LEUKAEMIAS	0	7	8	10	25	38.5	37.9	100.0	26.5	25.7	31.7	28.0	27.7	419	92.0
Acute lymphocytic	0	1	4	6	11	16.9	16.0	44.0	3.8	12.8	19.0	12.3	11.1	178	100.0
Other lymphocytic	0	0	1	0	1	1.5	1.4	4.0	-	3.2	-	1.1	1.0	16	100.0
Acute non-lymphocytic	0	2	1	4	7	10.8	10.6	28.0	7.6	3.2	12.7	7.8	7.6	117	100.0
Chronic myeloid	0	0	0	0	0	-	-	-	-	-	-	-	-	-	-
Other and unspecified	0	4	2	0	6	9.2	9.8	24.0	15.1	6.4	-	6.7	7.9	108	66.7
II. LYMPHOMAS	2	1	3	0	6	9.2	9.5	100.0	11.3	9.6	-	6.7	7.5	105	83.3
Hodgkin's disease	0	0	1	0	1	1.5	1.4	16.7	-	3.2	-	1.1	1.0	16	100.0
Non-Hodgkin lymphoma	0	1	2	0	3	4.6	4.6	50.0	3.8	6.4	-	3.4	3.5	51	100.0
Burkitt's lymphoma	0	0	0	0	0	-	-	-	-	-	-	-	-	-	-
Unspecified lymphoma	0	0	0	0	0	-	-	-	-	-	-	-	-	-	-
Histiocytosis X	1	0	0	0	1	1.5	1.7	16.7	3.8	-	-	1.1	1.5	19	-
Other reticuloendothelial	1	0	0	0	1	1.5	1.7	16.7	3.8	-	-	1.1	1.5	19	100.0
III. BRAIN AND SPINAL	0	3	5	1	9	13.8	13.8	100.0	11.3	16.1	3.2	10.1	10.5	153	55.6
Ependymoma	0	0	0	0	0	-	-	-	-	-	-	-	-	-	-
Astrocytoma	0	0	3	1	4	6.2	5.7	44.4	-	9.6	3.2	4.5	4.0	64	100.0
Medulloblastoma	0	0	0	0	0	-	-	-	-	-	-	-	-	-	-
Other glioma	0	0	1	0	1	1.5	1.4	11.1	-	3.2	-	1.1	1.0	16	100.0
Other and unspecified *	0	3	1	0	4	6.2	6.6	44.4	11.3	3.2	-	4.5	5.4	73	100.0
IV. SYMPATHETIC N.S.	1	2	0	1	4	6.2	6.6	100.0	11.3	-	3.2	4.5	5.3	73	100.0
Neuroblastoma	1	2	0	1	4	6.2	6.6	100.0	11.3	-	3.2	4.5	5.3	73	100.0
Other	0	0	0	0	0	-	-	-	-	-	-	-	-	-	-
V. RETINOBLASTOMA	0	0	0	0	0	-	-	-	-	-	-	-	-	-	-
VI. KIDNEY	0	3	1	0	4	6.2	6.6	100.0	11.3	3.2	-	4.5	5.4	73	50.0
Wilms' tumour	0	2	0	0	2	3.1	3.5	50.0	7.6	-	-	2.2	2.9	38	100.0
Renal carcinoma	0	0	0	0	0	-	-	-	-	-	-	-	-	-	-
Other and unspecified	0	1	1	0	2	3.1	3.2	50.0	3.8	3.2	-	2.2	2.5	35	50.0
VII. LIVER	1	0	1	0	2	3.1	3.2	100.0	3.8	3.2	-	2.2	2.5	35	50.0
Hepatoblastoma	0	0	1	0	1	1.5	1.7	50.0	-	3.2	-	1.1	1.5	19	100.0
Hepatic carcinoma	1	0	0	0	1	1.5	1.4	50.0	3.8	-	-	1.1	1.0	16	100.0
Other and unspecified	0	0	0	0	0	-	-	-	-	-	-	-	-	-	-
VIII. BONE	0	0	1	4	5	7.7	7.1	100.0	-	3.2	12.7	5.6	4.7	79	60.0
Osteosarcoma	0	0	1	1	2	3.1	2.9	40.0	-	3.2	3.2	2.2	2.0	32	100.0
Chondrosarcoma	0	0	0	1	1	1.5	1.4	20.0	-	-	3.2	1.1	0.9	16	100.0
Ewing's sarcoma	0	0	0	0	0	-	-	-	-	-	-	-	-	-	-
Other and unspecified	0	0	0	2	2	3.1	2.9	40.0	-	-	6.3	2.2	1.8	32	-
IX. SOFT TISSUE SARCOMAS	0	2	1	0	3	4.6	4.9	100.0	7.6	3.2	-	3.4	3.8	54	100.0
Rhabdomyosarcoma	0	0	1	0	1	1.5	1.4	33.3	-	3.2	-	1.1	0.9	16	100.0
Fibrosarcoma	0	1	0	0	1	1.5	1.7	33.3	3.8	-	-	1.1	1.1	19	100.0
Other and unspecified	0	1	0	0	1	1.5	1.7	33.3	3.8	-	-	1.1	1.5	19	100.0
X. GONADAL & GERM CELL	1	0	1	2	4	6.2	6.0	100.0	3.8	3.2	6.3	4.5	4.3	67	100.0
Non-gonadal germ cell	0	0	0	0	0	-	-	-	-	-	-	-	-	-	-
Gonadal germ cell	1	0	1	1	3	4.6	4.6	75.0	3.8	3.2	3.2	3.4	3.4	51	100.0
Gonadal carcinoma	0	0	0	1	1	1.5	1.4	25.0	-	-	3.2	1.1	0.9	16	100.0
Other and unspecified	0	0	0	0	0	-	-	-	-	-	-	-	-	-	-
XI. EPITHELIAL NEOPLASMS	0	0	0	1	1	1.5	1.4	100.0	-	-	3.2	1.1	0.9	16	100.0
Adrenocortical carcinoma	0	0	0	0	0	-	-	-	-	-	-	-	-	-	-
Thyroid carcinoma	0	0	0	0	0	-	-	-	-	-	-	-	-	-	-
Nasopharyngeal carcinoma	0	0	0	0	0	-	-	-	-	-	-	-	-	-	-
Melanoma	0	0	0	0	0	-	-	-	-	-	-	-	-	-	-
Other carcinoma	0	0	0	1	1	1.5	1.4	100.0	-	-	3.2	1.1	0.9	16	100.0
XII. OTHER	0	0	1	1	2	3.1	2.9	100.0	-	3.2	3.2	2.2	2.0	32	50.0
* Specified as malignant	0	3	1	0	4	6.2	6.6	100.0	11.3	3.2	-	4.5	5.4	73	-

group are the Malays (15% of the total), the great majority (89%) of whom come from Malaya and the remainder from other parts of Malaysia and from Indonesia; 19.6% overall, and 11.0% of those aged under 30, were born outside Singapore. Indians, including persons from Pakistan and Sri Lanka, accounted for 6% of the population; nearly two-thirds were Tamils.

Registry data have been used mainly to determine relative risks and incidence levels of cancers in Singapore by ethnic group, linguistic group, specific communities and migrant status. Such information has formed the basis of *ad hoc* surveys and studies on specific cancers.

Population

The average annual population at risk is derived from the data of the censuses of 1970 and 1980.

AVERAGE ANNUAL POPULATION: 1968–1982

Age	Male	Female
Chinese		
0–4	81571	75613
5–9	95712	89619
10–14	100005	94308
0–14	277288	259540
Malay		
0–4	18384	17638
5–9	21663	20761
10–14	21477	21063
0–14	61524	59462

Commentary

Tables are presented for children of Chinese origin (76% of the total registrations), and for Malays (15%).

In *Chinese* children, the incidence rates for many diagnostic groups were similar to those in Western populations. An unusually high proportion of leukaemias were chronic myeloid (8.5%). Hodgkin's disease was relatively uncommon, and from the few cases registered there appears to be a peak of incidence in the 5–9 age-group. Despite the fact that non-malignant CNS tumours are registered, the incidence of brain and spinal tumours was lower than in several other east Asian registries. Wilms' tumour and Ewing's sarcoma were relatively uncommon. There were high incidence rates for liver tumours (mostly hepatoblastoma) and thyroid carcinoma. Nasopharyngeal carcinoma was relatively common in boys.

The *Malay* population in general had lower incidence rates than the Chinese, with the deficit being most pronounced for retinoblastoma and soft-tissue sarcomas. However, the rates for leukaemia were similar for the two groups, and in fact the incidence of acute non-lymphocytic leukaemia seemed to be slightly higher in Malays (age-standardized rate 8.9 compared with 6.6 per million for Chinese).

References

Kwa, S.B., Seah, C.S., Hanam, E., Chen, B., Tham, N.B., Chan, S.K., Paul, F., Lee, S.K. & Tan, D. (1968) Leukaemia in Singapore. *Singapore med. J.*, *9*, 133

Muir, C.S. (1961) Cancer in Singapore children. *Cancer*, *14*, 534-538

Tan, K.H. & Tan, K.S. (1968) Chronic myeloid leukaemia in children. *Singapore med. J.*, *9*, 39-44

THAILAND

National Register: National Cancer Institute, 1971–1980

Sineenat Sontipong & Phisit Phanthumachinda

The National Cancer Institute of Thailand was established in 1968, one of its objectives being to act as the centre for the collection, study and dissemination of cancer statistics and data on cancer in Thailand. A cancer registry was established in 1971. Because of its national focus, the registry has recorded data on cases of cancer occurring throughout the country by receiving notifications of cases treated in hospital, both in the governmental and private sectors. The first target was to gain the co-operation of all Ministry of Public Health hospitals, followed by hospitals affiliated to medical schools or other governmental agencies, and finally from private hospitals and clinics. Data are collected both passively, from registration cards filled out and returned by the treating hospitals, and actively, by visits from registry personnel to collaborating hospitals at annual intervals.

Sources of data can be classified as follows:

— hospital records, for both out-patients and in-patients (about 60% of data);

— hospital cancer registries, which have been set up in the university medical schools, such as Siriraj Hospital in Bangkok, Maharaj Hospital in Chiengmai and Songkhla Nakarin Hospital in Songkhla, and which provide about 38% of all data;

— pathology departments of hospitals (about 1-2% of data).

Even cases diagnosed on the basis of clinical findings alone are registered. Many patients present at advanced stages of disease, and treatment may be started without waiting for the results of investigations. This happens in about 10-15% of cases in the major Bangkok hospitals and in about 40% in provincial hospitals.

Coding and processing of data is done manually.

Reporting of data is voluntary, and there has been a progressive increase in the number of hospitals participating in the registry programme during its first 10 years; the number of cases registered has risen accordingly:

	Notifying hospitals		Cases registered	
	Bangkok	Other	Total	With histology
1971	7	46	1785	765
1975	17	68	3428	1570
1980	24	119	12597	10040

Since the National Cancer Institute is in the governmental sector, funding is from central sources; however, the Institute is assisted by the Cancer Research Foundation for the National Cancer Institute, which subsidizes the personnel entering the data on the registry cards.

Thailand is located in South-east Asia, covering an area of about 513 115 square kilometres. On the north, it is bounded by Burma and Laos, on the east by Democratic Kampuchea and Laos, on the west by Burma and the Indian Ocean and on the south by Malaysia. Both the temperature and the humidity are rather high.

Thailand is divided into four geographical regions — the Central, the Northeastern, the Northern and the Southern Region — and 73 administrative provinces.

The population at the 1980 census was 44 824 540, of whom 38.3% were aged under 15 years. The population density was 3000 persons per square kilometre in Bangkok and ranged from 53 to 95 per square kilometre in the four regions. Urban and rural areas have not yet been clearly defined. Only 17% of the total population lived in municipal areas (roughly corresponding to urban areas).

In the country as a whole, the largest proportion of the working population was engaged in agriculture (72%), followed by services, commerce and manufacturing (8%, 7% and 6%, respectively).

Contd p. 216

Thailand 1971 – 1980 MALE

DIAGNOSTIC GROUP	NUMBER OF CASES					REL. FREQUENCY(%)			HV(%)
	0	1-4	5-9	10-14	All	Crude	Adj.	Group	
TOTAL	27	225	180	180	614¤	100.0	100.0	100.0	90.9
I. LEUKAEMIAS	8	89	85	54	236	38.4	38.6	100.0	92.6
Acute lymphocytic	6	59	65	24	154	25.1	25.2	65.3	92.1
Other lymphocytic	0	0	0	1	1	0.2	0.2	0.4	100.0
Acute non-lymphocytic	2	24	12	19	57	9.3	9.3	24.2	94.5
Chronic myeloid	0	1	1	4	6	1.0	1.0	2.5	83.3
Other and unspecified	0	5	7	6	18	2.9	3.0	7.6	93.8
II. LYMPHOMAS	0	27	27	32	87¤	14.2	14.1	100.0	96.5
Hodgkin's disease	0	2	7	10	20¤	3.3	3.2	23.0	100.0
Non-Hodgkin lymphoma	0	16	12	18	46	7.5	7.5	52.9	100.0
Burkitt's lymphoma	0	4	2	1	7	1.1	1.1	8.0	71.4
Unspecified lymphoma	0	5	6	2	13	2.1	2.1	14.9	92.3
Histiocytosis X	0	0	0	0	0	–	–	–	–
Other reticuloendothelial	0	0	0	1	1	0.2	0.2	1.1	100.0
III. BRAIN AND SPINAL	1	10	17	13	41	6.7	6.7	100.0	92.5
Ependymoma	0	3	3	1	7	1.1	1.1	17.1	100.0
Astrocytoma	0	2	6	5	13	2.1	2.2	31.7	100.0
Medulloblastoma	1	2	5	2	10	1.6	1.6	24.4	100.0
Other glioma	0	0	1	0	1	0.2	0.2	2.4	–
Other and unspecified *	0	3	2	5	10	1.6	1.6	24.4	80.0
IV. SYMPATHETIC N.S.	4	19	15	5	43	7.0	7.0	100.0	90.5
Neuroblastoma	4	19	15	5	43	7.0	7.0	100.0	90.5
Other	0	0	0	0	0	–	–	–	–
V. RETINOBLASTOMA	1	40	12	1	54	8.8	8.7	100.0	94.3
VI. KIDNEY	2	12	1	2	17	2.8	2.7	100.0	82.4
Wilms' tumour	2	10	1	2	15	2.4	2.4	88.2	80.0
Renal carcinoma	0	2	0	0	2	0.3	0.3	11.8	100.0
Other and unspecified	0	0	0	0	0	–	–	–	–
VII. LIVER	1	3	1	8	13	2.1	2.1	100.0	53.8
Hepatoblastoma	1	1	0	0	2	0.3	0.3	15.4	100.0
Hepatic carcinoma	1	0	1	3	5	0.8	0.8	38.5	100.0
Other and unspecified	0	2	0	4	6	1.0	1.0	46.2	–
VIII. BONE	0	2	2	30	34	5.5	5.7	100.0	87.9
Osteosarcoma	0	1	0	19	20	3.3	3.3	58.8	89.5
Chondrosarcoma	0	0	1	2	3	0.5	0.5	8.8	100.0
Ewing's sarcoma	0	1	0	8	9	1.5	1.5	26.5	100.0
Other and unspecified	0	0	1	1	2	0.3	0.3	5.9	–
IX. SOFT TISSUE SARCOMAS	5	9	10	12	36	5.9	5.9	100.0	100.0
Rhabdomyosarcoma	3	6	5	4	18	2.9	2.9	50.0	100.0
Fibrosarcoma	0	2	1	2	5	0.8	0.8	13.9	100.0
Other and unspecified	2	1	4	6	13	2.1	2.1	36.1	100.0
X. GONADAL & GERM CELL	2	8	0	2	13¤	2.1	1.9	100.0	100.0
Non-gonadal germ cell	1	3	0	1	6¤	1.0	0.8	46.2	100.0
Gonadal germ cell	1	2	0	1	4	0.7	0.6	30.8	100.0
Gonadal carcinoma	0	3	0	0	3	0.5	0.5	23.1	100.0
Other and unspecified	0	0	0	0	0	–	–	–	–
XI. EPITHELIAL NEOPLASMS	2	3	7	15	27	4.4	4.5	100.0	100.0
Adrenocortical carcinoma	0	0	0	0	0	–	–	–	–
Thyroid carcinoma	0	0	0	2	2	0.3	0.3	7.4	100.0
Nasopharyngeal carcinoma	0	0	2	6	8	1.3	1.3	29.6	100.0
Melanoma	2	0	0	0	2	0.3	0.3	7.4	100.0
Other carcinoma	0	3	5	7	15	2.4	2.5	55.6	100.0
XII. OTHER	1	3	3	6	13	2.1	2.1	100.0	7.7
* Specified as malignant	0	2	1	2	5	0.8	0.8	100.0	60.0

¤ Includes age unknown

Thailand   FEMALE

1971 - 1980

DIAGNOSTIC GROUP	NUMBER OF CASES					REL. FREQUENCY(%)			HV(%)
	0	1-4	5-9	10-14	All	Crude	Adj.	Group	
TOTAL	20	176	136	150	484¤	100.0	100.0	100.0	92.6
I. LEUKAEMIAS	3	71	45	34	155¤	32.0	31.8	100.0	94.1
Acute lymphocytic	1	48	21	15	85	17.6	17.6	54.8	96.4
Other lymphocytic	0	2	0	1	3	0.6	0.6	1.9	100.0
Acute non-lymphocytic	0	18	18	13	50¤	10.3	10.2	32.3	89.8
Chronic myeloid	2	1	4	3	11¤	2.3	2.1	7.1	100.0
Other and unspecified	0	2	2	2	6	1.2	1.2	3.9	83.3
II. LYMPHOMAS	4	16	16	19	55	11.4	11.4	100.0	96.1
Hodgkin's disease	0	0	2	2	4	0.8	0.8	7.3	100.0
Non-Hodgkin lymphoma	2	9	11	13	35	7.2	7.3	63.6	100.0
Burkitt's lymphoma	0	2	0	1	3	0.6	0.6	5.5	100.0
Unspecified lymphoma	2	3	2	2	9	1.9	1.9	16.4	75.0
Histiocytosis X	0	1	0	0	1	0.2	0.2	1.8	100.0
Other reticuloendothelial	0	1	1	1	3	0.6	0.6	5.5	100.0
III. BRAIN AND SPINAL	1	9	16	13	39	8.1	8.2	100.0	94.9
Ependymoma	0	2	2	3	7	1.4	1.4	17.9	100.0
Astrocytoma	0	2	7	4	13	2.7	2.8	33.3	100.0
Medulloblastoma	0	2	2	3	7	1.4	1.4	17.9	100.0
Other glioma	0	2	2	0	4	0.8	0.8	10.3	100.0
Other and unspecified *	1	1	3	3	8	1.7	1.7	20.5	75.0
IV. SYMPATHETIC N.S.	4	6	7	1	18	3.7	3.8	100.0	94.1
Neuroblastoma	4	6	7	1	18	3.7	3.8	100.0	94.1
Other	0	0	0	0	0	–	–	–	–
V. RETINOBLASTOMA	3	44	10	1	58	12.0	12.0	100.0	87.9
VI. KIDNEY	1	10	3	1	15	3.1	3.1	100.0	93.3
Wilms' tumour	1	10	3	1	15	3.1	3.1	100.0	93.3
Renal carcinoma	0	0	0	0	0	–	–	–	–
Other and unspecified	0	0	0	0	0	–	–	–	–
VII. LIVER	0	2	2	2	6	1.2	1.2	100.0	83.3
Hepatoblastoma	0	2	0	0	2	0.4	0.4	33.3	100.0
Hepatic carcinoma	0	0	2	1	3	0.6	0.6	50.0	100.0
Other and unspecified	0	0	0	1	1	0.2	0.2	16.7	–
VIII. BONE	1	0	5	18	24	5.0	4.9	100.0	87.5
Osteosarcoma	1	0	0	14	15	3.1	3.0	62.5	93.3
Chondrosarcoma	0	0	0	1	1	0.2	0.2	4.2	100.0
Ewing's sarcoma	0	0	3	1	4	0.8	0.9	16.7	100.0
Other and unspecified	0	0	2	2	4	0.8	0.8	16.7	50.0
IX. SOFT TISSUE SARCOMAS	2	11	12	7	32	6.6	6.7	100.0	100.0
Rhabdomyosarcoma	2	2	7	3	14	2.9	3.0	43.8	100.0
Fibrosarcoma	0	2	2	4	8	1.7	1.6	25.0	100.0
Other and unspecified	0	7	3	0	10	2.1	2.1	31.3	100.0
X. GONADAL & GERM CELL	0	4	10	28	42	8.7	8.6	100.0	90.2
Non-gonadal germ cell	0	2	0	1	3	0.6	0.6	7.1	100.0
Gonadal germ cell	0	1	6	20	27	5.6	5.5	64.3	100.0
Gonadal carcinoma	0	1	2	2	4	0.8	0.8	9.5	50.0
Other and unspecified	0	3	5	5	8	1.7	1.7	19.0	100.0
XI. EPITHELIAL NEOPLASMS	1	1	8	22	32	6.6	6.6	100.0	100.0
Adrenocortical carcinoma	0	0	0	0	0	–	–	–	–
Thyroid carcinoma	0	0	3	9	12	2.5	2.5	37.5	100.0
Nasopharyngeal carcinoma	0	0	3	3	3	0.6	0.6	9.4	100.0
Melanoma	0	0	0	0	0	–	–	–	–
Other carcinoma	1	1	5	10	17	3.5	3.5	53.1	100.0
XII. OTHER	0	2	2	4	8	1.7	1.6	100.0	37.5
* Specified as malignant	0	0	3	3	6	1.2	1.3	100.0	83.3
¤ Includes age unknown									

The tables show childhood registrations for a ten-year period, 1971–1980. Incidence rates, based on the national population, are not shown since they are very low, suggesting that registration has been far from complete.

Commentary

The ratio of acute lymphocytic to acute non-lymphocytic leukaemia was 2.2:1. Hodgkin's disease accounted for only 17% of lymphomas, and Burkitt's lymphoma for under 10%.

Slightly over 10% of all registrations (112/1098) were for retinoblastoma. Laterality was recorded in only 48 cases (43%), but of these only five were bilateral. Kidney tumours, nearly all of which were Wilms' tumour, were rare.

Among girls, 8% of all registrations were for gonadal tumours, predominantly of germ-cell type.

VIET NAM

Cancer Institute, Ho Chi Minh City, 1976–1980

Luong Tan Truong

The data reported here are the cases of cancer in children aged 0–14 years recorded by the registry of the Cancer Hospital in Ho Chi Minh City (formerly Saigon) in the five years 1976–1980. The hospital has 335 beds, and departments of clinical medicine, surgery, gynaecology and radiotherapy, and provides the only specialized oncology service for 10 provinces in the southern part of Viet Nam (the total population served is about 12 million). Cases of children's cancer treated in two paediatric hospitals, as well as the general medical service and the department of ophthalmology in two other hospitals of Ho Chi Minh City, are also registered.

Viet Nam has a total area of 335 000 square kilometres, and a population (1979) of 52.7 million, of whom 42% are aged under 15. The southern part of the country (Nam Phan) is occupied by the delta of the Mekong River, a rich agricultural plain used mainly for the cultivation of rice. The population density is low (under 100 per square kilometre). The climate is tropical, with high humidity and temperatures in Ho Chi Minh City ranging from 18° C to 33° C; annual rainfall is 200 cm, with a season of equatorial rains in June–October.

Commentary

The largest diagnostic group was the leukaemias, comprising 26% of all registrations. Of the leukaemias, 52% were acute lymphocytic and 38% acute non-lymphocytic. The second largest group was retinoblastoma (18% of the total). There were also substantial numbers of children with non-Hodgkin lymphoma, brain tumours and Wilms' tumour. There were only three cases of neuroblastoma and, unusually for countries of eastern Asia, no liver tumours.

Vietnam, Ho Chi Minh City   1976 - 1980   MALE

DIAGNOSTIC GROUP	NUMBER OF CASES				REL. FREQUENCY(%)			HV(%)
	0-4	5-9	10-14	All	Crude	Adj.	Group	
TOTAL	54	51	38	143	100.0	100.0	100.0	87.4
I. LEUKAEMIAS	11	20	12	43	30.1	29.4	100.0	100.0
Acute lymphocytic	5	9	8	22	15.4	15.3	51.2	100.0
Other lymphocytic	0	0	0	0	-	-	-	-
Acute non-lymphocytic	6	9	3	18	12.6	12.1	41.9	100.0
Chronic myeloid	0	1	1	2	1.4	1.4	4.7	100.0
Other and unspecified	0	1	0	1	0.7	0.6	2.3	100.0
II. LYMPHOMAS	3	7	7	17	11.9	11.9	100.0	100.0
Hodgkin's disease	0	1	3	4	2.8	3.0	23.5	100.0
Non-Hodgkin lymphoma	3	6	4	13	9.1	8.9	76.5	100.0
Burkitt's lymphoma	0	0	0	0	-	-	-	-
Unspecified lymphoma	0	0	0	0	-	-	-	-
Histiocytosis X	0	0	0	0	-	-	-	-
Other reticuloendothelial	0	0	0	0	-	-	-	-
III. BRAIN AND SPINAL	2	3	6	11	7.7	8.0	100.0	100.0
Ependymoma	1	0	0	1	0.7	0.7	9.1	100.0
Astrocytoma	1	2	5	8	5.6	5.9	72.7	100.0
Medulloblastoma	0	1	1	2	1.4	1.4	18.2	100.0
Other glioma	0	0	0	0	-	-	-	-
Other and unspecified *	0	0	0	0	-	-	-	-
IV. SYMPATHETIC N.S.	1	0	0	1	0.7	0.7	100.0	100.0
Neuroblastoma	1	0	0	1	0.7	0.7	100.0	100.0
Other	0	0	0	0	-	-	-	-
V. RETINOBLASTOMA	14	5	0	19	13.3	13.3	100.0	100.0
VI. KIDNEY	12	2	0	14	9.8	10.1	100.0	100.0
Wilms' tumour	11	2	0	13	9.1	9.3	92.9	92.9
Renal carcinoma	0	0	0	0	-	-	-	-
Other and unspecified	1	0	0	1	0.7	0.7	7.1	-
VII. LIVER	0	0	0	0	-	-	-	-
Hepatoblastoma	0	0	0	0	-	-	-	-
Hepatic carcinoma	0	0	0	0	-	-	-	-
Other and unspecified	0	0	0	0	-	-	-	-
VIII. BONE	1	7	3	11	7.7	7.2	100.0	45.5
Osteosarcoma	0	0	1	1	0.7	0.8	9.1	100.0
Chondrosarcoma	0	0	0	0	-	-	-	-
Ewing's sarcoma	0	2	2	4	2.8	2.8	36.4	100.0
Other and unspecified	1	5	0	6	4.2	3.7	54.5	-
IX. SOFT TISSUE SARCOMAS	1	1	2	4	2.8	2.9	100.0	100.0
Rhabdomyosarcoma	1	0	0	1	0.7	0.7	25.0	100.0
Fibrosarcoma	0	1	1	2	1.4	1.4	50.0	100.0
Other and unspecified	0	0	1	1	0.7	0.8	25.0	100.0
X. GONADAL & GERM CELL	3	1	0	4	2.8	2.8	100.0	100.0
Non-gonadal germ cell	0	0	0	0	-	-	-	-
Gonadal germ cell	3	1	0	4	2.8	2.8	100.0	100.0
Gonadal carcinoma	0	0	0	0	-	-	-	-
Other and unspecified	0	0	0	0	-	-	-	-
XI. EPITHELIAL NEOPLASMS	1	0	7	8	5.6	6.3	100.0	100.0
Adrenocortical carcinoma	0	0	0	0	-	-	-	-
Thyroid carcinoma	0	0	0	0	-	-	-	-
Nasopharyngeal carcinoma	0	0	3	3	2.1	2.4	37.5	100.0
Melanoma	0	0	0	0	-	-	-	-
Other carcinoma	1	0	4	5	3.5	3.9	62.5	100.0
XII. OTHER	5	5	1	11	7.7	7.4	100.0	-

* Specified as malignant

Vietnam, Ho Chi Minh City

1976 – 1980

FEMALE

DIAGNOSTIC GROUP	NUMBER OF CASES				REL. FREQUENCY(%)			HV(%)
	0-4	5-9	10-14	All	Crude	Adj.	Group	
TOTAL	47	30	20	97	100.0	100.0	100.0	95.9
I. LEUKAEMIAS	9	7	4	20	20.6	20.7	100.0	100.0
Acute lymphocytic	5	4	2	11	11.3	11.3	55.0	100.0
Other lymphocytic	0	0	0	0	-	-	-	-
Acute non-lymphocytic	3	2	1	6	6.2	6.1	30.0	100.0
Chronic myeloid	0	1	1	2	2.1	2.5	10.0	100.0
Other and unspecified	1	0	0	1	1.0	0.9	5.0	100.0
II. LYMPHOMAS	3	3	1	7	7.2	7.1	100.0	100.0
Hodgkin's disease	0	1	0	1	1.0	1.0	14.3	100.0
Non-Hodgkin lymphoma	3	2	1	6	6.2	6.1	85.7	100.0
Burkitt's lymphoma	0	0	0	0	-	-	-	-
Unspecified lymphoma	0	0	0	0	-	-	-	-
Histiocytosis X	0	0	0	0	-	-	-	-
Other reticuloendothelial	0	0	0	0	-	-	-	-
III. BRAIN AND SPINAL	2	2	4	8	8.2	9.7	100.0	100.0
Ependymoma	1	1	1	3	3.1	3.4	37.5	100.0
Astrocytoma	0	1	3	4	4.1	5.5	50.0	100.0
Medulloblastoma	1	0	0	1	1.0	0.9	12.5	100.0
Other glioma	0	0	0	0	-	-	-	-
Other and unspecified *	0	0	0	0	-	-	-	-
IV. SYMPATHETIC N.S.	1	1	0	2	2.1	1.9	100.0	100.0
Neuroblastoma	1	1	0	2	2.1	1.9	100.0	100.0
Other	0	0	0	0	-	-	-	-
V. RETINOBLASTOMA	17	6	0	23	23.7	20.5	100.0	100.0
VI. KIDNEY	8	3	1	12	12.4	11.3	100.0	100.0
Wilms' tumour	8	3	1	12	12.4	11.3	100.0	100.0
Renal carcinoma	0	0	0	0	-	-	-	-
Other and unspecified	0	0	0	0	-	-	-	-
VII. LIVER	0	0	0	0	-	-	-	-
Hepatoblastoma	0	0	0	0	-	-	-	-
Hepatic carcinoma	0	0	0	0	-	-	-	-
Other and unspecified	0	0	0	0	-	-	-	-
VIII. BONE	2	0	2	4	4.1	4.7	100.0	75.0
Osteosarcoma	1	0	1	2	2.1	2.4	50.0	100.0
Chondrosarcoma	0	0	0	0	-	-	-	-
Ewing's sarcoma	0	0	1	1	1.0	1.5	25.0	-
Other and unspecified	1	0	0	1	1.0	0.9	25.0	100.0
IX. SOFT TISSUE SARCOMAS	2	1	0	3	3.1	2.7	100.0	100.0
Rhabdomyosarcoma	1	0	0	1	1.0	0.9	33.3	100.0
Fibrosarcoma	1	1	0	2	2.1	1.9	66.7	100.0
Other and unspecified	0	0	0	0	-	-	-	-
X. GONADAL & GERM CELL	1	6	5	12	12.4	14.4	100.0	100.0
Non-gonadal germ cell	1	1	0	2	2.1	1.9	16.7	100.0
Gonadal germ cell	0	4	4	8	8.2	10.0	66.7	100.0
Gonadal carcinoma	0	1	1	2	2.1	2.5	16.7	100.0
Other and unspecified	0	0	0	0	-	-	-	-
XI. EPITHELIAL NEOPLASMS	0	1	2	3	3.1	4.0	100.0	100.0
Adrenocortical carcinoma	0	0	0	0	-	-	-	-
Thyroid carcinoma	0	0	0	0	-	-	-	-
Nasopharyngeal carcinoma	0	0	0	0	-	-	-	-
Melanoma	0	0	0	0	-	-	-	-
Other carcinoma	0	1	2	3	3.1	4.0	100.0	100.0
XII. OTHER	2	0	1	3	3.1	3.2	100.0	-

* Specified as malignant   0   0   0   0   -   -   -   -

EUROPE

CZECHOSLOVAKIA

National Cancer Registry of Slovakia, 1970-1979

I. Plesko, J. Somogyi & E. Dimitrova

Compulsory notification of oncological patients and persons dying from cancer was introduced throughout Czechoslovakia in 1952. On this basis, separate statistics for cancer incidence and mortality were published regularly for more than 20 years. During this period, cancer patients were treated at the Institute of Clinical Oncology in Bratislava and the departments of radiology in larger hospitals. In the last decade, a new network of specialized out-patient oncology clinics has been established in all districts of the country; the oncologists in charge of the clinics are responsible not only for medical care but also for the notification and follow-up of cancer patients. Meanwhile, hospital- and population-based cancer registries had been established in various parts of Czechoslovakia. In 1976, a population-based cancer registry, initially covering only western Slovakia, was established in the Cancer Epidemiology Department of the Cancer Research Institute of the Slovak Academy of Sciences in Bratislava. The data collected served mainly as a basis for epidemiological investigations and for international scientific projects, especially in countries belonging to the Council for Mutual Economic Assistance (CMEA).

In 1980, the population-based National Cancer Registry of Slovakia was established at the Oncological Centre in Bratislava. This comprehensive cancer centre consists of two independent institutes — the Cancer Research Institute of the Slovak Academy of Sciences and the Institute of Clinical Oncology. New, more detailed reporting forms had been introduced in 1977 and, when used with other sources of information, these allow the collection of the great majority of data items recommended for standardized population-based cancer registries.

Cancer registration takes place in two stages: (1) information about new cases is checked and compared with the list of registered cases; (2) abstracting and coding of individual data are done on a standard form. All death certificates are regularly reviewed and compared with the list of living patients, not only to ensure the inclusion of previously unregistered cases but also to complete the data on patients already registered. A system of cross-checking is used both to eliminate repeated registration of the same case and to ensure the proper registration of multiple primaries in the same patient.

The registry includes all malignant neoplasms, including skin tumours and histiocytosis X, and all benign and unspecified brain and spinal tumours. All cases notified and registered in the decade 1968-1977 were recoded using the ICD-O classification. Beginning with the year 1978, the ICD-O classification for coding topography and morphology of tumours has been used simultaneously with ICD-9. The data are stored on magnetic tape and all computations and analyses are performed at the State Computer Centre; confidentiality of the data in the registry is strictly preserved.

The registry now covers the entire territory of Slovakia (Slovak Socialist Republic). Administratively, Slovakia is divided into 38 districts, including two large cities, Bratislava and Kosice, having 381 165 and 203 109 inhabitants respectively in 1980. Some 20% of the population live either in these two cities or in six other cities with 50 000-100 000 inhabitants, and the remaining 80% in smaller towns or villages with under 50 000 inhabitants. The whole of Slovakia is characterized by a high degree of urbanization and the country has undergone extremely rapid industrialization since the Second World War. The major sources of employment are industry and building (some 44%) and agriculture and forestry (nearly 18%).

Most of the population are of Slovak nationality; the second most numerous group are Hungarians (11%).

Slovakia, which has an area of 49 014 square kilometres, can be divided into two main parts: the fertile lowlands irrigated by rivers situated mainly

Contd p. 224

Czechoslovakia, Slovakia   1970 – 1979   MALE

DIAGNOSTIC GROUP	NUMBER OF CASES 0	1-4	5-9	10-14	All	REL. FREQUENCY(%) Crude	Adj.	Group	RATES PER MILLION 0	1-4	5-9	10-14	Crude	Adj.	Cum	HV(%)
TOTAL	78	325	244	203	850	100.0	100.0	100.0	163.3	187.1	123.5	95.7	134.7	138.2	2008	94.7
I. LEUKAEMIAS	19	104	76	41	240	28.2	27.6	100.0	39.8	59.9	38.5	19.3	38.0	39.6	568	100.0
Acute lymphocytic	8	67	46	25	146	17.2	16.8	60.8	16.7	38.6	23.3	11.8	23.1	24.2	346	100.0
Other lymphocytic	0	0	0	0	0	-	-	-	-	-	-	-	-	-	-	-
Acute non-lymphocytic	5	14	8	7	34	4.0	3.9	14.2	10.5	8.1	4.1	3.3	5.4	5.6	79	100.0
Chronic myeloid	1	2	3	1	7	0.8	0.8	2.9	2.1	1.2	1.5	0.5	1.1	1.1	17	100.0
Other and unspecified	5	21	19	8	53	6.2	6.1	22.1	10.5	12.1	9.6	3.8	8.4	8.8	126	100.0
II. LYMPHOMAS	9	38	52	54	153	18.0	19.0	100.0	18.8	21.9	26.3	25.5	24.2	24.1	365	100.0
Hodgkin's disease	0	8	24	25	57	6.7	7.4	37.3	-	4.6	12.2	11.8	9.0	8.8	138	100.0
Non-Hodgkin lymphoma	3	13	18	21	55	6.5	6.9	35.9	6.3	7.5	9.1	9.9	8.7	8.6	131	100.0
Burkitt's lymphoma	0	1	1	1	3	0.4	0.4	2.0	-	0.6	0.5	0.5	0.5	0.4	7	100.0
Unspecified lymphoma	3	14	9	6	32	3.8	3.7	20.9	6.3	8.1	4.6	2.8	5.1	5.3	75	100.0
Histiocytosis X	2	1	0	1	4	0.5	0.4	2.6	4.2	0.6	-	0.5	0.6	0.6	9	100.0
Other reticuloendothelial	1	1	0	0	2	0.2	0.2	1.3	2.1	0.6	-	-	0.3	0.3	4	100.0
III. BRAIN AND SPINAL	8	49	54	50	161	18.9	19.7	100.0	16.7	28.2	27.3	23.6	25.5	25.7	384	93.0
Ependymoma	1	2	5	1	9	1.1	1.4	5.6	2.1	1.2	2.6	0.5	1.4	1.5	22	100.0
Astrocytoma	1	8	9	13	31	3.6	3.9	19.3	2.1	4.6	4.6	6.1	4.9	4.8	74	100.0
Medulloblastoma	3	9	10	7	29	3.4	3.5	18.0	6.3	5.2	5.1	3.3	4.6	4.7	69	100.0
Other glioma	3	24	20	21	68	8.0	8.2	42.2	6.3	13.8	10.1	9.9	10.8	10.9	162	100.0
Other and unspecified *	0	6	10	8	24	2.8	3.0	14.9	-	3.5	5.1	3.8	3.8	3.8	58	45.0
IV. SYMPATHETIC N.S.	4	20	3	0	27	3.2	2.8	100.0	8.4	11.5	1.5	-	4.3	4.7	62	100.0
Neuroblastoma	4	19	3	0	26	3.1	2.7	96.3	8.4	10.9	1.5	-	4.1	4.5	60	100.0
Other	0	1	0	0	1	0.1	0.1	3.7	-	0.6	-	-	0.2	0.2	2	100.0
V. RETINOBLASTOMA	5	24	1	1	31	3.6	3.1	100.0	10.5	13.8	0.5	0.5	4.9	5.4	71	100.0
VI. KIDNEY	10	37	12	0	59	6.9	6.1	100.0	20.9	21.3	6.1	-	9.3	10.2	137	93.2
Wilms' tumour	8	35	11	0	54	6.4	5.6	91.5	16.7	20.1	5.6	-	8.6	9.3	125	100.0
Renal carcinoma	1	0	0	0	1	0.1	0.1	1.7	2.1	-	-	-	0.2	0.2	2	100.0
Other and unspecified	1	2	1	0	4	0.5	0.4	6.8	2.1	1.2	0.5	-	0.6	0.7	9	-
VII. LIVER	1	6	1	3	11	1.3	1.3	100.0	2.1	3.5	0.5	1.4	1.7	1.8	26	100.0
Hepatoblastoma	1	4	0	2	7	0.8	0.8	63.6	2.1	2.3	-	0.9	1.1	1.1	16	100.0
Hepatic carcinoma	0	2	1	0	3	0.4	0.3	27.3	-	1.2	0.5	-	0.5	0.5	7	100.0
Other and unspecified	0	0	0	1	1	0.1	0.1	9.1	-	-	-	0.5	0.2	0.1	2	100.0
VIII. BONE	0	5	11	16	32	3.8	4.2	100.0	-	2.9	5.6	7.5	5.1	4.9	77	87.5
Osteosarcoma	0	0	3	8	11	1.3	1.6	34.4	-	-	1.5	3.8	1.7	1.6	26	100.0
Chondrosarcoma	0	0	0	0	0	-	-	-	-	-	-	-	-	-	-	-
Ewing's sarcoma	0	5	7	3	15	1.8	1.8	46.9	-	2.9	3.5	1.4	2.4	2.4	36	100.0
Other and unspecified	0	0	1	5	6	0.7	0.9	18.8	-	-	0.5	2.4	1.0	0.8	14	33.3
IX. SOFT TISSUE SARCOMAS	2	14	12	10	38	4.5	4.6	100.0	4.2	8.1	6.1	4.7	6.0	6.1	90	100.0
Rhabdomyosarcoma	0	6	2	1	9	1.1	1.0	23.7	-	3.5	1.0	0.5	1.4	1.1	21	100.0
Fibrosarcoma	0	2	2	3	7	0.8	0.9	18.4	-	1.2	1.0	1.4	1.1	1.1	17	100.0
Other and unspecified	2	6	8	6	22	2.6	2.7	57.9	4.2	3.5	4.1	2.8	3.5	3.5	52	100.0
X. GONADAL & GERM CELL	2	11	1	3	17	2.0	1.9	100.0	4.2	6.3	0.5	1.4	2.7	2.9	39	100.0
Non-gonadal germ cell	1	3	0	0	4	0.5	0.4	23.5	2.1	1.7	-	-	0.6	0.7	9	100.0
Gonadal germ cell	1	8	1	3	13	1.5	1.5	76.5	2.1	4.6	0.5	1.4	2.1	2.2	30	100.0
Gonadal carcinoma	0	0	0	0	0	-	-	-	-	-	-	-	-	-	-	-
Other and unspecified	0	0	0	0	0	-	-	-	-	-	-	-	-	-	-	-
XI. EPITHELIAL NEOPLASMS	7	6	11	16	40	4.7	5.0	100.0	14.7	3.5	5.6	7.5	6.3	6.2	94	100.0
Adrenocortical carcinoma	0	1	0	0	1	0.1	0.1	2.5	-	0.6	-	-	0.2	0.2	2	100.0
Thyroid carcinoma	0	0	0	1	1	0.1	0.1	2.5	-	-	-	0.5	0.2	0.1	2	100.0
Nasopharyngeal carcinoma	0	0	0	0	0	-	-	-	-	-	-	-	-	-	-	-
Melanoma	0	1	1	2	4	0.5	0.5	10.0	-	0.6	0.5	0.9	0.6	0.6	10	100.0
Other carcinoma	7	4	10	13	34	4.0	4.2	85.0	14.7	2.3	5.1	6.1	5.4	5.3	80	100.0
XII. OTHER	11	11	12	7	41	4.8	4.7	100.0	23.0	6.3	6.1	3.3	6.5	6.7	95	19.4
* Specified as malignant	0	4	7	7	18	2.1	2.3	100.0	-	2.3	3.5	3.3	2.9	2.8	43	21.4

Czechoslovakia, Slovakia

1970 – 1979

FEMALE

Diagnostic Group	Cases 0	Cases 1-4	Cases 5-9	Cases 10-14	Cases All	Rel.Freq Crude	Rel.Freq Adj.	Rel.Freq Group	Rate 0	Rate 1-4	Rate 5-9	Rate 10-14	Rate Crude	Rate Adj.	Cum	HV(%)
TOTAL	60	246	168	187	661	100.0	100.0	100.0	130.7	147.6	89.1	92.4	109.5	111.4	1628	93.4
I. LEUKAEMIAS	15	101	53	54	223	33.7	33.3	100.0	32.7	60.6	28.1	26.7	36.9	38.1	549	100.0
Acute lymphocytic	8	63	37	20	128	19.4	19.1	57.4	17.4	37.8	19.6	9.9	21.2	22.3	316	100.0
Other lymphocytic	0	0	0	0	0	–	–	–	–	–	–	–	–	–	–	–
Acute non-lymphocytic	2	20	6	16	44	6.7	6.5	19.7	4.4	12.0	3.2	7.9	7.3	7.4	108	100.0
Chronic myeloid	3	3	0	2	8	1.2	1.1	3.6	6.5	1.8	–	1.0	1.3	1.4	19	100.0
Other and unspecified	2	15	10	16	43	6.5	6.6	19.3	4.4	9.0	5.3	7.9	7.1	7.1	106	100.0
II. LYMPHOMAS	4	13	18	23	58	8.8	9.1	100.0	8.7	7.8	9.5	11.4	9.6	9.5	144	100.0
Hodgkin's disease	0	3	8	15	26	3.9	4.2	44.8	–	1.8	4.2	7.4	4.3	4.1	65	100.0
Non-Hodgkin lymphoma	4	4	4	3	15	2.3	2.2	25.9	8.7	2.4	2.1	1.5	2.5	2.5	36	100.0
Burkitt's lymphoma	0	0	0	0	0	–	–	–	–	–	–	–	–	–	–	–
Unspecified lymphoma	0	4	6	4	14	2.1	2.2	24.1	–	2.4	3.2	2.0	2.3	2.3	35	100.0
Histiocytosis X	0	1	0	0	1	0.2	0.1	1.7	–	0.6	–	–	0.2	0.2	2	100.0
Other reticuloendothelial	0	1	0	1	2	0.3	0.3	3.4	–	0.6	–	0.5	0.3	0.3	5	100.0
III. BRAIN AND SPINAL	6	32	43	38	119	18.0	18.7	100.0	13.1	19.2	22.8	18.8	19.7	19.8	298	89.5
Ependymoma	2	2	1	2	7	1.1	1.0	5.9	4.4	1.2	0.5	1.0	1.2	1.2	17	100.0
Astrocytoma	1	2	8	10	21	3.2	3.4	17.6	2.2	1.2	4.2	4.9	3.5	3.3	53	100.0
Medulloblastoma	0	5	6	5	16	2.4	2.4	13.4	–	3.0	3.2	2.5	2.7	2.7	40	100.0
Other glioma	3	16	18	10	47	7.1	7.3	39.5	6.5	9.6	9.5	4.9	7.8	8.0	117	100.0
Other and unspecified *	0	7	10	11	28	4.2	4.5	23.5	–	4.2	5.3	5.4	4.6	4.6	70	47.8
IV. SYMPATHETIC N.S.	4	22	3	5	34	5.1	4.7	100.0	8.7	13.2	1.6	2.5	5.6	6.0	82	100.0
Neuroblastoma	4	22	2	5	33	5.0	4.6	97.1	8.7	13.2	1.1	2.5	5.5	5.8	79	100.0
Other	0	0	1	0	1	0.2	0.2	2.9	–	–	0.5	–	0.2	0.2	3	–
V. RETINOBLASTOMA	6	19	1	1	27	4.1	3.6	100.0	13.1	11.4	0.5	0.5	4.5	4.9	64	100.0
VI. KIDNEY	4	29	12	1	46	7.0	6.6	100.0	8.7	17.4	6.4	0.5	7.6	8.3	113	97.8
Wilms' tumour	2	28	10	1	41	6.2	5.9	89.1	4.4	16.8	5.3	0.5	6.8	7.4	101	100.0
Renal carcinoma	0	0	2	0	2	0.3	0.4	4.3	–	–	1.1	–	0.3	0.3	5	100.0
Other and unspecified	2	1	0	0	3	0.5	0.4	6.5	4.4	0.6	–	–	0.5	0.5	7	66.7
VII. LIVER	0	2	2	1	5	0.8	0.8	100.0	–	1.2	1.1	0.5	0.8	0.9	13	100.0
Hepatoblastoma	0	2	2	1	5	0.8	0.8	100.0	–	1.2	1.1	0.5	0.8	0.9	13	100.0
Hepatic carcinoma	0	0	0	0	0	–	–	–	–	–	–	–	–	–	–	–
Other and unspecified	0	0	0	0	0	–	–	–	–	–	–	–	–	–	–	–
VIII. BONE	2	2	12	23	39	5.9	6.4	100.0	4.4	1.2	6.4	11.4	6.5	6.1	98	89.7
Osteosarcoma	0	0	3	12	15	2.3	2.5	38.5	–	–	1.6	5.9	2.5	2.2	38	100.0
Chondrosarcoma	0	0	0	2	2	0.3	0.3	5.1	–	–	–	1.0	0.3	0.3	5	100.0
Ewing's sarcoma	0	1	7	4	12	1.8	2.0	30.8	–	0.6	3.7	2.0	2.0	2.0	31	100.0
Other and unspecified	2	1	2	5	10	1.5	1.6	25.6	4.4	0.6	1.1	2.5	1.7	1.6	24	60.0
IX. SOFT TISSUE SARCOMAS	6	9	5	8	28	4.2	4.1	100.0	13.1	5.4	2.7	4.0	4.6	4.7	68	100.0
Rhabdomyosarcoma	0	3	0	0	3	0.5	0.4	10.7	–	1.8	–	–	0.5	0.6	7	100.0
Fibrosarcoma	1	2	3	1	7	1.1	1.1	25.0	2.2	1.2	1.6	0.5	1.2	1.2	17	100.0
Other and unspecified	5	4	2	7	18	2.7	2.7	64.3	10.9	2.4	1.1	3.5	3.0	2.9	43	100.0
X. GONADAL & GERM CELL	2	6	5	13	26	3.9	4.0	100.0	4.4	3.6	2.7	6.4	4.3	4.2	64	96.2
Non-gonadal germ cell	2	5	1	1	9	1.4	1.3	34.6	4.4	3.0	0.5	0.5	1.5	1.6	21	100.0
Gonadal germ cell	0	0	1	10	11	1.7	1.8	42.3	–	–	0.5	4.9	1.8	1.8	27	100.0
Gonadal carcinoma	0	0	2	1	3	0.5	0.5	11.5	–	–	1.1	0.5	0.5	0.5	8	100.0
Other and unspecified	0	1	1	1	3	0.5	0.5	11.5	–	0.6	0.5	0.5	0.5	0.5	8	66.7
XI. EPITHELIAL NEOPLASMS	4	2	7	12	25	3.8	4.0	100.0	8.7	1.2	3.7	5.9	4.1	4.0	62	100.0
Adrenocortical carcinoma	0	0	0	0	0	–	–	–	–	–	–	–	–	–	–	–
Thyroid carcinoma	0	0	0	3	3	0.5	0.5	12.0	–	–	–	1.5	0.5	0.4	7	100.0
Nasopharyngeal carcinoma	0	0	1	1	2	0.2	0.1	8.0	–	–	0.5	0.5	0.2	0.1	2	100.0
Melanoma	1	1	1	4	7	1.1	1.1	28.0	2.2	0.6	0.5	2.0	1.2	1.1	17	100.0
Other carcinoma	3	1	5	4	13	2.1	2.2	56.0	6.5	0.6	3.2	2.0	2.3	2.3	35	66.7
XII. OTHER	7	9	7	8	31	4.7	4.6	100.0	15.2	5.4	3.7	4.0	5.1	5.2	75	7.4
* Specified as malignant	0	5	5	8	18	2.7	2.8	100.0	–	3.0	2.7	4.0	3.0	2.9	45	7.7

in the south-western and eastern parts of the country with favourable climatic and geographical conditions for agriculture; and the major part of Slovakia, which is mountainous and covered with forests.

Population

The population at risk is derived from the 1970 census and mid-year estimates for 1975.

AVERAGE ANNUAL POPULATION: 1970–1979

Age	Male	Female
0	47774	45922
1–4	173708	166639
5–9	197497	188557
10–14	212120	202481
0–14	631099	603599

Commentary

The overall incidence rate and the relative frequencies of the principal categories of childhood cancer are typical of European populations and correspond closely to those published for the period 1968–1977 (Plesko et al., 1983). The 21% of leukaemias classified as 'other and unspecified' were nearly all of unspecified cell type; their age-distribution, at least among males, is consistent with their being, in fact, mostly acute lymphocytic leukaemia (ALL). Among the lymphomas, 22% were of unspecified type, but probably non-Hodgkin. The miscellaneous carcinomas and other unspecified tumours included 14 cases with sites in the oral cavity, etc; it is probable that some of these were nasopharyngeal tumours, particularly as only one case of nasopharyngeal carcinoma as such was recorded.

Reference

Plesko, I, Somogyi, J. & Dimitrova, E. (1983) Incidence of childhood tumors in Slovakia. Neoplasma, 30, 733-742

DENMARK

The Danish Cancer Registry, 1978-1982

O.M. Jensen & A. Prener

The Danish Cancer Registry is a research institute of the Danish Cancer Society (Kraeftens Bekaempelse). The Registry is subsidized by the Ministry of the Interior.

Since 1942, all cases of malignant neoplasms have been notified to the registry on a voluntary basis from the hospital departments treating cancer patients. In recent years, information on skin cancer has also been obtained from dermatologists in private practice. Non-malignant brain and spinal tumours are also registered routinely. Pathology institutes send separate reports on post mortems on cancer patients; this information is supplemented by a review of all death certificates. Since the start of the Registry, the policy has been to register a limited amount of data for each cancer patient notified by the staff of the treating hospital departments, supplementing this information on an *ad hoc* basis, if necessary, for epidemiological and clinical studies. Follow-up for cause of death and date of death is undertaken routinely by record-linkage with information from death certificates.

The introduction of a central personal number system in Denmark in 1968 provided a unique identification number for each person living in the country. This has been of great use in the organization of the Registry, which is now making extensive use of automated data processing in carrying out consistency checks and in eliminating errors. The identification number makes the checking of duplicate registration easy, and facilitates studies employing record-linkage.

All data from the period 1943-1977 were classified according to a modified version of the 7th revision of the *International Classification of Diseases*, expanded to include certain information on histology and tumour behaviour. Since 1978, all data have been classified according to the *International Classification of Diseases for Oncology* (ICD-O). After checks for completeness and coding, the data are stored in the Registry's data base.

The Danish population enjoys practically free primary medical care, and hospital treatment is provided free of charge to every member of the population. The Registry covers the Kingdom of Denmark, excluding the Faroe Islands, but including Greenland. Data for Greenland, with its Inuit population, are not included in the present tabulations. The total population of Denmark is approximately 5 million; it is of Caucasian stock and fairly homogeneous. Approximately 27% of the population lives in the Copenhagen area; 38% lives in provincial towns, ranging in size from 10 000 to about 200 000 inhabitants; and 35% lives in rural areas.

The Registry produces regular reports on cancer incidence in Denmark and routinely publishes regional and urban/rural comparisons, as well as publishing trends in cancer incidence since 1943. The Registry has been extensively used as an end-point in cohort studies of both environmental factors and medical procedures in relation to cancer risk.

Population

Annual population estimates are published by Danmarks Statistik (Statistics Denmark), and the data for 1978-1982 have been used.

AVERAGE ANNUAL POPULATION: 1978-1982

Age	Male	Female
0	29971	28624
1-4	133152	127330
5-9	185141	176997
10-14	202232	192327
0-14	550496	525278

Contd p. 228

Denmark   MALE

1978 - 1982

DIAGNOSTIC GROUP	NUMBER OF CASES					REL. FREQUENCY(%)			RATES PER MILLION						Cum	HV(%)
	0	1-4	5-9	10-14	All	Crude	Adj.	Group	0	1-4	5-9	10-14	Crude	Adj.		
TOTAL	30	119	112	117	378	100.0	100.0	100.0	200.2	178.7	121.0	115.7	137.3	143.5	2099	95.3
I. LEUKAEMIAS	3	49	29	30	111	29.4	29.4	100.0	20.0	73.6	31.3	29.7	40.3	43.1	619	100.0
Acute lymphocytic	1	39	24	24	88	23.3	23.3	79.3	6.7	58.6	25.9	23.7	32.0	33.9	489	100.0
Other lymphocytic	0	0	0	1	1	0.3	0.3	0.9	-	-	-	1.0	0.4	0.3	5	100.0
Acute non-lymphocytic	1	8	5	4	18	4.8	4.8	16.2	6.7	12.0	5.4	4.0	6.5	7.1	102	100.0
Chronic myeloid	0	2	0	0	2	0.5	0.5	1.8	-	3.0	-	-	0.7	0.9	12	100.0
Other and unspecified	1	0	0	1	2	0.5	0.5	1.8	6.7	-	-	1.0	0.7	0.8	12	100.0
II. LYMPHOMAS	1	8	18	24	51	13.5	13.4	100.0	6.7	12.0	19.4	23.7	18.5	17.4	271	100.0
Hodgkin's disease	0	1	2	11	14	3.7	3.6	27.5	-	1.5	2.2	10.9	5.1	4.3	71	100.0
Non-Hodgkin lymphoma	0	2	5	5	12	3.2	3.2	23.5	-	3.0	5.4	4.9	4.4	4.1	64	100.0
Burkitt's lymphoma	1	3	8	1	13	3.4	3.5	25.5	6.7	4.5	8.6	1.0	4.7	4.8	71	100.0
Unspecified lymphoma	0	1	2	6	9	2.4	2.4	17.6	-	1.5	2.2	4.9	3.3	3.1	48	100.0
Histiocytosis X	0	1	0	1	2	0.5	0.5	3.9	-	1.5	-	1.0	0.7	0.8	11	100.0
Other reticuloendothelial	0	0	1	0	1	0.3	0.3	2.0	-	-	1.1	-	0.4	0.3	5	100.0
III. BRAIN AND SPINAL	6	22	31	34	93	24.6	24.5	100.0	40.0	33.0	33.5	33.6	33.8	33.9	508	87.8
Ependymoma	2	3	3	5	13	3.4	3.4	14.0	13.3	4.5	3.2	4.9	4.7	4.9	72	100.0
Astrocytoma	1	7	10	14	32	8.5	8.4	34.4	6.7	10.5	10.8	13.8	11.6	11.3	172	100.0
Medulloblastoma	2	5	6	2	15	4.0	4.0	16.1	13.3	7.5	6.5	2.0	5.4	6.0	86	100.0
Other glioma	0	3	2	4	9	2.4	2.4	9.7	-	4.5	2.2	4.0	3.3	3.2	49	100.0
Other and unspecified *	1	4	10	9	24	6.3	6.3	25.8	6.7	6.0	10.8	8.9	8.7	8.4	129	47.6
IV. SYMPATHETIC N.S.	10	7	2	3	22	5.8	5.9	100.0	66.7	10.5	2.2	3.0	8.0	10.0	134	95.5
Neuroblastoma	9	7	2	2	20	5.3	5.3	90.9	60.1	10.5	2.2	2.0	7.3	9.2	123	95.0
Other	1	0	0	1	2	0.5	0.5	9.1	6.7	-	-	1.0	0.7	0.8	12	100.0
V. RETINOBLASTOMA	1	4	0	0	5	1.3	1.3	100.0	6.7	6.0	-	-	1.8	2.4	31	100.0
VI. KIDNEY	2	8	10	1	21	5.6	5.6	100.0	13.3	12.0	10.8	1.0	7.6	8.5	120	89.5
Wilms' tumour	2	8	6	1	17	4.5	4.5	81.0	13.3	12.0	6.5	1.0	6.2	6.8	97	100.0
Renal carcinoma	0	0	0	0	0	-	-	-	-	-	-	-	-	-	-	-
Other and unspecified	0	0	4	0	4	1.1	1.1	19.0	-	-	4.3	-	1.5	1.7	23	-
VII. LIVER	2	1	0	1	4	1.1	1.1	100.0	13.3	1.5	-	1.0	1.5	1.8	24	100.0
Hepatoblastoma	2	1	0	0	3	0.8	0.8	75.0	13.3	1.5	-	-	1.1	1.5	19	100.0
Hepatic carcinoma	0	0	0	1	1	0.3	0.3	25.0	-	-	-	1.0	0.4	0.3	5	100.0
Other and unspecified	0	0	0	0	0	-	-	-	-	-	-	-	-	-	-	-
VIII. BONE	0	2	3	8	13	3.4	3.4	100.0	-	3.0	3.2	7.9	4.7	4.3	68	92.3
Osteosarcoma	0	0	1	4	5	1.3	1.3	38.5	-	-	1.1	4.0	1.8	1.5	25	100.0
Chondrosarcoma	0	0	0	0	0	-	-	-	-	-	-	-	-	-	-	-
Ewing's sarcoma	0	2	1	4	7	1.9	1.8	53.8	-	3.0	1.1	4.0	2.5	2.4	37	100.0
Other and unspecified	0	0	1	0	1	0.3	0.3	7.7	-	-	1.1	-	0.4	0.3	5	-
IX. SOFT TISSUE SARCOMAS	3	11	7	2	23	6.1	6.1	100.0	20.0	16.5	7.6	2.0	8.4	9.7	134	100.0
Rhabdomyosarcoma	2	9	5	1	17	4.5	4.5	73.9	13.3	13.5	5.4	1.0	6.2	7.2	99	100.0
Fibrosarcoma	0	1	2	1	4	1.1	1.1	17.4	-	1.5	1.1	1.0	1.5	1.6	23	100.0
Other and unspecified	1	1	0	0	2	0.5	0.3	8.7	6.7	1.5	-	-	0.7	0.8	11	100.0
X. GONADAL & GERM CELL	1	2	0	1	4	1.1	1.1	100.0	6.7	3.0	-	1.0	1.5	1.7	24	100.0
Non-gonadal germ cell	1	0	0	1	2	0.5	0.5	50.0	6.7	-	-	1.0	0.7	0.8	12	100.0
Gonadal germ cell	0	2	0	0	2	0.5	0.5	50.0	-	3.0	-	-	0.7	0.9	12	100.0
Gonadal carcinoma	0	0	0	0	0	-	-	-	-	-	-	-	-	-	-	-
Other and unspecified	0	0	0	0	0	-	-	-	-	-	-	-	-	-	-	-
XI. EPITHELIAL NEOPLASMS	0	1	6	7	14	3.7	3.7	100.0	-	1.5	6.5	6.9	5.1	4.6	73	100.0
Adrenocortical carcinoma	0	0	0	0	0	-	-	-	-	-	-	-	-	-	-	-
Thyroid carcinoma	0	0	0	2	2	0.5	0.5	14.3	-	-	-	2.0	0.7	0.6	10	100.0
Nasopharyngeal carcinoma	0	0	2	0	2	-	-	-	-	-	2.0	-	-	-	-	100.0
Melanoma	0	0	2	3	5	1.3	1.3	35.7	-	-	2.2	3.0	1.8	1.6	26	100.0
Other carcinoma	0	1	3	2	7	1.9	1.9	50.0	-	1.5	4.3	2.0	2.5	2.4	38	100.0
XII. OTHER	1	4	6	6	17	4.5	4.5	100.0	6.7	6.0	6.5	5.9	6.2	6.2	93	81.8
* Specified as malignant	1	2	5	1	9	2.4	2.4	100.0	6.7	3.0	5.4	1.0	3.3	3.5	51	16.7

Denmark FEMALE

1978 - 1982

DIAGNOSTIC GROUP	NUMBER OF CASES					REL. FREQUENCY(%)			RATES PER MILLION						Cum	HV(%)
	0	1-4	5-9	10-14	All	Crude	Adj.	Group	0	1-4	5-9	10-14	Crude	Adj.		
TOTAL	21	97	75	82	275	100.0	100.0	100.0	146.7	152.4	84.7	85.3	104.7	110.6	1606	95.6
I. LEUKAEMIAS	7	34	23	18	82	29.8	29.7	100.0	48.9	53.4	26.0	18.7	31.2	34.1	486	100.0
Acute lymphocytic	3	29	20	10	62	22.5	22.5	75.6	21.0	45.6	22.6	10.4	23.6	26.0	368	100.0
Other lymphocytic	0	0	0	0	0	-	-	-	-	-	-	-	-	-	-	-
Acute non-lymphocytic	1	4	2	3	10	3.6	3.6	12.2	7.0	6.3	2.3	3.1	3.8	4.1	59	100.0
Chronic myeloid	0	0	0	4	4	1.5	1.5	4.9	-	-	-	4.2	1.5	1.2	21	100.0
Other and unspecified	3	1	1	1	6	2.2	2.1	7.3	21.0	1.6	1.1	1.0	2.3	2.8	38	100.0
II. LYMPHOMAS	2	3	4	14	23	8.4	8.4	100.0	14.0	4.7	4.5	14.6	8.8	8.2	128	95.7
Hodgkin's disease	0	0	2	10	12	4.4	4.5	52.2	-	-	2.3	10.4	4.6	3.7	63	100.0
Non-Hodgkin lymphoma	0	1	1	2	4	1.5	1.5	17.4	-	1.6	1.1	2.1	1.5	1.5	22	100.0
Burkitt's lymphoma	0	1	1	0	2	0.7	0.5	8.7	-	1.6	1.1	-	0.8	0.9	12	100.0
Unspecified lymphoma	1	0	0	2	3	1.1	1.1	13.0	7.0	-	-	2.1	1.1	1.1	17	66.7
Histiocytosis X	1	0	0	0	1	0.4	0.3	4.3	7.0	-	-	-	0.4	0.5	7	100.0
Other reticuloendothelial	0	1	0	0	1	0.4	0.3	4.3	-	1.6	-	-	0.4	0.5	6	100.0
III. BRAIN AND SPINAL	4	24	19	23	70	25.5	25.5	100.0	27.9	37.7	21.5	23.9	26.7	27.7	406	88.6
Ependymoma	2	5	2	2	11	4.0	3.9	15.7	14.0	7.9	2.3	2.1	4.2	4.8	67	100.0
Astrocytoma	0	9	7	15	31	11.3	11.3	44.3	-	14.1	7.9	15.6	11.8	11.5	174	96.8
Medulloblastoma	0	1	5	1	7	2.5	2.7	10.0	-	1.6	5.6	1.0	2.7	2.6	40	100.0
Other glioma	0	2	0	0	2	0.7	0.7	2.9	-	3.1	-	-	0.8	1.0	13	100.0
Other and unspecified *	2	7	5	5	19	6.9	6.9	27.1	14.0	11.0	5.6	5.2	7.2	7.8	112	63.2
IV. SYMPATHETIC N.S.	3	12	6	1	22	8.0	7.9	100.0	21.0	18.8	6.8	1.0	8.4	9.9	135	100.0
Neuroblastoma	3	12	6	1	22	8.0	7.9	100.0	21.0	18.8	6.8	1.0	8.4	9.9	135	100.0
Other	0	0	0	0	0	-	-	-	-	-	-	-	-	-	-	-
V. RETINOBLASTOMA	1	3	0	0	4	1.5	1.4	100.0	7.0	4.7	-	-	1.5	2.0	26	100.0
VI. KIDNEY	1	13	9	0	23	8.4	8.3	100.0	7.0	20.4	10.2	-	8.8	10.1	140	87.0
Wilms' tumour	0	10	8	0	18	6.5	6.6	78.3	-	15.7	9.0	-	6.9	7.8	108	100.0
Renal carcinoma	0	0	0	0	0	-	-	-	-	-	-	-	-	-	-	-
Other and unspecified	1	3	1	0	5	1.8	1.8	21.7	7.0	4.7	1.1	-	1.9	2.4	31	40.0
VII. LIVER	2	1	2	1	6	2.2	2.2	100.0	14.0	1.6	2.3	1.0	2.3	2.6	37	100.0
Hepatoblastoma	2	1	2	0	5	1.8	1.8	83.3	14.0	1.6	2.3	-	1.9	2.3	32	100.0
Hepatic carcinoma	0	0	0	1	1	0.4	0.4	16.7	-	-	-	1.0	0.4	0.3	5	100.0
Other and unspecified	0	0	0	0	0	-	-	-	-	-	-	-	-	-	-	-
VIII.BONE	0	1	8	9	18	6.5	6.8	100.0	-	1.6	9.0	9.4	6.9	6.1	98	100.0
Osteosarcoma	0	0	0	7	7	2.5	2.6	38.9	-	-	-	7.3	2.7	2.1	36	100.0
Chondrosarcoma	0	0	0	0	0	-	-	-	-	-	-	-	-	-	-	-
Ewing's sarcoma	0	1	8	2	11	4.0	4.3	61.1	-	1.6	9.0	2.1	4.2	4.0	62	100.0
Other and unspecified	0	0	0	0	0	-	-	-	-	-	-	-	-	-	-	-
IX. SOFT TISSUE SARCOMAS	0	1	4	3	8	2.9	3.0	100.0	-	1.6	4.5	3.1	3.0	2.9	44	100.0
Rhabdomyosarcoma	0	1	1	0	2	0.7	0.7	25.0	-	1.6	1.1	-	0.8	0.9	12	100.0
Fibrosarcoma	0	0	3	3	6	2.2	2.3	75.0	-	-	3.4	3.1	2.3	2.0	33	100.0
Other and unspecified	0	0	0	0	0	-	-	-	-	-	-	-	-	-	-	-
X. GONADAL & GERM CELL	1	1	0	5	7	2.5	2.5	100.0	7.0	1.6	-	5.2	2.7	2.5	39	100.0
Non-gonadal germ cell	1	0	0	0	1	0.4	0.3	14.3	7.0	-	-	-	0.4	0.5	7	100.0
Gonadal germ cell	0	1	0	5	6	2.2	2.2	85.7	-	1.6	-	5.2	2.3	2.0	32	100.0
Gonadal carcinoma	0	0	0	0	0	-	-	-	-	-	-	-	-	-	-	-
Other and unspecified	0	0	0	0	0	-	-	-	-	-	-	-	-	-	-	-
XI. EPITHELIAL NEOPLASMS	0	1	0	8	9	3.3	3.3	100.0	-	1.6	-	8.3	3.4	2.9	48	100.0
Adrenocortical carcinoma	0	0	0	0	0	-	-	-	-	-	-	-	-	-	-	-
Thyroid carcinoma	0	0	0	4	4	1.5	1.5	44.4	-	-	-	4.2	1.5	1.2	21	100.0
Nasopharyngeal carcinoma	0	0	0	0	0	-	-	-	-	-	-	-	-	-	-	-
Melanoma	0	1	0	1	2	0.7	0.7	22.2	-	1.6	-	1.0	0.8	0.8	11	100.0
Other carcinoma	0	0	0	3	3	1.1	1.1	33.3	-	-	-	3.1	1.1	0.9	16	100.0
XII. OTHER	0	3	0	0	3	1.1	1.0	100.0	-	4.7	-	-	1.1	1.5	19	100.0
* Specified as malignant	2	4	2	0	8	2.9	2.8	-	14.0	6.3	2.3	-	3.0	3.8	50	50.0

Commentary

In general, the incidence rates were typical of those for European registries. Leukaemia accounted for 30% of registrations, with a ratio of acute lymphocytic to acute non-lymphocytic of 5.4:1. The proportion of lymphomas (20%) categorized as Burkitt's was unusually high for a European population. Among embryonal tumours, retinoblastoma had a relatively low incidence rate and hepatoblastoma a relatively high one, but this latter observation is based on a small number of cases. The ratio of Ewing's sarcoma to osteosarcoma (1.5:1) was one of the highest in any registry.

Reference

Olsen, J.H. & Scheibel, E. (1984) Cancer i barnealderen i Danmark 1943-1980 (Childhood cancer in Denmark 1943-1980). *Ugeskr. Laeg.*, *146*, 3228-3230

FINLAND

Finnish Cancer Registry, 1970–1979

L. Teppo & E. Saxen

The Finnish Cancer Registry — the Institute for Statistical and Epidemiological Cancer Research — was established in 1952 on the initiative of the Cancer Society of Finland. Data on newly diagnosed cases of cancer have been collected since 1953.

All hospitals, pathological laboratories and practitioners are asked to report all cases of cancer, whether new or reported earlier. Reporting has been compulsory since 1961. Cases are reported from hospital in- and out-patient and radiotherapy departments by doctors, nurses or clerical staff; from pathological laboratories by laboratory staff; from death certificates mentioning cancer by the Central Statistical Office; and from all practising physicians. If a notification originates from a pathological laboratory or from a death certificate alone, further information is requested. Follow-up for death is done by checking all death certificates issued in Finland annually against the Cancer Registry files. Patients are never contacted. Case identification is based on the personal identification number used in Finland since 1967. If multiple primary tumours are diagnosed in the same person, each is recorded separately, except for skin tumours of the same histology occurring within one year. Information is coded by a physician (pathologist) usually two years after the initial diagnosis in order to collect additional information and thus obtain a good overview of the case.

In 1981, Finland had 9000 physicians (1.8 per 1000 inhabitants) and 74 000 hospital beds. The country is divided into 21 central hospital districts, five of which (Helsinki, Turku, Oulu, Kuopio, Tampere) have teaching hospitals. Diagnosis and treatment of cancer are only partly centralized; cancer surgery is practised in all central hospitals and also in many smaller units. Radiotherapy is available in nine of the central hospitals. There are facilities for paediatric oncology in five university hospitals.

The Registry covers the whole of Finland (area 338 000 square kilometres), which is bordered on the north by Norway, on the east by the USSR, on the west by Sweden and the Gulf of Bothnia and on the south by the Gulf of Finland. The average altitude is 150 m. Finland has 31 570 square kilometres of inland water and belongs to the coniferous forest zone. The population is 4.9 million (1986). Ethnically, the Finns are of mixed origin, including Baltic, Scandinavian and probably eastern elements; 89% are Lutherans. The official languages of the country are Finnish and Swedish; 6.1% of the population speak Swedish as their mother tongue (1986). The main occupation groups (1981) are services, business and communication 46%, industry, construction and mining 34%, and agriculture, forestry and fishing 11%. Some 60% of the population live in urban municipalities. The population of Helsinki with its suburbs accounts for 15.6% of the total.

Apart from providing routine statistics (annual incidence rates by sex, age, primary site, place of residence and province) and data for planning purposes, the Registry is engaged in active research on cancer epidemiology and provides material for clinical and pathological studies and follow-up data on cancer patients. The Registry also acts as a consultant body in Finland on cancer epidemiology problems. A report on cancer incidence in childhood during 1953–1970 was published in 1975 (Teppo *et al.*, 1975).

Population

The population of Finland is available from the national population registry as annual estimates by age and sex.

Contd p. 232

FINLAND

Finland

MALE

1970 - 1979

DIAGNOSTIC GROUP	NUMBER OF CASES 0	1-4	5-9	10-14	All	REL. FREQUENCY(%) Crude	Adj.	Group	RATES PER MILLION 0	1-4	5-9	10-14	Crude	Adj.	Cum	HV(%)
TOTAL	89	267	184	208	748	100.0	100.0	100.0	279.7	206.5	104.5	107.0	140.7	150.4	2163	97.1
I. LEUKAEMIAS	13	104	63	56	236	31.6	31.5	100.0	40.9	80.4	35.8	28.8	44.4	48.0	686	100.0
Acute lymphocytic	6	68	45	28	147	19.7	19.7	62.3	18.9	52.6	25.6	14.4	27.7	30.2	429	100.0
Other lymphocytic	0	0	1	1	2	0.3	0.3	0.8	-	-	0.6	0.5	0.4	0.3	-	100.0
Acute non-lymphocytic	1	12	5	12	30	4.0	4.0	12.7	3.1	9.3	2.8	6.2	5.6	5.8	85	100.0
Chronic myeloid	0	2	3	8	13	1.7	1.9	5.5	-	1.5	1.7	4.1	2.4	2.2	35	100.0
Other and unspecified	6	22	9	7	44	5.9	5.6	18.6	18.9	17.0	5.1	3.6	8.3	9.4	130	100.0
II. LYMPHOMAS	9	19	32	34	94	12.6	13.3	100.0	28.3	14.7	18.2	17.5	17.7	17.7	265	100.0
Hodgkin's disease	0	2	5	12	19	2.5	2.8	20.2	-	1.5	2.8	6.2	3.6	3.2	51	100.0
Non-Hodgkin lymphoma	6	7	12	16	41	5.5	5.7	43.6	18.9	5.4	6.8	8.2	7.7	7.7	116	100.0
Burkitt's lymphoma	0	0	0	0	0	-	-	-	-	-	-	-	-	-	-	-
Unspecified lymphoma	0	0	0	0	0	-	-	-	-	-	-	-	-	-	-	-
Histiocytosis X	3	10	15	6	34	4.5	4.8	36.2	9.4	7.7	8.5	3.1	6.4	6.8	98	100.0
Other reticuloendothelial	0	0	0	0	0	-	-	-	-	-	-	-	-	-	-	-
III. BRAIN AND SPINAL	13	55	53	51	172	23.0	23.6	100.0	40.9	42.5	30.1	26.2	32.4	33.7	493	87.8
Ependymoma	3	7	6	1	17	2.3	2.2	9.9	9.4	5.4	3.4	0.5	3.2	3.7	51	100.0
Astrocytoma	0	0	0	0	0	-	-	-	-	-	-	-	-	-	-	-
Medulloblastoma	2	17	12	4	35	4.7	4.7	20.3	6.3	13.1	6.8	2.1	6.6	7.4	103	100.0
Other glioma	6	15	26	24	71	9.5	10.1	41.3	18.9	11.6	14.8	12.3	13.4	13.4	201	100.0
Other and unspecified *	2	16	9	22	49	6.6	6.7	28.5	6.3	12.4	5.1	11.3	9.2	9.3	138	57.1
IV. SYMPATHETIC N.S.	14	17	6	4	41	5.5	5.0	100.0	44.0	13.1	3.4	2.1	7.7	9.2	124	100.0
Neuroblastoma	14	17	6	3	40	5.3	4.9	97.6	44.0	13.1	3.4	1.5	7.5	9.0	121	100.0
Other	0	0	0	1	1	0.1	0.1	2.4	-	-	-	0.5	0.2	0.1	3	100.0
V. RETINOBLASTOMA	6	17	4	1	28	3.7	3.4	100.0	18.9	13.1	2.3	0.5	5.3	6.4	85	100.0
VI. KIDNEY	13	27	11	0	51	6.8	6.3	100.0	40.9	20.9	6.2	-	9.6	11.6	156	100.0
Wilms' tumour	13	26	10	0	49	6.6	6.0	96.1	40.9	20.1	5.7	-	9.2	11.2	150	100.0
Renal carcinoma	0	0	0	0	0	-	-	-	-	-	-	-	-	-	-	-
Other and unspecified	0	1	1	0	2	0.3	0.3	3.9	-	0.8	0.6	-	0.4	0.4	6	100.0
VII. LIVER	3	2	0	1	6	0.8	0.7	100.0	9.4	1.5	-	0.5	1.1	1.4	18	100.0
Hepatoblastoma	3	2	0	0	5	0.7	0.6	83.3	9.4	1.5	-	-	0.9	1.2	16	100.0
Hepatic carcinoma	0	0	0	1	1	0.1	0.1	16.7	-	-	-	0.5	0.2	0.1	3	100.0
Other and unspecified	0	0	0	0	0	-	-	-	-	-	-	-	-	-	-	-
VIII. BONE	2	3	8	26	39	5.2	5.6	100.0	6.3	2.3	4.5	13.4	7.3	6.6	105	100.0
Osteosarcoma	0	0	6	16	22	2.9	3.3	56.4	-	-	3.4	8.2	4.1	3.5	58	100.0
Chondrosarcoma	1	2	1	1	5	0.7	0.6	12.8	3.1	1.5	0.6	0.5	0.9	1.1	15	100.0
Ewing's sarcoma	1	0	0	9	10	1.3	1.5	25.6	3.1	-	-	4.6	1.9	1.5	26	100.0
Other and unspecified	0	1	1	0	2	0.3	0.2	5.1	-	0.8	0.6	-	0.4	0.5	6	100.0
IX. SOFT TISSUE SARCOMAS	7	12	3	15	37	4.9	4.8	100.0	22.0	9.3	1.7	7.7	7.0	7.4	106	100.0
Rhabdomyosarcoma	2	3	0	4	9	1.2	1.1	24.3	6.3	2.3	-	2.1	1.7	1.8	26	100.0
Fibrosarcoma	2	4	1	6	13	1.7	1.7	35.1	6.3	3.1	0.6	3.1	2.4	2.5	37	100.0
Other and unspecified	3	5	2	5	15	2.0	1.9	40.5	9.4	3.9	1.1	2.6	2.8	3.0	43	100.0
X. GONADAL & GERM CELL	6	10	0	2	18	2.4	2.1	100.0	18.9	7.7	-	1.0	3.4	4.2	55	100.0
Non-gonadal germ cell	2	2	0	2	6	0.8	0.7	33.3	6.3	1.5	-	1.0	1.1	1.3	18	100.0
Gonadal germ cell	4	8	0	0	12	1.6	1.3	66.7	12.6	6.2	-	-	2.3	2.9	37	100.0
Gonadal carcinoma	0	0	0	0	0	-	-	-	-	-	-	-	-	-	-	-
Other and unspecified	0	0	0	0	0	-	-	-	-	-	-	-	-	-	-	-
XI. EPITHELIAL NEOPLASMS	3	0	3	18	24	3.2	3.4	100.0	9.4	-	1.7	9.3	4.5	4.0	64	100.0
Adrenocortical carcinoma	0	0	0	0	0	-	-	-	-	-	-	-	-	-	-	-
Thyroid carcinoma	0	0	0	4	4	0.5	0.6	16.7	-	-	-	2.1	0.8	0.6	10	100.0
Nasopharyngeal carcinoma	1	0	0	3	4	0.5	0.5	16.7	3.1	-	-	1.5	0.6	0.7	11	100.0
Melanoma	2	0	0	1	3	0.4	0.5	12.5	6.3	-	-	0.5	0.6	0.5	8	100.0
Other carcinoma	0	0	3	10	13	1.7	1.8	54.2	-	-	1.7	5.1	2.4	2.2	35	100.0
XII. OTHER	0	1	1	0	2	0.3	0.3	100.0	-	0.8	0.6	-	0.4	0.4	6	50.0
* Specified as malignant	2	15	6	12	35	4.7	4.6	100.0	6.3	11.6	3.4	6.2	6.6	7.0	101	40.0

Finland

1970 – 1979

FEMALE

DIAGNOSTIC GROUP	NUMBER OF CASES 0	1-4	5-9	10-14	All	REL. FREQUENCY(%) Crude	Adj.	Group	RATES PER MILLION 0	1-4	5-9	10-14	Crude	Adj.	Cum	HV(%)
TOTAL	51	201	147	171	570	100.0	100.0	100.0	168.0	162.8	87.0	91.5	111.9	118.1	1712	97.0
I. LEUKAEMIAS	10	72	52	38	172	30.2	30.3	100.0	32.9	58.3	30.8	20.3	33.8	36.4	522	100.0
Acute lymphocytic	4	47	35	19	105	18.4	18.6	61.0	13.2	38.1	20.7	10.2	20.6	22.4	320	100.0
Other lymphocytic	0	3	1	0	4	0.7	0.7	2.3	–	2.4	0.7	–	0.8	0.9	13	100.0
Acute non-lymphocytic	3	3	9	10	25	4.4	4.5	14.5	9.9	2.4	5.3	5.4	4.9	4.8	73	100.0
Chronic myeloid	0	0	1	3	4	0.7	0.7	2.3	–	–	0.6	1.6	0.8	0.7	11	100.0
Other and unspecified	3	19	6	6	34	6.0	5.8	19.8	9.9	15.4	3.6	3.2	6.7	7.6	105	100.0
II. LYMPHOMAS	4	12	9	19	44	7.7	7.7	100.0	13.2	9.7	5.3	10.2	8.6	8.7	130	97.7
Hodgkin's disease	0	0	1	10	11	1.9	2.0	25.0	–	–	0.6	5.4	2.2	1.7	30	90.9
Non-Hodgkin lymphoma	1	9	6	6	22	3.9	3.9	50.0	3.3	7.3	3.6	3.2	4.3	4.6	66	100.0
Burkitt's lymphoma	0	0	0	0	0	–	–	–	–	–	–	–	–	–	–	–
Unspecified lymphoma	3	3	2	3	11	1.9	1.9	25.0	9.9	2.4	1.2	1.6	2.2	2.4	34	100.0
Histiocytosis X	0	0	0	0	0	–	–	–	–	–	–	–	–	–	–	–
Other reticuloendothelial	0	0	0	0	0	–	–	–	–	–	–	–	–	–	–	–
III. BRAIN AND SPINAL	7	47	42	45	141	24.7	25.0	100.0	23.1	38.1	24.9	24.1	27.7	28.6	420	90.1
Ependymoma	1	8	6	6	21	3.7	3.7	14.9	3.3	6.5	3.6	3.2	4.1	4.3	63	100.0
Astrocytoma	0	0	0	0	0	–	–	–	–	–	–	–	–	–	–	–
Medulloblastoma	1	7	4	0	12	2.1	2.1	8.5	3.3	5.7	2.4	–	2.4	2.8	38	100.0
Other glioma	4	25	22	27	78	13.7	13.8	55.3	13.2	20.2	13.0	14.4	15.3	15.7	232	100.0
Other and unspecified *	1	7	10	12	30	5.3	5.4	21.3	3.3	5.7	5.9	6.4	5.9	5.8	88	53.3
IV. SYMPATHETIC N.S.	13	20	3	3	39	6.8	6.4	100.0	42.8	16.2	1.8	1.6	7.7	9.4	125	100.0
Neuroblastoma	13	20	3	3	39	6.8	6.4	100.0	42.8	16.2	1.8	1.6	7.7	9.4	125	100.0
Other	0	0	0	0	0	–	–	–	–	–	–	–	–	–	–	–
V. RETINOBLASTOMA	4	7	1	1	13	2.3	2.1	100.0	13.2	5.7	0.6	0.5	2.6	3.1	41	100.0
VI. KIDNEY	4	24	12	1	41	7.2	7.1	100.0	13.2	19.4	7.1	0.5	8.0	9.5	129	100.0
Wilms' tumour	3	24	11	0	38	6.7	6.5	92.7	9.9	19.4	6.5	–	7.5	8.9	120	100.0
Renal carcinoma	1	0	1	1	3	0.5	0.5	7.3	3.3	–	0.6	0.5	0.6	0.6	9	100.0
Other and unspecified	0	0	0	0	0	–	–	–	–	–	–	–	–	–	–	–
VII. LIVER	0	2	0	3	5	0.9	0.8	100.0	–	1.6	–	1.6	1.0	1.0	15	100.0
Hepatoblastoma	0	2	0	0	2	0.4	0.3	40.0	–	1.6	–	–	0.4	0.5	6	100.0
Hepatic carcinoma	0	0	0	3	3	0.5	0.5	60.0	–	–	–	1.6	0.6	0.5	8	100.0
Other and unspecified	0	0	0	0	0	–	–	–	–	–	–	–	–	–	–	–
VIII. BONE	0	3	8	16	27	4.7	4.9	100.0	–	2.4	4.7	8.6	5.3	4.8	76	96.3
Osteosarcoma	0	2	4	10	16	2.8	2.9	59.3	–	1.6	2.4	5.4	3.1	2.8	45	100.0
Chondrosarcoma	0	0	0	1	1	0.2	0.2	3.7	–	–	–	0.5	0.2	0.2	3	100.0
Ewing's sarcoma	0	1	2	4	7	1.2	1.3	25.9	–	0.8	1.2	2.1	1.4	1.3	20	100.0
Other and unspecified	0	0	2	1	3	0.5	0.6	11.1	–	–	1.2	0.5	0.6	0.5	9	66.7
IX. SOFT TISSUE SARCOMAS	3	8	4	17	32	5.6	5.5	100.0	9.9	6.5	2.4	9.1	6.3	6.2	93	96.9
Rhabdomyosarcoma	0	1	1	4	6	1.1	1.1	18.8	–	0.8	0.6	2.1	1.1	1.1	17	100.0
Fibrosarcoma	1	2	1	8	12	2.1	2.1	37.5	3.3	1.6	0.6	4.3	2.4	2.2	34	91.7
Other and unspecified	2	5	2	5	14	2.5	2.4	43.8	6.6	4.0	1.2	2.7	2.7	2.9	42	100.0
X. GONADAL & GERM CELL	4	4	1	7	16	2.8	2.7	100.0	13.2	3.2	0.6	3.7	3.1	3.3	48	100.0
Non-gonadal germ cell	4	4	1	2	11	1.9	1.8	68.8	13.2	3.2	0.6	1.1	2.2	2.5	34	100.0
Gonadal germ cell	0	0	0	2	2	0.4	0.4	12.5	–	–	–	1.1	0.4	0.3	5	100.0
Gonadal carcinoma	0	0	0	2	2	0.4	0.4	12.5	–	–	–	1.1	0.4	0.3	5	100.0
Other and unspecified	0	0	0	1	1	0.2	0.2	6.3	–	–	–	0.5	0.2	0.2	3	100.0
XI. EPITHELIAL NEOPLASMS	2	2	13	19	36	6.3	6.6	100.0	6.6	1.6	7.7	10.2	7.1	6.4	102	100.0
Adrenocortical carcinoma	0	1	2	1	4	0.7	0.7	11.1	–	0.8	1.2	0.5	0.8	0.8	12	100.0
Thyroid carcinoma	0	0	2	2	4	0.7	0.8	11.1	–	–	1.2	1.1	0.8	0.7	11	100.0
Nasopharyngeal carcinoma	0	0	0	1	1	0.2	0.2	2.8	–	–	–	0.5	0.2	0.2	3	100.0
Melanoma	0	1	1	5	7	1.2	1.2	19.4	–	0.8	0.6	2.7	1.4	1.2	20	100.0
Other carcinoma	2	0	8	10	20	3.5	3.7	55.6	6.6	–	4.7	5.4	3.9	3.6	57	100.0
XII. OTHER	0	0	2	2	4	0.7	0.8	100.0	–	–	1.2	1.1	0.8	0.7	11	100.0
* Specified as malignant	1	4	10	8	23	4.0	4.2	100.0	3.3	3.2	5.9	4.3	4.5	4.4	67	39.1

232   FINLAND

AVERAGE ANNUAL POPULATION: 1970-1979

Age	Male	Female
0	31817	30362
1-4	129305	123466
5-9	176044	168871
10-14	194350	186856
0-14	531516	509555

Commentary

The total incidence rate was among the highest for any Western registry. The relative frequencies of major diagnostic groups were similar to those in other European countries. Leukaemia was the largest group and accounted for 31% of registrations. Among lymphomas, Hodgkin's disease was relatively infrequent. The incidence of brain and spinal tumours was among the highest in any registry; astrocytomas were not allocated a separate morphology code, but were subsumed under 'other glioma'. There were particularly high incidence rates in boys for retinoblastoma and Wilms' tumour. Of Wilms' tumours with known laterality, 4.5% (4/88) were bilateral. Osteosarcoma was more than twice as frequent as Ewing's sarcoma. About 5% of all registrations were for carcinoma.

Compared with the incidence rates for 1953-1970 reported by Teppo et al. (1975), those for 1970-1979 were higher by 18% in males and 10% in females. Because of the different classification schemes used in the two periods, it is difficult to make comparisons for most individual diagnostic groups; this may account for the apparent doubling of the incidence of neuroblastoma.

Reference

Teppo, L., Salonen, T. & Hakulinen, T. (1975) Incidence of childhood cancer in Finland. *J. natl Cancer Inst.*, *55*, 1065-1067

FRANCE

Cancer registration in France has developed in recent years at the level of the department. Because of the relatively small population size (approx. 600 000), most registries are too recent to provide sufficient childhood cancer cases for calculating reliable incidence rates. However, the oldest registry, that of Bas-Rhin, had recorded over 240 cases in its first 10 years, and the results are included here.

Recently, specialized paediatric cancer registries have been established covering the populations of two regions, those of Lorraine (four departments) and Provence-Alpes-Côte d'Azur and Corse (PACA-Corse) (eight departments). Tables have been prepared showing numbers of cases and incidence rates for the 12 major diagnostic groupings for each of these two paediatric registries. A total of 197 cases were recorded in Lorraine for the three-year period 1983-1985, and 203 in PACA-Corse for the two-year period 1984-1985. In addition, because these registries use almost identical methodology, the data have been pooled and incidence rates calculated for 'France, Paediatric Registries', using the combined populations at risk, for the full range of tumour types.

FRANCE — PAEDIATRIC REGISTRIES:
AVERAGE ANNUAL POPULATION: 1983-1985

Age	Male	Female
0	35519	34867
1–4	136146	131375
5–9	177539	168376
10–14	200737	190131
0–14	549941	524749

Cancer Registry of Bas-Rhin, 1975–1984

P. Schaffer

The Cancer Registry of the French Department of Bas-Rhin was established in 1975. Cases are collected by the doctors working in the Registry from hospital services, laboratories, administrative services, etc. At the same time, the information necessary to complete epidemiological questionnaires is abstracted.

In 1982, the total population of the Department was 915 676. The population is slightly younger than that of France as a whole, with 22% aged under 15. In 1982, 61 152 foreigners (6.7% of the population) were resident in the Department. The area covered by the Department is 4755 square kilometres and the population density is 193 inhabitants per square kilometre. The Department is situated between the Rhine to the east, of which it forms the left bank, and the Lower Vosges to the west. The maximum altitude (1100 m) is reached in the Vosges, the minimum altitude (115 m) in the Rhine valley. The climate is temperate with a slight continental influence.

Bas-Rhin is an industrialized department characterized by a diversity of manufacturing activities; it is without mineral resources and does not produce any raw materials. Agriculture plays an important role in spite of the low percentage of the working population employed in this sector. As well as cereals (wheat and corn), sugar-beet, potatoes and vines, there are areas of specialized cultivation, such as the cabbage (for choucroute), hops and tobacco.

The data reproduced here represent the cases of childhood cancer recorded during the first 10 years of the registry, 1975-1984.

Population

The population at risk has been calculated from the data of the censuses of 1975 and 1982 (Institut National de la Statistique et des Etudes Economiques).

AVERAGE ANNUAL POPULATION: 1975–1984

Age	Male	Female
0–4	30884	29642
5–9	33382	32087
10–14	37875	36376
0–14	102141	98105

Childhood Cancer Registry of Lorraine, 1983-1985

M.C. L'Huillier, D. Steschenko & D. Olive

The population-based Childhood Cancer Registry of Lorraine was started on 1 January 1983. In parallel to the Registry, a retrospective case-control study on the risk factors for cancer in childhood was undertaken from the same date.

The concentration of a great proportion of the childhood cancers in the region in one paediatric oncology centre (Nancy) was a compelling reason for the creation of such a registry. This centre also recruits cases from an area very much larger than that covered by the Registry.

Data are collected from medical and administrative sources. Registration is active, and every source is recontacted annually; new cases are notified using a standard notification form.

The Registry contacts all doctors practising in the Lorraine area who might include children among their patients (general practitioners and hospital personnel in the public and private sector), and the laboratories of pathology and cytology. In addition, the University Hospital Centres and Anti-Cancer Centres in adjacent regions, as well as in Paris, are contacted. Death certificates for children aged less than 15 years dying of a malignant neoplasm are sent to the Registry by the Departments of Health of four departments; social security statistics are communicated annually, but without personal identifying information.

All malignant neoplasms are included as well as all cerebral tumours (irrespective of malignancy grade) and certain conditions of borderline malignancy, such as aggressive fibromatoses, disseminated histiocytosis X and lymphohistiocytoses.

The data items collected are as follows: name, age, sex, address, date of diagnosis, method of diagnosis, histological diagnosis, anatomical site, stage, treatment, any relapses and the sources of information. In addition, it is planned to carry out a regular follow-up of the children.

The geographical region covered is the Lorraine area, consisting of four departments (Meurthe-et-Moselle, Meuse, Moselle, Vosges), of which three are located on the frontiers of Belgium, Luxembourg, and Germany.

The population of the area totals 2 319 905 inhabitants, of whom 535 236 are children aged 0–14 (23%). The average population density is 101 per square kilometre, although this density varies greatly in the different departments. Lorraine has a rural tradition but industrialization in the 19th century has given rise to a very high proportion of urban population (72.7% on average). There is a relatively high percentage of foreigners (8.2%; the percentage for the whole of France is 6.8%). The working population accounts for 41% of the total, with a socioprofessional structure characterized by a very high proportion of labourers.

Population

The population at risk is that of the 1982 census (Institut National de la Statistique et des Etudes Economiques).

AVERAGE ANNUAL POPULATION: 1983–1985

Age	Male	Female
0	17976	18192
1–4	69248	65468
5–9	87460	82528
10–14	99168	95196
0–14	273852	261384

The Childhood Cancer Registry of
Provence-Alpes-Côte d'Azur and Corse, 1984–1985

J.L. Bernard

The Childhood Cancer Registry was set up in the regions of Provence-Alpes-Côte d'Azur (PACA) and Corse on 1 January 1984. It is a population-based registry and aims at registering every new case of cancer appearing in the childhood population living at the time of diagnosis in one of the eight departments of the two regions. The choice of this geographical basis is justified by the relative concentration of paediatric centres, essentially in Marseille and Nice. The peripheral hospital centres outside these regions and likely to receive cases eligible for the Registry are well defined (Lyon, Grenoble, Montpellier). The Registry also carries out etiological research.

All doctors and hospital centres who might make a diagnosis of cancer in a child or undertake the child's treatment, have been invited to participate in the Registry by voluntarily notifying their cases. The sources of information are :

— hospital centres, universities and the anti-cancer centres in Marseille and Nice;
— the regional hospital centres of PACA and Corse;
— doctors in private practice (paediatricians, surgeons, radiotherapists, cancer specialists, anatomopathologists and neurosurgeons);
— haematology and paediatric oncology departments in University Hospital Centres and Anti-Cancer Centres of neighbouring areas (Montpellier, Lyon and Grenoble).

As well as this passive collection of information, some groups (anatomopathologists, neurosurgeons, heads of paediatric services, etc.) are contacted actively every six months.

The treatment of nearly all childhood cancer is undertaken by the Departments of Paediatric Oncology and Haematology of the Regional University Hospital Centre of Marseille and by the Anti-Cancer Centre of Nice. Very few cases are treated in the private sector or outside the area.

It is not possible to use death certificates as a source, since the data communicated by the administrative services are not linked to specific individuals; for childhood cancer, the utility of this source is, in any case, very limited.

The population of the regions of PACA and Corse totalled 4 182 992 at the 1982 census, of whom 809 196 were children aged 0–14 (19.4% of the total).

The majority of the population is urban, concentrated on the coast in the three large urban centres: Marseille, Nice and Toulon. The northern area of the PACA region is mountainous, sparsely populated and essentially rural.

Data on ethnicity and religion are not collected, as this is not legally permitted. A fairly large proportion of the population consists of immigrants, mainly from the Maghreb countries (Algeria, Morocco, Tunisia).

Population

The population at risk is that of the 1982 census (Institut National de la Statistique et des Etudes Economiques).

AVERAGE ANNUAL POPULATION: 1984–1985

Age	Male	Female
0	26315	25013
1–4	100349	98863
5–9	135121	128775
10–14	152356	142404
0–14	414141	395055

Commentary

Incidence rates overall were similar to those in other Western countries. Leukaemia was the commonest diagnostic group, accounting for around 30% of total incidence in all three registries. Incidence rates were generally high for lymphomas other than Hodgkin's disease. The incidence of neuroblastoma was very high in PACA-Corse. Wilms' tumour was relatively infrequent in the two paediatric registries; in Bas-Rhin, the rate was the highest in Europe, but this was based on a total of only 19 cases. PACA-Corse also had an unusually large number of soft-tissue sarcomas, most of which were rhabdomyosarcoma.

France, Bas Rhin   1975 - 1984   MALE

DIAGNOSTIC GROUP	NUMBER OF CASES					REL. FREQUENCY(%)			RATES PER MILLION						HV(%)
	0	1-4	5-9	10-14	All	Crude	Adj.	Group	0-4	5-9	10-14	Crude	Adj.	Cum	
TOTAL	12	46	39	34	131	100.0	100.0	100.0	187.8	116.8	89.8	128.3	136.4	1972	96.2
I. LEUKAEMIAS	2	16	10	6	34	26.0	25.4	100.0	58.3	30.0	15.8	33.3	36.8	520	97.1
Acute lymphocytic	2	12	5	3	22	16.8	16.1	64.7	45.3	15.0	7.9	21.5	24.7	341	95.5
Other lymphocytic	0	1	1	1	3	2.3	2.3	8.8	3.2	3.0	2.6	2.9	3.0	44	100.0
Acute non-lymphocytic	0	0	4	1	5	3.8	4.0	14.7	-	12.0	2.6	4.9	4.6	73	100.0
Chronic myeloid	0	0	0	0	0										
Other and unspecified	0	3	0	1	4	3.1	3.0	11.8	9.7	-	2.6	3.9	4.5	62	100.0
II. LYMPHOMAS	1	7	6	7	21	16.0	16.3	100.0	25.9	18.0	18.5	20.6	21.2	312	100.0
Hodgkin's disease	0	1	2	1	4	3.1	3.1	19.0	3.2	6.0	2.6	3.9	4.0	59	100.0
Non-Hodgkin lymphoma	0	2	3	5	10	7.6	8.1	47.6	6.5	9.0	13.2	9.8	9.2	143	100.0
Burkitt's lymphoma	0	0	1	0	1	0.8	0.8	4.8	-	3.0	-	1.0	1.0	15	100.0
Unspecified lymphoma	0	1	0	1	2	1.5	1.6	9.5	3.2	-	2.6	2.0	2.0	29	100.0
Histiocytosis X	1	0	0	0	1	0.8	0.7	4.8	3.2	-	-	1.0	1.3	16	100.0
Other reticuloendothelial	0	3	0	0	3	2.3	2.1	14.3	9.7	-	-	2.9	3.8	49	100.0
III. BRAIN AND SPINAL	2	4	11	9	26	19.8	20.5	100.0	19.4	33.0	23.8	25.5	25.0	381	88.5
Ependymoma	2	1	1	0	4	3.1	3.0	15.4	9.7	-	-	3.9	4.5	62	100.0
Astrocytoma	0	2	5	4	11	8.4	8.8	42.3	-	15.0	10.6	10.8	10.4	160	100.0
Medulloblastoma	0	1	2	1	4	3.1	3.1	15.4	6.5	6.0	2.6	3.9	4.0	59	100.0
Other glioma	0	0	2	1	3	2.3	2.4	11.5	3.2	6.0	2.6	2.9	2.7	43	66.7
Other and unspecified *	0	0	2	2	4	3.1	3.3	15.4	-	6.0	5.3	3.9	3.5	56	50.0
IV. SYMPATHETIC N.S.	3	6	4	2	15	11.5	11.0	100.0	29.1	12.0	5.3	14.7	16.7	232	100.0
Neuroblastoma	3	6	4	2	15	11.5	11.0	100.0	29.1	12.0	5.3	14.7	16.7	232	100.0
Other	0	0	0	0	0										
V. RETINOBLASTOMA	1	0	0	0	1	0.8	0.7	100.0	3.2	-	-	1.0	1.3	16	100.0
VI. KIDNEY	3	7	3	0	13	9.9	9.2	100.0	32.4	9.0	-	12.7	15.4	207	92.3
Wilms' tumour	3	7	3	0	13	9.9	9.2	100.0	32.4	9.0	-	12.7	15.4	207	92.3
Renal carcinoma	0	0	0	0	0										
Other and unspecified	0	0	0	0	0										
VII. LIVER	0	0	0	1	1	0.8	0.9	100.0	-	-	2.6	1.0	0.8	13	100.0
Hepatoblastoma	0	0	0	1	1	0.8	0.9	100.0	-	-	2.6	1.0	0.8	13	100.0
Hepatic carcinoma	0	0	0	0	0										
Other and unspecified	0	0	0	0	0										
VIII. BONE	0	0	2	3	5	3.8	4.2	100.0	-	6.0	7.9	4.9	4.2	70	100.0
Osteosarcoma	0	0	0	1	1	0.8	0.9	20.0	-	-	2.6	1.0	0.8	13	100.0
Chondrosarcoma	0	0	0	0	0										
Ewing's sarcoma	0	0	2	2	4	3.1	3.3	80.0	-	6.0	5.3	3.9	3.5	56	100.0
Other and unspecified	0	0	0	0	0										
IX. SOFT TISSUE SARCOMAS	0	3	3	3	9	6.9	7.0	100.0	9.7	9.0	7.9	8.8	9.0	133	100.0
Rhabdomyosarcoma	0	2	3	1	6	4.6	4.6	66.7	6.5	9.0	2.6	5.9	6.2	91	100.0
Fibrosarcoma	0	0	0	1	1	0.8	0.9	11.1	-	-	2.6	1.0	0.8	13	100.0
Other and unspecified	0	1	0	1	2	1.5	1.6	22.2	3.2	-	2.6	2.0	2.0	29	100.0
X. GONADAL & GERM CELL	0	2	0	0	2	1.5	1.4	100.0	6.5	-	-	2.0	2.5	32	100.0
Non-gonadal germ cell	0	1	0	0	1	0.8	0.7	50.0	3.2	-	-	1.0	1.3	16	100.0
Gonadal germ cell	0	1	0	0	1	0.8	0.7	50.0	3.2	-	-	1.0	1.3	16	100.0
Gonadal carcinoma	0	0	0	0	0										
Other and unspecified	0	0	0	0	0										
XI. EPITHELIAL NEOPLASMS	0	0	0	2	2	1.5	1.8	100.0	-	-	5.3	2.0	1.5	26	100.0
Adrenocortical carcinoma	0	0	0	0	0										
Thyroid carcinoma	0	0	0	0	0										
Nasopharyngeal carcinoma	0	0	0	1	1	0.8	0.9	50.0	-	-	2.6	1.0	0.8	13	100.0
Melanoma	0	0	0	0	0										
Other carcinoma	0	0	0	1	1	0.8	0.9	50.0	-	-	2.6	1.0	0.8	13	100.0
XII. OTHER	0	1	0	1	2	1.5	1.6	100.0	3.2	-	2.6	2.0	2.0	29	100.0
* Specified as malignant	0	0	2	1	3	2.3	2.4	100.0	-	6.0	2.6	2.9	2.7	43	33.3

France, Bas Rhin

1975 – 1984

FEMALE

DIAGNOSTIC GROUP	NUMBER OF CASES					REL. FREQUENCY(%)			RATES PER MILLION					Cum	HV(%)
	0	1-4	5-9	10-14	All	Crude	Adj.	Group	0-4	5-9	10-14	Crude	Adj.		
TOTAL	9	48	25	30	112	100.0	100.0	100.0	192.3	77.9	82.5	114.2	123.5	1763	94.6
I. LEUKAEMIAS	2	18	8	7	35	31.3	30.6	100.0	67.5	24.9	19.2	35.7	39.7	558	100.0
Acute lymphocytic	2	10	7	6	25	22.3	22.8	71.4	40.5	21.8	16.5	25.5	27.5	394	100.0
Other lymphocytic	0	2	0	0	2	1.8	1.4	5.7	6.7	-	-	2.0	2.6	34	100.0
Acute non-lymphocytic	0	3	0	0	3	2.7	2.1	8.6	10.1	-	-	3.1	3.9	51	100.0
Chronic myeloid	0	0	0	0	0	-	-	-	-	-	-	-	-	-	-
Other and unspecified	0	3	1	1	5	4.5	4.3	14.3	10.1	3.1	2.7	5.1	5.7	80	100.0
II. LYMPHOMAS	1	5	4	4	14	12.5	13.0	100.0	20.2	12.5	11.0	14.3	15.0	219	100.0
Hodgkin's disease	0	0	0	2	2	1.8	1.8	14.3	-	-	5.5	2.0	1.6	27	100.0
Non-Hodgkin lymphoma	0	2	4	2	8	7.1	8.2	57.1	6.7	12.5	5.5	8.2	8.2	124	100.0
Burkitt's lymphoma	0	0	0	0	0	-	-	-	-	-	-	-	-	-	-
Unspecified lymphoma	0	2	0	0	2	1.8	1.4	14.3	6.7	-	-	2.0	2.6	34	100.0
Histiocytosis X	1	0	0	0	1	0.9	0.7	7.1	3.4	-	-	1.0	1.3	17	100.0
Other reticuloendothelial	0	1	0	0	1	0.9	0.7	7.1	3.4	-	-	1.0	1.3	17	100.0
III. BRAIN AND SPINAL	1	11	6	9	27	24.1	24.6	100.0	40.5	18.7	24.7	27.5	28.9	420	85.2
Ependymoma	1	0	3	0	4	3.6	4.3	14.8	3.4	9.3	-	4.1	4.3	64	100.0
Astrocytoma	0	6	1	5	12	10.7	10.4	44.4	20.2	3.1	13.7	12.2	12.8	186	100.0
Medulloblastoma	0	1	1	1	3	2.7	2.9	11.1	3.4	3.1	2.7	3.1	3.4	46	100.0
Other glioma	0	1	0	0	1	0.9	0.7	3.7	3.4	-	-	1.0	1.3	17	42.9
Other and unspecified *	0	3	1	3	7	6.3	6.3	25.9	10.1	3.1	8.2	7.1	7.3	107	100.0
IV. SYMPATHETIC N.S.	2	3	0	0	5	4.5	3.5	100.0	16.9	-	-	5.1	6.5	84	100.0
Neuroblastoma	2	3	0	0	5	4.5	3.5	100.0	16.9	-	-	5.1	6.5	84	100.0
Other	0	0	0	0	0	-	-	-	-	-	-	-	-	-	-
V. RETINOBLASTOMA	0	3	0	0	3	2.7	2.1	100.0	10.1	-	-	3.1	3.9	51	66.7
VI. KIDNEY	0	6	0	1	7	6.3	5.2	100.0	20.2	-	2.7	7.1	8.6	115	100.0
Wilms' tumour	0	6	0	0	6	5.4	4.2	85.7	20.2	-	-	6.1	7.8	101	100.0
Renal carcinoma	0	0	0	1	1	0.9	1.0	14.3	-	-	2.7	1.0	0.8	14	100.0
Other and unspecified	0	0	0	0	0	-	-	-	-	-	-	-	-	-	-
VII. LIVER	0	0	0	0	0	-	-	-	-	-	-	-	-	-	-
Hepatoblastoma	0	0	0	0	0	-	-	-	-	-	-	-	-	-	-
Hepatic carcinoma	0	0	0	0	0	-	-	-	-	-	-	-	-	-	-
Other and unspecified	0	0	0	0	0	-	-	-	-	-	-	-	-	-	-
VIII. BONE	0	0	4	3	7	6.3	7.8	100.0	-	12.5	8.2	7.1	6.4	104	100.0
Osteosarcoma	0	0	2	3	5	4.5	5.4	71.4	-	6.2	8.2	5.1	4.4	72	100.0
Chondrosarcoma	0	0	0	0	0	-	-	-	-	-	-	-	-	-	-
Ewing's sarcoma	0	0	2	0	2	1.8	2.4	28.6	-	6.2	-	2.0	2.0	31	100.0
Other and unspecified	0	0	0	0	0	-	-	-	-	-	-	-	-	-	-
IX. SOFT TISSUE SARCOMAS	1	2	0	2	5	4.5	4.1	100.0	10.1	-	5.5	5.1	5.5	78	100.0
Rhabdomyosarcoma	1	2	0	1	4	3.6	3.1	80.0	10.1	-	2.7	4.1	4.7	64	100.0
Fibrosarcoma	0	0	0	0	0	-	-	-	-	-	-	-	-	-	-
Other and unspecified	0	0	0	1	1	0.9	1.0	20.0	-	-	2.7	1.0	0.8	14	100.0
X. GONADAL & GERM CELL	1	0	0	2	3	2.7	2.7	100.0	3.4	-	5.5	3.1	2.9	44	100.0
Non-gonadal germ cell	1	0	0	1	2	1.8	1.7	66.7	3.4	-	2.7	2.0	2.1	31	100.0
Gonadal germ cell	0	0	0	1	1	0.9	1.0	33.3	-	-	2.7	1.0	0.8	14	100.0
Gonadal carcinoma	0	0	0	0	0	-	-	-	-	-	-	-	-	-	-
Other and unspecified	0	0	0	0	0	-	-	-	-	-	-	-	-	-	-
XI. EPITHELIAL NEOPLASMS	0	0	2	1	3	2.7	3.4	100.0	-	6.2	2.7	3.1	2.8	45	100.0
Adrenocortical carcinoma	0	0	0	0	0	-	-	-	-	-	-	-	-	-	-
Thyroid carcinoma	0	0	0	0	0	-	-	-	-	-	-	-	-	-	-
Nasopharyngeal carcinoma	0	0	0	0	0	-	-	-	-	-	-	-	-	-	-
Melanoma	0	0	1	0	1	0.9	1.2	33.3	-	3.1	-	1.0	1.0	16	100.0
Other carcinoma	0	0	1	1	2	1.8	2.2	66.7	-	3.1	2.7	2.0	1.8	29	100.0
XII. OTHER	1	0	1	1	3	2.7	2.9	100.0	3.4	3.1	2.7	3.1	3.1	46	66.7
* Specified as malignant	0	1	1	2	4	3.6	3.9	100.0	3.4	3.1	5.5	4.1	3.9	60	-

France, Paediatric Registries   1983 - 1985   MALE

DIAGNOSTIC GROUP	\[NUMBER OF CASES\] 0	1-4	5-9	10-14	All	\[REL. FREQUENCY (%)\] Crude	Adj.	Group	\[RATES PER MILLION\] 0	1-4	5-9	10-14	Crude	Adj.	Cum	HV (%)
TOTAL	19	93	55	60	227	100.0	100.0	100.0	178.3	227.7	103.3	99.6	137.6	146.6	2104	96.5
I. LEUKAEMIAS	4	28	14	13	59	26.0	25.6	100.0	37.5	68.6	26.3	21.6	35.8	38.9	551	100.0
Acute lymphocytic	3	22	14	10	49	21.6	21.6	83.1	28.2	53.9	26.3	16.6	29.7	32.2	458	100.0
Other lymphocytic																
Acute non-lymphocytic	1	5	0	2	8	3.5	3.1	13.6	9.4	12.2		3.3	4.8	5.5	75	100.0
Chronic myeloid	0	1	0	0	1	0.4	0.4	1.7		2.4			0.6	0.8	10	100.0
Other and unspecified	0	0	0	1	1	0.4	0.5	1.7				1.7	0.6	0.5	8	100.0
II. LYMPHOMAS	2	7	8	14	31	13.7	14.6	100.0	18.8	17.1	15.0	23.2	18.8	18.4	279	100.0
Hodgkin's disease	0	1	2	6	9	4.0	4.4	29.0		2.4	3.8	10.0	5.5	4.9	78	100.0
Non-Hodgkin lymphoma	0	0	5	2	7	3.1	3.7	22.6			9.4	3.3	4.2	4.0	64	100.0
Burkitt's lymphoma	0	4	1	6	11	4.8	5.0	35.5		9.8	1.9	10.0	6.7	6.5	98	100.0
Unspecified lymphoma																
Histiocytosis X	1	2	0	0	3	1.3	1.1	9.7	9.4	4.9			1.8	2.2	29	100.0
Other reticuloendothelial	1	0	0	0	1	0.4	0.4	3.2	9.4				0.6	0.7	9	100.0
III. BRAIN AND SPINAL	3	17	20	14	54	23.8	25.1	100.0	28.2	41.6	37.6	23.2	32.7	33.9	499	85.2
Ependymoma	1	2	2	0	5	2.2	2.2	9.3	9.4	4.9	3.8		3.0	3.5	48	100.0
Astrocytoma	1	9	4	8	22	9.7	9.8	40.7	9.4	22.0	7.5	13.3	13.3	13.8	201	100.0
Medulloblastoma	0	3	5	2	10	4.4	4.8	18.5		7.3	9.4	3.3	6.1	6.3	93	95.5
Other glioma	0	2	2	0	4	1.8	1.8	7.4		4.9	3.8		2.4	2.7	38	50.0
Other and unspecified *	1	1	7	4	13	5.7	6.5	24.1	9.4	2.4	13.1	6.6	7.9	7.7	118	61.5
IV. SYMPATHETIC N.S.	7	15	2	0	24	10.6	8.9	100.0	65.7	36.7	3.8		14.5	17.7	231	100.0
Neuroblastoma	7	14	2	0	23	10.1	8.6	95.8	65.7	34.3	3.8		13.9	16.9	222	100.0
Other	0	1	0	0	1	0.4	0.4	4.2		2.4			0.6	0.8	10	100.0
V. RETINOBLASTOMA	0	6	0	0	6	2.6	2.1	100.0		14.7			3.6	4.5	59	100.0
VI. KIDNEY	0	6	0	3	9	4.0	3.6	100.0		14.7		5.0	5.5	6.0	84	100.0
Wilms' tumour	0	6	0	2	8	3.5	3.1	88.9		14.7		3.3	4.8	5.5	75	100.0
Renal carcinoma	0	0	0	1	1	0.4	0.5	11.1				1.7	0.6	0.5	8	100.0
Other and unspecified																
VII. LIVER	1	1	1	0	3	1.3	1.3	100.0	9.4	2.4	1.9		1.8	2.1	29	100.0
Hepatoblastoma	1	1	1	0	3	1.3	1.3	100.0	9.4	2.4	1.9		1.8	2.1	29	100.0
Hepatic carcinoma																
Other and unspecified																
VIII. BONE	0	0	2	6	8	3.5	4.1	100.0			3.8	10.0	4.8	4.1	69	100.0
Osteosarcoma	0	0	2	5	7	3.1	3.6	87.5			3.8	8.3	4.2	3.6	60	100.0
Chondrosarcoma																
Ewing's sarcoma	0	0	0	1	1	0.4	0.5	12.5				1.7	0.6	0.5	8	100.0
Other and unspecified																
IX. SOFT TISSUE SARCOMAS	1	8	7	5	21	9.3	9.5	100.0	9.4	19.6	13.1	8.3	12.7	13.4	195	100.0
Rhabdomyosarcoma	1	6	6	2	15	6.6	6.8	71.4	9.4	14.7	11.3	3.3	9.1	9.9	141	100.0
Fibrosarcoma	0	1	1	1	3	1.3	1.4	14.3		2.4	1.9	1.7	1.8	1.8	27	100.0
Other and unspecified	0	1	0	2	3	1.3	1.4	14.3		2.4		3.3	1.8	1.7	26	100.0
X. GONADAL & GERM CELL	0	3	0	0	3	1.3	1.1	100.0		7.3			1.8	2.3	29	100.0
Non-gonadal germ cell	0	3	0	0	3	1.3	1.1	100.0		7.3			1.8	2.3	29	100.0
Gonadal germ cell																
Gonadal carcinoma																
Other and unspecified																
XI. EPITHELIAL NEOPLASMS	1	1	1	5	8	3.5	3.8	100.0	9.4	2.4	1.9	8.3	4.8	4.5	70	100.0
Adrenocortical carcinoma	1	0	0	0	1	0.4	0.4	12.5	9.4				0.6	0.8	10	100.0
Thyroid carcinoma																
Nasopharyngeal carcinoma																
Melanoma	0	0	0	2	2	0.9	1.0	25.0				3.3	1.2	1.0	17	100.0
Other carcinoma	0	1	1	3	5	2.2	2.4	62.5		2.4	1.9	5.0	3.0	2.8	44	100.0
XII. OTHER	0	1	0	0	1	0.4	0.4	100.0		2.4			0.6	1.2	10	100.0
* Specified as malignant	1	0	0	1	2	0.9	0.9	100.0	9.4			1.7	1.2	1.2	18	50.0

France, Paediatric Registries

1983 – 1985

FEMALE

DIAGNOSTIC GROUP	NUMBER OF CASES 0	1-4	5-9	10-14	All	REL. FREQUENCY(%) Crude	Adj.	Group	RATES PER MILLION 0	1-4	5-9	10-14	Crude	Adj.	Cum	HV(%)
TOTAL	15	67	40	51	173	100.0	100.0	100.0	143.4	170.0	79.2	89.4	109.9	115.2	1666	94.2
I. LEUKAEMIAS	5	28	14	14	61	35.3	34.8	100.0	47.8	71.0	27.7	24.5	38.7	41.8	593	100.0
Acute lymphocytic	1	27	13	10	51	29.5	29.3	83.6	9.6	68.5	25.7	17.5	32.4	35.3	500	100.0
Other lymphocytic	0	0	0	0	0	-	-	-	-	-	-	-	-	-	-	-
Acute non-lymphocytic	4	1	1	4	10	5.8	5.5	16.4	38.2	2.5	2.0	7.0	6.4	6.4	93	100.0
Chronic myeloid	0	0	0	0	0	-	-	-	-	-	-	-	-	-	-	-
Other and unspecified	0	0	0	0	0	-	-	-	-	-	-	-	-	-	-	-
II. LYMPHOMAS	3	5	3	8	19	11.0	10.9	100.0	28.7	12.7	5.9	14.0	12.1	12.1	179	100.0
Hodgkin's disease	0	0	1	5	6	3.5	3.7	31.6	-	-	2.0	8.8	3.8	3.2	54	100.0
Non-Hodgkin lymphoma	0	1	0	3	4	2.3	2.4	21.1	-	2.5	-	5.3	2.5	2.4	38	100.0
Burkitt's lymphoma	0	1	0	0	1	0.6	0.5	5.3	-	2.5	-	-	0.6	0.8	10	100.0
Unspecified lymphoma	0	0	0	0	0	-	-	-	-	-	-	-	-	-	-	-
Histiocytosis X	2	2	1	0	5	2.9	1.6	26.3	19.1	5.1	2.0	-	3.2	2.0	49	100.0
Other reticuloendothelial	1	1	1	0	3	1.7	1.4	15.8	9.6	2.5	2.0	-	1.9	2.0	28	100.0
III. BRAIN AND SPINAL	2	5	11	14	32	18.5	19.9	100.0	19.1	12.7	21.8	24.5	20.3	19.6	301	81.3
Ependymoma	1	0	1	0	2	1.2	1.2	6.3	9.6	-	2.0	-	1.2	1.4	19	50.0
Astrocytoma	0	4	4	8	16	9.2	9.7	50.0	-	10.1	7.9	14.0	10.2	9.8	150	93.8
Medulloblastoma	0	1	2	3	6	3.5	3.8	18.8	-	2.5	4.0	5.3	3.8	3.6	56	100.0
Other glioma	0	0	1	0	1	0.6	0.8	3.1	-	-	2.0	-	0.6	0.6	10	-
Other and unspecified *	1	0	3	3	7	4.0	4.5	21.9	9.6	-	5.9	5.3	4.4	4.2	66	57.1
IV. SYMPATHETIC N.S.	1	12	1	0	14	8.1	7.1	100.0	9.6	30.4	2.0	-	8.9	10.8	141	85.7
Neuroblastoma	1	11	1	0	13	7.5	6.6	92.9	9.6	27.9	2.0	-	8.3	10.0	131	84.6
Other	0	1	0	0	1	0.6	0.5	7.1	-	2.5	-	-	0.6	0.8	10	100.0
V. RETINOBLASTOMA	1	3	0	0	4	2.3	2.0	100.0	9.6	7.6	-	-	2.5	3.1	40	100.0
VI. KIDNEY	0	6	2	0	8	4.6	4.4	100.0	-	15.2	4.0	-	5.1	6.0	81	100.0
Wilms' tumour	0	6	2	0	8	4.6	4.4	100.0	-	15.2	4.0	-	5.1	6.0	81	100.0
Renal carcinoma	0	0	0	0	0	-	-	-	-	-	-	-	-	-	-	-
Other and unspecified	0	0	0	0	0	-	-	-	-	-	-	-	-	-	-	-
VII. LIVER	1	2	0	1	4	2.3	2.1	100.0	9.6	5.1	-	1.8	2.5	2.8	39	50.0
Hepatoblastoma	1	1	0	0	2	1.2	1.0	50.0	9.6	2.5	-	-	1.3	1.5	20	100.0
Hepatic carcinoma	0	1	0	1	2	1.2	1.1	50.0	-	2.5	-	1.8	1.3	1.3	19	-
Other and unspecified	0	0	0	0	0	-	-	-	-	-	-	-	-	-	-	-
VIII. BONE	0	0	4	5	9	5.2	5.9	100.0	-	-	7.9	8.8	5.7	5.1	83	100.0
Osteosarcoma	0	0	2	3	5	2.9	3.3	55.6	-	-	4.0	5.3	3.2	2.8	46	100.0
Chondrosarcoma	0	0	1	0	1	0.6	0.8	11.1	-	-	2.0	-	0.6	0.6	10	100.0
Ewing's sarcoma	0	0	1	2	3	1.7	1.9	33.3	-	-	2.0	3.5	1.9	1.7	27	100.0
Other and unspecified	0	0	0	0	0	-	-	-	-	-	-	-	-	-	-	-
IX. SOFT TISSUE SARCOMAS	1	3	3	1	8	4.6	4.8	100.0	9.6	7.6	5.9	1.8	5.1	5.5	78	100.0
Rhabdomyosarcoma	1	3	0	1	5	2.9	3.0	62.5	9.6	7.6	-	1.8	3.2	3.6	50	100.0
Fibrosarcoma	0	0	1	0	1	0.6	0.5	12.5	-	-	2.0	-	0.6	0.7	10	100.0
Other and unspecified	0	0	2	0	2	1.2	1.3	25.0	-	-	4.0	-	1.3	1.1	19	100.0
X. GONADAL & GERM CELL	1	3	1	1	6	3.5	3.3	100.0	9.6	7.6	2.0	1.8	3.8	4.2	59	100.0
Non-gonadal germ cell	1	3	1	0	5	2.9	2.7	83.3	9.6	7.6	2.0	-	3.2	3.7	50	100.0
Gonadal germ cell	0	0	0	1	1	0.6	0.6	16.7	-	-	-	1.8	0.6	0.5	9	100.0
Gonadal carcinoma	0	0	0	0	0	-	-	-	-	-	-	-	-	-	-	-
Other and unspecified	0	0	0	0	0	-	-	-	-	-	-	-	-	-	-	-
XI. EPITHELIAL NEOPLASMS	0	0	1	7	8	4.6	4.9	100.0	-	-	2.0	12.3	5.1	4.2	71	100.0
Adrenocortical carcinoma	0	0	1	1	2	1.2	1.3	25.0	-	-	2.0	1.8	1.3	1.1	19	100.0
Thyroid carcinoma	0	0	0	3	3	1.7	1.8	37.5	-	-	-	5.3	1.9	1.5	26	100.0
Nasopharyngeal carcinoma	0	0	0	2	2	1.2	1.2	25.0	-	-	-	3.5	1.3	1.0	18	100.0
Melanoma	0	0	0	1	1	0.6	0.6	12.5	-	-	-	1.8	0.6	0.5	9	100.0
Other carcinoma	0	0	0	0	0	-	-	-	-	-	-	-	-	-	-	-
XII. OTHER	0	0	0	0	0	-	-	-	-	-	-	-	-	-	-	-
* Specified as malignant	1	0	1	1	3	1.7	1.8	100.0	9.6	-	2.0	1.8	1.9	1.9	28	33.3

France, Lorraine

1983 – 1985 MALE

DIAGNOSTIC GROUP	NUMBER OF CASES					REL. FREQUENCY(%)			RATES PER MILLION							HV(%)
	0	1-4	5-9	10-14	All	Crude	Adj.	Group	0	1-4	5-9	10-14	Crude	Adj.	Cum	
TOTAL	15	49	23	33	120	100.0	100.0	100.0	278.1	235.9	87.7	110.9	146.1	155.1	2215	96.6
I. LEUKAEMIAS	4	14	4	6	28	23.3	21.9	100.0	74.2	67.4	15.2	20.2	34.1	37.4	521	100.0
II. LYMPHOMAS	1	4	5	7	17	14.2	16.0	100.0	18.5	19.3	19.1	23.5	20.7	20.4	308	100.0
III. BRAIN AND SPINAL	3	10	9	9	31	25.8	28.0	100.0	55.6	48.1	34.3	30.3	37.7	39.1	571	87.1
IV. SYMPATHETIC N.S.	5	5	0	0	10	8.3	6.3	100.0	92.7	24.1	-	-	12.2	14.6	189	100.0
V. RETINOBLASTOMA	0	3	0	0	3	2.5	1.9	100.0	-	14.4	-	-	3.7	4.5	58	100.0
VI. KIDNEY	0	4	0	2	6	5.0	4.3	100.0	-	19.3	-	6.7	7.3	7.9	111	100.0
VII. LIVER	1	1	1	0	3	2.5	2.6	100.0	18.5	4.8	-	-	3.7	4.2	57	100.0
VIII. BONE	0	0	1	4	5	4.2	4.9	100.0	-	-	3.8	13.4	6.1	5.1	86	100.0
IX. SOFT TISSUE SARCOMAS	1	5	2	1	9	7.5	7.3	100.0	18.5	24.1	7.6	3.4	11.0	12.3	170	100.0
X. GONADAL & GERM CELL	0	1	0	0	1	0.8	0.6	100.0	-	4.8	-	-	1.2	1.5	19	100.0
XI. EPITHELIAL NEOPLASMS	0	1	1	4	6	5.0	5.6	100.0	-	4.8	3.8	13.4	7.3	6.6	106	100.0
XII. OTHER	0	1	0	0	1	0.8	0.6	100.0	-	4.8	-	-	1.2	1.5	19	100.0

France, Lorraine

1983 – 1985 FEMALE

DIAGNOSTIC GROUP	NUMBER OF CASES					REL. FREQUENCY(%)			RATES PER MILLION							HV(%)
	0	1-4	5-9	10-14	All	Crude	Adj.	Group	0	1-4	5-9	10-14	Crude	Adj.	Cum	
TOTAL	9	27	16	25	77	100.0	100.0	100.0	164.9	137.5	64.6	87.5	98.2	101.6	1476	88.3
I. LEUKAEMIAS	5	11	7	7	30	39.0	39.3	100.0	91.6	56.0	28.3	24.5	38.3	40.7	580	100.0
II. LYMPHOMAS	1	3	2	7	13	16.9	16.6	100.0	18.3	15.3	8.1	24.5	16.6	15.9	242	100.0
III. BRAIN AND SPINAL	1	3	6	4	14	18.2	20.5	100.0	18.3	15.3	24.2	14.0	17.9	18.0	271	64.3
IV. SYMPATHETIC N.S.	0	5	0	0	5	6.5	5.6	100.0	-	25.5	-	-	6.4	7.9	102	60.0
V. RETINOBLASTOMA	1	1	0	0	2	2.6	2.2	100.0	18.3	5.1	-	-	2.6	3.0	39	100.0
VI. KIDNEY	0	1	1	0	2	2.6	3.0	100.0	-	5.1	4.0	-	2.6	2.9	41	100.0
VII. LIVER	0	2	0	1	3	3.9	3.4	100.0	-	10.2	-	3.5	3.8	4.2	58	33.3
VIII. BONE	0	0	0	4	4	5.2	4.8	100.0	-	-	-	14.0	5.1	4.1	70	100.0
IX. SOFT TISSUE SARCOMAS	0	1	0	0	1	1.3	1.1	100.0	-	5.1	-	-	1.3	1.6	20	100.0
X. GONADAL & GERM CELL	1	0	0	0	1	1.3	1.1	100.0	18.3	-	-	-	1.3	1.4	18	100.0
XI. EPITHELIAL NEOPLASMS	0	0	0	2	2	2.6	2.4	100.0	-	-	-	7.0	2.6	2.0	35	100.0
XII. OTHER	0	0	0	0	0	-	-	-	-	-	-	-	-	-	-	-

France, PACA and Corsica — MALE — 1984 – 1985

DIAGNOSTIC GROUP	NUMBER OF CASES 0	1-4	5-9	10-14	All	REL. FREQUENCY(%) Crude	Adj.	Group	RATES PER MILLION 0	1-4	5-9	10-14	Crude	Adj.	Cum	HV(%)
TOTAL	4	44	32	27	107	100.0	100.0	100.0	76.0	219.2	118.4	88.6	129.2	137.7	1988	96.3
I. LEUKAEMIAS	0	14	10	7	31	29.0	28.8	100.0	-	69.8	37.0	23.0	37.4	40.2	579	100.0
II. LYMPHOMAS	1	3	3	7	14	13.1	13.9	100.0	19.0	14.9	11.1	23.0	16.9	16.4	249	100.0
III. BRAIN AND SPINAL	0	7	11	5	23	21.5	21.7	100.0	-	34.9	40.7	16.4	27.8	28.7	425	82.6
IV. SYMPATHETIC N.S.	2	10	2	0	14	13.1	11.9	100.0	38.0	49.8	7.4	-	16.9	20.8	274	100.0
V. RETINOBLASTOMA	0	3	0	0	3	2.8	2.5	100.0	-	14.9	-	-	3.6	4.6	60	100.0
VI. KIDNEY	0	2	0	1	3	2.8	2.8	100.0	-	10.0	-	3.3	3.6	4.0	56	100.0
VII. LIVER	0	0	0	0	0	-	-	-	-	-	-	-	-	-	-	-
VIII. BONE	0	0	1	2	3	2.8	3.2	100.0	-	-	3.7	6.6	3.6	3.1	51	100.0
IX. SOFT TISSUE SARCOMAS	0	3	5	4	12	11.2	11.6	100.0	-	14.9	18.5	13.1	14.5	14.4	218	100.0
X. GONADAL & GERM CELL	0	2	0	0	2	1.9	1.7	100.0	-	10.0	-	-	2.4	3.1	40	100.0
XI. EPITHELIAL NEOPLASMS	1	0	0	1	2	1.9	1.9	100.0	19.0	-	-	3.3	2.4	2.4	35	100.0
XII. OTHER	0	0	0	0	0	-	-	-	-	-	-	-	-	-	-	-

France, PACA and Corsica — FEMALE — 1984 – 1985

DIAGNOSTIC GROUP	NUMBER OF CASES 0	1-4	5-9	10-14	All	REL. FREQUENCY(%) Crude	Adj.	Group	RATES PER MILLION 0	1-4	5-9	10-14	Crude	Adj.	Cum	HV(%)
TOTAL	6	40	24	26	96	100.0	100.0	100.0	119.9	202.3	93.2	91.3	121.5	128.5	1852	99.0
I. LEUKAEMIAS	0	17	7	7	31	32.3	31.6	100.0	-	86.0	27.2	24.6	39.2	42.5	603	100.0
II. LYMPHOMAS	2	2	1	1	6	6.3	5.9	100.0	40.0	10.1	3.9	3.5	7.6	8.5	117	94.4
III. BRAIN AND SPINAL	1	2	5	10	18	18.8	20.4	100.0	20.0	10.1	19.4	35.1	22.8	21.1	333	100.0
IV. SYMPATHETIC N.S.	1	7	1	0	9	9.4	8.2	100.0	20.0	35.4	3.9	-	11.4	13.8	181	100.0
V. RETINOBLASTOMA	0	2	0	0	2	2.1	1.7	100.0	-	10.1	-	-	2.5	3.1	40	100.0
VI. KIDNEY	0	5	1	0	6	6.3	5.6	100.0	-	25.3	3.9	-	7.6	9.1	121	100.0
VII. LIVER	1	0	0	0	1	1.0	0.9	100.0	20.0	-	-	-	1.3	1.5	20	100.0
VIII. BONE	0	0	4	1	5	5.2	6.2	100.0	-	-	15.5	3.5	6.3	6.0	95	100.0
IX. SOFT TISSUE SARCOMAS	1	2	3	1	7	7.3	7.5	100.0	20.0	10.1	11.6	3.5	8.9	9.5	136	100.0
X. GONADAL & GERM CELL	0	3	1	1	5	5.2	5.0	100.0	-	15.2	3.9	3.5	6.3	7.0	98	100.0
XI. EPITHELIAL NEOPLASMS	0	0	1	5	6	6.3	7.0	100.0	-	-	3.9	17.6	7.6	6.3	107	100.0
XII. OTHER	0	0	0	0	0	-	-	-	-	-	-	-	-	-	-	-

GERMAN DEMOCRATIC REPUBLIC

National Cancer Registry, 1976–1980

W. Staneczek & W. Mehnert

A nation-wide, obligatory system of cancer case reporting was established in the German Democratic Republic (GDR) in 1953 to help optimize care for patients with malignant disease. The cancer reporting system is an integral part of a network of medical and social services for cancer patients. Such services are provided or co-ordinated by Cancer Control Agencies (CCAs) located in each of the 227 counties. Whereas the CCAs are part of the National Health Service, the National Cancer Registry (NCR) is a branch of the Central Institute for Cancer Research of the Academy of Sciences of the GDR.

A 'report of a new case' form must be completed by the physician or institution responsible for the patient's initial treatment and sent to the CCA in the patient's county of residence. The form is reviewed and a copy forwarded to the NCR. Each additional course of treatment (including that for recurrent or metastatic disease) must be similarly reported. Pathological institutes performing an autopsy on a deceased person with cancer must submit a copy of the report to the NCR via the CCA. The overall autopsy rate as of 1981 was 22%, as compared with 55% for persons with cancer, reflecting recommendations that such cases undergo post mortem examination whenever possible. Death certificates for all persons dying in the catchment area are reviewed by the CCA. If a diagnosis of cancer is found on a death certificate of a person not previously known to the CCA, the case is investigated and the required reporting forms are completed on the basis of the medical report.

Reporting forms sent to the NCR are edited and selected information is coded and prepared for computer entry. Data are entered at an associated computer centre and stored on magnetic tape.

Anatomical site of tumour is coded by an internal code wholly compatible with the ICD-O topography codes. Since 1976, histology has been coded according to the ICD-O morphology classification.

The NCR covers the entire territory of the GDR. The population density is 154 per square kilometre. The population in 1980 was 16.7 million, of whom 3.3 million (19.7%) were aged 0–14. The country is highly industrialized, but there is a substantial agricultural and forestry sector. The population is stable with a high average level of education and is fairly homogeneous.

NCR data are used for health services planning, evaluation of medical services and epidemiological research. Data on childhood incidence by site and histology for periods in the 1970s have been published elsewhere (Staneczek, 1984, 1985).

Population

The population is derived from annual estimates, prepared using census data from 1971 and 1981, and information on births, deaths and migration (Staatliche Zentralverwaltung fur Statistik, Berlin, DDR).

AVERAGE ANNUAL POPULATION: 1976–1980

Age	Male	Female
0	112400	106400
1–4	396200	375700
5–9	558100	531400
10–14	677400	645000
0–14	1744100	1658500

Commentary

Leukaemia accounted for 26% of all registrations. There was an unusually low acute lymphocytic:acute non-lymphocytic ratio of 3.1:1. Incidence rates were relatively high for lymphomas, both Hodgkin's disease and others. There was also a very high incidence of soft-tissue sarcomas. This group contained roughly one-third each of rhabdomyosarcoma, fibrosarcoma and other and unspecified

Contd p. 246

German Democratic Republic　　　　　1976 - 1980　　　　　MALE

DIAGNOSTIC GROUP	NUMBER OF CASES 0	1-4	5-9	10-14	All	REL. FREQUENCY(%) Crude	Adj.	Group	RATES PER MILLION 0	1-4	5-9	10-14	Crude	Adj.	Cum	HV(%)
TOTAL	107	340	321	325	1093	100.0	100.0	100.0	190.4	171.6	115.0	96.0	125.3	132.9	1932	92.7
I. LEUKAEMIAS	14	116	94	61	285	26.1	26.0	100.0	24.9	58.6	33.7	18.0	32.7	36.2	518	97.9
Acute lymphocytic	8	88	67	32	195	17.8	17.8	68.4	14.2	44.4	24.0	9.4	22.4	25.3	359	97.9
Other lymphocytic	1	0	0	0	1	0.1	0.1	0.4	1.8	-	-	-	0.1	0.1	-	100.0
Acute non-lymphocytic	5	18	18	18	59	5.4	5.4	20.7	8.9	9.1	6.5	5.3	6.8	7.1	104	96.6
Chronic myeloid	0	5	4	5	14	1.3	1.3	4.9	-	2.5	1.4	1.5	1.6	1.7	25	100.0
Other and unspecified	0	5	5	6	16	1.5	1.5	5.6	-	2.5	1.8	1.8	1.8	1.9	28	100.0
II. LYMPHOMAS	10	33	65	91	199	18.2	18.3	100.0	17.8	16.7	23.3	26.9	22.8	21.9	335	97.5
Hodgkin's disease	0	8	25	43	76	7.0	7.0	38.2	-	4.0	9.0	12.7	8.7	7.8	124	98.7
Non-Hodgkin lymphoma	3	12	33	40	88	8.1	8.1	44.2	5.3	6.1	11.8	11.8	10.1	9.5	148	95.5
Burkitt's lymphoma	0	5	4	3	12	1.1	1.1	6.0	-	2.5	1.4	0.9	1.4	1.4	21	100.0
Unspecified lymphoma	0	0	0	3	3	0.3	0.3	1.5	-	-	-	0.9	0.3	0.3	4	100.0
Histiocytosis X	4	6	1	0	11	1.0	1.0	5.5	7.1	3.0	0.4	-	1.3	1.6	21	100.0
Other reticuloendothelial	3	2	2	2	9	0.8	0.8	4.5	5.3	1.0	0.7	0.6	1.0	1.2	17	100.0
III. BRAIN AND SPINAL	15	61	86	74	236	21.6	21.7	100.0	26.7	30.8	30.8	21.8	27.1	27.9	413	74.4
Ependymoma	5	17	11	10	43	3.9	3.9	18.2	8.9	8.6	3.9	3.0	4.9	5.5	78	72.5
Astrocytoma	2	19	33	30	84	7.7	7.7	35.6	3.6	9.6	11.8	8.9	9.6	9.9	145	78.4
Medulloblastoma	6	13	22	18	59	5.4	5.4	25.0	10.7	6.6	7.9	5.3	6.8	6.9	103	70.9
Other glioma	0	4	3	2	9	0.8	0.8	3.8	-	2.0	1.1	0.6	1.0	1.1	16	62.5
Other and unspecified *	2	8	17	14	41	3.8	3.8	17.4	3.6	4.0	6.1	4.1	4.7	4.7	71	76.9
IV. SYMPATHETIC N.S.	20	34	11	5	70	6.4	6.3	100.0	35.6	17.2	3.9	1.5	8.0	9.8	131	91.4
Neuroblastoma	20	34	11	5	70	6.4	6.3	100.0	35.6	17.2	3.9	1.5	8.0	9.8	131	91.4
Other	0	0	0	0	0	-	-	-	-	-	-	-	-	-	-	-
V. RETINOBLASTOMA	8	15	0	0	23	2.1	2.1	100.0	14.2	7.6	-	-	2.6	3.4	45	100.0
VI. KIDNEY	10	27	8	4	49	4.5	4.4	100.0	17.8	13.6	2.9	1.2	5.6	6.9	93	95.9
Wilms' tumour	10	26	7	4	47	4.3	4.2	95.9	17.8	13.1	2.5	1.2	5.4	6.6	89	97.9
Renal carcinoma	0	0	1	0	1	0.1	0.1	2.0	-	-	0.4	-	0.1	0.1	2	100.0
Other and unspecified	0	1	0	0	1	0.1	0.1	2.0	-	0.5	-	-	0.1	0.1	2	-
VII. LIVER	2	3	3	1	9	0.8	0.8	100.0	3.6	1.5	1.1	0.3	1.0	1.2	16	88.9
Hepatoblastoma	0	0	0	0	0	-	-	-	-	-	-	-	-	-	-	-
Hepatic carcinoma	2	2	3	1	8	0.7	0.7	88.9	3.6	1.0	1.1	0.3	0.9	1.0	14	87.5
Other and unspecified	0	1	0	0	1	0.1	0.1	11.1	-	0.5	-	-	0.1	0.2	2	100.0
VIII. BONE	0	9	24	42	75	6.9	6.9	100.0	-	4.5	8.6	12.4	8.6	7.8	123	98.7
Osteosarcoma	0	0	11	15	26	2.4	2.4	34.7	-	-	3.9	4.4	3.0	2.6	42	100.0
Chondrosarcoma	0	0	1	4	5	0.5	0.5	6.7	-	-	0.4	1.2	0.6	0.5	8	100.0
Ewing's sarcoma	0	6	8	16	30	2.7	2.8	40.0	-	3.0	2.9	4.7	3.4	3.2	50	96.7
Other and unspecified	0	3	4	7	14	1.3	1.3	18.7	-	1.5	1.4	2.1	1.6	1.5	24	100.0
IX. SOFT TISSUE SARCOMAS	18	20	18	24	80	7.3	7.3	100.0	32.0	10.1	6.5	7.1	9.2	9.7	140	98.7
Rhabdomyosarcoma	2	12	10	5	29	2.7	2.6	36.3	3.6	6.1	3.6	1.5	3.3	3.7	53	96.6
Fibrosarcoma	8	4	7	8	27	2.5	2.5	33.8	14.2	2.0	2.5	2.4	3.1	3.2	47	100.0
Other and unspecified	8	4	1	11	24	2.2	2.2	30.0	14.2	2.0	0.4	3.2	2.8	2.8	40	100.0
X. GONADAL & GERM CELL	6	15	1	5	27	2.5	2.4	100.0	10.7	7.6	0.4	1.5	3.1	3.7	50	96.3
Non-gonadal germ cell	2	2	1	1	6	0.5	0.5	22.2	3.6	1.0	0.4	0.3	0.7	0.7	10	100.0
Gonadal germ cell	4	13	0	3	20	1.8	1.8	74.1	7.1	6.6	-	0.9	2.3	2.9	38	100.0
Gonadal carcinoma	0	0	0	1	1	0.1	0.1	3.7	-	-	-	0.3	0.1	0.2	2	95.0
Other and unspecified	0	0	0	0	0	-	-	-	-	-	-	-	-	-	-	-
XI. EPITHELIAL NEOPLASMS	3	6	9	13	31	2.8	2.8	100.0	5.3	3.0	3.2	3.8	3.6	3.5	53	100.0
Adrenocortical carcinoma	1	3	0	0	4	0.4	0.4	12.9	1.8	1.5	-	-	0.5	0.6	8	100.0
Thyroid carcinoma	0	0	2	2	4	0.4	0.4	12.9	-	-	0.7	0.6	0.5	0.4	7	100.0
Nasopharyngeal carcinoma	0	0	1	1	2	0.2	0.2	6.5	-	-	0.4	0.3	0.2	0.2	3	100.0
Melanoma	1	0	2	4	7	0.6	0.6	22.6	1.8	-	0.7	1.2	0.8	0.7	11	100.0
Other carcinoma	1	3	4	6	14	1.3	1.3	45.2	1.8	1.5	1.4	1.8	1.6	1.6	24	100.0
XII. OTHER	1	1	2	5	9	0.8	0.8	100.0	1.8	0.5	0.7	1.5	1.0	1.0	15	75.0
* Specified as malignant	0	6	11	6	23	2.1	2.1		-	3.0	3.9	1.8	2.6	2.7	41	54.5

German Democratic Republic

1976 – 1980 FEMALE

DIAGNOSTIC GROUP	NUMBER OF CASES					REL. FREQUENCY(%)			RATES PER MILLION							HV(%)
	0	1-4	5-9	10-14	All	Crude	Adj.	Group	0	1-4	5-9	10-14	Crude	Adj.	Cum	
TOTAL	85	285	217	312	899	100.0	100.0	100.0	159.8	151.7	81.7	96.7	108.4	113.8	1659	93.1
I. LEUKAEMIAS	13	102	69	56	240	26.7	27.4	100.0	24.4	54.3	26.0	17.4	28.9	32.1	458	97.1
Acute lymphocytic	7	80	49	28	164	18.2	18.9	68.3	13.2	42.6	18.4	8.7	19.8	22.7	319	98.8
Other lymphocytic	0	0	0	0	0											
Acute non-lymphocytic	5	16	15	20	56	6.2	6.3	23.3	9.4	8.5	5.6	6.2	6.8	7.0	103	92.9
Chronic myeloid	0	0	0	0	0											
Other and unspecified	1	6	5	8	20	2.2	2.2	8.3	1.9	3.2	1.9	2.5	2.4	2.5	36	95.0
II. LYMPHOMAS	4	23	23	59	109	12.1	11.8	100.0	7.5	12.2	8.7	18.3	13.1	12.5	191	98.2
Hodgkin's disease	0	3	10	39	52	5.8	5.5	47.7		1.6	3.8	12.1	6.3	5.2	86	100.0
Non-Hodgkin lymphoma	1	8	11	19	39	4.3	4.3	35.8	1.9	4.3	4.1	5.9	4.7	4.5	69	97.4
Burkitt's lymphoma	0	3	1	0	4	0.4	0.5	3.7		1.6	0.4		0.5	0.6	8	100.0
Unspecified lymphoma	0	0	0	1	1	0.1	0.1	0.9				0.3	0.1	0.1	2	100.0
Histiocytosis X	2	7	1	0	10	1.1	1.1	9.2	3.8	3.7	0.4		1.2	1.6	21	90.0
Other reticuloendothelial	1	2	0	0	3	0.3	0.3	2.8	1.9	1.1			0.4	0.5	6	100.0
III. BRAIN AND SPINAL	8	49	69	65	191	21.2	22.0	100.0	15.0	26.1	26.0	20.2	23.0	23.5	350	78.3
Ependymoma	2	12	8	6	28	3.1	3.2	14.7	3.8	6.4	3.0	1.9	3.4	3.8	54	76.9
Astrocytoma	2	19	34	27	82	9.1	9.6	42.9	3.8	10.1	12.8	8.4	9.9	10.0	150	82.9
Medulloblastoma	3	9	10	8	30	3.3	3.4	15.7	5.6	4.8	3.8	1.6	3.6	3.9	56	76.0
Other glioma	0	1	3	5	9	1.0	1.0	4.7		0.5	1.1	1.6	1.1	1.0	16	66.7
Other and unspecified *	1	8	14	19	42	4.7	4.7	22.0	1.9	4.3	5.3	5.9	5.1	4.9	75	74.1
IV. SYMPATHETIC N.S.	16	22	3	8	49	5.5	5.3	100.0	30.1	11.7	1.1	2.5	5.9	7.0	95	87.8
Neuroblastoma	16	21	2	8	47	5.2	5.0	95.9	30.1	11.2	0.8	2.5	5.7	6.8	91	87.2
Other	0	1	1	0	2	0.2	0.2	4.1		0.5	0.4		0.2	0.3	4	100.0
V. RETINOBLASTOMA	7	16	2	0	25	2.8	2.8	100.0	13.2	8.5	0.8		3.0	3.9	51	100.0
VI. KIDNEY	9	33	9	8	59	6.6	6.6	100.0	16.9	17.6	3.4	2.5	7.1	8.6	117	96.5
Wilms' tumour	9	33	9	6	57	6.3	6.4	96.6	16.9	17.6	3.4	1.9	6.9	8.4	113	96.4
Renal carcinoma	0	0	0	2	2	0.2	0.2	3.4				0.6	0.2	0.2	3	100.0
Other and unspecified	0	0	0	0	0											
VII. LIVER	0	2	0	1	3	0.3	0.3	100.0		1.1		0.3	0.4	0.4	6	100.0
Hepatoblastoma	0	1	0	0	1	0.1	0.1	33.3		0.5			0.1	0.1	2	100.0
Hepatic carcinoma	0	1	0	1	2	0.2	0.2	66.7		0.5		0.3	0.2	0.2	4	100.0
Other and unspecified	0	0	0	0	0											
VIII. BONE	1	2	14	39	56	6.2	6.0	100.0	1.9	1.1	5.3	12.1	6.8	5.7	93	84.4
Osteosarcoma	0	2	7	22	31	3.4	3.3	55.4		1.1	2.6	6.8	3.7	3.2	52	100.0
Chondrosarcoma	0	0	1	1	2	0.2	0.2	3.6			0.4	0.3	0.2	0.2	3	100.0
Ewing's sarcoma	0	0	3	10	13	1.4	1.4	23.2			1.1	3.1	1.6	1.3	21	100.0
Other and unspecified	1	0	3	6	10	1.1	1.1	17.9	1.9		1.1	1.9	1.2	1.0	17	100.0
IX. SOFT TISSUE SARCOMAS	16	19	13	24	72	8.0	7.9	100.0	30.1	10.1	4.9	7.4	8.7	9.2	132	100.0
Rhabdomyosarcoma	3	10	3	8	24	2.7	2.6	33.3	5.6	5.3	1.1	2.5	2.9	3.2	45	100.0
Fibrosarcoma	7	5	6	4	22	2.4	2.5	30.6	13.2	2.7	2.3	1.2	2.7	2.9	41	100.0
Other and unspecified	6	4	4	12	26	2.9	2.8	36.1	11.3	2.1	1.5	3.7	3.1	3.1	46	100.0
X. GONADAL & GERM CELL	10	4	9	22	45	5.0	4.9	100.0	18.8	2.1	3.4	6.8	5.4	5.2	78	84.4
Non-gonadal germ cell	10	4	3	3	20	2.2	2.2	44.4	18.8	2.1	1.1	0.9	2.4	2.7	38	65.0
Gonadal germ cell	0	0	6	11	17	1.9	1.9	37.8			2.3	3.4	2.1	1.7	28	100.0
Gonadal carcinoma	0	0	0	2	2	0.2	0.2	4.4				0.6	0.2	0.2	3	100.0
Other and unspecified	0	0	0	6	6	0.7	0.6	13.3				1.9	0.7	0.5	9	100.0
XI. EPITHELIAL NEOPLASMS	1	8	6	29	44	4.9	4.6	100.0	1.9	4.3	2.3	9.0	5.3	4.8	75	97.7
Adrenocortical carcinoma	0	0	0	1	1	0.1	0.1	2.3				0.3	0.1	0.1	2	100.0
Thyroid carcinoma	0	1	3	7	11	1.2	1.2	25.0		0.5	1.1	2.2	1.3	1.2	19	100.0
Nasopharyngeal carcinoma	0	0	0	2	2	0.2	0.2	4.5				0.6	0.2	0.2	3	100.0
Melanoma	0	2	0	5	7	0.8	0.7	15.9		1.1		1.6	0.8	0.8	12	85.7
Other carcinoma	1	5	3	14	23	2.6	2.4	52.3	1.9	2.7	1.1	4.3	2.8	2.6	40	100.0
XII. OTHER	0	5	0	1	6	0.7	0.6	100.0		2.7		0.3	0.7	0.9	12	100.0
* Specified as malignant	0	3	7	10	20	2.2	2.3	100.0		1.6	2.6	3.1	2.4	2.2	35	37.5

sarcomas. Of the last category, 30% (15/50) were classified as angiosarcoma, etc; this is an extremely high frequency for such tumours in childhood and it seems possible that haemangioendotheliomas and haemangiopericytomas of unknown malignancy are routinely coded as malignant. Carcinoma of the thyroid had a relatively high incidence, with a characteristic excess of females to males. Nearly half (17/37 = 46%) of the miscellaneous carcinomas were skin tumours.

References

Staneczek, W. (1984) Neubildungen bei Kindern in der DDR. *Arch. Geschwultsforsch.*, *54*, 357-364

Staneczek, W. (1985) Neubildungen nach histologischen Typen bei Kindern in der DDR. *Arch. Geschwultsforsch.*, *55*, 375-386

GERMANY, FEDERAL REPUBLIC OF

Co-operative Register of Childhood Malignancies, 1982–1984

J. Michaelis & P. Kaatsch

In 1980, a co-operative effort was started in the Federal Republic of Germany in order to register all newly diagnosed childhood malignancies. This project was initiated by the two German societies for paediatric oncology (GPO) and leukaemia treatment (DAL). The first five years of the project were financed by the Stiftung Volkswagenwerk as a pilot phase but the Federal Government and the Government of the Land of Rheinland-Pfalz, where the registry is physically located, are now supporting the registry on a continuous basis. Since there is no legislation making reporting of cancer compulsory, and information is provided on a voluntary basis by both the participating clinicians and the patient's parents. Less than 1% of parents have refused their consent to storage of the data; such consent is required by the legislation on data privacy and security.

After diagnosis, a basic questionnaire including identification data and a tentative diagnosis is filled in by the attending physician and sent to the Institut für Medizinische Statistik und Dokumentation (IMSD), where coding of site and histology (ICD-O) is performed. The IMSD sends back a set of tumour-specific questionnaires for collecting information about the patient's history, stage of disease, diagnostic and therapeutic procedures. Collection of these data is in accordance with the recommendations of the working party on cancer centres. These questionnaires are completed by the co-operating clinicians at the end of the first therapeutic cycle.

In the first three years of the project, a co-operative relationship was built up with over 90 hospitals in the Federal Republic of Germany. The number of registrations increased successively in the first three years, but the incidence of new cancers was more or less constant by 1983, and estimated to be over 90% complete. However, until 1985, certain neuropaediatric and neurosurgical hospitals did not participate in the project, so that there is a relative deficit of brain tumours in the period (1982–1984) reported here.

The precise basis of diagnosis is not recorded by the Register for all cases. For cases enrolled in clinical trials, histological data are always available, and the percentage of such cases out of the total for each diagnostic group is shown in the tables, under HV (%). However, the percentage of cases with histology available is likely to be considerably higher than this (perhaps 95%).

More than 60% of the patients are also enrolled into controlled clinical trials of cancer therapy. These trials — of which there are currently 15 — are organized jointly by the DAL, GPO and the International Society of Paediatric Oncology. All related questionnaires are structured in modular form, so that no information has to be given twice by the clinicians. Basic data are collected within the general documentation system; trial-specific data are collected on additional forms.

Population

The populations used for the calculation of incidence are the annual estimates for the Federal Republic of Germany, for 1982–1984 *(Statistisches Jahrbuch für die Bundesrepublik Deutschland*, Statistisches Bundesamt, 1984, 1985, 1986).

AVERAGE ANNUAL POPULATION: 1982–1984

Age	Male	Female
0	309200	293300
1–4	1228165	1169332
5–9	1513598	1450333
10–14	2047032	1951431
0–14	5097995	4864396

Commentary

For the reasons explained in the above description of the Registry, the apparent incidence of brain
Contd. p. 250

FRG, Children's Tumour Registry   1982 – 1984   MALE

DIAGNOSTIC GROUP	Cases 0	Cases 1–4	Cases 5–9	Cases 10–14	Cases All	Rel.Freq Crude	Rel.Freq Adj	Rel.Freq Group	Rate 0	Rate 1–4	Rate 5–9	Rate 10–14	Rate Crude	Rate Adj	Rate Cum	HV(%)
TOTAL	170	640	419	476	1705	100.0	100.0	100.0	183.3	173.7	92.3	77.5	111.5	120.2	1727	68.9
I. LEUKAEMIAS	33	303	165	151	652	38.2	37.9	100.0	35.6	82.2	36.3	24.6	42.6	47.1	669	85.3
Acute lymphocytic	15	265	141	117	538	31.6	31.3	82.5	16.2	71.9	31.1	19.1	35.2	39.1	554	91.1
Other lymphocytic	0	0	0	0	0	–	–	–	–	–	–	–	–	–	–	–
Acute non-lymphocytic	12	27	21	25	85	5.0	5.0	13.0	12.9	7.3	4.6	4.1	5.6	5.9	86	74.1
Chronic myeloid	4	7	3	6	20	1.2	1.1	3.1	4.3	1.9	0.7	1.0	1.3	1.4	20	5.0
Other and unspecified	2	4	0	3	9	0.5	0.5	1.4	2.2	1.1	–	0.5	0.6	0.6	9	22.2
II. LYMPHOMAS	18	61	91	146	316	18.5	19.6	100.0	19.4	16.6	20.0	23.8	20.7	20.0	305	69.9
Hodgkin's disease	0	14	32	69	115	6.7	7.3	36.4	–	3.8	7.0	11.2	7.5	6.7	107	83.5
Non-Hodgkin lymphoma	1	19	42	57	119	7.0	7.6	37.7	1.1	5.2	9.2	9.3	7.8	7.4	114	75.6
Burkitt's lymphoma	0	0	0	1	1	0.1	0.2	0.3	–	–	–	0.3	0.1	0.2	1	100.0
Unspecified lymphoma	0	1	1	2	4	0.2	0.2	1.3	–	0.3	0.2	0.3	0.3	0.2	4	50.0
Histiocytosis X	14	26	16	14	70	4.1	4.0	22.2	15.1	7.1	3.5	2.3	4.6	5.2	72	40.0
Other reticuloendothelial	3	1	0	3	7	0.4	0.4	2.2	3.2	0.3	–	0.5	0.5	0.4	7	57.1
III. BRAIN AND SPINAL	16	68	61	60	205	12.0	12.3	100.0	17.2	18.5	13.4	9.8	13.4	14.2	207	21.0
Ependymoma	3	9	4	5	21	1.2	1.2	10.2	3.2	2.4	0.9	0.8	1.4	1.5	21	14.3
Astrocytoma	1	15	14	21	51	3.0	3.1	24.9	1.1	4.1	3.1	3.4	3.3	3.3	50	–
Medulloblastoma	4	29	27	15	75	4.4	4.5	36.6	4.3	7.9	5.9	2.4	4.9	5.4	78	52.0
Other glioma	1	1	0	2	4	0.2	0.2	2.0	1.1	0.3	–	0.3	0.3	0.3	4	–
Other and unspecified *	7	14	16	17	54	3.2	3.3	26.3	7.5	3.8	3.5	2.8	3.5	3.7	54	1.9
IV. SYMPATHETIC N.S.	46	63	16	2	127	7.4	6.7	100.0	49.6	17.1	3.5	0.3	8.3	10.4	137	78.0
Neuroblastoma	46	63	16	2	127	7.4	6.7	100.0	49.6	17.1	3.5	0.3	8.3	10.4	137	78.0
Other	0	0	0	0	0	–	–	–	–	–	–	–	–	–	–	–
V. RETINOBLASTOMA	17	17	0	0	34	2.0	1.7	100.0	18.3	4.6	–	–	2.2	2.8	37	–
VI. KIDNEY	20	53	18	2	93	5.5	5.0	100.0	21.6	14.4	4.0	0.3	6.1	7.5	101	73.1
Wilms' tumour	20	53	16	2	91	5.3	4.9	97.8	21.6	14.4	3.5	0.3	6.0	7.4	98	74.7
Renal carcinoma	0	0	2	0	2	0.1	0.1	2.2	–	–	0.4	–	0.1	0.1	2	–
Other and unspecified	0	0	0	0	0	–	–	–	–	–	–	–	–	–	–	–
VII. LIVER	2	11	1	1	15	0.9	0.8	100.0	2.2	3.0	0.2	0.2	1.0	1.2	16	–
Hepatoblastoma	2	9	0	0	11	0.6	0.5	73.3	2.2	2.4	–	–	0.7	0.9	12	–
Hepatic carcinoma	0	2	1	1	4	0.2	0.2	26.7	–	0.5	0.2	0.2	0.3	0.3	4	–
Other and unspecified	0	0	0	0	0	–	–	–	–	–	–	–	–	–	–	–
VIII. BONE	1	10	24	63	98	5.7	6.2	100.0	1.1	2.7	5.3	10.3	6.4	5.6	90	75.5
Osteosarcoma	1	2	12	33	48	2.8	3.1	49.0	1.1	0.5	2.6	5.4	3.1	2.7	43	77.1
Chondrosarcoma	0	0	0	3	3	0.2	0.2	3.1	–	–	–	0.5	0.2	0.1	3	33.3
Ewing's sarcoma	0	3	11	26	40	2.3	2.6	40.8	–	0.8	2.4	4.2	2.6	2.3	37	85.0
Other and unspecified	0	5	1	1	7	0.4	0.4	7.1	–	1.4	0.2	0.2	0.5	0.5	7	28.6
IX. SOFT TISSUE SARCOMAS	11	43	34	32	120	7.0	7.1	100.0	11.9	11.7	7.5	5.2	7.8	8.5	122	80.0
Rhabdomyosarcoma	6	37	25	20	88	5.2	5.2	73.3	6.5	10.0	5.5	3.3	5.8	6.3	90	90.9
Fibrosarcoma	3	2	1	7	13	0.8	0.8	10.8	3.2	0.5	0.2	1.1	0.9	0.8	13	46.2
Other and unspecified	2	4	8	5	19	1.1	1.2	15.8	2.2	1.1	1.8	0.8	1.2	1.3	19	52.6
X. GONADAL & GERM CELL	5	8	3	9	25	1.5	1.4	100.0	5.4	2.2	0.7	1.5	1.6	1.7	25	60.0
Non-gonadal germ cell	2	7	2	8	19	1.1	1.1	76.0	2.2	1.9	0.4	–	1.2	1.3	18	63.2
Gonadal germ cell	3	1	1	1	6	0.4	0.3	24.0	3.2	0.3	0.2	0.2	0.4	0.5	6	50.0
Gonadal carcinoma	0	0	0	0	0	–	–	–	–	–	–	–	–	–	–	–
Other and unspecified	0	0	0	0	0	–	–	–	–	–	–	–	–	–	–	–
XI. EPITHELIAL NEOPLASMS	0	2	5	10	17	1.0	1.1	100.0	–	0.5	1.1	1.6	1.1	1.0	16	5.9
Adrenocortical carcinoma	0	1	1	0	2	0.1	0.1	11.8	–	0.3	0.2	–	0.1	0.2	2	–
Thyroid carcinoma	0	0	3	2	5	0.3	0.3	29.4	–	–	0.7	0.3	0.3	0.3	5	–
Nasopharyngeal carcinoma	0	0	0	5	5	0.3	0.3	29.4	–	–	–	0.7	0.3	0.3	4	20.0
Melanoma	0	0	0	1	1	0.1	0.1	5.9	–	–	–	0.2	0.1	–	1	–
Other carcinoma	0	1	1	3	4	0.2	0.2	23.5	–	0.3	0.2	0.5	0.3	0.2	4	–
XII. OTHER	1	1	1	0	3	0.2	0.2	100.0	1.1	0.3	0.2	–	0.2	0.2	3	33.3
* Specified as malignant	7	10	10	9	36	2.1	2.1	100.0	7.5	2.7	2.2	1.5	2.4	2.6	37	2.8

FRG, Children's Tumour Registry   1982 - 1984   FEMALE

DIAGNOSTIC GROUP	\#0	\#1-4	\#5-9	\#10-14	\#All	RF Crude	RF Adj.	RF Group	R 0	R 1-4	R 5-9	R 10-14	R Crude	R Adj.	Cum	HV(%)
TOTAL	142	532	298	315	1287	100.0	100.0	100.0	161.4	151.7	68.5	53.8	88.2	97.2	1379	70.1
I. LEUKAEMIAS	19	255	138	104	516	40.1	40.1	100.0	21.6	72.7	31.7	17.8	35.4	39.6	560	86.2
Acute lymphocytic	12	229	117	72	430	33.4	32.9	83.3	13.6	65.3	26.9	12.3	29.5	33.5	471	90.5
Other lymphocytic	0	0	0	0	0	-	-	-	-	-	-	-	-	-	-	-
Acute non-lymphocytic	7	21	17	28	73	5.7	6.0	14.1	8.0	6.0	3.9	4.8	5.0	5.1	75	72.6
Chronic myeloid	0	3	1	3	7	0.5	0.6	1.4	-	0.9	0.2	0.5	0.5	0.5	7	-
Other and unspecified	0	2	3	1	6	0.5	0.5	1.2	-	0.6	0.7	0.2	0.4	0.4	7	50.0
II. LYMPHOMAS	14	29	34	64	141	11.0	12.1	100.0	15.9	8.3	7.8	10.9	9.7	9.5	143	73.0
Hodgkin's disease	0	2	14	41	57	4.4	5.4	40.4	-	0.6	3.2	7.0	3.9	3.2	53	87.7
Non-Hodgkin lymphoma	0	9	14	13	36	2.8	3.2	25.5	-	2.6	3.2	2.2	2.5	2.5	37	80.6
Burkitt's lymphoma	0	0	0	0	0	-	-	-	-	-	-	-	-	-	-	-
Unspecified lymphoma	0	0	1	2	3	0.2	0.3	2.1	-	-	0.2	0.3	0.2	0.2	3	66.7
Histiocytosis X	11	17	5	4	37	2.9	2.5	26.2	12.5	4.8	1.1	0.7	2.5	3.0	41	43.2
Other reticuloendothelial	3	1	0	4	8	0.6	0.6	5.7	3.4	0.3	-	0.7	0.5	0.6	8	75.0
III. BRAIN AND SPINAL	15	60	50	43	168	13.1	13.6	100.0	17.0	17.1	11.5	7.3	11.5	12.5	180	15.5
Ependymoma	2	15	6	3	26	2.0	1.9	15.5	2.3	4.3	1.4	0.5	1.8	2.1	29	3.8
Astrocytoma	6	15	16	17	54	4.2	4.5	32.1	6.8	4.3	3.7	2.9	3.7	3.9	57	-
Medulloblastoma	4	23	13	5	45	3.5	3.4	26.8	4.5	6.6	3.0	0.9	3.1	3.6	50	53.3
Other glioma	0	0	1	3	4	0.3	0.4	2.4	-	-	0.2	0.5	0.3	0.2	4	-
Other and unspecified *	3	7	14	15	39	3.0	3.4	23.2	3.4	2.0	3.2	2.6	2.7	2.7	40	2.6
IV. SYMPATHETIC N.S.	43	54	17	2	116	9.0	7.7	100.0	48.9	15.4	3.9	0.3	7.9	9.9	132	84.5
Neuroblastoma	43	53	17	2	115	8.9	7.6	99.1	48.9	15.1	3.9	0.3	7.9	9.8	131	85.2
Other	0	1	0	0	1	0.1	0.1	0.9	-	0.3	-	-	0.1	0.1	1	-
V. RETINOBLASTOMA	17	23	3	1	44	3.4	2.8	100.0	19.3	6.6	0.7	0.2	3.0	3.8	50	76.9
VI. KIDNEY	17	65	19	3	104	8.1	7.1	100.0	19.3	18.5	4.4	0.5	7.1	8.7	118	77.7
Wilms' tumour	17	64	19	3	103	8.0	7.0	99.0	19.3	18.2	4.4	0.5	7.1	8.7	117	77.7
Renal carcinoma	0	0	0	0	0	-	-	-	-	-	-	-	-	-	-	-
Other and unspecified	0	1	0	0	1	0.1	0.1	1.0	-	0.3	-	-	0.1	0.1	1	-
VII. LIVER	3	7	1	1	12	0.9	0.8	100.0	3.4	2.0	0.2	0.2	0.8	1.0	13	16.7
Hepatoblastoma	3	7	1	0	11	0.9	0.7	91.7	3.4	2.0	0.2	-	0.8	1.0	13	9.1
Hepatic carcinoma	0	0	0	1	1	0.1	0.1	8.3	-	-	-	0.2	0.1	-	1	100.0
Other and unspecified	0	0	0	0	0	-	-	-	-	-	-	-	-	-	-	-
VIII. BONE	0	8	15	55	78	6.1	7.2	100.0	-	2.3	3.4	9.4	5.3	4.5	73	85.9
Osteosarcoma	0	1	6	34	41	3.2	3.9	52.6	-	0.3	1.4	5.8	2.8	2.2	37	87.8
Chondrosarcoma	0	0	0	1	1	0.1	0.1	1.3	-	-	-	0.2	0.1	-	1	-
Ewing's sarcoma	0	6	9	20	35	2.7	3.2	44.9	-	1.7	2.1	3.4	2.4	2.2	34	88.6
Other and unspecified	0	1	0	0	1	0.1	0.1	1.3	-	0.3	-	-	0.1	0.1	1	-
IX. SOFT TISSUE SARCOMAS	10	18	14	26	68	5.3	5.5	100.0	11.4	5.1	3.2	4.4	4.7	4.8	70	80.9
Rhabdomyosarcoma	7	13	8	11	39	3.0	3.0	57.4	8.0	3.7	1.8	1.9	2.7	2.9	41	92.3
Fibrosarcoma	2	1	1	6	10	0.8	0.9	14.7	2.3	0.3	0.2	1.3	0.7	0.6	10	60.0
Other and unspecified	1	4	5	9	19	1.5	1.7	27.9	1.1	1.1	1.1	1.5	1.3	1.3	19	68.4
X. GONADAL & GERM CELL	3	12	4	9	28	2.2	2.2	100.0	3.4	3.4	0.9	1.5	1.9	2.1	29	82.1
Non-gonadal germ cell	3	10	1	2	16	1.2	1.1	57.1	3.4	2.9	0.2	0.3	1.1	1.3	18	75.0
Gonadal germ cell	0	2	3	6	11	0.9	1.0	39.3	-	0.6	0.7	1.0	0.8	0.7	11	100.0
Gonadal carcinoma	0	0	0	0	0	-	-	-	-	-	-	-	-	-	-	-
Other and unspecified	0	0	0	1	1	0.1	-	3.6	-	-	-	0.2	0.1	-	1	-
XI. EPITHELIAL NEOPLASMS	1	1	2	6	10	0.8	0.9	100.0	1.1	0.3	0.5	1.0	0.7	0.6	10	10.0
Adrenocortical carcinoma	0	0	0	1	1	0.1	0.1	10.0	-	-	-	0.2	0.1	0.1	1	-
Thyroid carcinoma	0	0	0	1	1	0.1	0.1	10.0	-	-	-	0.2	0.1	-	1	-
Nasopharyngeal carcinoma	0	0	1	2	3	0.2	0.3	30.0	-	-	0.2	0.5	0.2	0.1	3	-
Melanoma	1	1	0	0	2	0.1	0.1	20.0	1.1	0.3	-	-	0.2	0.2	2	-
Other carcinoma	0	0	1	2	3	0.2	0.3	30.0	-	-	0.2	0.3	0.2	0.2	3	33.3
XII. OTHER	0	0	1	1	2	0.2	0.2	100.0	-	-	0.2	0.2	0.1	0.1	2	100.0
* Specified as malignant	3	4	9	8	24	1.9	2.1	100.0	3.4	1.1	2.1	1.4	1.6	1.7	25	4.2

tumours is low. Most of the other rates are similar to those from other European registries. The rate tumours is low. Most of the other rates are similar to those from other European registries. The rate for histiocytosis X is high, presumably as a result of good ascertainment for this condition.

References

Kaatsch, P. & Michaelis, J. (1983) *Cooperative documentation of childhood malignancies in the FRG, Combination of a population-based and hospital-based registry.* In: Van Bemmel J.H., Ball, M.J. & Wigert, O., eds, *Medinfo 83*, Amsterdam, New York, Oxford, North-Holland, pp. 1226-1229

Michaelis, J. (1985) *Multizentrische Krankheitsregister — Erfahrungen am Beispiel eines bundesweiten Registers für Malignome im Kindesalter.* In: Abt, K., Giere, W. & Leiber, B., eds, *Krankendaten, Krankheitsregister, Datenschutz*, Berlin, Heidelberg, New York, Springer Verlag, pp. 219-282

Michaelis, J. & Kaatsch, P. (1985) *Cooperative documentation of childhood malignancies in the FRG — system design and five-year results.* In: Riehm, H., ed., *Monographs in Paediatrics 18*, Basel, Karger, pp. 56-67

Michaelis, J., Kaatsch, P. & Schicketanz, K.H. (1983) Zwei Jahre kooperative Dokumentation von Malignomen im Kindesalter — Erfahrungen und erste Ergebnisse. *Verh. Dtsch. Krebs Ges., 4,* 183-191

Cancer Registry of Saarland, 1967–1982

H. Ziegler

The Cancer Registry of Saarland was established in 1966, the funding being shared equally between the Government of the Federal Republic of Germany and the Government of the Saarland. Special legal provisions have existed since 1979 to permit cases of cancer to be notified to the Registry; nevertheless, problems of confidentiality still exist. In October 1979, a new council of medical advisers was appointed to secure a further improvement in the efficiency of the Registry.

Notification of cases to the Registry is voluntary. The main sources of information are the records of hospital in-patients and out-patients, pathology and radiotherapy departments, medical practitioners and death certificates. These sources are used in such a manner as to minimize under-registration. About 50% of all new cases are reported to the Registry by the pathology departments in Saarland. Cases coming to the notice of the Registry for the first time through death certificates are the subject of further enquiries. If, after several months, no additional data are available, they are registered using the basic data on the death certificate. Cases reported from death certificates only have decreased in recent years to 10–12%. A study of incidence rates by time period showed a general increase during the initial years of registration (1968–1972), since when rates have been more or less stable.

Patients' records are filed by birth date. Each individual is counted only once, even if there is more than one neoplasm in the same person. It is intended to follow up all cases until the death of the patient.

The Registry covers the whole of Saarland, which has an area of 2567 square kilometres; altitudes range from 150 to 695 m above sea level.

About 48% of the territory of Saarland is used for agricultural purposes, 33% is covered with forests, and the remaining 19% comprises built-up and industrial areas, water, areas used for recreation, etc.

The total population of Saarland in 1982 was 1 057 543, of whom some 54% live in conurbations of more than 20 000 inhabitants. The population density is 411 per square kilometre. Some 74% are Roman Catholics, 24% Protestants and 2% others. The working population, 38% of the total, is employed in industry (49%), commerce and transport (18%), agriculture (2%), and services (32%).

Population

The source of the population at risk is the census of 1970 together with figures for 1974 and 1982 derived from the census plus records of births, deaths and migration (Statistisches Amt des Saarlandes).

AVERAGE ANNUAL POPULATION: 1967–1982

Age	Male	Female
0–4	34116	32754
5–9	41859	40013
10–14	45214	43273
0–14	121189	116040

Commentary

The incidence rates overall and for most diagnostic groups were similar to those in other European registries. A third of registrations were for leukaemia, with acute lymphocytic 5.3 times as frequent as acute non-lymphocytic. The peak in incidence of acute lymphocytic leukaemia in young children was less marked than in many other Western countries, and a relatively large proportion of leukaemias (35%) were of 'other and unspecified' type. There was an unusually low incidence of retinoblastoma. Ewing's sarcoma had a higher incidence than in any other registry. There were four adenocarcinomas of the appendix, and two of the colon.

FRG, Saarland   1967 – 1982   MALE

DIAGNOSTIC GROUP	NUMBER OF CASES					REL. FREQUENCY(%)			RATES PER MILLION						HV(%)
	0	1-4	5-9	10-14	All	Crude	Adj.	Group	0-4	5-9	10-14	Crude	Adj.	Cum	
TOTAL	19	70	69	64	222	100.0	100.0	100.0	163.0	103.0	88.5	114.5	122.0	1773	90.2
I. LEUKAEMIAS	6	30	30	11	77	34.7	34.4	100.0	66.0	44.8	15.2	39.7	44.4	630	98.5
Acute lymphocytic	1	16	19	4	40	18.0	17.8	51.9	31.1	28.4	5.5	20.6	22.8	325	100.0
Other lymphocytic	0	1	1	2	4	1.8	1.8	5.2	1.8	1.5	2.8	2.1	2.0	30	100.0
Acute non-lymphocytic	0	4	3	0	7	3.2	3.1	9.1	7.3	4.5	–	3.6	4.3	59	100.0
Chronic myeloid	0	0	0	1	1	0.5	0.4	1.3	1.8	–	–	0.5	0.7	9	–
Other and unspecified	5	8	7	5	25	11.3	11.2	32.5	23.8	10.5	6.9	12.9	14.6	206	95.5
II. LYMPHOMAS	2	4	11	14	31	14.0	14.0	100.0	11.0	16.4	19.4	16.0	15.2	234	100.0
Hodgkin's disease	0	0	3	6	9	4.1	4.1	29.0	–	4.5	8.3	4.6	3.9	64	100.0
Non-Hodgkin lymphoma	2	2	6	5	15	6.8	6.8	48.4	7.3	9.0	6.9	7.7	7.7	116	100.0
Burkitt's lymphoma	0	1	2	0	3	1.4	1.3	9.7	1.8	3.0	–	1.5	1.7	24	100.0
Unspecified lymphoma	0	1	0	3	4	1.8	1.9	12.9	–	–	4.1	2.1	1.9	30	100.0
Histiocytosis X	0	0	0	0	0	–	–	–	–	–	–	–	–	–	–
Other reticuloendothelial	0	0	0	0	0	–	–	–	–	–	–	–	–	–	–
III. BRAIN AND SPINAL	1	19	9	14	43	19.4	19.5	100.0	36.6	13.4	19.4	22.2	24.1	347	60.5
Ependymoma	0	1	2	0	3	1.4	1.3	7.0	1.8	3.0	–	1.5	1.7	24	66.7
Astrocytoma	0	7	0	4	11	5.0	5.0	25.6	12.8	–	5.5	5.7	6.6	92	90.9
Medulloblastoma	0	4	3	2	9	4.1	4.0	20.9	7.3	4.5	2.8	4.6	5.1	73	88.9
Other glioma	0	1	0	0	1	0.5	0.4	2.3	1.8	–	–	0.5	0.7	9	–
Other and unspecified *	1	6	4	8	19	8.6	8.6	44.2	12.8	6.0	11.1	9.8	10.1	149	21.4
IV. SYMPATHETIC N.S.	0	6	2	1	9	4.1	4.0	100.0	11.0	3.0	1.4	4.6	5.6	77	77.8
Neuroblastoma	0	6	2	1	9	4.1	4.0	100.0	11.0	3.0	1.4	4.6	5.6	77	77.8
Other	0	0	0	0	0	–	–	–	–	–	–	–	–	–	–
V. RETINOBLASTOMA	2	1	0	0	3	1.4	1.3	100.0	5.5	–	–	1.5	2.1	27	100.0
VI. KIDNEY	4	5	3	2	14	6.3	6.3	100.0	16.5	4.5	2.8	7.2	8.6	119	100.0
Wilms' tumour	3	4	2	1	10	4.5	4.5	71.4	12.8	3.0	1.4	5.2	6.3	86	100.0
Renal carcinoma	1	1	1	1	4	1.8	1.8	28.6	3.7	1.5	1.4	2.1	2.3	33	100.0
Other and unspecified	0	0	0	0	0	–	–	–	–	–	–	–	–	–	–
VII. LIVER	0	0	0	1	1	0.5	0.5	100.0	–	–	1.4	0.5	0.4	7	100.0
Hepatoblastoma	0	0	0	0	0	–	–	–	–	–	–	–	–	–	–
Hepatic carcinoma	0	0	0	1	1	0.5	0.5	100.0	–	–	1.4	0.5	0.4	7	100.0
Other and unspecified	0	0	0	0	0	–	–	–	–	–	–	–	–	–	–
VIII. BONE	0	0	7	11	18	8.1	8.2	100.0	–	10.5	15.2	9.3	7.8	128	94.4
Osteosarcoma	0	0	3	4	7	3.2	3.2	38.9	–	4.5	5.5	3.6	3.1	50	85.7
Chondrosarcoma	0	0	0	0	0	–	–	–	–	–	–	–	–	–	–
Ewing's sarcoma	0	0	3	4	7	3.2	3.2	38.9	–	4.5	5.5	3.6	3.1	50	100.0
Other and unspecified	0	0	1	3	4	1.8	1.8	22.2	–	1.5	4.1	2.1	1.7	28	100.0
IX. SOFT TISSUE SARCOMAS	1	3	4	4	12	5.4	5.4	100.0	7.3	6.0	5.5	6.2	6.4	94	100.0
Rhabdomyosarcoma	0	3	1	1	5	2.3	2.3	41.7	5.5	1.5	1.4	2.6	3.0	42	100.0
Fibrosarcoma	0	0	0	1	1	0.5	0.5	8.3	–	–	1.4	0.5	0.4	7	100.0
Other and unspecified	1	0	3	2	6	2.7	2.7	50.0	1.8	4.5	2.8	3.1	3.0	45	100.0
X. GONADAL & GERM CELL	2	0	0	1	3	1.4	1.4	100.0	3.7	–	1.4	1.5	1.8	25	100.0
Non-gonadal germ cell	0	0	0	0	0	–	–	–	–	–	–	–	–	–	–
Gonadal germ cell	1	0	0	1	2	0.9	0.9	66.7	1.8	–	1.4	1.0	1.1	16	100.0
Gonadal carcinoma	1	0	0	0	1	0.5	0.4	33.3	1.8	–	–	0.5	0.7	9	100.0
Other and unspecified	0	0	0	0	0	–	–	–	–	–	–	–	–	–	–
XI. EPITHELIAL NEOPLASMS	1	1	3	4	9	4.1	4.1	100.0	3.7	4.5	5.5	4.6	4.5	68	100.0
Adrenocortical carcinoma	0	0	0	0	0	–	–	–	–	–	–	–	–	–	–
Thyroid carcinoma	0	0	0	0	0	–	–	–	–	–	–	–	–	–	–
Nasopharyngeal carcinoma	0	0	0	0	0	–	–	–	–	–	–	–	–	–	–
Melanoma	0	1	1	1	3	1.4	1.4	33.3	1.8	1.5	1.4	1.5	1.6	24	100.0
Other carcinoma	1	0	2	3	6	2.7	2.7	66.7	1.8	3.0	4.1	3.1	2.9	45	100.0
XII. OTHER	0	1	0	1	2	0.9	0.9	100.0	1.8	–	1.4	1.0	1.1	16	50.0
* Specified as malignant	1	6	4	4	15	6.8	6.8	100.0	12.8	6.0	5.5	7.7	8.5	122	10.0

FRG, Saarland

FEMALE

1967 – 1982

DIAGNOSTIC GROUP	NUMBER OF CASES					REL. FREQUENCY(%)			RATES PER MILLION						HV(%)
	0	1-4	5-9	10-14	All	Crude	Adj.	Group	0-4	5-9	10-14	Crude	Adj.	Cum	
TOTAL	11	60	58	50	179	100.0	100.0	100.0	135.5	90.6	72.2	96.4	102.6	1491	94.2
I. LEUKAEMIAS	2	24	21	12	59	33.0	32.7	100.0	49.6	32.8	17.3	31.8	34.8	499	98.2
Acute lymphocytic	1	15	11	2	29	16.2	15.9	49.2	30.5	17.2	2.9	15.6	18.2	253	100.0
Other lymphocytic	0	0	2	0	2	1.1	1.0	3.4	-	3.1	-	1.1	1.0	16	100.0
Acute non-lymphocytic	0	4	1	1	6	3.4	3.4	10.2	7.6	1.6	1.4	3.2	3.9	53	100.0
Chronic myeloid	0	0	0	0	0	-	-	-	-	-	-	-	-	-	-
Other and unspecified	1	5	7	9	22	12.3	12.4	37.3	11.4	10.9	13.0	11.8	11.7	177	95.2
II. LYMPHOMAS	0	3	3	6	12	6.7	6.8	100.0	5.7	4.7	8.7	6.5	6.2	95	100.0
Hodgkin's disease	0	1	1	4	6	3.4	3.5	50.0	1.9	1.6	5.8	3.2	2.9	46	100.0
Non-Hodgkin lymphoma	0	1	1	2	4	2.2	2.3	33.3	1.9	1.6	2.9	2.2	2.1	32	100.0
Burkitt's lymphoma	0	1	1	0	2	1.1	1.1	16.7	1.9	1.6	-	1.1	1.2	17	100.0
Unspecified lymphoma	0	0	0	0	0	-	-	-	-	-	-	-	-	-	-
Histiocytosis X	0	0	0	0	0	-	-	-	-	-	-	-	-	-	-
Other reticuloendothelial	0	0	0	0	0	-	-	-	-	-	-	-	-	-	-
III. BRAIN AND SPINAL	1	10	18	7	36	20.1	19.7	100.0	21.0	28.1	10.1	19.4	20.1	296	91.2
Ependymoma	1	1	0	0	2	1.1	1.1	5.6	3.8	-	-	1.1	1.5	19	100.0
Astrocytoma	0	3	8	3	14	7.8	7.6	38.9	5.7	12.5	4.3	7.5	7.5	113	92.9
Medulloblastoma	0	3	4	2	9	5.0	5.0	25.0	5.7	6.2	2.9	4.8	5.1	74	88.9
Other glioma	0	3	6	2	11	6.1	6.0	30.6	5.7	9.4	2.9	5.9	6.1	90	88.9
Other and unspecified *	0	0	0	0	0	-	-	-	-	-	-	-	-	-	-
IV. SYMPATHETIC N.S.	6	4	2	0	12	6.7	6.7	100.0	19.1	3.1	-	6.5	8.4	111	83.3
Neuroblastoma	6	4	2	0	12	6.7	6.7	100.0	19.1	3.1	-	6.5	8.4	111	83.3
Other	0	0	0	0	0	-	-	-	-	-	-	-	-	-	-
V. RETINOBLASTOMA	0	1	0	0	1	0.6	0.6	100.0	1.9	-	-	0.5	0.7	10	100.0
VI. KIDNEY	1	6	2	1	10	5.6	5.6	100.0	13.4	3.1	1.4	5.4	6.6	90	90.0
Wilms' tumour	1	6	2	0	9	5.0	5.0	90.0	13.4	3.1	-	4.8	6.2	82	88.9
Renal carcinoma	0	0	0	1	1	0.6	0.6	10.0	-	-	1.4	0.5	0.4	7	100.0
Other and unspecified	0	0	0	0	0	-	-	-	-	-	-	-	-	-	-
VII. LIVER	0	0	0	0	0	-	-	-	-	-	-	-	-	-	-
Hepatoblastoma	0	0	0	0	0	-	-	-	-	-	-	-	-	-	-
Hepatic carcinoma	0	0	0	0	0	-	-	-	-	-	-	-	-	-	-
Other and unspecified	0	0	0	0	0	-	-	-	-	-	-	-	-	-	-
VIII. BONE	0	4	6	12	22	12.3	12.6	100.0	7.6	9.4	17.3	11.8	11.0	172	85.7
Osteosarcoma	0	1	3	5	9	5.0	5.1	40.9	1.9	4.7	7.2	4.8	4.3	69	77.8
Chondrosarcoma	0	0	0	0	0	-	-	-	-	-	-	-	-	-	-
Ewing's sarcoma	0	1	3	5	9	5.0	5.1	40.9	1.9	4.7	7.2	4.8	4.3	69	88.9
Other and unspecified	0	2	0	2	4	2.2	2.3	18.2	3.8	-	2.9	2.2	2.3	34	100.0
IX. SOFT TISSUE SARCOMAS	1	5	4	2	12	6.7	6.6	100.0	11.4	6.2	2.9	6.5	7.3	103	100.0
Rhabdomyosarcoma	0	1	1	0	2	1.1	1.1	16.7	1.9	1.6	-	1.1	1.2	17	100.0
Fibrosarcoma	0	1	1	2	4	2.2	2.3	33.3	1.9	1.6	2.9	2.2	2.1	32	100.0
Other and unspecified	1	3	2	0	6	3.4	3.3	50.0	7.6	3.1	-	3.2	4.0	54	100.0
X. GONADAL & GERM CELL	0	0	0	4	4	2.2	2.4	100.0	-	-	5.8	2.2	1.7	29	100.0
Non-gonadal germ cell	0	0	0	1	1	0.6	0.6	25.0	-	-	1.4	0.5	0.4	7	100.0
Gonadal germ cell	0	0	0	3	3	1.7	1.8	75.0	-	-	4.3	1.6	1.3	22	100.0
Gonadal carcinoma	0	0	0	0	0	-	-	-	-	-	-	-	-	-	-
Other and unspecified	0	0	0	0	0	-	-	-	-	-	-	-	-	-	-
XI. EPITHELIAL NEOPLASMS	0	2	1	4	7	3.9	4.0	100.0	3.8	1.6	5.8	3.8	3.7	56	100.0
Adrenocortical carcinoma	0	1	0	0	1	0.6	0.6	14.3	1.9	-	-	0.5	0.7	10	100.0
Thyroid carcinoma	0	0	0	0	0	-	-	-	-	-	-	-	-	-	-
Nasopharyngeal carcinoma	0	0	0	0	0	-	-	-	-	-	-	-	-	-	-
Melanoma	0	1	0	0	1	0.6	0.6	14.3	1.9	-	-	0.5	0.7	10	100.0
Other carcinoma	0	0	1	4	5	2.8	2.9	71.4	-	1.6	5.8	2.7	2.2	37	100.0
XII. OTHER	0	1	1	2	4	2.2	2.3	100.0	1.9	1.6	2.9	2.2	2.1	32	100.0
* Specified as malignant	0	3	5	1	9	5.0	4.9	100.0	5.7	7.8	1.4	4.8	5.2	75	85.7

HUNGARY

Paediatric Tumour Registry, 1975-1984

T. Révész & D. Schüler

The Registry was originally established for the purpose of collecting clinical data on all patients diagnosed with leukaemia in Hungary. Ten treatment centres have participated in this study since 1971. At the time of diagnosis, bone marrow smears and a registration form are sent to the paediatric oncology section in the National Institute of Paediatrics, Budapest. Collection of data is voluntary, but compliance is good as uniform treatment schedules are followed and most cytotoxic drugs are distributed cost-free from the paediatric oncology section. Data are entered in a computer and the data base is updated each year.

In 1975, the system was expanded to collect data on all other childhood malignancies as well. Most of these come from the same paediatric departments that participate in the leukaemia study but, in addition, some other treatment centres, such as those of neurosurgery, ophthalmology, etc., are involved. Data are collected on a very simple information sheet that is filled in for each patient at the end of the year. In 1984, the National Institute of Oncology introduced compulsory registration of all childhood and adult malignancies, so that registration forms are completed for all paediatric patients and are sent to the national registry. Despite the fact that a national registry has been established, the separate registration of childhood cases will be continued, since it is possible to obtain more clinically relevant information by this means.

The liaison between the paediatric oncology section and the participating treatment centres is thought to be good. Members of a working party meet every six months, and once a year there is also a meeting of paediatric oncology nurses involved in various aspects of care. Although it is difficult to estimate the completeness of registration, this is thought to be between 85 and 90%.

The whole of Hungary is covered by the registry. Approximately one-fifth of the population lives in or around Budapest and the majority of the population lives in towns. Children with malignancies are treated in specialized units, usually the one nearest to their home.

Although there is a sizeable gipsy population in the country, no data are available on ethnic differences in incidence or mortality. Treatment can usually be given to these children without any difficulty.

The Registry includes all childhood malignant disease except for squamous and basal-cell carcinomas of the skin. Benign and unspecified tumours of the central nervous system and most other sites are also included. Death certificates are not used as a source of cases for the registry, but cases where the malignancy was discovered at post mortem at the paediatric unit are included.

Population

The size of the paediatric population is based on annual estimates provided by the National Institute of Statistics.

AVERAGE ANNUAL POPULATION: 1975-1984

Age	Male	Female
0	81399	77478
1-4	333922	316603
5-9	402040	379242
10-14	354490	334073
0-14	1171851	1107396

Commentary

The incidence of childhood cancer overall and in the principal diagnostic groups is similar to that observed in other European countries.

Of the children with retinoblastoma, 19/34 (56%) had unilateral and 15/34 (44%) had bilateral tumours. Laterality was recorded for all but two of

Contd p. 258

Hungary

1975 – 1984   MALE

DIAGNOSTIC GROUP	NUMBER OF CASES					REL. FREQUENCY(%)			RATES PER MILLION						Cum	HV(%)
	0	1-4	5-9	10-14	All	Crude	Adj.	Group	0	1-4	5-9	10-14	Crude	Adj.		
TOTAL	126	527	406	245	1305¤	100.0	100.0	100.0	154.8	157.8	101.0	69.1	111.4	113.5	1637	94.5
I. LEUKAEMIAS	20	224	130	73	448¤	34.3	33.5	100.0	24.6	67.1	32.3	20.6	38.2	39.1	558	100.0
Acute lymphocytic	7	192	103	51	353	27.0	26.0	78.8	8.6	57.5	25.6	14.4	30.1	30.9	439	100.0
Other lymphocytic	0	0	0	0	0	-	-	-	-	-	-	-	-	-	-	-
Acute non-lymphocytic	10	27	24	18	79	6.1	6.2	17.6	12.3	8.1	6.0	5.1	6.7	6.9	100	100.0
Chronic myeloid	3	2	3	3	11	0.8	0.9	2.5	3.7	0.6	0.7	0.8	0.9	1.0	14	100.0
Other and unspecified	0	3	0	1	5¤	0.4	0.3	1.1	-	0.9	-	0.3	0.4	0.4	5	100.0
II. LYMPHOMAS	6	51	97	70	224	17.2	19.2	100.0	7.4	15.3	24.1	19.7	19.1	18.8	288	100.0
Hodgkin's disease	0	11	38	25	74	5.7	6.5	33.0	-	3.3	9.5	7.1	6.3	6.1	96	100.0
Non-Hodgkin lymphoma	2	1	3	1	7	0.5	0.5	3.1	2.5	0.3	0.7	0.3	0.6	0.6	6	100.0
Burkitt's lymphoma	0	8	12	5	25	1.9	2.0	11.2	-	2.4	3.0	1.4	2.1	2.1	32	100.0
Unspecified lymphoma	3	21	38	35	97	7.4	8.6	43.3	3.7	6.3	9.5	9.9	8.3	8.1	125	100.0
Histiocytosis X	1	8	5	4	18	1.4	1.4	8.0	1.2	2.4	1.2	1.1	1.5	1.6	23	100.0
Other reticuloendothelial	0	2	1	0	3	0.2	0.2	1.3	-	0.6	0.2	-	0.3	0.2	4	100.0
III. BRAIN AND SPINAL	14	83	95	45	237	18.2	18.5	100.0	17.2	24.9	23.6	12.7	20.2	20.3	298	73.0
Ependymoma	3	17	12	5	37	2.8	2.7	15.6	3.7	5.1	3.0	1.4	3.2	3.2	46	100.0
Astrocytoma	5	23	27	22	77	5.9	6.4	32.5	6.1	6.9	6.7	6.2	6.6	6.6	98	100.0
Medulloblastoma	1	10	26	3	40	3.1	3.0	16.9	1.2	3.0	6.5	0.8	3.4	3.4	50	98.7
Other glioma	1	1	0	0	2	0.2	0.1	0.8	1.2	0.3	-	-	0.2	0.2	2	100.0
Other and unspecified *	4	32	30	15	81	6.2	6.3	34.2	4.9	9.6	7.5	4.2	6.9	7.0	102	22.2
IV. SYMPATHETIC N.S.	32	67	20	5	124	9.5	8.2	100.0	39.3	20.1	5.0	1.4	10.6	11.3	151	100.0
Neuroblastoma	32	66	18	5	121	9.3	7.9	97.6	39.3	19.8	4.5	1.4	10.3	11.0	148	100.0
Other	0	1	2	0	3	0.2	0.2	2.4	-	0.3	0.5	-	0.3	0.3	4	100.0
V. RETINOBLASTOMA	4	9	0	0	13	1.0	0.8	100.0	4.9	2.7	-	-	1.1	1.2	16	100.0
VI. KIDNEY	22	39	18	2	81	6.2	5.3	100.0	27.0	11.7	4.5	0.6	6.9	7.3	99	100.0
Wilms' tumour	21	39	17	1	78	6.0	5.1	96.3	25.8	11.7	4.2	0.3	6.7	7.1	95	100.0
Renal carcinoma	1	0	1	1	3	0.2	0.3	3.7	1.2	-	0.2	0.3	0.3	0.3	4	100.0
Other and unspecified	0	0	0	0	0	-	-	-	-	-	-	-	-	-	-	-
VII. LIVER	4	1	2	3	10	0.8	0.8	100.0	4.9	0.3	0.5	0.8	0.9	0.9	13	100.0
Hepatoblastoma	3	0	1	1	5	0.4	0.4	50.0	3.7	-	0.2	0.3	0.4	0.4	6	100.0
Hepatic carcinoma	1	1	1	2	5	0.4	0.4	50.0	1.2	0.3	0.2	0.6	0.4	0.4	6	100.0
Other and unspecified	0	0	0	0	0	-	-	-	-	-	-	-	-	-	-	-
VIII. BONE	0	8	12	26	46	3.5	4.6	100.0	-	2.4	3.0	7.3	3.9	3.8	61	100.0
Osteosarcoma	0	0	5	10	15	1.1	1.6	32.6	-	-	1.2	2.8	1.3	1.2	20	100.0
Chondrosarcoma	0	0	1	2	3	0.2	0.3	6.5	-	-	0.2	0.6	0.3	0.2	4	100.0
Ewing's sarcoma	0	7	6	12	25	1.9	2.3	54.3	-	2.1	1.5	3.4	2.1	2.1	33	100.0
Other and unspecified	0	1	0	2	3	0.2	0.3	6.5	-	0.3	-	0.6	0.3	0.3	4	33.3
IX. SOFT TISSUE SARCOMAS	17	25	22	10	74	5.7	5.4	100.0	20.9	7.5	5.5	2.8	6.3	6.5	92	100.0
Rhabdomyosarcoma	6	16	13	1	36	2.8	2.4	48.6	7.4	4.8	3.2	0.3	3.1	3.2	44	100.0
Fibrosarcoma	1	3	0	3	7	0.5	0.6	9.5	1.2	0.9	-	0.8	0.6	0.6	9	100.0
Other and unspecified	10	6	9	6	31	2.4	2.4	41.9	12.3	1.8	2.2	1.7	2.6	2.7	39	100.0
X. GONADAL & GERM CELL	6	18	2	3	29	2.2	2.0	100.0	7.4	5.4	0.5	0.8	2.5	2.6	36	100.0
Non-gonadal germ cell	3	7	2	2	14	1.1	1.0	48.3	3.7	2.1	0.5	0.6	1.2	1.3	17	95.7
Gonadal germ cell	3	11	0	1	15	1.1	1.0	51.7	3.7	3.3	-	0.3	1.3	1.4	18	100.0
Gonadal carcinoma	0	0	0	0	0	-	-	-	-	-	-	-	-	-	-	100.0
Other and unspecified	0	0	0	0	0	-	-	-	-	-	-	-	-	-	-	-
XI. EPITHELIAL NEOPLASMS	0	0	5	6	11	0.8	1.1	100.0	-	-	1.2	1.7	0.9	0.9	15	100.0
Adrenocortical carcinoma	0	0	1	0	1	0.1	0.1	9.1	-	-	0.2	-	0.1	0.1	1	100.0
Thyroid carcinoma	0	0	1	1	2	0.2	0.2	18.2	-	-	0.2	0.3	0.2	0.1	3	100.0
Nasopharyngeal carcinoma	0	0	0	2	2	0.2	0.2	18.2	-	-	-	0.6	0.2	0.2	3	100.0
Melanoma	0	0	0	0	0	-	-	-	-	-	-	-	-	-	-	-
Other carcinoma	0	0	3	3	6	0.5	0.6	54.5	-	-	0.7	0.8	0.5	0.5	8	100.0
XII. OTHER	1	2	3	2	8	0.6	0.7	100.0	1.2	0.6	0.7	0.6	0.7	0.7	10	25.0
* Specified as malignant	3	26	26	8	63	4.8	4.7	100.0	3.7	7.8	6.5	2.3	5.4	5.4	78	-
¤ Includes age unknown																

Hungary FEMALE

1975 - 1984

DIAGNOSTIC GROUP	NUMBER OF CASES 0	1-4	5-9	10-14	All	REL. FREQUENCY(%) Crude	Adj.	Group	RATES PER MILLION 0	1-4	5-9	10-14	Crude	Adj.	Cum	HV(%)
TOTAL	93	390	239	166	888	100.0	100.0	100.0	120.0	123.2	63.0	49.7	80.2	82.2	1176	95.8
I. LEUKAEMIAS	24	164	74	52	314	35.4	34.3	100.0	31.0	51.8	19.5	15.6	28.4	29.3	414	100.0
Acute lymphocytic	15	147	62	37	261	29.4	27.9	83.1	19.4	46.4	16.3	11.1	23.6	24.4	342	100.0
Other lymphocytic	0	0	0	0	0	-	-	-	-	-	-	-	-	-	-	-
Acute non-lymphocytic	7	15	11	12	45	5.1	5.4	14.3	9.0	4.7	2.9	3.6	4.1	4.1	60	100.0
Chronic myeloid	1	1	0	1	3	0.3	0.3	1.0	1.3	0.3	-	0.3	0.3	0.3	4	100.0
Other and unspecified	1	1	1	2	5	0.6	0.7	1.6	1.3	0.3	0.3	0.6	0.5	0.5	7	100.0
II. LYMPHOMAS	6	21	28	21	76	8.6	9.5	100.0	7.7	6.6	7.4	6.3	6.9	6.9	103	100.0
Hodgkin's disease	0	3	4	13	20	2.3	3.1	26.3	-	0.9	1.1	3.9	1.8	1.8	29	100.0
Non-Hodgkin lymphoma	0	1	1	1	3	0.3	0.6	3.9	-	0.6	0.5	0.3	0.3	0.5	4	100.0
Burkitt's lymphoma	0	2	2	1	5	0.6	0.6	6.6	-	0.6	0.5	-	0.5	0.5	7	100.0
Unspecified lymphoma	0	7	19	5	31	3.5	3.9	40.8	-	2.2	5.0	1.5	2.8	2.7	41	100.0
Histiocytosis X *	6	7	1	1	15	1.7	1.4	19.7	7.7	2.2	0.3	0.3	1.4	1.5	19	100.0
Other reticuloendothelial	0	1	1	0	2	0.3	0.3	2.6	-	0.6	0.3	-	0.2	0.2	3	100.0
III. BRAIN AND SPINAL	11	55	74	42	182	20.5	22.3	100.0	14.2	17.4	19.5	12.6	16.4	16.4	244	81.3
Ependymoma	3	17	7	4	31	3.5	3.3	17.0	3.9	5.4	1.8	1.2	2.8	2.9	41	100.0
Astrocytoma	3	18	32	15	68	7.7	8.5	37.4	3.9	5.7	8.4	4.5	6.1	6.1	91	100.0
Medulloblastoma	1	7	13	6	27	3.0	3.4	14.8	1.3	2.2	3.4	1.8	2.4	2.4	36	100.0
Other glioma	1	0	0	1	2	0.2	0.3	1.1	1.3	-	-	0.3	0.2	0.2	3	100.0
Other and unspecified *	3	13	22	16	54	6.1	7.0	29.7	3.9	4.1	5.8	4.8	4.9	4.8	73	37.0
IV. SYMPATHETIC N.S.	23	53	12	6	94	10.6	8.9	100.0	29.7	16.7	3.2	1.8	8.5	9.0	121	100.0
Neuroblastoma	23	51	11	6	91	10.2	8.6	96.8	29.7	16.1	2.9	1.8	8.2	8.7	118	100.0
Other	0	2	1	0	3	0.3	0.3	3.2	-	0.6	0.3	-	0.3	0.3	4	100.0
V. RETINOBLASTOMA	5	16	0	0	21	2.4	1.7	100.0	6.5	5.1	-	-	1.9	2.1	27	100.0
VI. KIDNEY	11	44	9	3	67	7.5	6.2	100.0	14.2	13.9	2.4	0.9	6.1	6.4	86	100.0
Wilms' tumour	11	44	8	2	65	7.3	5.9	97.0	14.2	13.9	2.1	0.6	5.9	6.3	83	100.0
Renal carcinoma	0	0	1	1	2	0.2	0.3	3.0	-	-	0.3	0.3	0.2	0.2	3	100.0
Other and unspecified	0	0	0	0	0	-	-	-	-	-	-	-	-	-	-	-
VII. LIVER	7	3	0	1	11	1.2	1.0	100.0	9.0	0.9	-	0.3	1.0	1.1	14	100.0
Hepatoblastoma	5	0	0	0	5	0.6	0.4	45.5	6.5	-	-	-	0.5	0.5	6	100.0
Hepatic carcinoma	2	3	0	1	6	0.7	0.6	54.5	2.6	0.9	-	0.3	0.5	0.6	8	100.0
Other and unspecified	0	0	0	0	0	-	-	-	-	-	-	-	-	-	-	-
VIII. BONE	0	4	12	22	38	4.3	5.8	100.0	-	1.3	3.2	6.6	3.4	3.3	54	97.4
Osteosarcoma	0	1	3	16	20	2.3	3.4	52.6	-	0.3	0.8	4.8	1.8	1.7	29	100.0
Chondrosarcoma	0	0	1	1	2	0.2	0.3	5.3	-	-	0.3	0.3	0.2	0.2	3	100.0
Ewing's sarcoma	0	2	8	5	15	1.7	2.1	39.5	-	0.6	2.1	1.5	1.4	1.3	21	100.0
Other and unspecified	0	1	0	0	1	0.1	0.1	2.6	-	0.3	-	-	0.1	0.1	1	100.0
IX. SOFT TISSUE SARCOMAS	3	17	14	11	45	5.1	5.4	100.0	3.9	5.4	3.7	3.3	4.1	4.1	60	100.0
Rhabdomyosarcoma	1	11	4	4	20	2.2	2.2	44.4	1.3	3.5	1.1	1.2	1.8	1.9	26	100.0
Fibrosarcoma	2	4	5	1	12	1.4	1.3	26.7	2.6	1.3	1.3	0.3	1.1	1.1	16	100.0
Other and unspecified	0	2	5	6	13	1.5	1.9	28.9	-	0.6	1.3	1.8	1.2	1.1	18	100.0
X. GONADAL & GERM CELL	2	11	12	4	29	3.3	3.3	100.0	2.6	3.5	3.2	1.2	2.6	2.6	38	100.0
Non-gonadal germ cell	2	10	4	1	17	1.9	1.7	58.6	2.6	3.2	1.1	0.3	1.5	1.6	22	100.0
Gonadal germ cell	0	1	6	3	10	1.1	1.4	34.5	-	0.3	1.6	0.9	0.9	0.9	14	100.0
Gonadal carcinoma	0	0	1	0	1	0.1	0.1	3.4	-	-	0.3	-	0.1	0.1	1	100.0
Other and unspecified	0	0	1	0	1	0.1	0.1	3.4	-	-	0.3	-	0.1	0.1	1	100.0
XI. EPITHELIAL NEOPLASMS	0	1	2	3	6	0.7	0.9	100.0	-	0.3	0.5	0.9	0.5	0.5	8	100.0
Adrenocortical carcinoma	0	0	0	0	0	-	-	-	-	-	-	-	-	-	-	-
Thyroid carcinoma	0	0	0	1	1	0.1	0.2	16.7	-	-	-	0.3	0.1	0.1	1	100.0
Nasopharyngeal carcinoma	0	0	0	1	1	0.1	-	16.7	-	-	-	0.3	0.1	-	1	100.0
Melanoma	0	1	0	0	1	0.2	0.3	33.3	-	0.3	-	-	0.2	0.3	3	100.0
Other carcinoma	0	0	2	1	3	0.3	0.4	50.0	-	-	0.5	0.3	0.3	0.3	4	100.0
XII. OTHER	1	1	2	1	5	0.6	0.6	100.0	1.3	0.3	0.5	0.3	0.5	0.5	7	60.0
* Specified as malignant	3	9	17	8	37	4.2	4.6	100.0	3.9	2.8	4.5	2.4	3.3	3.3	50	10.8

* Specified as malignant
¤ Includes age unknown

the children with Wilms' tumour; of these, 5/141 (4%) had bilateral tumours.

Among soft-tissue sarcomas, 44/119 (37%) were in the 'other and unspecified' group. The most numerous types were synovial sarcoma (12 cases), angiosarcoma (11) and sarcoma not otherwise specified (10).

ITALY

Childhood Cancer Registry of the Province of Torino, 1967–1981

G. Pastore, C. Magnani, M.L. Mosso, S. Rosso, B. Terracini & R. Zanetti

The Childhood Cancer Registry (Registro dei Tumori Infantili della Provincia di Torino, RTIPT) is operated by the Chair of Cancer Epidemiology of the Department of Biomedical Sciences and Human Oncology of the University of Torino. Originally, it developed as an *ad hoc* activity of the Cancer Registry of Piedmont (RTP). The latter, since 1972, only collected mortality data for the whole of Piedmont and — in some years only — incidence data for the city of Torino. As an additional exercise, RTIPT has also registered cancer in children in the other five provinces of Piedmont since 1976.

Cases are identified in the paediatric, haematology, neurology, orthopaedic and radiotherapy units of hospitals in the Province. In 1981–1983, a retrospective check with units of medicine in other small hospitals of the Province did not identify any missing case. The search for cases has included a number of major institutions located outside the Province.

With the exception of a few sources (see below), registration has been active, by systematic survey of the relevant files (clinical records and/or registry of diagnoses at admission/discharge and/or files of the radiotherapy units). This has been done retrospectively at intervals of 2–3 years. The files of the pathology departments were surveyed until 1978, when it became obvious that no new cases were being identified through this source, since pathology reports were included in the clinical records of all hospitals. Since 1976, the hospital admission/discharge files (including diagnoses at discharge) established by the Piedmont Region have been used in order to verify completeness of registration.

With the exception of cancer of the central nervous system (for which there is no specialized paediatric service in the Province), around two-thirds of the cases under age nine are hospitalized in the Unit of Paediatric Oncology of the Children's Hospital in Torino.

For eight major treatment centres or cancer registries outside the Province (including Paris and Geneva), a system of passive registration was adopted, i.e., a request by letter to provide information on patients with cancer, aged 0–14 at diagnosis, living in any of the 315 municipalities of the Province of Torino. Information requested included, among other items, data on method of diagnosis. Deceased children have been identified both from clinical records and through the lists of residents dying with cancer regularly sent from the 315 towns of the Piedmont Region to the RTP.

The registered cases of cancer have been coded by the Registry using a topography code which is an adaptation of ICD-8, and for morphology a specialized code developed for paediatric oncology by the Registry. For the present study, the morphology codes were converted to the ICD-O equivalent by a special computer program; where an ICD-O code equivalent to the Torino code could not be allocated automatically, the records were reviewed and a code appropriate to the histology was given.

Histiocytosis X was not registered.

The Registry covers the Province of Torino (6830 square kilometres). At the 1981 census, 47.6% of the population lived in the city of Torino and 78.6% in the metropolitan area (city of Torino and 53 suburbs). The rest of the Province includes a few partially industrialized towns and a relatively large mountain area with a low population density.

The total population at the 1981 census was 2 345 771, of whom 19% were children aged 0–14. The occupationally active population was 1 036 814, 42% of whom were engaged in industrial activities (mainly related to automobile production).

Less than 1% of the population is non-Catholic (Jews and Protestants).

Data on incidence and survival have been published (Pastore *et al.*, 1981; Magnani *et al.*,

Contd p. 262

Italy, Torino   MALE   1967 – 1981

DIAGNOSTIC GROUP	NUMBER OF CASES 0	1-4	5-9	10-14	All	REL. FREQUENCY(%) Crude	Adj.	Group	RATES PER MILLION 0	1-4	5-9	10-14	Crude	Adj.	Cum	HV(%)
TOTAL	47	213	179	145	584	100.0	100.0	100.0	196.6	210.6	134.4	114.3	151.6	157.0	2282	88.9
I. LEUKAEMIAS	14	85	60	40	199	34.1	33.6	100.0	58.6	84.0	45.0	31.5	51.7	54.2	778	97.5
Acute lymphocytic	4	63	34	22	123	21.1	20.6	61.8	16.7	62.3	25.5	17.3	31.9	33.9	480	100.0
Other lymphocytic	0	1	1	1	3	0.5	0.5	1.5	-	-	0.8	0.8	0.5	0.8	12	100.0
Acute non-lymphocytic	3	5	8	7	23	3.9	4.0	11.6	12.5	4.9	6.0	5.5	6.0	6.0	90	100.0
Chronic myeloid	1	1	1	0	3	0.5	0.5	1.5	4.2	1.0	0.8	-	0.8	0.9	12	100.0
Other and unspecified	6	15	16	10	47	8.0	8.0	23.6	25.1	14.8	12.0	7.9	12.2	12.7	184	89.4
II. LYMPHOMAS	5	13	41	28	87	14.9	15.4	100.0	20.9	12.9	30.8	22.1	22.6	21.9	337	95.4
Hodgkin's disease	1	5	14	14	34	5.8	6.2	39.1	4.2	4.9	10.5	11.0	8.8	8.4	132	100.0
Non-Hodgkin lymphoma	2	7	21	8	38	6.5	6.6	43.7	8.4	6.9	15.8	6.3	9.9	9.7	146	97.4
Burkitt's lymphoma	0	0	0	0	0	-	-	-	-	-	-	-	-	-	-	-
Unspecified lymphoma	0	0	5	3	8	1.4	1.5	9.2	-	-	3.8	2.4	2.1	1.9	31	62.5
Histiocytosis X	0	0	0	0	0	-	-	-	-	-	-	-	-	-	-	-
Other reticuloendothelial	2	1	1	3	7	1.2	1.2	8.0	8.4	1.0	0.8	2.4	1.8	1.9	28	100.0
III. BRAIN AND SPINAL	4	40	42	29	115	19.7	19.8	100.0	16.7	39.6	31.5	22.9	29.9	30.4	447	68.7
Ependymoma	0	4	1	1	6	1.0	1.0	5.2	-	4.0	0.8	0.8	1.6	1.7	24	100.0
Astrocytoma	1	19	9	8	37	6.3	6.2	32.2	4.2	18.8	6.8	6.3	9.6	10.2	145	94.6
Medulloblastoma	2	8	13	6	29	5.0	5.0	25.2	8.4	7.9	9.8	4.7	7.5	7.6	112	96.6
Other glioma	0	0	1	1	2	0.3	0.4	1.7	-	-	0.8	0.8	0.5	0.5	8	50.0
Other and unspecified *	1	9	18	13	41	7.0	7.2	35.7	4.2	8.9	13.5	10.2	10.6	10.4	159	22.0
IV. SYMPATHETIC N.S.	9	26	3	3	41	7.0	6.5	100.0	37.6	25.7	2.3	2.4	10.6	12.3	164	100.0
Neuroblastoma	9	26	3	3	41	7.0	6.5	100.0	37.6	25.7	2.3	2.4	10.6	12.3	164	100.0
Other	0	0	0	0	0	-	-	-	-	-	-	-	-	-	-	-
V. RETINOBLASTOMA	4	12	1	0	14	2.4	2.2	100.0	4.2	11.9	0.8	-	3.6	4.2	55	78.6
VI. KIDNEY	4	16	2	2	24	4.1	3.8	100.0	16.7	15.8	1.5	1.6	6.2	7.1	95	87.5
Wilms' tumour	4	16	2	2	24	4.1	3.8	100.0	16.7	15.8	1.5	1.6	6.2	7.1	95	87.5
Renal carcinoma	0	0	0	0	0	-	-	-	-	-	-	-	-	-	-	-
Other and unspecified	0	0	0	0	0	-	-	-	-	-	-	-	-	-	-	-
VII. LIVER	3	3	1	1	8	1.4	1.3	100.0	12.5	3.0	0.8	0.8	2.1	2.4	32	87.5
Hepatoblastoma	2	3	0	1	6	1.0	1.0	75.0	8.4	3.0	-	0.8	1.6	1.8	24	100.0
Hepatic carcinoma	0	0	1	0	1	0.2	0.2	12.5	-	-	0.8	-	0.3	0.2	4	100.0
Other and unspecified	1	0	0	0	1	0.2	0.2	12.5	4.2	-	-	-	0.3	0.3	4	-
VIII. BONE	0	2	6	19	27	4.6	5.2	100.0	-	2.0	4.5	15.0	7.0	6.4	105	92.6
Osteosarcoma	0	0	6	6	12	2.1	2.2	44.4	-	-	4.5	4.7	3.1	2.8	46	100.0
Chondrosarcoma	0	0	0	1	1	0.2	0.2	3.7	-	-	-	0.8	0.3	0.2	4	100.0
Ewing's sarcoma	0	2	0	9	11	1.9	2.2	40.7	-	2.0	-	7.1	2.9	2.7	43	90.9
Other and unspecified	0	0	0	3	3	0.5	0.6	11.1	-	-	-	2.4	0.8	0.7	12	66.7
IX. SOFT TISSUE SARCOMAS	4	10	11	9	34	5.8	5.9	100.0	16.7	9.9	8.3	7.1	8.8	9.1	133	91.2
Rhabdomyosarcoma	1	6	3	2	12	2.1	2.0	35.3	4.2	5.9	2.3	1.6	3.1	3.3	47	100.0
Fibrosarcoma	1	3	2	2	8	1.4	1.4	23.5	4.2	3.0	1.5	1.6	2.1	2.2	31	87.5
Other and unspecified	2	1	6	5	14	2.4	2.5	41.2	8.4	1.0	4.5	3.9	3.6	3.6	55	85.7
X. GONADAL & GERM CELL	2	1	4	0	7	1.2	1.1	100.0	8.4	1.0	3.0	-	1.8	1.9	27	100.0
Non-gonadal germ cell	1	1	0	0	2	0.3	0.3	28.6	4.2	1.0	-	-	0.5	0.6	8	100.0
Gonadal germ cell	1	0	4	0	5	0.9	0.8	71.4	4.2	-	3.0	-	1.3	1.3	19	100.0
Gonadal carcinoma	0	0	0	0	0	-	-	-	-	-	-	-	-	-	-	-
Other and unspecified	0	0	0	0	0	-	-	-	-	-	-	-	-	-	-	-
XI. EPITHELIAL NEOPLASMS	0	0	6	12	18	3.1	3.5	100.0	-	-	4.5	9.5	4.7	4.2	70	100.0
Adrenocortical carcinoma	0	0	1	1	2	0.3	0.4	11.1	-	-	0.8	0.8	0.5	0.5	8	100.0
Thyroid carcinoma	0	0	2	4	6	1.0	1.2	33.3	-	-	1.5	3.2	1.6	1.4	23	100.0
Nasopharyngeal carcinoma	0	0	0	3	3	0.5	0.6	16.7	-	-	-	2.4	0.8	0.7	12	100.0
Melanoma	0	0	3	1	4	0.7	0.7	22.2	-	-	2.3	0.8	1.0	1.0	15	100.0
Other carcinoma	0	0	0	3	3	0.5	0.6	16.7	-	-	-	2.4	0.8	0.6	12	100.0
XII. OTHER	1	5	2	2	10	1.7	1.7	-	4.2	4.9	1.5	1.6	2.6	2.8	39	20.0

* Specified as malignant

Italy, Torino   1967 – 1981   FEMALE

DIAGNOSTIC GROUP	NUMBER OF CASES					REL. FREQUENCY(%)			RATES PER MILLION						Cum	HV(%)
	0	1-4	5-9	10-14	All	Crude	Adj.	Group	0	1-4	5-9	10-14	Crude	Adj.		
TOTAL	47	151	130	111	439	100.0	100.0	100.0	211.5	157.3	102.3	92.4	120.1	124.9	1814	84.3
I. LEUKAEMIAS	12	64	52	24	152	34.6	33.8	100.0	54.0	66.7	40.9	20.0	41.6	43.8	625	94.1
Acute lymphocytic	4	45	27	10	86	19.6	18.8	56.6	18.0	46.9	21.2	8.3	23.5	25.2	353	98.8
Other lymphocytic	1	2	1	0	4	0.9	0.8	2.6	4.5	2.1	0.8	-	1.1	1.2	17	50.0
Acute non-lymphocytic	0	2	7	6	15	3.4	3.6	9.9	-	2.1	5.5	5.0	4.1	3.9	61	100.0
Chronic myeloid	0	0	4	1	5	1.1	1.2	3.3	-	-	3.1	0.8	1.4	1.3	20	100.0
Other and unspecified	7	15	13	7	42	9.6	9.3	27.6	31.5	15.6	10.2	5.8	11.5	12.3	174	85.7
II. LYMPHOMAS	2	8	8	20	38	8.7	9.3	100.0	9.0	8.3	6.3	16.7	10.4	10.1	157	94.7
Hodgkin's disease	1	2	2	16	21	4.8	5.4	55.3	4.5	2.1	1.6	13.3	5.7	5.4	87	95.2
Non-Hodgkin lymphoma	0	4	6	4	14	3.2	3.3	36.8	-	4.2	4.7	3.3	3.8	3.8	57	92.9
Burkitt's lymphoma	0	0	0	0	0	-	-	-	-	-	-	-	-	-	-	-
Unspecified lymphoma	0	1	0	0	1	0.2	0.2	2.6	-	1.0	-	-	0.3	0.3	4	100.0
Histiocytosis X	0	0	0	0	0	-	-	-	-	-	-	-	-	-	-	-
Other reticuloendothelial	1	1	0	0	2	0.5	0.4	5.3	4.5	1.0	-	-	0.5	0.7	9	100.0
III. BRAIN AND SPINAL	6	19	34	28	87	19.8	20.5	100.0	27.0	19.8	26.8	23.3	23.8	23.6	357	62.1
Ependymoma	1	0	3	3	7	1.6	1.7	8.0	4.5	-	2.4	2.5	1.9	1.8	29	100.0
Astrocytoma	0	6	14	2	22	5.0	5.0	25.3	-	6.3	11.0	1.7	6.0	6.0	88	100.0
Medulloblastoma	2	4	5	5	16	3.6	3.7	18.4	9.0	4.2	3.9	4.2	4.4	4.5	66	100.0
Other glioma	1	1	1	3	6	1.4	1.4	6.9	4.5	1.0	0.8	2.5	1.6	1.6	25	33.3
Other and unspecified *	2	8	11	15	36	8.2	8.6	41.4	9.0	8.3	8.7	12.5	9.9	9.7	148	19.4
IV. SYMPATHETIC N.S.	6	17	8	2	33	7.5	7.0	100.0	27.0	17.7	6.3	1.7	9.0	10.1	138	84.8
Neuroblastoma	6	17	8	2	33	7.5	7.0	100.0	27.0	17.7	6.3	1.7	9.0	10.1	138	84.8
Other	0	0	0	0	0	-	-	-	-	-	-	-	-	-	-	-
V. RETINOBLASTOMA	6	5	2	0	13	3.0	2.7	100.0	27.0	5.2	1.6	-	3.6	4.2	56	61.5
VI. KIDNEY	7	17	1	0	25	5.7	5.1	100.0	31.5	17.7	0.8	-	6.8	8.2	106	92.0
Wilms' tumour	6	17	1	0	24	5.5	4.9	96.0	27.0	17.7	0.8	-	6.6	7.8	102	91.7
Renal carcinoma	1	0	0	0	1	0.2	0.2	4.0	4.5	-	-	-	0.3	0.3	4	100.0
Other and unspecified	0	0	0	0	0	-	-	-	-	-	-	-	-	-	-	-
VII. LIVER	1	2	1	2	6	1.4	1.4	100.0	4.5	2.1	0.8	1.7	1.6	1.7	25	83.3
Hepatoblastoma	1	2	0	0	3	0.7	0.6	50.0	4.5	2.1	-	-	0.8	1.0	13	100.0
Hepatic carcinoma	0	0	0	2	2	0.5	0.5	33.3	-	-	-	1.7	0.5	0.5	8	100.0
Other and unspecified	0	0	1	0	1	0.2	0.2	16.7	-	-	0.8	-	0.3	0.3	4	-
VIII. BONE	2	1	11	17	31	7.1	7.7	100.0	9.0	1.0	8.7	14.2	8.5	7.9	127	83.9
Osteosarcoma	1	0	6	12	19	4.3	4.8	61.3	4.5	-	4.7	10.0	5.2	4.8	78	94.7
Chondrosarcoma	0	0	1	0	1	0.2	0.3	3.2	-	-	0.8	-	0.3	0.2	4	100.0
Ewing's sarcoma	0	0	2	3	5	1.1	1.3	16.1	-	-	1.6	2.5	1.4	1.2	20	100.0
Other and unspecified	1	1	2	2	6	1.4	1.4	19.4	4.5	1.0	1.6	1.7	1.6	1.7	25	33.3
IX. SOFT TISSUE SARCOMAS	1	9	8	2	20	4.6	4.4	100.0	4.5	9.4	6.3	1.7	5.5	5.8	82	100.0
Rhabdomyosarcoma	0	5	5	0	10	2.3	2.2	50.0	-	5.2	3.9	-	2.7	2.9	41	100.0
Fibrosarcoma	0	3	1	1	5	1.1	1.1	25.0	-	3.1	0.8	0.8	1.4	1.5	21	100.0
Other and unspecified	1	1	2	1	5	1.1	1.1	25.0	4.5	1.0	1.6	0.8	1.4	1.4	21	100.0
X. GONADAL & GERM CELL	1	6	2	7	16	3.6	3.8	100.0	4.5	6.3	1.6	5.8	4.4	4.5	67	100.0
Non-gonadal germ cell	1	5	0	1	7	1.6	1.5	43.8	4.5	5.2	-	0.8	1.9	2.2	30	100.0
Gonadal germ cell	0	1	2	6	9	2.1	2.3	56.3	-	1.0	1.6	5.0	2.5	2.3	37	100.0
Gonadal carcinoma	0	0	0	0	0	-	-	-	-	-	-	-	-	-	-	-
Other and unspecified	0	0	0	0	0	-	-	-	-	-	-	-	-	-	-	-
XI. EPITHELIAL NEOPLASMS	0	0	3	7	10	2.3	2.6	100.0	-	-	2.4	5.8	2.7	2.5	41	100.0
Adrenocortical carcinoma	0	0	0	0	0	-	-	-	-	-	-	-	-	-	-	-
Thyroid carcinoma	0	0	1	4	5	1.1	1.3	50.0	-	-	0.8	3.3	1.4	1.2	21	100.0
Nasopharyngeal carcinoma	0	0	0	0	0	-	-	-	-	-	-	-	-	-	-	-
Melanoma	0	0	1	1	2	0.5	0.5	20.0	-	-	0.8	0.8	0.5	0.5	8	100.0
Other carcinoma	0	0	1	2	3	0.7	0.8	30.0	-	-	0.8	1.7	0.8	0.7	12	100.0
XII. OTHER	3	3	0	2	8	1.8	1.8	100.0	13.5	3.1	-	1.7	2.2	2.5	34	12.5

* Specified as malignant

1983; Pastore *et al.*, 1986) and a case-control study on risk factors for leukaemias and soft-tissue sarcomas is under way.

Population

Annual estimates of the childhood population of the Province by sex and single year of age are available from local sources.

AVERAGE ANNUAL POPULATION: 1967–1981

Age	Male	Female
0	15936	14817
1–4	67420	63984
5–9	88814	84728
10–14	84569	80066
0–14	256739	243595

Commentary

The total incidence rate was the highest for any European registry. As the rates for many individual diagnostic groups were also high, this may well be largely due to unusually complete ascertainment and to the routine registration of cases from death certificates (46 cases) and post mortem findings. The incidence rates for liver tumours (mostly hepatoblastoma) and thyroid carcinoma were particularly high, but both these groups of rare tumours nevertheless contained small numbers of cases. The frequencies of brain and spinal tumours and of neuroblastoma were relatively low.

References

Pastore, G., Magnani, C., Zanetti, R. & Terracini, B. (1981) Incidence of cancer in the Province of Torino (Italy) 1967-68. *Eur. J. Cancer Oncol., 17,* 1337-1341

Magnani, C., Pastore, G., Cesana, B., Di Prima, S., Stalleri, D. & Terracini, B. (1983) Survival of children with cancer in Torino. *Med. Pediatr. Oncol., 11,* 263-268

Pastore, G., Magnani, C., Ghisetti, V., Terracini, B., Mosso, M.L. & Zanetti, R. (1986) Childhood cancer registry of the province of Torino: Survival patterns since 1967 and update of incidence rates. *Pediatr. Hematol. Oncol., 3,* 195-204

NETHERLANDS

Dutch Childhood Leukaemia Study Group (DCLSG), 1973–1982

J.W.W. Coebergh, A. van der Does-van den Berg, H.A. van Steensel-Moll,
E.R. van Wering & G.E. van Zanen

The DCLSG, which was set up by the Dutch Paediatric Society in 1972, aims to optimize and co-ordinate treatment of childhood leukaemia in the Netherlands and to stimulate research. Almost all paediatricians (98%) participate on a voluntary basis. The DCLSG is responsible for a central laboratory, registration of patients and collection of data during treatment and follow-up, as well as distributing protocols for treatment, supportive care and follow-up. The DCLSG was financed by a grant from the Ministry of Health and Environmental Hygiene from 1972 to 1975 and from private funds, through the Queen Wilhelmina Cancer Foundation, from 1975 to 1980. Since 1980, health insurance has provided a stable source of funding.

New registrations and regular updates of clinical data are recorded in the central office. The data are analysed by the European Organisation for the Research and Treatment of Cancer (EORTC) in Brussels. Cytomorphological examination of bone-marrow and blood smears and, recently, spinal fluid samples of every patient, is performed at diagnosis and regularly during treatment and follow-up. The French-American-British (FAB) classification has been used since 1975. Immunological phenotyping of leukaemia cells has been performed in collaboration with the Central Laboratory of the Red Cross Blood Transfusion Service in Amsterdam since 1979. Cytogenetic analysis of leukaemic cells has been carried out since 1984 through collaboration with specialized laboratories. Co-ordination of treatment has resulted in centralization of allogeneic bone-marrow transplantation for children with leukaemia in the Department of Paediatrics in the University Hospital in Leiden.

A nation-wide childhood leukaemia register was established in 1973. Its coverage proved to be about 97% complete in an evaluation study performed in 1980. The number of new cases of childhood leukaemia has varied between 100 and 125 per year, among a decreasing childhood population (0–14 years) of approximately 3.5 million. Incidence rates in urban areas are slightly higher than those in rural areas.

Access to medical care is excellent in all parts of the Netherlands. Patients are generally referred to paediatricians via general practitioners, of whom there were about one for every 3000 inhabitants in 1975. The 70% of the population in the lower income bracket are insured through sickness funds; the other 30% are nearly all privately insured.

The registry of the DCLSG covers the whole of the Netherlands, a densely populated country with about 400 inhabitants per square kilometre. Differences between urban and rural areas are, in general, not very large. They have been further reduced as a result of extensive migration out of the larger cities in the 1960s and 1970s.

In the 1970s, about 600 000 people migrated to the Netherlands from the Mediterranean region and from the former colony of Suriname. Until about 1970, approximately 40% of the population was Roman Catholic by birth, and the same percentage was Protestant. A strong trend towards secularization has occurred since that time.

Several epidemiological studies have been carried out, descriptive as well as etiological, in collaboration with the Department of Epidemiology, Erasmus University, Rotterdam (see references). These include a time trend analysis of incidence rates and a study of the geographical distribution. In addition to the leukaemia registration, a retrospective survey of children with malignant lymphoma has recently started.

Population

The population at risk has been calculated from the estimates for the Netherlands of 1973, 1976 and 1980, which are available as a result of continuous registration of the population (Central Bureau of Statistics).

AVERAGE ANNUAL POPULATION: 1973-1982

Age	Male	Female
0–4	495949	478508
5–9	583102	557012
10–14	624532	596623
0–14	1703583	1632143

Commentary

The rates are similar to those for other European registries.

References

Coebergh, J.W.W., van Steensel-Moll, H.A., van Wering, E.R. & van 't Veer, M.B. (1985) Epidemiological and immunological characteristics of childhood leukaemia in The Netherlands: population-based data from a nationwide co-operative group of paediatricians. *Leukaemia Res., 9,* 683-688

Van Steensel-Moll, H.A., Valkenburg, H.A. & van Zanen, G.E. (1983) Incidence of childhood leukaemia in the Netherlands (1973-1980). *Br. J. Cancer, 47,* 471-475

Van Steensel-Moll, H.A., Valkenburg, H.A., Vandenbroucke, J.P. & van Zanen, G.E. (1983) Time space distribution of childhood leukaemia in The Netherlands (1973-1980). *J. Epidemiol. comm. Health, 37,* 145-148

Netherlands, DCLSG

1973 – 1982

FEMALE

DIAGNOSTIC GROUP	NUMBER OF CASES					REL. FREQUENCY(%)			RATES PER MILLION						HV(%)
	0	1-4	5-9	10-14	All	Crude	Adj.	Group	0-4	5-9	10-14	Crude	Adj.	Cum	
I. LEUKAEMIAS	28	235	147	91	501	100.0	100.0	100.0	55.0	26.4	15.3	30.7	34.2	483	100.0
Acute lymphocytic	21	204	125	65	415	82.8	81.2	82.8	47.0	22.4	10.9	25.4	28.6	402	100.0
Other lymphocytic	0	0	0	0	0	-	-	-	-	-	-	-	-	-	
Acute non-lymphocytic	5	22	17	20	64	12.8	14.2	12.8	5.6	3.1	3.4	3.9	4.1	60	100.0
Chronic myeloid	0	5	5	4	14	2.8	3.1	2.8	1.0	0.9	0.7	0.9	0.9	13	100.0
Other and unspecified	2	4	0	2	8	1.6	1.6	1.6	1.3	-	0.3	0.5	0.6	8	100.0

Netherlands, DCLSG

1973 – 1982

MALE

DIAGNOSTIC GROUP	NUMBER OF CASES					REL. FREQUENCY(%)			RATES PER MILLION						HV(%)
	0	1-4	5-9	10-14	All	Crude	Adj.	Group	0-4	5-9	10-14	Crude	Adj.	Cum	
I. LEUKAEMIAS	30	292	187	117	626	100.0	100.0	100.0	64.9	32.1	18.7	36.7	40.9	579	100.0
Acute lymphocytic	19	255	150	85	509	81.3	79.9	81.3	55.2	25.7	13.6	29.9	33.6	473	100.0
Other lymphocytic	0	0	0	0	0	-	-	-	-	-	-	-	-	-	
Acute non-lymphocytic	6	21	29	23	79	12.6	13.9	12.6	5.4	5.0	3.7	4.6	4.8	71	100.0
Chronic myeloid	2	13	5	5	25	4.0	3.9	4.0	3.0	0.9	0.8	1.5	1.7	23	100.0
Other and unspecified	3	3	3	4	13	2.1	2.3	2.1	1.2	0.5	0.6	0.8	0.8	12	100.0

South-East Registry (IKZ/SOOZ), Eindhoven, 1973–1983

J.W.W. Coebergh, D. Bakker, M.A. Crommelin,
L. van der Heyden & M. Verhagen-Teulings

This regional cancer registry began operation in 1955 as part of a national cancer registration programme. It started as an oncological documentation project in three hospitals in Eindhoven, a major city in the south-eastern part of the Netherlands. In 1979, the continuation of the registry was assured by the setting up of a cancer organization for the region — the Cooperative Association of Hospitals in Oncology Care (Fig. 4.)

Fig. 4. The Netherlands, showing the SOOZ Cancer Registry area

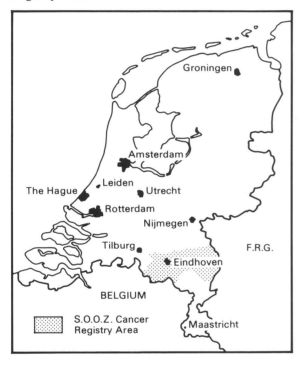

An evaluation of the registry during 1981-1983 revealed that completeness had largely been attained since 1976 for most tumour sites in the greater part of the region. For epidemiological reasons, the registration area was divided into a central 'core' area covering about 85% of the inhabitants (6% of the total Dutch population) and a peripheral 'peel' area. The registration of childhood cancer appeared to be somewhat incomplete, as quite a few patients are directly referred to major

oncological centres, all of them located outside the area. Neurosurgical and ophthalmological treatment of children takes place entirely outside the area. Additional data have therefore been collected on patients from the core area in the major centres, and have been taken into account in the data presented here.

There is virtually free access to medical care as a result of the relatively short distances that patients have to travel, adequate health services and the existence of a health insurance system. The childhood population is served by about 20 paediatricians working in 11 general hospitals. Specialized cancer centres are located elsewhere. The Radiotherapy Department in Eindhoven serves all the hospitals. The diagnosis of leukaemia has been confirmed in all patients through a review of bone marrow slides in the Central Laboratory of the Dutch Childhood Leukaemia Study Group in The Hague.

During the period 1973–1983, the sources of data were voluntary reporting by doctors; regular, active and personal collection of data from patient files in the hospitals by the registration staff; and miscellaneous sources, including reports from radiotherapy, pathology and medical records departments, and regular checks in three hospitals located just outside the region and in university hospitals.

For the present publication, searches for additional cases were carried out in several other hospitals and organizations. Approximately 80% of the patients were already known to the registry. It can be estimated that ascertainment is virtually complete for leukaemia from 1973 and for solid tumours from 1976.

The registry covers an area of more than 2000 square kilometres at an altitude of 20–30 metres above sea-level. The total population is slightly more than 800 000 inhabitants, with an average density of 400 per square kilometre. The average number of children was about 200 000. The population as a whole was largely (over 80%) Roman Catholic, this percentage being higher in the more rural areas. The region consists to a large extent of industrial and agricultural areas.

Contd. p. 270

Netherlands, SOOZ, Eindhoven   1973 - 1983   MALE

DIAGNOSTIC GROUP	NUMBER OF CASES					REL. FREQUENCY(%)			RATES PER MILLION					Cum	HV(%)
	0	1-4	5-9	10-14	All	Crude	Adj.	Group	0-4	5-9	10-14	Crude	Adj.		
TOTAL	16	47	36	39	138	100.0	100.0	100.0	212.7	95.8	95.5	127.7	141.0	2020	96.4
I. LEUKAEMIAS	3	25	13	6	47	34.1	33.2	100.0	94.5	34.6	14.7	43.5	52.0	719	97.9
Acute lymphocytic	0	16	12	4	32	23.2	23.2	68.1	54.0	31.9	9.8	29.6	34.1	479	100.0
Other lymphocytic	0	1	0	1	2	1.4	1.4	4.3	3.4	-	2.4	1.9	2.0	29	100.0
Acute non-lymphocytic	1	5	1	1	8	5.8	5.4	17.0	20.3	2.7	2.4	7.4	9.4	127	100.0
Chronic myeloid	1	3	0	0	4	2.9	2.5	8.5	13.5	-	-	3.7	5.2	68	100.0
Other and unspecified	1	0	0	0	1	0.7	0.6	2.1	3.4	-	-	0.9	1.3	17	-
II. LYMPHOMAS	4	4	9	5	22	15.9	16.4	100.0	27.0	24.0	12.2	20.4	21.7	316	100.0
Hodgkin's disease	0	1	1	1	3	2.2	2.2	13.6	3.4	2.7	2.4	2.8	2.9	42	100.0
Non-Hodgkin lymphoma	1	2	7	4	14	10.1	10.8	63.6	10.1	18.6	9.8	13.0	12.8	193	100.0
Burkitt's lymphoma	0	0	0	0	0	-	-	-	-	-	-	-	-	-	-
Unspecified lymphoma	0	1	0	0	1	0.7	0.6	4.5	3.4	-	-	0.9	1.3	17	100.0
Histiocytosis X	2	0	0	0	2	1.4	1.3	9.1	6.8	-	-	1.9	2.6	34	100.0
Other reticuloendothelial	1	0	1	0	2	1.4	1.5	9.1	3.4	2.7	-	1.9	2.2	30	100.0
III. BRAIN AND SPINAL	3	5	6	7	21	15.2	15.5	100.0	27.0	16.0	17.1	19.4	20.6	301	85.7
Ependymoma	0	1	0	0	1	0.7	0.6	4.8	3.4	-	-	0.9	1.3	17	100.0
Astrocytoma	0	2	2	5	9	6.5	6.8	42.9	6.8	5.3	12.2	8.3	7.9	122	100.0
Medulloblastoma	1	1	1	0	3	2.2	2.1	14.3	6.8	2.7	-	2.8	3.5	47	100.0
Other glioma	1	0	2	1	4	2.9	2.9	19.0	3.4	5.3	2.4	3.7	3.7	56	100.0
Other and unspecified *	1	1	1	1	4	2.9	2.9	19.0	6.8	2.7	2.4	3.7	4.2	59	25.0
IV. SYMPATHETIC N.S.	2	3	1	0	6	4.3	4.0	100.0	16.9	2.7	-	5.6	7.4	98	100.0
Neuroblastoma	2	3	1	0	6	4.3	4.0	100.0	16.9	2.7	-	5.6	7.4	98	100.0
Other	0	0	0	0	0	-	-	-	-	-	-	-	-	-	-
V. RETINOBLASTOMA	0	0	1	0	1	0.7	0.8	100.0	-	2.7	-	0.9	0.9	13	100.0
VI. KIDNEY	1	4	1	0	6	4.3	4.0	100.0	16.9	2.7	-	5.6	7.4	98	100.0
Wilms' tumour	1	4	1	0	6	4.3	4.0	100.0	16.9	2.7	-	5.6	7.4	98	100.0
Renal carcinoma	0	0	0	0	0	-	-	-	-	-	-	-	-	-	-
Other and unspecified	0	0	0	0	0	-	-	-	-	-	-	-	-	-	-
VII. LIVER	0	1	0	0	1	0.7	0.6	100.0	3.4	-	-	0.9	1.3	17	100.0
Hepatoblastoma	0	1	0	0	1	0.7	0.6	100.0	3.4	-	-	0.9	1.3	17	100.0
Hepatic carcinoma	0	0	0	0	0	-	-	-	-	-	-	-	-	-	-
Other and unspecified	0	0	0	0	0	-	-	-	-	-	-	-	-	-	-
VIII. BONE	0	0	1	7	8	5.8	6.2	100.0	-	2.7	17.1	7.4	5.8	99	100.0
Osteosarcoma	0	0	0	4	4	2.9	3.1	50.0	-	-	9.8	3.7	2.8	49	100.0
Chondrosarcoma	0	0	0	1	1	0.7	0.8	12.5	-	-	2.4	0.9	0.7	12	100.0
Ewing's sarcoma	0	0	1	2	3	2.2	2.4	37.5	-	2.7	4.9	2.8	2.3	38	100.0
Other and unspecified	0	0	0	0	0	-	-	-	-	-	-	-	-	-	-
IX. SOFT TISSUE SARCOMAS	0	2	3	2	7	5.1	5.3	100.0	6.8	8.0	4.9	6.5	6.6	98	100.0
Rhabdomyosarcoma	0	2	2	0	4	2.9	2.9	57.1	6.8	5.3	-	3.7	4.3	60	100.0
Fibrosarcoma	0	0	1	0	1	0.7	0.8	14.3	-	2.7	-	0.9	0.9	13	100.0
Other and unspecified	0	0	0	2	2	1.4	1.5	28.6	-	-	4.9	1.9	1.4	24	100.0
X. GONADAL & GERM CELL	2	3	0	0	5	3.6	3.2	100.0	16.9	-	-	4.6	6.5	84	100.0
Non-gonadal germ cell	1	0	0	0	1	0.7	0.6	20.0	3.4	-	-	0.9	1.3	17	100.0
Gonadal germ cell	1	3	0	0	4	2.9	2.5	80.0	13.5	-	-	3.7	5.2	68	100.0
Gonadal carcinoma	0	0	0	0	0	-	-	-	-	-	-	-	-	-	-
Other and unspecified	0	0	0	0	0	-	-	-	-	-	-	-	-	-	-
XI. EPITHELIAL NEOPLASMS	1	0	1	12	14	10.1	10.7	100.0	3.4	2.7	29.4	13.0	10.7	177	92.9
Adrenocortical carcinoma	0	0	0	0	0	-	-	-	-	-	-	-	-	-	-
Thyroid carcinoma	0	0	0	0	0	-	-	-	-	-	-	-	-	-	-
Nasopharyngeal carcinoma	0	0	0	0	0	-	-	-	-	-	-	-	-	-	-
Melanoma	0	0	1	1	2	1.4	1.6	14.3	-	2.7	2.4	1.9	1.6	26	100.0
Other carcinoma	1	0	0	11	12	8.7	9.1	85.7	3.4	-	26.9	11.1	9.1	151	91.7
XII. OTHER	0	0	0	0	0	-	-	-	-	-	-	-	-	-	-
* Specified as malignant	1	1	1	0	3	2.2	2.1	100.0	6.8	2.7	-	2.8	3.5	47	-

Netherlands, SOOZ, Eindhoven

1973 - 1983

FEMALE

DIAGNOSTIC GROUP	NUMBER OF CASES					REL. FREQUENCY(%)			RATES PER MILLION						HV(%)
	0	1-4	5-9	10-14	All	Crude	Adj.	Group	0-4	5-9	10-14	Crude	Adj.	Cum	
TOTAL	11	30	22	34	97	100.0	100.0	100.0	145.5	61.5	85.9	93.7	101.1	1465	95.9
I. LEUKAEMIAS	1	14	8	8	31	32.0	32.6	100.0	53.2	22.4	20.2	29.9	33.7	479	100.0
Acute lymphocytic	1	12	8	4	25	25.8	27.1	80.6	46.1	22.4	10.1	24.1	28.0	393	100.0
Other lymphocytic	0	0	0	1	1	1.0	0.9	3.2	-	-	2.5	1.0	0.7	13	100.0
Acute non-lymphocytic	0	2	0	3	5	5.2	4.6	16.1	7.1	-	7.6	4.8	4.9	73	100.0
Chronic myeloid	0	0	0	0	0	-	-	-	-	-	-	-	-	-	-
Other and unspecified	0	0	0	0	0	-	-	-	-	-	-	-	-	-	-
II. LYMPHOMAS	0	3	2	4	9	9.3	9.2	100.0	10.6	5.6	10.1	8.7	8.9	132	100.0
Hodgkin's disease	0	0	1	3	4	4.1	4.0	44.4	-	2.8	7.6	3.9	3.1	52	100.0
Non-Hodgkin lymphoma	0	2	1	1	4	4.1	4.2	44.4	7.1	2.8	2.5	3.9	4.4	62	100.0
Burkitt's lymphoma	0	0	0	0	0	-	-	-	-	-	-	-	-	-	-
Unspecified lymphoma	0	0	0	0	0	-	-	-	-	-	-	-	-	-	-
Histiocytosis X	0	0	0	0	0	-	-	-	-	-	-	-	-	-	-
other reticuloendothelial	0	1	0	0	1	1.0	1.0	11.1	3.5	-	-	1.0	1.4	18	100.0
III. BRAIN AND SPINAL	0	2	4	5	11	11.3	11.8	100.0	7.1	11.2	12.6	10.6	10.0	155	81.8
Ependymoma	0	1	0	0	1	1.0	1.0	9.1	3.5	-	-	1.0	1.0	18	100.0
Astrocytoma	0	0	2	4	6	6.2	6.3	54.5	-	5.6	10.1	5.8	4.7	78	100.0
Medulloblastoma	0	1	1	0	2	2.1	2.3	18.2	3.5	2.8	-	1.9	2.3	32	100.0
other glioma	0	0	0	0	0	-	-	-	-	-	-	-	-	-	-
Other and unspecified *	0	0	1	1	2	2.1	2.2	18.2	-	2.8	2.5	1.9	1.6	27	-
IV. SYMPATHETIC N.S.	2	4	0	0	6	6.2	5.9	100.0	21.3	-	-	5.8	8.2	106	100.0
Neuroblastoma	2	4	0	0	6	6.2	5.9	100.0	21.3	-	-	5.8	8.2	106	100.0
Other	0	0	0	0	0	-	-	-	-	-	-	-	-	-	-
V. RETINOBLASTOMA	6	1	0	0	7	7.2	6.8	100.0	24.8	-	-	6.8	9.6	124	100.0
VI. KIDNEY	0	2	1	0	3	3.1	3.3	100.0	7.1	2.8	-	2.9	3.6	49	100.0
Wilms' tumour	0	2	1	0	3	3.1	3.3	100.0	7.1	2.8	-	2.9	3.6	49	100.0
Renal carcinoma	0	0	0	0	0	-	-	-	-	-	-	-	-	-	-
Other and unspecified	0	0	0	0	0	-	-	-	-	-	-	-	-	-	-
VII. LIVER	0	0	0	0	0	-	-	-	-	-	-	-	-	-	-
Hepatoblastoma	0	0	0	0	0	-	-	-	-	-	-	-	-	-	-
Hepatic carcinoma	0	0	0	0	0	-	-	-	-	-	-	-	-	-	-
Other and unspecified	0	0	0	0	0	-	-	-	-	-	-	-	-	-	-
VIII. BONE	0	0	4	5	9	9.3	9.9	100.0	-	11.2	12.6	8.7	7.3	119	100.0
Osteosarcoma	0	0	2	4	6	6.2	6.3	66.7	-	5.6	10.1	5.8	4.7	78	100.0
Chondrosarcoma	0	0	0	0	0	-	-	-	-	-	-	-	-	-	-
Ewing's sarcoma	0	0	2	1	3	3.1	3.6	33.3	-	5.6	2.5	2.9	2.5	41	100.0
Other and unspecified	0	0	0	0	0	-	-	-	-	-	-	-	-	-	-
IX. SOFT TISSUE SARCOMAS	1	4	3	2	10	10.3	10.7	100.0	17.7	8.4	5.1	9.7	11.0	156	100.0
Rhabdomyosarcoma	0	3	1	1	5	5.2	5.1	50.0	7.1	2.8	5.1	4.8	5.1	75	100.0
Fibrosarcoma	0	0	0	0	0	-	-	-	-	-	-	-	-	-	-
Other and unspecified	1	2	2	0	5	5.2	5.7	50.0	10.6	5.6	-	4.8	5.9	81	100.0
X. GONADAL & GERM CELL	0	0	0	2	2	2.1	1.8	100.0	-	-	5.1	1.9	1.5	25	100.0
Non-gonadal germ cell	0	0	0	0	0	-	-	-	-	-	-	-	-	-	-
Gonadal germ cell	0	0	0	2	2	2.1	1.8	100.0	-	-	5.1	1.9	1.5	25	100.0
Gonadal carcinoma	0	0	0	0	0	-	-	-	-	-	-	-	-	-	-
Other and unspecified	0	0	0	0	0	-	-	-	-	-	-	-	-	-	-
XI. EPITHELIAL NEOPLASMS	1	0	0	7	8	8.2	7.2	100.0	3.5	-	17.7	7.7	6.5	106	87.5
Adrenocortical carcinoma	0	0	0	0	0	-	-	-	-	-	-	-	-	-	-
Thyroid carcinoma	0	0	0	1	1	1.0	0.9	12.5	-	-	2.5	1.0	0.7	13	100.0
Nasopharyngeal carcinoma	0	0	0	1	1	1.0	0.9	12.5	-	-	2.5	1.0	0.7	13	100.0
Melanoma	0	0	0	2	2	2.1	1.8	25.0	-	-	5.1	1.9	1.5	25	100.0
Other carcinoma	1	0	0	3	4	4.1	3.6	50.0	3.5	-	7.6	3.9	3.6	56	75.0
XII. OTHER	0	0	0	1	1	1.0	0.9	100.0	-	-	2.5	1.0	0.7	13	-
* Specified as malignant	0	0	1	1	2	2.1	2.2	100.0	-	2.8	2.5	1.9	1.6	27	-

Population

The population at risk has been calculated from estimates for 1977 and 1982, available as a result of continuous recording in all communities in the Netherlands (Central Bureau of Statistics).

AVERAGE ANNUAL POPULATION: 1973–1983

Age	Male	Female
0–4	26928	25609
5–9	34155	32526
10–14	37144	35982
0–14	98227	94117

Commentary

The rates are generally similar to those for other European registries except that those for brain tumours are rather low, possibly because tumours of unspecified nature are not registered.

NORWAY

The Cancer Registry of Norway, 1970–1979

F. Langmark

The Cancer Registry of Norway has been in operation since 1952. Based on compulsory notification, registration covers the whole of Norway and aims at complete ascertainment of all cases of cancer. According to the rules laid down by the Ministry of Social Affairs, reports are required from all hospital departments and institutes of pathology. Every new cancer patient must be reported, whether treated or not, whether in hospital or seen only as an out-patient. A new report, filled in and signed by a physician, must be submitted each time a cancer patient is readmitted or re-examined for his malignant disease. Instead of submitting reports, some hospitals prefer to send original patient records for abstracting in the Cancer Registry.

Most cases are reported several times from different institutions (the average number of reports per case registered is over six), increasing the probability that a case will eventually be registered and resulting in more accurate and complete information. The quality and completeness of cancer registration has been assessed by means of a national survey covering all patients in hospitals or other institutions for cancer or other diseases on a given date. Results show that reporting from these sources is very nearly complete. Reporting from pathologists is excellent and increasingly tends to cover not only the definitely malignant but also a broad spectrum of semi-malignant and borderline cases. Histiocytosis X, however, is not registered. Approximately 1% of all cancer cases are registered on the basis of death certificates only.

Data from the Registry have been used for a variety of epidemiological studies, including several on childhood cancer (Bjelke, 1964a,b, 1970).

Norway, 324 000 square kilometres in area, is bounded on the north by the Arctic Ocean, on the west and south by the North Sea, and on the east by Finland, Sweden and the USSR. The population in 1975 was 4.02 million, of whom 24% were children aged 0–14. Approximately 0.5% of the population are Lapps, the remainder being Caucasian. The main occupations for males over 15 years were (1970): industry 31%, public and personal services 15%, construction 14%, commerce 13%, transport 12%, agriculture and forestry 11% and fishing 4%. Of the total population, 19% live in conurbations of more than 100 000 inhabitants.

Population

Annual population estimates by single year of age are available from the Central Bureau of Statistics.

AVERAGE ANNUAL POPULATION: 1970–1979

Age	Male	Female
0	29417	27961
1–4	125970	120123
5–9	166600	158079
10–14	162171	153919
0–14	484158	460082

Commentary

In general the rates were typical of those for most European registries. Among the leukaemias, 28% were in the 'other and unspecified' category. The age-distribution of these cases suggests that they were predominantly acute lymphocytic.

The rates for lymphomas, both Hodgkin's disease and others, were the lowest in any European registry.

There was a high incidence of liver tumours in boys, though this is based on only 14 cases; over half these tumours were carcinomas.

The rate for Ewing's sarcoma was very low, but 11 out of 50 bone tumours were 'other and unspeci-

Contd p. 274

1970 – 1979

Values are grouped as: NUMBER OF CASES (0, 1-4, 5-9, 10-14, All) | REL. FREQUENCY(%) (Crude, Adj., Group) | RATES PER MILLION (0, 1-4, 5-9, 10-14, Crude, Adj., Cum) | HV(%)

DIAGNOSTIC GROUP	Cases 0	1-4	5-9	10-14	All	RF Crude	RF Adj.	RF Group	Rate 0	1-4	5-9	10-14	Crude	Adj.	Cum	HV(%)
TOTAL	57	243	184	155	639	100.0	100.0	100.0	193.8	192.9	110.4	95.6	132.0	138.1	1995	95.9
I. LEUKAEMIAS	12	111	63	42	228	35.7	34.8	100.0	40.8	88.1	37.8	25.9	47.1	50.2	712	99.1
Acute lymphocytic	3	59	33	15	110	17.2	16.6	48.2	10.2	46.8	19.8	9.2	22.7	24.4	343	100.0
Other lymphocytic	-	1	1	-	2	0.3	0.3	0.9	-	0.8	0.6	-	0.4	0.4	6	100.0
Acute non-lymphocytic	2	9	7	20	38	5.9	6.5	16.7	6.8	7.1	4.2	12.3	7.8	7.7	118	100.0
Chronic myeloid	-	4	-	1	5	0.8	0.7	2.2	-	3.2	-	0.6	1.0	1.2	16	80.0
Other and unspecified	7	38	22	6	73	11.4	10.7	32.0	23.8	30.2	13.2	3.7	15.1	16.5	229	98.6
II. LYMPHOMAS	-	10	24	25	59	9.2	10.1	100.0	-	7.9	14.4	15.4	12.2	11.6	181	100.0
Hodgkin's disease	-	-	8	8	16	2.5	2.9	27.1	-	-	4.8	4.9	3.3	3.0	49	100.0
Non-Hodgkin lymphoma	-	4	8	14	26	4.1	4.5	44.1	-	3.2	4.8	8.6	5.4	5.0	80	100.0
Burkitt's lymphoma	-	-	3	2	5	0.8	0.9	8.5	-	-	1.8	1.2	1.0	0.9	15	100.0
Unspecified lymphoma	-	6	5	1	12	1.9	1.8	20.3	-	4.8	3.0	0.6	2.5	2.6	37	100.0
Histiocytosis X	-	-	-	-	-	-	-	-	-	-	-	-	-	-	-	-
Other reticuloendothelial	-	-	-	-	-	-	-	-	-	-	-	-	-	-	-	-
III. BRAIN AND SPINAL	10	42	53	39	144	22.5	23.1	100.0	34.0	33.3	31.8	24.0	29.7	30.2	447	87.5
Ependymoma	-	4	1	2	7	1.1	1.1	4.9	-	3.2	0.6	1.2	1.4	1.5	22	100.0
Astrocytoma	2	13	25	15	55	8.6	9.0	38.2	6.8	10.3	15.0	9.2	11.4	11.5	169	98.2
Medulloblastoma	2	8	12	6	28	4.4	4.5	19.4	6.8	6.4	7.2	3.7	5.8	5.9	87	100.0
Other glioma	2	6	5	11	24	3.8	4.0	16.7	6.8	4.8	3.0	6.8	5.0	4.9	75	100.0
Other and unspecified *	4	11	10	5	30	4.7	4.6	20.8	13.6	8.7	6.0	3.1	6.2	6.6	94	43.3
IV. SYMPATHETIC N.S.	11	9	10	2	32	5.0	4.7	100.0	37.4	7.1	6.0	1.2	6.6	7.4	102	96.9
Neuroblastoma	11	9	10	2	32	5.0	4.7	100.0	37.4	7.1	6.0	1.2	6.6	7.4	102	96.9
Other	-	-	-	-	-	-	-	-	-	-	-	-	-	-	-	-
V. RETINOBLASTOMA	4	9	1	-	14	2.2	1.9	100.0	13.6	7.1	0.6	-	2.9	3.5	45	100.0
VI. KIDNEY	7	23	10	-	40	6.3	5.6	100.0	23.8	18.3	6.0	-	8.3	9.4	127	97.5
Wilms' tumour	7	20	9	-	36	5.6	5.1	90.0	23.8	15.9	5.4	-	7.4	8.5	114	100.0
Renal carcinoma	-	1	-	-	1	0.2	0.2	2.5	-	0.8	-	-	0.2	0.2	4	100.0
Other and unspecified	-	2	1	-	3	0.5	0.4	7.5	-	1.6	0.6	-	0.6	0.7	9	66.7
VII. LIVER	5	5	3	1	14	2.2	2.1	100.0	17.0	4.0	1.8	0.6	2.9	3.3	45	92.9
Hepatoblastoma	5	-	-	-	5	0.8	0.9	35.7	17.0	-	-	-	1.0	1.2	16	100.0
Hepatic carcinoma	-	5	2	1	8	1.3	1.2	57.1	-	4.0	1.2	0.6	1.7	1.8	26	100.0
Other and unspecified	-	-	1	-	1	0.2	0.1	7.1	-	-	0.6	-	0.2	0.2	3	-
VIII. BONE	-	-	9	22	31	4.9	5.4	100.0	-	-	5.4	13.6	6.4	6.0	95	96.8
Osteosarcoma	-	-	7	12	19	3.0	3.5	61.3	-	-	4.2	7.4	3.9	3.5	58	100.0
Chondrosarcoma	-	-	-	1	1	0.2	0.2	3.2	-	-	-	0.6	0.2	0.2	3	100.0
Ewing's sarcoma	-	-	-	2	2	0.3	0.2	6.5	-	-	-	1.2	0.4	0.4	6	100.0
Other and unspecified	-	-	2	7	9	1.4	1.4	29.0	-	-	1.2	4.3	1.9	2.0	28	88.9
IX. SOFT TISSUE SARCOMAS	2	6	5	7	20	3.1	3.2	100.0	6.8	4.8	3.0	4.3	4.1	4.2	62	100.0
Rhabdomyosarcoma	1	3	2	-	6	0.9	0.9	30.0	3.4	2.4	1.2	-	1.2	1.4	19	100.0
Fibrosarcoma	1	2	2	2	7	1.1	1.2	35.0	3.4	1.6	1.2	1.2	1.4	1.5	22	100.0
Other and unspecified	-	1	1	5	7	1.1	1.1	35.0	-	0.8	0.6	3.1	1.4	1.3	22	100.0
X. GONADAL & GERM CELL	6	11	-	5	22	3.4	3.2	100.0	20.4	8.7	-	3.1	4.5	5.2	71	100.0
Non-gonadal germ cell	4	-	-	-	4	0.6	0.7	18.2	13.6	-	-	-	0.8	0.9	13	100.0
Gonadal germ cell	2	8	-	5	15	2.3	2.2	68.2	6.8	6.4	-	3.1	3.1	3.6	48	100.0
Gonadal carcinoma	-	-	-	-	-	-	-	-	-	-	-	-	-	-	-	-
Other and unspecified	-	3	-	-	3	0.5	0.4	13.6	-	2.4	-	-	0.6	0.8	10	100.0
XI. EPITHELIAL NEOPLASMS	-	2	6	11	19	3.0	3.4	100.0	-	1.6	3.6	6.8	3.9	3.6	58	100.0
Adrenocortical carcinoma	-	1	-	1	2	0.3	0.3	10.5	-	0.8	-	0.6	0.4	0.4	6	100.0
Thyroid carcinoma	-	-	1	1	2	0.3	0.4	10.5	-	-	0.6	0.6	0.4	0.4	6	100.0
Nasopharyngeal carcinoma	-	-	-	1	1	0.2	0.2	5.3	-	-	-	0.6	0.2	0.2	3	100.0
Melanoma	-	1	3	3	7	1.1	1.2	36.8	-	0.8	1.8	1.8	1.4	1.3	21	100.0
Other carcinoma	-	-	2	5	7	1.1	1.3	36.8	-	-	1.2	3.1	1.4	1.3	21	100.0
XII. OTHER	-	10	2	4	16	2.5	2.4	100.0	-	7.9	1.2	2.5	3.3	3.6	50	87.5
* Specified as malignant	4	11	10	4	29	4.5	4.4	100.0	13.6	8.7	6.0	2.5	6.0	6.4	91	41.4

Norway

FEMALE

1970 – 1979

DIAGNOSTIC GROUP	NUMBER OF CASES					REL. FREQUENCY(%)			RATES PER MILLION							HV(%)
	0	1-4	5-9	10-14	All	Crude	Adj.	Group	0	1-4	5-9	10-14	Crude	Adj.	Cum	
TOTAL	48	173	127	117	465	100.0	100.0	100.0	171.7	144.0	80.3	76.0	101.1	105.9	1529	97.0
I. LEUKAEMIAS	13	84	45	23	165	35.5	34.1	100.0	46.5	69.9	28.5	14.9	35.9	38.8	543	99.4
Acute lymphocytic	4	53	17	11	85	18.3	17.2	51.5	14.3	44.1	10.8	7.1	18.5	20.3	280	100.0
Other lymphocytic	0	1	0	0	1	0.2	0.2	0.6	–	0.8	–	–	0.2	0.3	3	100.0
Acute non-lymphocytic	4	9	15	10	38	8.2	8.5	23.0	14.3	7.5	9.5	6.5	8.2	8.3	124	100.0
Chronic myeloid	1	1	1	0	3	0.6	0.6	1.8	3.6	0.8	0.6	–	0.7	0.7	10	100.0
Other and unspecified	4	20	12	2	38	8.2	7.7	23.0	14.3	16.6	7.6	1.3	8.3	9.1	125	97.4
II. LYMPHOMAS	2	6	6	8	22	4.7	4.9	100.0	7.2	5.0	3.8	5.2	4.8	4.8	72	100.0
Hodgkin's disease	0	1	2	6	9	1.9	2.2	40.9	–	0.8	1.3	3.9	2.0	1.8	29	100.0
Non-Hodgkin lymphoma	1	4	3	1	9	1.9	1.9	40.9	3.6	3.3	1.9	0.6	2.0	2.1	30	100.0
Burkitt's lymphoma	0	0	1	0	1	0.2	0.2	4.5	–	–	0.6	–	0.2	0.2	1	100.0
Unspecified lymphoma	0	1	0	1	2	0.4	0.4	9.1	–	0.8	–	0.6	0.4	0.5	6	100.0
Histiocytosis X	1	0	0	0	1	0.2	0.2	4.5	3.6	–	–	–	0.2	0.3	4	100.0
Other reticuloendothelial	0	0	0	0	0	–	–	–	–	–	–	–	–	–	–	–
III. BRAIN AND SPINAL	7	23	40	35	105	22.6	23.9	100.0	25.0	19.1	25.3	22.7	22.8	22.6	342	88.6
Ependymoma	0	2	2	0	4	0.9	0.8	3.8	–	1.7	1.3	–	0.9	0.8	13	100.0
Astrocytoma	3	12	24	20	59	12.7	13.5	56.2	10.7	10.0	15.2	13.0	12.8	12.6	192	100.0
Medulloblastoma	2	2	2	5	11	2.4	2.5	10.5	7.2	1.7	1.3	3.2	2.4	2.4	36	100.0
Other glioma	2	2	5	4	13	2.8	3.1	12.4	7.2	1.7	3.2	2.6	2.8	2.7	42	100.0
Other and unspecified *	0	5	7	6	18	3.9	3.9	17.1	–	4.2	4.4	3.9	3.9	4.0	59	33.3
IV. SYMPATHETIC N.S.	10	11	5	0	26	5.6	5.0	100.0	35.8	9.2	3.2	–	5.7	6.6	88	100.0
Neuroblastoma	10	11	5	0	26	5.6	5.0	100.0	35.8	9.2	3.2	–	5.7	6.6	88	100.0
Other	0	0	0	0	0	–	–	–	–	–	–	–	–	–	–	–
V. RETINOBLASTOMA	5	7	0	0	12	2.6	2.2	100.0	17.9	5.8	–	–	2.6	3.2	41	100.0
VI. KIDNEY	2	18	8	1	29	6.2	5.8	100.0	7.2	15.0	5.1	0.6	6.3	7.0	96	96.6
Wilms' tumour	2	17	5	1	25	5.4	4.9	86.2	7.2	14.2	3.2	0.6	5.4	6.1	83	100.0
Renal carcinoma	0	1	3	0	4	0.9	0.9	13.8	–	0.8	1.9	–	0.9	0.9	13	75.0
Other and unspecified	0	0	0	0	0	–	–	–	–	–	–	–	–	–	–	–
VII. LIVER	1	1	0	0	2	0.4	0.4	100.0	3.6	0.8	–	–	0.4	0.5	7	100.0
Hepatoblastoma	1	0	0	0	1	0.2	0.2	50.0	3.6	–	–	–	0.2	0.3	3	100.0
Hepatic carcinoma	0	1	0	0	1	0.2	0.2	50.0	–	0.8	–	–	0.2	0.2	4	100.0
Other and unspecified	0	0	0	0	0	–	–	–	–	–	–	–	–	–	–	–
VIII. BONE	0	1	6	12	19	4.1	4.7	100.0	–	0.8	3.8	7.8	4.1	3.7	61	100.0
Osteosarcoma	0	0	5	6	11	2.4	2.7	57.9	–	–	3.2	3.9	2.4	2.2	35	100.0
Chondrosarcoma	0	0	1	2	3	0.6	0.7	15.8	–	–	0.6	1.3	0.6	0.6	10	100.0
Ewing's sarcoma	0	0	0	3	3	0.6	0.8	15.8	–	–	–	1.9	0.6	0.4	10	100.0
Other and unspecified	0	1	0	1	2	0.4	0.4	10.5	–	0.8	–	0.6	0.4	0.4	7	100.0
IX. SOFT TISSUE SARCOMAS	6	10	10	8	34	7.3	7.3	100.0	21.5	8.3	6.3	5.2	7.4	7.8	112	100.0
Rhabdomyosarcoma	3	6	5	2	16	3.4	3.3	47.1	10.7	5.0	3.2	1.3	3.5	3.8	53	100.0
Fibrosarcoma	2	0	4	2	8	1.7	1.8	23.5	7.2	–	2.5	1.3	1.7	1.7	26	100.0
Other and unspecified	1	4	1	4	10	2.2	2.2	29.4	3.6	3.3	0.6	2.6	2.2	2.3	33	100.0
X. GONADAL & GERM CELL	1	3	0	11	15	3.2	3.5	100.0	3.6	2.5	–	7.1	3.3	3.1	49	100.0
Non-gonadal germ cell	1	2	0	1	4	0.9	0.8	26.7	3.6	1.7	–	0.6	0.9	1.0	13	100.0
Gonadal germ cell	0	1	0	9	10	2.2	2.6	66.7	–	0.8	–	6.5	2.2	1.9	32	100.0
Gonadal carcinoma	0	0	0	1	1	0.2	0.2	6.7	–	–	–	0.6	0.2	0.3	3	100.0
Other and unspecified	0	0	0	0	0	–	–	–	–	–	–	–	–	–	–	–
XI. EPITHELIAL NEOPLASMS	0	4	4	14	22	4.7	5.3	100.0	–	3.3	2.5	9.1	4.8	4.5	71	100.0
Adrenocortical carcinoma	0	0	0	0	0	–	–	–	–	–	–	–	–	–	–	–
Thyroid carcinoma	0	0	0	6	6	1.3	1.5	27.3	–	–	–	3.9	1.3	1.1	19	100.0
Nasopharyngeal carcinoma	0	0	1	0	1	0.2	0.3	4.5	–	–	0.6	–	0.2	0.2	3	100.0
Melanoma	0	3	3	4	10	2.2	2.3	45.5	–	2.5	1.9	2.6	2.2	2.2	32	100.0
Other carcinoma	0	1	0	4	5	1.1	1.2	22.7	–	0.8	–	2.6	1.1	1.0	16	100.0
XII. OTHER	1	5	3	5	14	3.0	3.1	100.0	3.6	4.2	1.9	3.2	3.0	3.1	46	100.0
* Specified as malignant	2	5	7	4	18	3.9	3.9	100.0	7.2	4.2	4.4	2.6	3.9	4.0	59	33.3

fied'. There was an unusual excess of girls with rhabdomyosarcoma.

References

Bjelke, E. (1964a) Leukaemia in children and young adults in Norway. *Cancer*, *17*, 248-255

Bjelke, E. (1964b) Malignant neoplasms of the kidney in children. *Cancer*, *17*, 318-321

Bjelke, E. (1970) Maligne sykdommer hos barn i Norge (Malignant tumours in children in Norway). *Tidsskr. nor. Laegeforen.*, *90*, 837-842

POLAND

Warsaw City Cancer Registry, 1970–1979

H. Gadomska & M. Zwierko

The Warsaw Cancer Registry was established in 1963 in collaboration with the National Cancer Institute, USA, to conduct comparative studies on the incidence of gastric cancer in Poland and among Americans of Polish origin.

In subsequent years, these studies were extended to cancer of other organs, and registration now embraces all sites. The Registry is located in the Institute of Oncology, which is responsible for the organization of epidemiological activities, scientific research and therapeutic services in relation to cancer for the whole country.

National reporting of cancer has been compulsory in Poland since 1952.
Individual doctors as well as medical centres must report all cases of malignant neoplasms, and are obliged to fill in a special notification card.

New notification cards are immediately checked for consistency of their identification data. The Registry contains an alphabetical file of patients' names with cancer site, date of birth, date of first diagnosis and, if applicable, date of death. A card file is maintained by site; it contains the information received at first notification and from subsequent follow-up.

When more than one neoplasm is observed in the same person, a new card is prepared for each different site.

Warsaw, the capital of Poland, lies on the river Vistula, in the eastern part of central Poland, i.e., in the Mazowian Lowlands. The area of registration amounts to 445 square kilometres. The average altitude is 100 m above sea level. In 1975, the population was about 1.4 million.

In addition to its administrative role as the capital city, Warsaw is an industrial centre with automobile, machine, chemical, textile, printing, metallurgical and food industries. The main occupational groups are industry 30%, construction 13%, trade 12%, transport and communications 7%.

The number of physicians in 1975 was 7047. There were 13 768 hospital beds. There are no special facilities for paediatric oncology.

The Cancer Registry, together with its file of notification cards, is used as a basis for research work on the epidemiology of cancer. It is also used as a basis for planning new hospitals, oncological centres and medical schools.

Population

Population data by single year of age are available from the censuses of 1970, 1975 and 1979 (Central Statistical Office, Warsaw).

AVERAGE ANNUAL POPULATION: 1970–1979

Age	Male	Female
0	12200	11308
1–4	43886	41658
5–9	50604	48214
10–14	60324	58107
0–14	167014	159287

Commentary

Incidence rates overall and for most major diagnostic groups were low compared with those for nearly all other European registries despite the fact that registration is compulsory and non-malignant CNS tumours are included. The cell type was not generally specified for leukaemia. However, the pattern of increased incidence in the 1–4 age-group suggests that the ratio of acute lymphocytic to acute non-lymphocytic would probably be similar to that observed elsewhere in Europe. Within the overall pattern of rather low incidence, there were relatively high frequencies of retinoblastoma, Wilms' tumour and rhabdomyosarcoma.

Poland, Warsaw City

1970 - 1979   MALE

DIAGNOSTIC GROUP	NUMBER OF CASES					REL. FREQUENCY(%)			RATES PER MILLION							
	0	1-4	5-9	10-14	All	Crude	Adj.	Group	0	1-4	5-9	10-14	Crude	Adj.	Cum	HV(%)
TOTAL	9	72	49	41	171	100.0	100.0	100.0	73.8	164.1	96.8	68.0	102.4	107.5	1554	90.1
I. LEUKAEMIAS	1	29	15	13	58	33.9	33.5	100.0	8.2	66.1	29.6	21.5	34.7	36.9	528	100.0
Acute lymphocytic	0	0	0	0	0	-	-	-	-	-	-	-	-	-	-	-
Other lymphocytic	0	0	0	0	0	-	-	-	-	-	-	-	-	-	-	-
Acute non-lymphocytic	0	1	1	3	5	2.9	3.3	8.6	-	2.3	2.0	5.0	3.0	2.8	44	100.0
Chronic myeloid	0	0	0	1	1	0.7	0.7	1.7	-	-	-	1.7	0.6	0.5	8	100.0
Other and unspecified	1	28	14	9	52	30.4	29.5	89.7	8.2	63.8	27.7	14.9	31.0	33.6	476	100.0
II. LYMPHOMAS	1	5	6	8	20	11.7	12.5	100.0	8.2	11.4	11.9	13.3	12.0	11.8	179	100.0
Hodgkin's disease	0	2	2	2	6	3.5	3.7	30.0	-	4.6	4.0	3.3	3.6	3.6	55	100.0
Non-Hodgkin lymphoma	1	1	1	3	6	3.5	3.8	30.0	8.2	2.3	2.0	5.0	3.6	3.4	52	100.0
Burkitt's lymphoma	0	0	0	0	0	-	-	-	-	-	-	-	-	-	-	-
Unspecified lymphoma	0	0	2	3	5	2.9	3.4	25.0	-	-	4.0	5.0	3.0	2.7	45	100.0
Histiocytosis X	0	2	1	0	3	1.8	1.6	15.0	-	4.6	2.0	-	1.8	2.0	28	100.0
Other reticuloendothelial	0	0	0	0	0	-	-	-	-	-	-	-	-	-	-	-
III. BRAIN AND SPINAL	0	8	12	8	28	16.4	17.2	100.0	-	18.2	23.7	13.3	16.8	17.1	258	62.5
Ependymoma	0	2	0	0	2	1.2	1.0	7.1	-	4.6	-	-	1.2	1.4	18	100.0
Astrocytoma	0	2	2	0	4	2.3	2.7	14.3	-	4.6	4.0	-	2.3	2.2	36	100.0
Medulloblastoma	0	2	5	1	8	4.7	4.8	28.6	-	4.6	9.9	1.7	4.8	5.1	76	100.0
Other glioma	0	0	0	0	0	-	-	-	-	-	-	-	-	-	-	-
Other and unspecified *	0	2	5	5	14	8.2	8.7	50.0	-	4.6	9.9	8.3	8.4	8.4	127	10.0
IV. SYMPATHETIC N.S.	0	10	3	1	14	8.2	7.5	100.0	-	22.8	5.9	1.7	8.4	9.4	129	84.6
Neuroblastoma	0	10	3	1	14	8.2	7.5	100.0	-	22.8	5.9	1.7	8.4	9.4	129	84.6
Other	0	0	0	0	0	-	-	-	-	-	-	-	-	-	-	-
V. RETINOBLASTOMA	3	7	0	0	10	5.8	4.9	100.0	24.6	15.9	-	-	6.0	6.8	88	90.0
VI. KIDNEY	1	8	4	0	13	7.6	6.9	100.0	8.2	18.2	7.9	-	7.8	8.8	121	100.0
Wilms' tumour	1	8	3	0	12	7.0	6.3	92.3	8.2	18.2	5.9	-	7.2	8.2	111	100.0
Renal carcinoma	0	0	1	0	1	0.6	0.6	7.7	-	-	2.0	-	0.6	0.6	10	100.0
Other and unspecified	0	0	0	0	0	-	-	-	-	-	-	-	-	-	-	-
VII. LIVER	1	0	0	1	2	1.2	1.1	100.0	8.2	-	-	1.7	1.2	1.1	18	50.0
Hepatoblastoma	1	0	0	0	1	0.6	0.6	50.0	8.2	-	-	-	0.6	0.6	10	100.0
Hepatic carcinoma	0	0	0	1	1	0.6	0.5	50.0	-	-	-	1.7	0.6	0.5	8	100.0
Other and unspecified	0	0	0	0	0	-	-	-	-	-	-	-	-	-	-	-
VIII. BONE	0	0	1	6	7	4.1	5.0	100.0	-	-	2.0	9.9	4.2	3.5	60	85.7
Osteosarcoma	0	0	0	4	4	2.3	2.9	57.1	-	-	-	6.6	2.4	1.9	33	75.0
Chondrosarcoma	0	0	0	0	0	-	-	-	-	-	-	-	-	-	-	-
Ewing's sarcoma	0	0	1	1	2	1.2	1.3	28.6	-	-	2.0	1.7	1.2	1.1	18	100.0
Other and unspecified	0	0	0	1	1	0.6	0.7	14.3	-	-	-	1.7	0.6	0.5	8	100.0
IX. SOFT TISSUE SARCOMAS	2	4	3	2	11	6.4	6.3	100.0	16.4	9.1	5.9	3.3	6.6	7.0	99	100.0
Rhabdomyosarcoma	2	3	3	1	9	5.3	5.0	81.8	16.4	6.8	5.9	1.7	5.4	5.4	82	100.0
Fibrosarcoma	0	1	0	0	1	0.6	0.5	9.1	-	2.3	-	-	0.6	0.7	9	100.0
Other and unspecified	0	0	0	1	1	0.6	0.7	9.1	-	-	-	1.7	0.6	0.5	8	100.0
X. GONADAL & GERM CELL	0	0	0	0	0	-	-	-	-	-	-	-	-	-	-	-
Non-gonadal germ cell	0	0	0	0	0	-	-	-	-	-	-	-	-	-	-	-
Gonadal germ cell	0	0	0	0	0	-	-	-	-	-	-	-	-	-	-	-
Gonadal carcinoma	0	0	0	0	0	-	-	-	-	-	-	-	-	-	-	-
Other and unspecified	0	0	0	0	0	-	-	-	-	-	-	-	-	-	-	-
XI. EPITHELIAL NEOPLASMS	0	0	1	2	3	1.8	2.1	100.0	-	-	2.0	3.3	1.8	1.6	26	66.7
Adrenocortical carcinoma	0	0	0	0	0	-	-	-	-	-	-	-	-	-	-	-
Thyroid carcinoma	0	0	1	1	2	1.2	1.3	66.7	-	-	2.0	1.7	1.2	1.1	18	100.0
Nasopharyngeal carcinoma	0	0	0	0	0	-	-	-	-	-	-	-	-	-	-	-
Melanoma	0	0	0	1	1	0.6	0.7	33.3	-	-	-	1.7	0.6	0.5	8	-
Other carcinoma	0	0	0	0	0	-	-	-	-	-	-	-	-	-	-	-
XII. OTHER	0	1	3	1	5	2.9	3.1	100.0	-	2.3	5.9	1.7	3.0	3.1	47	75.0
* Specified as malignant	0	4	4	5	13	7.6	8.1	-	-	9.1	7.9	8.3	7.8	7.8	117	-

Poland, Warsaw City   1970 - 1979   FEMALE

DIAGNOSTIC GROUP	NUMBER OF CASES					REL. FREQUENCY(%)			RATES PER MILLION							HV(%)
	0	1-4	5-9	10-14	All	Crude	Adj.	Group	0	1-4	5-9	10-14	Crude	Adj.	Cum	
TOTAL	5	58	32	38	133	100.0	100.0	100.0	44.2	139.2	66.4	65.4	83.5	86.9	1260	84.3
I. LEUKAEMIAS	0	18	11	8	37	27.8	28.1	100.0	-	43.2	22.8	13.8	23.2	24.7	356	100.0
Acute lymphocytic	0	1	0	0	1	0.8	0.6	2.7	-	2.4	-	-	0.6	0.7	10	100.0
Other lymphocytic	0	1	1	1	3	2.3	2.4	8.1	-	2.4	2.1	1.7	1.9	1.9	29	100.0
Acute non-lymphocytic	0	1	1	2	4	3.0	3.2	10.8	-	2.4	2.1	3.4	2.5	2.4	37	100.0
Chronic myeloid	0	0	0	0	0	-	-	-	-	-	-	-	-	-	-	-
Other and unspecified	0	15	9	5	29	21.8	21.9	78.4	-	36.0	18.7	8.6	18.2	19.7	280	100.0
II. LYMPHOMAS	1	2	8	1	12	9.0	10.2	100.0	8.8	4.8	16.6	1.7	7.5	8.0	120	91.7
Hodgkin's disease	1	1	2	0	4	3.0	3.1	33.3	8.8	2.4	4.1	-	2.5	2.8	39	75.0
Non-Hodgkin lymphoma	0	1	2	0	3	2.3	2.5	25.0	-	2.4	4.1	-	1.9	2.1	30	100.0
Burkitt's lymphoma	0	0	0	1	1	0.8	0.9	8.3	-	-	-	1.7	0.6	0.6	10	100.0
Unspecified lymphoma	0	0	3	0	3	2.3	2.7	25.0	-	-	6.2	-	1.9	1.8	29	100.0
Histiocytosis X	0	0	1	0	1	0.8	0.9	8.3	-	-	2.1	-	0.6	0.7	10	100.0
Other reticuloendothelial	0	0	0	0	0	-	-	-	-	-	-	-	-	-	-	-
III. BRAIN AND SPINAL	0	16	4	11	31	23.3	22.6	100.0	-	38.4	8.3	18.9	19.5	20.1	290	50.0
Ependymoma	0	0	0	2	2	1.5	1.6	6.5	-	-	-	3.4	1.3	1.0	17	100.0
Astrocytoma	0	4	1	1	6	4.5	4.3	19.4	-	9.6	2.1	1.7	3.8	4.1	57	100.0
Medulloblastoma	0	1	1	0	2	1.5	1.6	6.5	-	2.4	2.1	-	1.3	1.4	20	100.0
Other glioma	0	0	1	0	1	0.8	0.9	3.2	-	-	2.1	-	0.6	0.7	10	100.0
Other and unspecified *	0	11	1	8	20	15.0	14.2	64.5	-	26.4	2.1	13.8	12.6	12.8	185	-
IV. SYMPATHETIC N.S.	1	3	1	2	7	5.3	5.1	100.0	8.8	7.2	2.1	3.4	4.4	4.6	65	71.4
Neuroblastoma	1	3	1	2	7	5.3	5.1	100.0	8.8	7.2	2.1	3.4	4.4	4.6	65	71.4
Other	0	0	0	0	0	-	-	-	-	-	-	-	-	-	-	-
V. RETINOBLASTOMA	1	1	0	0	2	1.5	1.3	100.0	8.8	2.4	-	-	1.3	1.4	18	100.0
VI. KIDNEY	0	9	2	2	13	9.8	9.2	100.0	-	21.6	4.1	3.4	8.2	9.0	124	100.0
Wilms' tumour	0	9	2	2	13	9.8	9.2	100.0	-	21.6	4.1	3.4	8.2	9.0	124	100.0
Renal carcinoma	0	0	0	0	0	-	-	-	-	-	-	-	-	-	-	-
Other and unspecified	0	0	0	0	0	-	-	-	-	-	-	-	-	-	-	-
VII. LIVER	1	1	0	0	2	1.5	1.3	100.0	8.8	2.4	-	-	1.3	1.5	19	100.0
Hepatoblastoma	1	1	0	0	2	1.5	1.3	100.0	8.8	2.4	-	-	1.3	1.5	19	100.0
Hepatic carcinoma	0	0	0	0	0	-	-	-	-	-	-	-	-	-	-	-
Other and unspecified	0	0	0	0	0	-	-	-	-	-	-	-	-	-	-	-
VIII. BONE	0	1	1	5	7	5.3	5.2	100.0	-	2.4	2.1	8.6	4.4	3.9	61	66.7
Osteosarcoma	0	1	0	2	3	2.3	2.2	42.9	-	2.4	-	3.4	1.9	1.7	27	66.7
Chondrosarcoma	0	0	1	0	1	0.8	0.8	14.3	-	-	2.1	-	0.6	0.5	9	-
Ewing's sarcoma	0	0	0	1	1	0.8	0.8	14.3	-	-	-	1.7	0.6	0.6	9	100.0
Other and unspecified	0	0	0	2	2	1.5	1.4	28.6	-	-	-	3.4	1.3	1.2	17	100.0
IX. SOFT TISSUE SARCOMAS	0	5	1	6	12	9.0	8.8	100.0	-	12.0	2.1	10.3	7.5	7.4	110	91.7
Rhabdomyosarcoma	0	4	0	4	8	6.0	5.7	66.7	-	9.6	-	6.9	5.0	5.0	73	100.0
Fibrosarcoma	0	0	1	0	1	0.8	0.9	8.3	-	-	2.1	-	0.6	0.7	10	100.0
Other and unspecified	0	1	0	2	3	2.3	2.2	25.0	-	2.4	-	3.4	1.9	1.7	27	66.7
X. GONADAL & GERM CELL	0	2	1	3	6	4.5	4.9	100.0	-	4.8	2.1	5.2	3.8	3.6	56	100.0
Non-gonadal germ cell	0	2	1	2	5	3.8	4.2	83.3	-	4.8	2.1	3.4	3.1	2.8	47	100.0
Gonadal germ cell	0	0	0	0	0	-	-	-	-	-	-	-	-	-	-	-
Gonadal carcinoma	0	0	0	0	0	-	-	-	-	-	-	-	-	-	-	-
Other and unspecified	0	0	0	1	1	0.8	0.6	16.7	-	-	-	1.7	0.6	0.7	10	100.0
XI. EPITHELIAL NEOPLASMS	0	0	2	0	2	1.5	1.9	100.0	-	-	4.1	-	1.3	1.3	21	100.0
Adrenocortical carcinoma	0	0	0	0	0	-	-	-	-	-	-	-	-	-	-	-
Thyroid carcinoma	0	0	1	0	1	0.8	0.9	50.0	-	-	2.1	-	0.6	0.7	10	100.0
Nasopharyngeal carcinoma	0	0	0	0	0	-	-	-	-	-	-	-	-	-	-	-
Melanoma	0	0	0	0	0	-	-	-	-	-	-	-	-	-	-	-
Other carcinoma	0	0	1	0	1	0.8	0.9	50.0	-	-	2.1	-	0.6	0.7	10	100.0
XII. OTHER	1	0	1	0	2	1.5	1.6	100.0	8.8	-	2.1	-	1.3	1.4	19	-
* Specified as malignant	0	10	1	8	19	14.3	13.6	100.0	-	24.0	2.1	13.8	11.9	12.1	175	-

SPAIN

National Childhood Cancer Registry, 1980–1984

R. Peris-Bonet, F. Abad García & F. Taberner Alberola[1]

The National Childhood Cancer Registry (NCCR) has been developed as a joint project involving the Sección de Oncología of the Asociación Espanola de Pediatría and the Centro de Documentación e Informatica Biomedica, which has now been incorporated into the Instituto de Estudios Documentales e Históricos sobre la Ciencia (Consejo Superior de Investigaciones Cientificas — Universidad de Valencia).

The NCCR aims to provide information on the dimensions of the problem of cancer in children, to make possible the active follow-up of patients, to facilitate the study of preventive measures, the rate and quality of survival, and to contribute to clinical investigation and the improvement of medical care.

It is based on the following principles: the voluntary commitment of a highly motivated network of collaborating hospital departments; notification of all cases to a central register; useful feedback to the collaborating centres; control of the quality of diagnosis; the retention of the identity of each individual collaborating centre; and the fact that the majority of patients obtain medical care in highly specialized centres.

The collaborating centres of the NCCR[2] are the hospital departments represented in the Sección de Oncología, and some others that have joined the Registry (see above). The collaborating hospital departments are responsible for notification and active follow-up. The data processing is carried out in the central registry.

ICD-O has been used as a list of notifiable tumours, but excluding those with behaviour code /0. The set of data collected for each case is based on the core data proposed by the *WHO Handbook for standardized cancer registries* (1976). The ICD-O is used for the classification and coding of site and morphology.

The case registry was begun in 1980.

The NCCR is not population-based. Completeness is affected by several factors, and the following should be taken into account: (1) the age of paediatric hospitalization is not the same in all the collaborating centres. It is up to 14 years in the university centres, but only up to seven years in the majority of the centres which come under the National Social Security Service (INSALUD); (2) childhood cancer cases are distributed among different specialized departments in the hospitals, which are not always in contact with the local collaborating centre. This clearly affects several tumour types which are therefore under-represented, for example leukaemias; (3) some tumours, such as the group of miscellaneous reticuloendothelial neoplasms, are rarely registered because of the absence of essential data on patient identifi-

Contd p. 282

[1]Unidad de Información y Documentación Médicosanitaria y Centro de Documentación e Informática Biomedica, Instituto de Estudios Documentales e Historicós sobre la Ciencia (CSIC — Universidad de Valencia), Valencia, España.

[2]*Contributors from the collaborating centres*

B. Agra Cadarso (Madrid); V. Alvarez Angel (Valencia); M.J. Antuña (Oviedo); A.M. Badía Torroella (Barcelona); J.L. Bezanilla Regato (Baracaldo); V. Castel Sánchez (Valencia); J.M. Couselo (Santiago de Compostela); J. Donat Colomer (Valencia); C. Estellés Valls (Madrid); M.T. García Muñoz (Riaño-Langreo); S. Gonzalez Huambos (Sevilla); F.J. Guisasola (Valladolid); T. Hurtado Ruano (Madrid); J.M. Indiano Arce (Bilbao); C. Jiménez Alvarez (Granada); J. López Muñoz (Almeria); F.J. Molina Garicano (Pamplona); J. Mulet Ferragut (Barcelona); A. Muñoz Villa (Madrid); F. Negro López (Oviedo); N. Pardo García (Barcelona); R. Pérez de Sobrino (Córdoba); G. Pineda Cuevas (Sevilla); F.J. Pisón Garcés (Zaragoza); J. Rodriguez Luis (Santa Cruz de Tenerife); J.L. Ruiz Gimenez (Murcia); J. Sánchez de Toledo (Barcelona); A. Sancho Vendrell (Barcelona); Serra y Chacartegui (Palma de Mallorca); L. Sierrasesumaga Ariznavarrete (Pamplona); M.A. Suñol (San Sebastian); A. Urda Cardona (Málaga).

Spain, Childhood Cancer Registry   1980 – 1984   MALE

DIAGNOSTIC GROUP	NUMBER OF CASES					REL. FREQUENCY(%)			HV(%)
	0	1-4	5-9	10-14	All	Crude	Adj.	Group	
TOTAL	129	525	405	164	1223	100.0	100.0	100.0	92.2
I. LEUKAEMIAS	11	142	88	25	266	21.7	20.4	100.0	100.0
Acute lymphocytic	6	116	77	18	217	17.7	16.5	81.6	100.0
Other lymphocytic	0	0	0	0	0	-	-	-	-
Acute non-lymphocytic	2	19	8	5	34	2.8	2.8	12.8	100.0
Chronic myeloid	0	3	1	0	4	0.3	0.3	1.5	100.0
Other and unspecified	3	4	2	2	11	0.9	0.9	4.1	100.0
II. LYMPHOMAS	2	72	114	45	233	19.1	21.2	100.0	98.7
Hodgkin's disease	0	6	18	22	46	3.8	5.7	19.7	100.0
Non-Hodgkin lymphoma	0	29	58	15	102	8.3	8.8	43.8	100.0
Burkitt's lymphoma	0	29	30	7	66	5.4	5.3	28.3	98.5
Unspecified lymphoma	0	5	8	1	14	1.1	1.1	6.0	92.3
Histiocytosis X	0	1	0	0	1	0.1	0.1	0.4	100.0
Other reticuloendothelial	2	2	0	0	4	0.3	0.2	1.7	66.7
III. BRAIN AND SPINAL	5	76	91	35	207	16.9	18.1	100.0	78.9
Ependymoma	0	10	5	1	16	1.3	1.2	7.7	100.0
Astrocytoma	4	24	30	9	67	5.5	5.6	32.4	87.9
Medulloblastoma	1	21	27	11	60	4.9	5.4	29.0	98.3
Other glioma	0	4	4	6	14	1.1	1.6	6.8	64.3
Other and unspecified *	0	17	25	8	50	4.1	4.4	24.2	40.8
IV. SYMPATHETIC N.S.	53	69	15	0	137	11.2	8.6	100.0	81.6
Neuroblastoma	52	69	15	0	136	11.1	8.5	99.3	81.5
Other	1	0	0	0	1	0.1	0.1	0.7	100.0
V. RETINOBLASTOMA	9	21	3	0	33	2.7	2.1	100.0	81.8
VI. KIDNEY	19	62	21	6	108	8.8	7.6	100.0	95.3
Wilms' tumour	16	60	21	6	103	8.4	7.3	95.4	95.1
Renal carcinoma	0	0	0	0	0	-	-	-	-
Other and unspecified	3	2	0	0	5	0.4	0.3	4.6	100.0
VII. LIVER	7	12	3	1	23	1.9	1.6	100.0	73.9
Hepatoblastoma	6	9	2	1	18	1.5	1.2	78.3	83.3
Hepatic carcinoma	0	0	1	0	1	0.1	0.1	4.3	100.0
Other and unspecified	1	3	0	0	4	0.3	0.2	17.4	25.0
VIII. BONE	0	8	29	26	63	5.2	7.4	100.0	100.0
Osteosarcoma	0	0	6	12	18	1.5	2.6	28.6	100.0
Chondrosarcoma	0	0	1	1	1	0.1	0.1	1.6	100.0
Ewing's sarcoma	0	8	22	13	43	3.5	4.5	68.3	100.0
Other and unspecified	0	0	1	0	1	0.1	0.1	1.6	100.0
IX. SOFT TISSUE SARCOMAS	14	42	31	17	104	8.5	8.8	100.0	99.0
Rhabdomyosarcoma	6	37	24	12	79	6.5	6.6	76.0	98.7
Fibrosarcoma	4	3	1	1	9	0.7	0.7	8.7	100.0
Other and unspecified	4	2	6	4	16	1.3	1.5	15.4	100.0
X. GONADAL & GERM CELL	6	14	0	3	23	1.9	1.8	100.0	95.5
Non-gonadal germ cell	2	3	0	3	8	0.7	0.9	34.8	87.5
Gonadal germ cell	4	11	0	0	15	1.2	0.9	65.2	100.0
Gonadal carcinoma	0	0	0	0	0	-	-	-	-
Other and unspecified	0	0	0	0	0	-	-	-	-
XI. EPITHELIAL NEOPLASMS	0	3	8	5	16	1.3	1.7	100.0	100.0
Adrenocortical carcinoma	0	0	0	0	0	-	-	-	-
Thyroid carcinoma	0	0	0	3	6	0.5	0.8	37.5	100.0
Nasopharyngeal carcinoma	0	0	0	2	2	0.2	0.4	12.5	100.0
Melanoma	0	0	0	0	0	-	-	-	-
Other carcinoma	0	3	5	0	8	0.7	0.6	50.0	100.0
XII. OTHER	3	4	2	1	10	0.8	0.8	100.0	50.0
* Specified as malignant	0	13	18	4	35	2.9	2.9	100.0	20.6

Spain, Childhood Cancer Registry   1980 – 1984   FEMALE

DIAGNOSTIC GROUP	NUMBER OF CASES					REL. FREQUENCY(%)			HV(%)
	0	1-4	5-9	10-14	All	Crude	Adj.	Group	
TOTAL	110	368	297	113	888	100.0	100.0	100.0	89.9
I. LEUKAEMIAS	11	104	73	24	212	23.9	23.4	100.0	100.0
Acute lymphocytic	6	93	69	17	185	20.8	19.8	87.3	100.0
Other lymphocytic	0	0	0	0	0	-	-	-	-
Acute non-lymphocytic	5	8	4	5	22	2.5	2.8	10.4	100.0
Chronic myeloid	0	1	0	2	3	0.3	0.6	1.4	100.0
Other and unspecified	0	2	0	0	2	0.2	0.2	0.9	100.0
II. LYMPHOMAS	5	22	39	23	89	10.0	12.3	100.0	100.0
Hodgkin's disease	0	0	11	10	21	2.4	3.8	23.6	100.0
Non-Hodgkin lymphoma	1	9	16	7	33	3.7	4.3	37.1	100.0
Burkitt's lymphoma	0	4	9	3	16	1.8	2.0	18.0	100.0
Unspecified lymphoma	0	5	3	3	11	1.2	1.5	12.4	100.0
Histiocytosis X	2	3	0	0	5	0.6	0.4	5.6	100.0
Other reticuloendothelial	2	1	0	0	3	0.3	0.3	3.4	100.0
III. BRAIN AND SPINAL	10	57	85	23	175	19.7	20.3	100.0	74.0
Ependymoma	1	8	2	1	12	1.4	1.2	6.9	91.7
Astrocytoma	6	25	32	9	72	8.1	8.2	41.1	94.4
Medulloblastoma	2	5	16	2	25	2.8	2.7	14.3	100.0
Other glioma	0	6	5	1	12	1.4	1.3	6.9	50.0
Other and unspecified *	1	13	30	10	54	6.1	6.9	30.9	35.8
IV. SYMPATHETIC N.S.	35	52	19	3	109	12.3	10.0	100.0	78.5
Neuroblastoma	34	52	17	3	106	11.9	9.7	97.2	77.9
Other	1	0	2	0	3	0.3	0.3	2.8	100.0
V. RETINOBLASTOMA	10	13	2	0	25	2.8	2.1	100.0	72.0
VI. KIDNEY	8	57	26	3	94	10.6	8.9	100.0	89.2
Wilms' tumour	7	54	23	3	87	9.8	8.2	92.6	89.5
Renal carcinoma	0	0	0	0	0	-	-	-	-
Other and unspecified	1	3	3	0	7	0.8	0.6	7.4	85.7
VII. LIVER	3	6	0	2	11	1.2	1.3	100.0	90.9
Hepatoblastoma	2	5	0	1	8	0.9	0.9	72.7	100.0
Hepatic carcinoma	0	1	0	1	2	0.2	0.3	18.2	100.0
Other and unspecified	1	0	0	0	1	0.1	0.1	9.1	-
VIII.BONE	2	5	20	18	45	5.1	7.4	100.0	100.0
Osteosarcoma	0	4	10	7	21	2.4	3.2	46.7	100.0
Chondrosarcoma	0	0	0	0	0	-	-	-	-
Ewing's sarcoma	2	1	10	10	23	2.6	3.9	51.1	100.0
Other and unspecified	0	0	0	1	1	0.1	0.3	2.2	100.0
IX. SOFT TISSUE SARCOMAS	12	29	23	7	71	8.0	7.6	100.0	100.0
Rhabdomyosarcoma	7	21	14	2	44	5.0	4.3	62.0	100.0
Fibrosarcoma	1	5	5	2	13	1.5	1.5	18.3	100.0
Other and unspecified	4	3	4	3	14	1.6	1.8	19.7	100.0
X. GONADAL & GERM CELL	10	13	5	5	33	3.7	3.8	100.0	100.0
Non-gonadal germ cell	10	13	1	0	24	2.7	2.9	72.7	100.0
Gonadal germ cell	0	0	4	4	8	0.9	1.5	24.2	100.0
Gonadal carcinoma	0	0	0	1	1	0.1	0.3	3.0	100.0
Other and unspecified	0	0	0	0	0	-	-	-	-
XI. EPITHELIAL NEOPLASMS	2	5	4	4	15	1.7	2.1	100.0	93.3
Adrenocortical carcinoma	1	3	0	0	4	0.5	0.3	26.7	100.0
Thyroid carcinoma	0	0	1	1	2	0.2	0.4	13.3	100.0
Nasopharyngeal carcinoma	0	0	0	2	2	0.2	0.5	13.3	100.0
Melanoma	0	0	0	0	0	-	-	-	-
Other carcinoma	1	2	3	1	7	0.8	0.8	46.7	85.7
XII. OTHER	2	5	1	1	9	1.0	1.0	100.0	77.8
* Specified as malignant	0	11	25	5	41	4.6	4.8	100.0	20.0

cation or about the tumour itself; (4) information from death certificates has not been obtained.

Commentary

As would be expected from the nature of ascertainment for this Registry, relatively few cases were aged 10—14. Within the 0—9 age range there were, in comparison with other European registries, markedly high relative frequencies of lymphomas and soft tissue sarcomas. Among the lymphomas there was a high proportion of Burkitt's lymphoma. Leukaemias and brain tumours had low relative frequencies, which probably reflects under-ascertainment rather than a low underlying incidence for these groups.

References

Registro Nacional de Tumores Infantiles (1983) Anuario de estadisticas basicas del RNTI.1. (1980-1982). *An. esp. Pediatr.*, *20*, 187-342

Peris-Bonet, R. *et al.* (1986) *Estadisticas basicas del Registro Nacional de Tumores Infantiles 2 (1980-1984)*, Valencia, Conselleria de Sanitat i Consum (*Monografies Sanitaries*, Serie C, Num. 3)

Cancer Registry of Zaragoza, 1973-1982

A. Zubiri, L. Zubiri, A. Vergara, C. Martos,

P. Moreo & V. Hernandez

The Cancer Registry of Zaragoza began activities in 1960 with the support of the Spanish Association Against Cancer, and was the first registry to be established in Spain. It published the first results in 1966 (for the period 1960-1974) and annual and quinquennial reports have been published since then.

The Registry was set up to obtain systematic data on the incidence of cancer by site and histology, and to maintain interest among both physicians and the public in malignant tumours in order to ensure early diagnosis and immediate treatment.

The area covered by the Registry corresponds to the Province of Zaragoza; only those patients domiciled in the Province and who have a diagnosis of malignant tumour are registered.

For each patient the following data are recorded: identity (name, sex, age, residence), source of information, topographical and morphological diagnosis, treatment, clinical course and, if applicable, date of death.

The principal sources of data for the registry are: primary care physicians, the Tumour Registry of the Ciudad Sanitaria Miguel Servet (Social Security), the Department of Preventive Medicine in the Hospital clinico Universitario, the Regional Centre of Oncology, the Provincial Hospital and the Provincial Delegation of Statistics, which provides the death certificates. Notification is not compulsory but in general there is a willingness to provide data for the Registry.

Altogether, there are 4381 hospital beds in the capital and 342 in hospitals situated in villages within the region (5.5 per 1000 inhabitants). There is a Faculty of Medicine and 3800 physicians (4.4 per 1000 inhabitants).

The Registry obtains data from the whole region of Zaragoza, which is situated in the northeast of Spain and has an area of 17 194 square kilometres and an altitude ranging from 50 to 2313 metres. The average temperature is 26° C in summer and 6° C in winter; there are more than 200 clear and sunny days a year; rainfall is 341 mm per year. A prevailing north-west wind blows at an average speed of 40 kilometres per hour and, as a result, the air is clean. There are about 30 days a year with industrial atmospheric contamination, but only in the capital, Zaragoza, when there is mist.

There is little variation in religious, racial or language groups in both the capital and Province of Zaragoza; almost everybody is Roman Catholic, belongs to the Mediterranean white race and speaks Spanish.

The total number of inhabitants is 828 588 (1981 census) and of these 571 855 live in Zaragoza, which is a predominantly industrial city. The remainder live in 297 towns and villages, for most of which the economy depends on agriculture, and whose population is decreasing.

The economically active population (16 years of age and over) accounts for 33.8% of the total and is mainly engaged in industry (chemicals, metallurgy) agriculture, building, and services.

The Registry includes cases ascertained from death certificate only but excludes neoplasms found incidentally at post mortem. All malignant neoplasms except histiocytosis X are included, as well as benign and unspecified tumours of the CNS, pineal and pituitary (except craniopharyngioma).

Population

The population has been estimated from data from the censuses of 1975 and 1980.

AVERAGE ANNUAL POPULATION: 1973-1982

Age	Male	Female
0	6408	5936
1–4	25619	23816
5–9	32885	30823
10–14	31201	29670
0–14	96113	90245

Commentary

The incidence rates for most diagnostic groups are similar to those in other European countries. The rate for lymphoma was among the highest in Europe. No cases of retinoblastoma were recorded in the 10-year period reported here (indeed, only one case has been registered since 1960) and it is possible that this is due to under-ascertainment.

Spain, Zaragoza　　　　　　　　1973 - 1982　　　　　　　　MALE

DIAGNOSTIC GROUP	NUMBER OF CASES					REL. FREQUENCY(%)			RATES PER MILLION						Cum	HV(%)
	0	1-4	5-9	10-14	All	Crude	Adj.	Group	0	1-4	5-9	10-14	Crude	Adj.		
TOTAL	9	52	61	39	161	100.0	100.0	100.0	140.4	203.0	185.5	125.0	167.5	169.9	2505	96.8
I. LEUKAEMIAS	1	18	20	7	46	28.6	27.7	100.0	15.6	70.3	60.8	22.4	47.9	49.1	713	97.6
Acute lymphocytic	0	8	11	4	23	14.3	13.7	50.0		31.2	33.4	12.8	23.9	24.2	356	95.5
Other lymphocytic	0	1	0	1	2	1.2	1.4	4.3		3.9		3.2	2.1	2.1	32	100.0
Acute non-lymphocytic	0	1	1	0	2	1.2	1.1	4.3		3.9	3.0		2.1	2.2	31	100.0
Chronic myeloid	0	0	0	0	0											
Other and unspecified	1	8	8	2	19	11.8	11.4	41.3	15.6	31.2	24.3	6.4	19.8	20.6	294	100.0
II. LYMPHOMAS	0	5	19	6	30	18.6	17.2	100.0		19.5	57.8	19.2	31.2	30.3	463	100.0
Hodgkin's disease	0	2	3	3	8	5.0	5.1	26.7		7.8	9.1	9.6	8.3	8.2	125	100.0
Non-Hodgkin lymphoma	0	3	14	2	19	11.8	10.4	63.3		11.7	42.6	6.4	19.8	19.2	292	100.0
Burkitt's lymphoma	0	0	2	1	3	1.9	1.8	10.0			6.1	3.2	3.1	2.9	46	100.0
Unspecified lymphoma	0	0	0	0	0											
Histiocytosis X	0	0	0	0	0											
Other reticuloendothelial	0	0	0	0	0											
III. BRAIN AND SPINAL	0	12	10	7	29	18.0	18.2	100.0		46.8	30.4	22.4	30.2	30.8	452	70.0
Ependymoma	0	0	0	0	0											
Astrocytoma	0	1	0	2	3	1.9	2.2	10.3		3.9		6.4	3.1	3.1	48	100.0
Medulloblastoma	0	2	1	1	4	2.5	2.6	13.8		7.8	3.0	3.2	4.2	4.3	62	100.0
Other glioma	0	0	0	2	2	1.2	1.3	6.9			3.0	3.2	2.1	1.9	31	100.0
Other and unspecified *	0	9	8	3	20	12.4	12.1	69.0		35.1	24.3	9.6	20.8	21.5	310	25.0
IV. SYMPATHETIC N.S.	2	6	1	1	10	6.2	6.5	100.0	31.2	23.4	3.0	3.2	10.4	11.6	156	100.0
Neuroblastoma	2	6	1	1	10	6.2	6.5	100.0	31.2	23.4	3.0	3.2	10.4	11.6	156	100.0
Other	0	0	0	0	0											
V. RETINOBLASTOMA	0	0	0	0	0											
VI. KIDNEY	0	5	3	0	8	5.0	4.8	100.0		19.5	9.1		8.3	9.0	124	100.0
Wilms' tumour	0	5	3	0	8	5.0	4.8	100.0		19.5	9.1		8.3	9.0	124	100.0
Renal carcinoma	0	0	0	0	0											
Other and unspecified	0	0	0	0	0											
VII. LIVER	2	1	2	2	7	4.3	4.5	100.0	31.2	3.9	6.1	6.4	7.3	7.4	109	100.0
Hepatoblastoma	2	0	2	0	4	2.5	2.3	57.1	31.2		6.1		4.2	4.4	62	100.0
Hepatic carcinoma	0	1	0	0	1	0.6	0.7	14.3		3.9			1.0	1.2	16	
Other and unspecified	0	0	0	2	2	1.2	1.5	28.6				6.4	2.1	1.9	32	
VIII. BONE	0	0	2	10	12	7.5	8.7	100.0			6.1	32.1	12.5	11.3	191	100.0
Osteosarcoma	0	0	0	8	8	5.0	6.2	66.7				25.6	8.3	7.4	128	100.0
Chondrosarcoma	0	0	0	0	0											
Ewing's sarcoma	0	0	2	2	4	2.5	2.5	33.3			6.1	6.4	4.2	3.8	62	100.0
Other and unspecified	0	0	0	0	0											
IX. SOFT TISSUE SARCOMAS	0	3	4	6	13	8.1	8.5	100.0		11.7	12.2	19.2	13.5	13.1	204	100.0
Rhabdomyosarcoma	0	2	3	0	5	3.1	2.8	38.5		7.8	9.1		5.2	5.4	77	100.0
Fibrosarcoma	0	0	0	5	5	3.1	3.8	38.5				16.0	5.2	4.7	80	100.0
Other and unspecified	0	1	1	1	3	1.9	1.9	23.1		3.9	3.0	3.2	3.1	3.1	47	100.0
X. GONADAL & GERM CELL	0	0	0	0	0											
Non-gonadal germ cell	0	0	0	0	0											
Gonadal germ cell	0	0	0	0	0											
Gonadal carcinoma	0	0	0	0	0											
Other and unspecified	0	0	0	0	0											
XI. EPITHELIAL NEOPLASMS	0	0	0	0	0											
Adrenocortical carcinoma	0	0	0	0	0											
Thyroid carcinoma	0	0	0	0	0											
Nasopharyngeal carcinoma	0	0	0	0	0											
Melanoma	0	0	0	0	0											
Other carcinoma	0	0	0	0	0											
XII. OTHER	4	2	0	0	6	3.7	3.9	100.0	62.4	7.8			6.2	7.3	94	-
* Specified as malignant	0	8	8	3	19	11.8	11.5	100.0		31.2	24.3	9.6	19.8	20.3	295	-

Spain, Zaragoza

1973 – 1982

FEMALE

DIAGNOSTIC GROUP	NUMBER OF CASES					REL. FREQUENCY(%)			RATES PER MILLION						Cum	HV(%)
	0	1-4	5-9	10-14	All	Crude	Adj.	Group	0	1-4	5-9	10-14	Crude	Adj.		
TOTAL	7	34	24	24	89	100.0	100.0	100.0	117.9	142.8	77.9	80.9	98.6	101.9	1483	94.8
I. LEUKAEMIAS	0	19	7	12	38	42.7	42.3	100.0	-	79.8	22.7	40.4	42.1	43.8	635	97.2
Acute lymphocytic	0	14	7	5	26	29.2	28.7	68.4	-	58.8	22.7	16.9	28.8	30.4	433	96.2
Other lymphocytic	0	0	0	0	0	-	-	-	-	-	-	-	-	-	-	-
Acute non-lymphocytic	0	3	0	4	7	7.9	7.9	18.4	-	12.6	-	13.5	7.8	7.8	118	100.0
Chronic myeloid	0	0	0	0	0	-	-	-	-	-	-	-	-	-	-	-
Other and unspecified	0	2	0	3	5	5.6	5.7	13.2	-	8.4	-	10.1	5.5	5.5	84	100.0
II. LYMPHOMAS	0	4	4	3	11	12.4	12.7	100.0	-	16.8	13.0	10.1	12.2	12.3	183	100.0
Hodgkin's disease	0	0	1	1	2	2.2	2.5	18.2	-	-	3.2	3.4	2.2	2.0	33	100.0
Non-Hodgkin lymphoma	0	3	1	2	6	6.7	6.7	54.5	-	12.6	3.2	6.7	6.6	6.9	100	100.0
Burkitt's lymphoma	0	1	1	0	2	2.2	2.2	18.2	-	4.2	3.2	-	2.2	2.3	33	100.0
Unspecified lymphoma	0	0	1	0	1	1.1	1.3	9.1	-	-	3.2	-	1.1	1.0	16	100.0
Histiocytosis X	0	0	0	0	0	-	-	-	-	-	-	-	-	-	-	-
Other reticuloendothelial	0	0	0	0	0	-	-	-	-	-	-	-	-	-	-	-
III. BRAIN AND SPINAL	1	2	8	5	16	18.0	19.2	100.0	16.8	8.4	26.0	16.9	17.7	17.2	264	83.3
Ependymoma	0	0	0	0	0	-	-	-	-	-	-	-	-	-	-	-
Astrocytoma	0	0	2	1	3	3.4	3.8	18.8	-	-	6.5	3.4	3.3	3.1	49	100.0
Medulloblastoma	0	1	0	1	2	2.2	2.2	12.5	-	4.2	-	3.4	2.2	2.3	34	100.0
Other glioma	0	0	1	0	1	1.1	1.3	6.3	-	-	3.2	-	1.1	1.0	16	100.0
Other and unspecified *	1	1	5	3	10	11.2	12.0	62.5	16.8	4.2	16.2	10.1	11.1	10.8	165	-
IV. SYMPATHETIC N.S.	5	1	0	0	6	6.7	5.9	100.0	84.2	4.2	-	-	6.6	7.8	101	83.3
Neuroblastoma	5	1	0	0	6	6.7	5.9	100.0	84.2	4.2	-	-	6.6	7.8	101	83.3
Other	0	0	0	0	0	-	-	-	-	-	-	-	-	-	-	-
V. RETINOBLASTOMA	0	0	0	0	0	-	-	-	-	-	-	-	-	-	-	-
VI. KIDNEY	1	1	2	0	4	4.5	4.5	100.0	16.8	4.2	6.5	-	4.4	4.7	66	75.0
Wilms' tumour	1	1	2	0	4	4.5	4.5	100.0	16.8	4.2	6.5	-	4.4	4.7	66	75.0
Renal carcinoma	0	0	0	0	0	-	-	-	-	-	-	-	-	-	-	-
Other and unspecified	0	0	0	0	0	-	-	-	-	-	-	-	-	-	-	-
VII. LIVER	0	0	0	0	0	-	-	-	-	-	-	-	-	-	-	-
Hepatoblastoma	0	0	0	0	0	-	-	-	-	-	-	-	-	-	-	-
Hepatic carcinoma	0	0	0	0	0	-	-	-	-	-	-	-	-	-	-	-
Other and unspecified	0	0	0	0	0	-	-	-	-	-	-	-	-	-	-	-
VIII. BONE	0	1	1	2	4	4.5	3.5	100.0	-	4.2	3.2	6.7	4.4	4.3	67	100.0
Osteosarcoma	0	1	0	2	3	3.4	2.2	75.0	-	4.2	-	6.7	3.3	3.3	50	100.0
Chondrosarcoma	0	0	0	0	0	-	-	-	-	-	-	-	-	-	-	-
Ewing's sarcoma	0	0	1	0	1	1.1	1.3	25.0	-	-	3.2	-	1.1	1.0	16	100.0
Other and unspecified	0	0	0	0	0	-	-	-	-	-	-	-	-	-	-	-
IX. SOFT TISSUE SARCOMAS	0	5	2	1	8	9.0	8.6	100.0	-	21.0	6.5	3.4	8.9	9.6	133	100.0
Rhabdomyosarcoma	0	5	2	0	7	7.9	7.4	87.5	-	21.0	6.5	-	7.8	8.6	116	100.0
Fibrosarcoma	0	0	0	0	0	-	-	-	-	-	-	-	-	-	-	-
Other and unspecified	0	0	0	1	1	1.1	1.3	12.5	-	-	-	3.4	1.1	1.0	17	100.0
X. GONADAL & GERM CELL	0	1	0	1	2	2.2	2.2	100.0	-	4.2	-	3.4	2.2	2.3	34	100.0
Non-gonadal germ cell	0	1	0	0	1	1.1	1.0	50.0	-	4.2	-	-	1.1	1.3	17	100.0
Gonadal germ cell	0	0	0	1	1	1.1	1.3	50.0	-	-	-	3.4	1.1	1.0	17	100.0
Gonadal carcinoma	0	0	0	0	0	-	-	-	-	-	-	-	-	-	-	-
Other and unspecified	0	0	0	0	0	-	-	-	-	-	-	-	-	-	-	-
XI. EPITHELIAL NEOPLASMS	0	0	0	0	0	-	-	-	-	-	-	-	-	-	-	-
Adrenocortical carcinoma	0	0	0	0	0	-	-	-	-	-	-	-	-	-	-	-
Thyroid carcinoma	0	0	0	0	0	-	-	-	-	-	-	-	-	-	-	-
Nasopharyngeal carcinoma	0	0	0	0	0	-	-	-	-	-	-	-	-	-	-	-
Melanoma	0	0	0	0	0	-	-	-	-	-	-	-	-	-	-	-
Other carcinoma	0	0	0	0	0	-	-	-	-	-	-	-	-	-	-	-
XII. OTHER	0	0	0	0	0	-	-	-	-	-	-	-	-	-	-	-
* Specified as malignant	1	1	5	3	10	11.2	12.0	100.0	16.8	4.2	16.2	10.1	11.1	10.8	165	-

SWEDEN

Swedish Cancer Registry, 1970–1982

T. Gunnarson

The Swedish Cancer Registry was established in 1958 on the initiative of the National Board of Health. It now functions under the National Board of Health and Welfare and is financed by the Government.

The registration of newly-detected tumour cases is based on compulsory reporting by all physicians responsible for in-patient and out-patient departments in all public and private establishments for medical treatment. Private practitioners have been required to report such cases since 1983. In Sweden, nearly every cancer case will sooner or later be seen at a hospital. Hospital and forensic pathologists make independent compulsory reports on every cancer diagnosis made from surgical biopsies, cytological specimens and autopsies.

During the last ten years Swedish cancer registration has been reorganized. Regional registries have been started in the six medical regions and all registration is now performed at these institutions. The National Registry has overall responsibility for registration and for the reporting of all cancer cases for the whole country.

The data in the Registry are supplemented by information on cause and date of death by computerized matching against death certificates obtained from Statistics Sweden. No case with the diagnosis of cancer based on a death certificate alone is accepted.

Information concerning occupation, industry, domicile, etc., is obtained by transferring data from the 1960 census to the Cancer Registry. Religion, race and language group are not asked for or coded.

In addition to malignant neoplasms, reports are received on a variety of benign or potentially malignant tumours. These are registered, but are not included in the regular reports of incidence (except for benign epithelial urinary tract neoplasms and benign intracranial and intraspinal tumours). Basal-cell carcinomas of the skin are excluded. The 7th Revision of the ICD is mainly used for coding site, with the exception of leukaemia, where the ICD-8 classification is followed. Histology is coded according to the recommendations of the WHO Expert Committee on Health Statistics (WHO, 1956). For the purposes of the present study, these codes were translated into their ICD-O equivalents. For most histological types, this was straightforward; however, almost all central nervous system tumours required review of the histological diagnosis and recoding, and a rather high percentage of leukaemias remained unallocated to a specific cell type.

The Registry covers the whole of Sweden, which is bordered on the north and west by Norway, on the east by Finland and on the east, south and west by the Baltic. The total area is 449 964 square kilometres.

The total population in 1980 was 8.32 million, of whom 20% were children aged 0–14. Virtually the whole population is Caucasian and Protestant. The main occupations of the economically active population in 1980 were services 33%, mining, manufacturing and production of electricity 26% and commerce 20%.

A report on the incidence of childhood cancer in Sweden has been published (Ericsson *et al.*, 1978).

Population

Population estimates by age and sex are available for each year from the National Central Bureau of Statistics, and the average for 1970–1982 has been calculated.

AVERAGE ANNUAL POPULATION: 1970–1982

Age	Male	Female
0	52367	49683
1–4	219740	208935
5–9	292228	277773
10–14	289399	274773
0–14	853734	811164

Contd p. 290

Sweden   1970 – 1982   MALE

DIAGNOSTIC GROUP	NUMBER OF CASES					REL. FREQUENCY(%)			RATES PER MILLION						Cum	HV(%)
	0	1-4	5-9	10-14	All	Crude	Adj.	Group	0	1-4	5-9	10-14	Crude	Adj.		
TOTAL	154	586	432	417	1589	100.0	100.0	100.0	226.2	205.1	113.7	110.8	143.2	149.9	2170	89.4
I. LEUKAEMIAS	22	224	147	86	479	30.1	29.7	100.0	32.3	78.4	38.7	22.9	43.2	45.9	654	73.7
Acute lymphocytic	10	150	88	43	291	18.3	17.9	60.8	14.7	52.5	23.2	11.4	26.2	28.2	398	74.9
Other lymphocytic	0	5	2	3	10	0.6	0.6	2.1		1.8	0.5	0.8	0.9	0.9	14	100.0
Acute non-lymphocytic	4	18	14	18	54	3.4	3.5	11.3	5.9	6.3	3.7	4.8	4.9	5.0	73	79.6
Chronic myeloid	0	1	5	6	12	0.8	0.8	2.5		0.4	1.3	1.6	1.1	1.0	16	83.3
Other and unspecified	8	50	38	16	112	7.0	6.9	23.4	11.8	17.5	10.0	4.3	10.1	10.8	153	64.3
II. LYMPHOMAS	4	36	78	81	199	12.5	13.4	100.0	5.9	12.6	20.5	21.5	17.9	17.2	267	99.5
Hodgkin's disease	0	7	22	33	62	3.9	4.3	31.2		2.5	5.8	8.8	5.6	5.2	83	98.4
Non-Hodgkin lymphoma	4	22	39	34	99	6.2	6.6	49.7	5.9	7.7	10.3	9.0	8.9	8.8	133	100.0
Burkitt's lymphoma	0	0	0	0	0											
Unspecified lymphoma	0	7	17	14	38	2.4	2.6	19.1		2.5	4.5	3.7	3.4	3.3	51	100.0
Histiocytosis X	0	0	0	0	0											
Other reticuloendothelial	0	0	0	0	0											
III. BRAIN AND SPINAL	23	135	121	123	402	25.3	25.8	100.0	33.8	47.3	31.9	32.7	36.2	37.0	546	91.8
Ependymoma	8	21	13	6	48	3.0	2.9	11.9	11.8	7.4	3.4	1.6	4.3	4.8	66	100.0
Astrocytoma	5	58	43	61	167	10.5	10.8	41.5	7.3	20.3	11.3	16.2	15.2	15.2	226	100.0
Medulloblastoma	5	34	32	13	84	5.3	5.3	20.9	7.3	11.9	8.4	3.5	7.6	8.0	114	100.0
Other glioma	0	10	10	12	32	2.0	2.1	8.0		3.5	2.6	3.2	2.9	2.9	43	96.9
Other and unspecified *	5	12	23	31	71	4.5	4.7	17.7	7.3	4.2	6.1	8.2	6.4	6.2	96	54.9
IV. SYMPATHETIC N.S.	36	46	11	4	97	6.1	5.5	100.0	52.9	16.1	2.9	1.1	8.7	10.3	137	100.0
Neuroblastoma	36	46	10	4	96	6.0	5.4	99.0	52.9	16.1	2.6	1.1	8.6	10.2	136	100.0
Other	0	0	1	0	1	0.1	0.1	1.0			0.3		0.1	0.1	1	100.0
V. RETINOBLASTOMA	14	29	2	0	45	2.8	2.5	100.0	20.6	10.2	0.5		4.1	4.9	64	100.0
VI. KIDNEY	12	55	17	4	88	5.5	5.1	100.0	17.6	19.3	4.5	1.1	7.9	9.1	122	100.0
Wilms' tumour	11	54	16	4	85	5.3	4.9	96.6	16.2	18.9	4.2	1.1	7.7	8.8	118	100.0
Renal carcinoma	1	1	1	0	3	0.2	0.2	3.4	1.5	0.4	0.3		0.3	0.3	4	100.0
Other and unspecified	0	0	0	0	0											
VII. LIVER	6	2	3	4	15	0.9	0.9	100.0	8.8	0.7	0.8	1.1	1.4	1.5	21	100.0
Hepatoblastoma	3	2	0	0	5	0.3	0.3	33.3	4.4	0.7			0.5	0.6	7	100.0
Hepatic carcinoma	3	0	3	4	10	0.6	0.7	66.7	4.4		0.8	1.1	0.9	0.9	14	100.0
Other and unspecified	0	0	0	0	0											
VIII. BONE	0	5	15	52	72	4.5	5.1	100.0		1.8	3.9	13.8	6.5	5.8	96	94.4
Osteosarcoma	0	0	8	24	34	2.1	2.4	47.2		0.7	2.1	6.4	3.1	2.7	45	100.0
Chondrosarcoma	0	0	0	3	3	0.2	0.2	4.2				0.3	0.3	0.2	4	100.0
Ewing's sarcoma	0	2	7	19	28	1.8	2.0	38.9		0.7	1.8	5.1	2.5	2.3	37	100.0
Other and unspecified	0	1	0	6	7	0.4	0.5	9.7		0.4		1.6	0.6	0.6	9	42.9
IX. SOFT TISSUE SARCOMAS	16	22	22	18	78	4.9	4.9	100.0	23.5	7.7	5.8	4.8	7.0	7.5	107	100.0
Rhabdomyosarcoma	2	4	11	7	24	1.5	1.6	30.8	2.9	1.4	2.9	1.9	2.2	2.1	32	100.0
Fibrosarcoma	7	7	3	3	20	1.3	1.2	25.6	10.3	2.5	0.8	0.8	1.8	2.0	28	100.0
Other and unspecified	7	11	8	8	34	2.1	2.1	43.6	10.3	3.9	2.1	2.1	3.1	3.3	47	100.0
X. GONADAL & GERM CELL	17	19	3	4	43	2.7	2.4	100.0	25.0	6.7	0.8	1.1	3.9	4.6	61	100.0
Non-gonadal germ cell	5	5	0	1	11	0.7	0.6	25.6	7.3	1.8		0.3	1.0	1.2	16	100.0
Gonadal germ cell	12	13	3	3	31	2.0	1.8	72.1	17.6	4.6	0.8	0.8	2.8	3.3	44	100.0
Gonadal carcinoma	0	0	0	0	0											
Other and unspecified	0	1	0	0	1	0.1	0.1	2.3		0.4			0.1	0.1	1	100.0
XI. EPITHELIAL NEOPLASMS	3	4	7	33	47	3.0	3.2	100.0	4.4	1.4	1.8	8.8	4.2	3.9	63	100.0
Adrenocortical carcinoma	0	1	0	1	2	0.1	0.1	4.3		0.4		0.3	0.2	0.2	3	100.0
Thyroid carcinoma	0	0	1	4	5	0.3	0.4	10.6			0.3	0.5	0.4	0.4	7	100.0
Nasopharyngeal carcinoma	0	0	2	2	4	0.3	0.3	8.5			0.5	0.5	0.4	0.3	5	100.0
Melanoma	0	2	0	4	6	0.4	0.4	12.8		0.7		1.1	0.5	0.5	8	100.0
Other carcinoma	3	1	4	22	30	1.9	2.1	63.8	4.4	0.4	1.1	5.8	2.7	2.5	40	100.0
XII. OTHER	1	9	6	8	24	1.5	1.5	100.0	1.5	3.2	1.6	2.1	2.2	2.2	33	83.3
* Specified as malignant	4	7	12	13	36	2.3	2.4	100.0	5.9	2.5	3.2	3.5	3.2	3.2	49	11.1

Sweden   FEMALE

1970 – 1982

DIAGNOSTIC GROUP	NUMBER OF CASES					REL. FREQUENCY(%)			RATES PER MILLION							HV(%)
	0	1-4	5-9	10-14	All	Crude	Adj.	Group	0	1-4	5-9	10-14	Crude	Adj.	Cum	
TOTAL	137	468	363	341	1309	100.0	100.0	100.0	212.1	172.3	100.5	95.5	124.1	129.9	1881	89.5
I. LEUKAEMIAS	16	209	124	72	421	32.2	31.5	100.0	24.8	76.9	34.3	20.2	39.9	42.7	605	74.3
Acute lymphocytic	5	128	88	33	254	19.4	19.0	60.3	7.7	47.1	24.4	9.2	24.1	25.7	364	78.3
Other lymphocytic	0	6	2	0	8	0.6	0.6	1.9	-	2.2	0.6	-	0.8	0.9	12	87.5
Acute non-lymphocytic	7	19	9	18	53	4.0	4.0	12.6	10.8	7.0	2.5	5.0	5.0	5.3	76	75.5
Chronic myeloid	0	1	2	7	10	0.8	0.8	2.4	-	0.4	0.6	2.0	0.9	0.9	14	90.0
Other and unspecified	4	55	23	14	96	7.3	7.0	22.8	6.2	20.2	6.4	3.9	9.1	9.9	139	60.4
II. LYMPHOMAS	10	11	24	28	73	5.6	5.8	100.0	15.5	4.0	6.6	7.8	6.9	6.9	104	100.0
Hodgkin's disease	0	0	3	12	15	1.1	1.3	20.5	-	-	0.8	3.4	1.4	1.2	21	100.0
Non-Hodgkin lymphoma	7	7	15	12	41	3.1	3.2	56.2	10.8	2.6	4.2	3.4	3.9	4.0	59	100.0
Burkitt's lymphoma	0	0	0	0	0	-	-	-	-	-	-	-	-	-	-	-
Unspecified lymphoma	3	4	6	4	17	1.3	1.3	23.3	4.6	1.5	1.7	1.1	1.6	1.7	24	100.0
Histiocytosis X	0	0	0	0	0	-	-	-	-	-	-	-	-	-	-	-
Other reticuloendothelial	0	0	0	0	0	-	-	-	-	-	-	-	-	-	-	-
III. BRAIN AND SPINAL	18	97	98	102	315	24.1	24.7	100.0	27.9	35.7	27.1	28.6	29.9	30.3	449	94.0
Ependymoma	5	12	9	14	40	3.1	3.1	12.7	7.7	4.4	2.5	3.9	3.8	3.9	57	100.0
Astrocytoma	4	55	58	52	169	12.9	13.2	53.7	6.2	20.2	16.1	14.3	16.0	16.2	243	99.4
Medulloblastoma	1	13	16	21	51	3.9	4.0	16.2	1.5	4.8	4.4	5.9	4.8	4.8	73	100.0
Other glioma	3	5	3	2	13	1.0	1.0	4.1	4.6	1.8	0.8	0.6	1.2	1.3	19	100.0
Other and unspecified *	5	12	12	13	42	3.2	3.3	13.3	7.7	4.4	3.3	3.6	4.0	4.0	60	57.1
IV. SYMPATHETIC N.S.	32	31	13	0	76	5.8	5.2	100.0	49.5	11.4	3.6	-	7.2	8.5	113	100.0
Neuroblastoma	31	31	13	0	75	5.7	5.2	98.7	48.0	11.4	3.6	-	7.1	8.4	112	100.0
Other	1	0	0	0	1	0.1	0.1	1.3	1.5	-	-	-	0.1	0.1	2	100.0
V. RETINOBLASTOMA	21	19	2	0	42	3.2	2.8	100.0	32.5	7.0	0.6	-	4.0	4.9	63	97.6
VI. KIDNEY	10	49	31	3	93	7.1	6.7	100.0	15.5	18.0	8.6	0.8	8.8	9.8	135	98.9
Wilms' tumour	10	48	31	3	92	7.0	6.7	98.9	15.5	17.7	8.6	0.8	8.7	9.7	133	100.0
Renal carcinoma	0	0	0	0	0	-	-	-	-	-	-	-	-	-	-	-
Other and unspecified	0	1	0	0	1	0.1	0.1	1.1	-	0.4	-	-	0.1	0.1	1	-
VII. LIVER	4	6	3	3	16	1.2	1.2	100.0	6.2	2.2	0.8	0.8	1.5	1.7	23	100.0
Hepatoblastoma	2	3	0	0	5	0.4	0.3	31.3	3.1	1.1	-	-	0.5	0.6	8	100.0
Hepatic carcinoma	2	3	3	3	11	0.8	0.8	68.8	3.1	1.1	0.8	0.8	1.0	1.1	16	100.0
Other and unspecified	0	0	0	0	0	-	-	-	-	-	-	-	-	-	-	-
VIII. BONE	0	9	18	44	71	5.4	6.0	100.0	-	3.3	5.0	12.3	6.7	6.2	100	98.6
Osteosarcoma	0	0	7	21	28	2.1	2.4	39.4	-	-	1.9	5.9	2.7	2.3	39	100.0
Chondrosarcoma	0	0	1	4	5	0.4	0.4	7.0	-	-	0.3	1.1	0.5	0.4	7	100.0
Ewing's sarcoma	0	2	8	17	27	2.1	2.3	38.0	-	0.7	2.2	4.8	2.6	2.3	38	100.0
Other and unspecified	0	7	2	2	11	0.8	0.8	15.5	-	2.6	0.6	0.6	1.0	1.1	16	90.9
IX. SOFT TISSUE SARCOMAS	15	22	16	19	72	5.5	5.4	100.0	23.2	8.1	4.4	5.3	6.8	7.3	104	100.0
Rhabdomyosarcoma	8	6	5	2	21	1.6	1.5	29.2	12.4	2.2	1.4	0.6	2.0	2.3	31	100.0
Fibrosarcoma	5	1	7	2	15	1.1	1.1	20.8	7.7	0.4	1.9	0.6	1.4	1.5	22	100.0
Other and unspecified	2	15	4	15	36	2.8	2.8	50.0	3.1	5.5	1.1	4.2	3.4	3.6	52	100.0
X. GONADAL & GERM CELL	7	7	12	14	40	3.1	3.1	100.0	10.8	2.6	3.3	3.9	3.8	3.8	57	100.0
Non-gonadal germ cell	5	6	1	1	13	1.0	0.9	32.5	7.7	2.2	0.3	0.3	1.2	1.5	19	100.0
Gonadal germ cell	0	0	9	6	15	1.1	1.3	37.5	-	-	2.5	1.7	1.4	1.3	21	100.0
Gonadal carcinoma	1	0	0	2	3	0.2	0.2	7.5	1.5	-	-	0.6	0.3	0.3	4	100.0
Other and unspecified	1	1	2	5	9	0.7	0.7	22.5	1.5	0.4	0.6	1.4	0.9	0.8	13	100.0
XI. EPITHELIAL NEOPLASMS	2	2	17	51	72	5.5	6.2	100.0	3.1	0.7	4.7	14.3	6.8	6.1	101	100.0
Adrenocortical carcinoma	0	0	1	1	2	0.2	0.1	2.8	-	-	0.3	0.3	0.2	0.2	3	100.0
Thyroid carcinoma	0	0	1	18	19	1.5	1.7	26.4	-	-	0.3	5.0	1.8	1.6	27	100.0
Nasopharyngeal carcinoma	0	0	0	1	1	0.1	0.1	1.4	-	-	-	0.3	0.1	0.1	2	100.0
Melanoma	0	1	2	4	7	0.5	0.6	9.7	-	0.4	0.6	1.1	0.7	0.6	10	100.0
Other carcinoma	2	1	13	27	43	3.3	3.6	59.7	3.1	0.4	3.6	7.6	4.1	3.7	60	100.0
XII. OTHER	2	6	5	5	18	1.4	1.4	100.0	3.1	2.2	1.4	1.4	1.7	1.8	26	61.1
* Specified as malignant	2	9	9	3	23	1.8	1.7		3.1	3.3	2.5	0.8	2.2	2.3	33	21.7

Commentary

Overall, the incidence rate was one of the highest in Europe. Of the leukaemias, 23% were of 'other and unspecified' type but the age-distribution in this subgroup, with a peak in 1—4-year-olds, suggests that within this group the ratio of acute lymphocytic to acute non-lymphocytic would not differ markedly from that for the leukaemias of specified type (5.1:1). The incidence rates were particularly high for brain and spinal tumours, retinoblastomas, germ-cell tumours and thyroid carcinoma. The large number of cases classified as malignant mesenchymoma — 38/150 = 25% of all soft-tissue sarcomas — is probably an artefact of the coding system. The 49 miscellaneous carcinomas in colorectal sites were all malignant carcinoid tumours of the appendix.

References

World Health Organization (1956) *Statistical code for human tumours*, Geneva (unpublished document WHO/HS/-CANC/24.1)

Ericsson, J.L.E., Karnstrom, L. & Mattsson, B. (1978) Childhood cancer in Sweden, 1958-1974. I. Incidence and mortality. *Acta Paediatr. Scand.*, 67, 425-432

SWITZERLAND

Cancer Registries of three western Cantons: Geneva, Neuchâtel and Vaud, 1974–1983

F. Levi (Vaud)

L. Raymond, M. Obradovic, & P. Vassilakos (Geneva)

S. Pellaux, A.M. Mean & R.P. Baumann (Neuchâtel)

Cancer registration in Switzerland has developed at the level of the Canton. There are currently six cancer registries (Tuyns et *al.*, 1985), which form the Swiss Association of Cancer Registries and have agreed on standardized definitions, codes and procedures. However, they have a relatively small population base, and several have collected data for quite short periods of time. In consequence, the Association agreed that, for the present volume, the data from the three most western Cantons — Geneva, Neuchâtel and Vaud — could be pooled for the longest time period possible, in order to provide sufficient cases to allow calculation of reliable incidence rates. The three registries are described below. The Cantons are all French-speaking and relatively homogeneous socially and culturally, with a combined population of 1.03 million in 1980, of whom 17% were children aged 0–14. The time period analysed (1974-1983) was determined by the date of establishment of the most recent registry.

The Geneva Cancer Registry was set up in 1970 primarily to evaluate the results of screening for cervical cancer and was thus attached to the Cytology Centre, an official organization under the auspices of the public health authorities of the Canton of Geneva. The Neuchatel Registry, which started in 1972, is located in the Institute of Pathology at Neuchatel. The Vaud Registry began in 1973 as a constituent part of the Department of Epidemiology at the Institute for Social and Preventive Medicine, University of Lausanne. All three registries are funded mainly by the Public Health Departments of the cantons in which they are situated. Additional support is given by the Federal Ministry of Health through the Swiss Association of Cancer Registries.

Mechanisms of case ascertainment vary from one registry to another, but all three receive notifications from pathology departments (including a private laboratory in Geneva), hospital departments and, in the case of Vaud, from medical practitioners. A few cases (fewer than 5%) are ascertained from death certificates alone. Reporting of cases to the registries is voluntary, but it is felt that ascertainment is very nearly complete. All skin cancers are eligible, as is Letterer-Siwe disease.

The three cantons have a total of around 6500 public hospital beds, one per 160 inhabitants. There are no special facilities for paediatric oncology but many patients are treated at the university hospitals in Geneva and Lausanne.

The cantons are all in the westernmost part of Switzerland. The total areas are: Geneva, 282 square kilometres (including 36 square kilometres of Lake Geneva); Neuchâtel, 800 square kilometres; Vaud, 3219 square kilometres. The Canton of Geneva is dominated by the city of the same name. The Canton of Neuchâtel is more rural, with only two towns of approximately 40 000 inhabitants. Although Lausanne, the capital of the Canton of Vaud, and its suburbs represent only 4% of the total area, 43% of the Canton's population lives there; the rest of the Canton is predominantly rural. The climate throughout is temperate.

The populations of the three cantons in the Federal Census of 1980 were 349 040 (Geneva), 157 143 (Neuchâtel) and 529 000 (Vaud). Virtually all of the population is white Caucasian, but 23% is of foreign origin, mostly from European Mediterranean countries. Most of the working population are employed in service and manufacturing industries. With the reduction in land under cultivation and increased mechanization, fewer than 10% are agricultural workers.

Routine cancer incidence data are published by all three registries. The Geneva and Vaud Registries also publish regular analyses of cancer mortality and survival rates. Cases recorded in the Geneva

Contd p. 294

Switzerland, Three Western Cantons 1974 - 1983 MALE

DIAGNOSTIC GROUP	NUMBER OF CASES 0	1-4	5-9	10-14	All	REL. FREQUENCY(%) Crude	Adj.	Group	RATES PER MILLION 0	1-4	5-9	10-14	Crude	Adj.	Cum	HV(%)
TOTAL	13	37	44	30	124	100.0	100.0	100.0	238.4	158.8	135.3	85.2	128.5	136.0	1976	100.0
I. LEUKAEMIAS	3	14	17	8	42	33.9	33.2	100.0	55.0	60.1	52.3	22.7	43.5	46.3	670	100.0
Acute lymphocytic	2	14	16	6	38	30.6	29.7	90.5	36.7	60.1	49.2	17.0	39.4	42.3	608	100.0
Other lymphocytic	0	0	0	0	0	-	-	-	-	-	-	-	-	-	-	-
Acute non-lymphocytic	0	0	1	1	2	1.6	1.7	4.8	-	-	3.1	2.8	2.1	1.8	30	100.0
Chronic myeloid	0	0	0	1	1	0.8	1.0	2.4	-	-	-	2.8	1.0	0.8	14	100.0
Other and unspecified	1	0	0	0	1	0.8	0.8	2.4	18.3	-	-	-	1.0	1.4	18	100.0
II. LYMPHOMAS	1	4	6	8	19	15.3	16.1	100.0	18.3	17.2	18.5	22.7	19.7	19.3	293	100.0
Hodgkin's disease	0	0	2	3	5	4.0	4.4	26.3	-	-	6.2	8.5	5.2	4.5	73	100.0
Non-Hodgkin lymphoma	0	1	3	3	7	5.6	5.8	36.8	-	4.3	9.2	8.5	7.3	6.8	106	100.0
Burkitt's lymphoma	0	0	1	1	2	1.6	1.8	10.5	-	-	3.1	2.8	2.1	2.2	31	100.0
Unspecified lymphoma	0	0	0	1	1	0.8	1.0	5.3	-	-	-	2.8	1.0	0.8	14	100.0
Histiocytosis X	1	1	0	0	2	1.6	1.6	10.5	18.3	4.3	-	-	2.1	2.7	36	100.0
Other reticuloendothelial	0	1	0	1	2	1.6	1.5	10.5	-	4.3	-	2.8	2.1	2.3	33	100.0
III. BRAIN AND SPINAL	1	6	7	2	16	12.9	12.4	100.0	18.3	25.8	21.5	5.7	16.6	18.0	257	100.0
Ependymoma	0	2	0	0	2	1.6	1.6	12.5	-	8.6	-	-	2.1	2.7	34	100.0
Astrocytoma	1	2	5	1	9	7.3	6.8	56.3	18.3	8.6	15.4	2.8	9.3	9.9	144	100.0
Medulloblastoma	0	1	1	1	3	2.4	2.5	18.8	-	4.3	3.1	2.8	3.1	3.1	47	100.0
Other glioma	0	0	1	0	1	0.8	0.7	6.3	-	-	3.1	-	1.0	1.0	15	100.0
Other and unspecified *	0	1	0	0	1	0.8	0.8	6.3	-	4.3	-	-	1.0	1.3	17	100.0
IV. SYMPATHETIC N.S.	5	6	0	1	12	9.7	9.8	100.0	91.7	25.8	-	2.8	12.4	15.9	209	100.0
Neuroblastoma	5	6	0	1	12	9.7	9.8	100.0	91.7	25.8	-	2.8	12.4	15.9	209	100.0
Other	0	0	0	0	0	-	-	-	-	-	-	-	-	-	-	-
V. RETINOBLASTOMA	0	0	0	0	0	-	-	-	-	-	-	-	-	-	-	-
VI. KIDNEY	0	2	3	0	5	4.0	3.6	100.0	-	8.6	9.2	-	5.2	5.6	80	100.0
Wilms' tumour	0	2	3	0	5	4.0	3.6	100.0	-	8.6	9.2	-	5.2	5.6	80	100.0
Renal carcinoma	0	0	0	0	0	-	-	-	-	-	-	-	-	-	-	-
Other and unspecified	0	0	0	0	0	-	-	-	-	-	-	-	-	-	-	-
VII. LIVER	1	0	0	0	1	0.8	0.8	100.0	18.3	-	-	-	1.0	1.4	18	100.0
Hepatoblastoma	1	0	0	0	1	0.8	0.8	100.0	18.3	-	-	-	1.0	1.4	18	100.0
Hepatic carcinoma	0	0	0	0	0	-	-	-	-	-	-	-	-	-	-	-
Other and unspecified	0	0	0	0	0	-	-	-	-	-	-	-	-	-	-	-
VIII. BONE	0	0	4	5	9	7.3	7.7	100.0	-	-	12.3	14.2	9.3	8.1	132	100.0
Osteosarcoma	0	0	3	2	5	4.0	4.0	55.6	-	-	9.2	5.7	5.2	4.6	75	100.0
Chondrosarcoma	0	0	0	0	0	-	-	-	-	-	-	-	-	-	-	-
Ewing's sarcoma	0	0	1	3	4	3.2	3.7	44.4	-	-	3.1	8.5	4.1	3.5	58	100.0
Other and unspecified	0	0	0	0	0	-	-	-	-	-	-	-	-	-	-	-
IX. SOFT TISSUE SARCOMAS	1	3	4	2	10	8.1	7.9	100.0	18.3	12.9	12.3	5.7	10.4	11.0	160	100.0
Rhabdomyosarcoma	1	3	3	0	7	5.6	5.2	70.0	18.3	12.9	9.2	-	7.3	8.4	116	100.0
Fibrosarcoma	0	0	0	1	1	0.8	1.0	10.0	-	-	-	2.8	1.0	0.8	14	100.0
Other and unspecified	0	0	1	1	2	1.6	1.7	20.0	-	-	3.1	2.8	2.1	1.8	30	100.0
X. GONADAL & GERM CELL	1	2	0	1	4	3.2	3.4	100.0	18.3	8.6	-	2.8	4.1	4.9	67	100.0
Non-gonadal germ cell	0	0	0	0	0	-	-	-	-	-	-	-	-	-	-	-
Gonadal germ cell	1	2	0	1	4	3.2	3.4	100.0	18.3	8.6	-	2.8	4.1	4.9	67	100.0
Gonadal carcinoma	0	0	0	0	0	-	-	-	-	-	-	-	-	-	-	-
Other and unspecified	0	0	0	0	0	-	-	-	-	-	-	-	-	-	-	-
XI. EPITHELIAL NEOPLASMS	0	0	3	2	5	4.0	4.0	100.0	-	-	9.2	5.7	5.2	4.6	75	100.0
Adrenocortical carcinoma	0	0	0	0	0	-	-	-	-	-	-	-	-	-	-	-
Thyroid carcinoma	0	0	0	0	0	-	-	-	-	-	-	-	-	-	-	-
Nasopharyngeal carcinoma	0	0	0	1	1	0.8	1.0	20.0	-	-	-	2.8	1.0	0.8	14	100.0
Melanoma	0	0	0	0	0	-	-	-	-	-	-	-	-	-	-	-
Other carcinoma	0	0	3	1	4	3.2	3.0	80.0	-	-	9.2	2.8	4.1	3.8	60	100.0
XII. OTHER	0	0	0	1	1	0.8	1.0	100.0	-	-	-	2.8	1.0	1.0	14	100.0
* Specified as malignant	0	1	0	0	1	0.8	0.8	100.0	-	4.3	-	-	1.0	1.3	17	100.0

Switzerland, Three Western Cantons   1974 - 1983   FEMALE

DIAGNOSTIC GROUP	NUMBER OF CASES 0	1-4	5-9	10-14	All	REL. FREQ.(%) Crude	Adj.	Group	RATES PER MILLION 0	1-4	5-9	10-14	Crude	Adj.	Cum	HV(%)
TOTAL	5	47	22	22	96	100.0	100.0	100.0	96.3	210.5	71.1	64.8	103.8	114.4	1617	98.9
I. LEUKAEMIAS	2	16	12	4	34	35.4	35.7	100.0	38.5	71.7	38.8	11.8	36.8	41.1	578	100.0
Acute lymphocytic	0	14	10	3	27	28.1	28.5	79.4	-	62.7	32.3	8.8	29.2	32.4	456	100.0
Other lymphocytic	0	0	0	0	0	-	-	-	-	-	-	-	-	-	-	-
Acute non-lymphocytic	1	2	2	1	6	6.3	6.4	17.6	19.3	9.0	6.5	2.9	6.5	7.2	102	100.0
Chronic myeloid	0	0	0	0	0	-	-	-	-	-	-	-	-	-	-	-
Other and unspecified	1	0	0	0	1	1.0	0.8	2.9	19.3	-	-	-	1.1	1.5	19	100.0
II. LYMPHOMAS	1	1	0	5	7	7.3	8.4	100.0	19.3	4.5	-	14.7	7.6	7.2	111	100.0
Hodgkin's disease	0	0	0	4	4	4.2	5.5	57.1	-	-	-	11.8	4.3	3.4	59	100.0
Non-Hodgkin lymphoma	0	1	0	1	2	2.1	2.1	28.6	-	4.5	-	2.9	2.2	2.2	33	100.0
Burkitt's lymphoma	0	0	0	0	0	-	-	-	-	-	-	-	-	-	-	-
Unspecified lymphoma	1	0	0	0	1	1.0	0.8	14.3	19.3	-	-	-	1.1	1.5	19	-
Histiocytosis X	0	0	0	0	0	-	-	-	-	-	-	-	-	-	-	-
Other reticuloendothelial	0	0	0	0	0	-	-	-	-	-	-	-	-	-	-	-
III. BRAIN AND SPINAL	0	12	4	5	21	21.9	21.5	100.0	-	53.7	12.9	14.7	22.7	25.1	353	95.2
Ependymoma	0	1	0	0	1	1.0	0.8	4.8	-	4.5	-	-	1.1	1.4	18	100.0
Astrocytoma	0	6	3	2	11	11.5	11.4	52.4	-	26.9	9.7	5.9	11.9	13.2	185	100.0
Medulloblastoma	0	1	0	1	2	2.1	2.2	9.5	-	4.5	-	2.9	2.2	2.2	33	100.0
Other glioma	0	1	1	1	3	3.1	3.5	14.3	-	4.5	3.2	2.9	3.2	3.3	49	100.0
Other and unspecified *	0	3	0	1	4	4.2	3.7	19.0	-	13.4	-	2.9	4.3	5.0	68	75.0
IV. SYMPATHETIC N.S.	1	5	1	0	7	7.3	6.0	100.0	19.3	22.4	3.2	-	7.6	9.5	125	100.0
Neuroblastoma	1	5	0	0	6	6.3	4.6	85.7	19.3	22.4	-	-	6.5	8.4	109	100.0
Other	0	0	1	0	1	1.0	1.4	14.3	-	-	3.2	-	1.1	1.0	16	100.0
V. RETINOBLASTOMA	0	4	0	0	4	4.2	3.1	100.0	-	17.9	-	-	4.3	5.5	72	100.0
VI. KIDNEY	0	6	2	0	8	8.3	7.3	100.0	-	26.9	6.5	-	8.7	10.4	140	100.0
Wilms' tumour	0	6	2	0	8	8.3	7.3	100.0	-	26.9	6.5	-	8.7	10.4	140	100.0
Renal carcinoma	0	0	0	0	0	-	-	-	-	-	-	-	-	-	-	-
Other and unspecified	0	0	0	0	0	-	-	-	-	-	-	-	-	-	-	-
VII. LIVER	0	0	0	0	0	-	-	-	-	-	-	-	-	-	-	-
Hepatoblastoma	0	0	0	0	0	-	-	-	-	-	-	-	-	-	-	-
Hepatic carcinoma	0	0	0	0	0	-	-	-	-	-	-	-	-	-	-	-
Other and unspecified	0	0	0	0	0	-	-	-	-	-	-	-	-	-	-	-
VIII. BONE	0	1	0	3	4	4.2	4.9	100.0	-	4.5	-	8.8	4.3	4.0	62	100.0
Osteosarcoma	0	0	0	1	1	1.0	1.4	25.0	-	-	-	2.9	1.1	0.9	15	100.0
Chondrosarcoma	0	0	0	0	0	-	-	-	-	-	-	-	-	-	-	-
Ewing's sarcoma	0	0	0	1	1	1.0	1.4	25.0	-	-	-	2.9	1.1	2.2	15	100.0
Other and unspecified	0	1	0	1	2	2.1	2.1	50.0	-	4.5	-	2.9	2.2	2.9	33	100.0
IX. SOFT TISSUE SARCOMAS	1	1	1	2	5	5.2	5.6	100.0	19.3	4.5	3.2	5.9	5.4	5.6	83	100.0
Rhabdomyosarcoma	1	1	0	0	2	2.1	1.5	40.0	19.3	4.5	-	-	2.2	2.9	37	100.0
Fibrosarcoma	0	0	0	1	1	1.0	2.7	20.0	-	-	-	2.9	1.1	2.8	15	100.0
Other and unspecified	0	0	1	1	2	2.1	1.4	40.0	-	-	3.2	2.9	2.2	2.2	31	100.0
X. GONADAL & GERM CELL	0	1	0	1	2	2.1	2.1	100.0	-	4.5	-	2.9	2.2	2.2	33	100.0
Non-gonadal germ cell	0	1	0	0	1	1.0	1.4	50.0	-	4.5	-	-	1.1	1.4	18	100.0
Gonadal germ cell	0	0	0	1	1	1.0	0.8	50.0	-	-	-	2.9	1.1	0.9	15	100.0
Gonadal carcinoma	0	0	0	0	0	-	-	-	-	-	-	-	-	-	-	-
Other and unspecified	0	0	0	0	0	-	-	-	-	-	-	-	-	-	-	-
XI. EPITHELIAL NEOPLASMS	0	0	2	1	3	3.1	4.1	100.0	-	-	6.5	2.9	3.2	2.9	47	100.0
Adrenocortical carcinoma	0	0	0	0	0	-	-	-	-	-	-	-	-	-	-	-
Thyroid carcinoma	0	0	0	0	0	-	-	-	-	-	-	-	-	-	-	-
Nasopharyngeal carcinoma	0	0	1	1	2	2.1	2.7	66.7	-	-	3.2	2.9	2.2	1.9	31	100.0
Melanoma	0	0	1	0	1	1.0	1.4	33.3	-	-	3.2	-	1.1	1.0	16	100.0
Other carcinoma	0	0	0	0	0	-	-	-	-	-	-	-	-	-	-	-
XII. OTHER	0	0	0	1	1	1.0	1.4	100.0	-	-	-	2.9	1.1	0.9	15	100.0
* Specified as malignant	0	3	0	1	4	4.2	3.7	100.0	-	13.4	-	2.9	4.3	5.0	68	75.0

and Vaud Registries have been used in epidemiological investigations, including case-control studies.

Population

The population data represent the mean population for the period 1977-1980, derived from estimates based on the Federal Censuses of 1970 and 1980.

AVERAGE ANNUAL POPULATION: 1974–1983

Age	Male	Female
0	5453	5190
1–4	23296	22328
5–9	32509	30956
10–14	35224	33974
0–14	96482	92448

Commentary

Overall, the incidence rates are similar to those observed in other European countries. The rate for brain and spinal tumours seems low but this may be due to some under-reporting, since only one of the cases was not histologically confirmed. Letterer-Siwe disease is the only form of histiocytosis X to be registered.

Reference

Tuyns, A., Levi, F., Raymond, L., Baumann, R.P., Enderlin, F., Schuler, G. & Tornhost, J. (1985) Incidence des cancers en Suisse (1979-1981). *Schweiz. Arzteztg.*, *66*, 1900-1906

UNITED KINGDOM — ENGLAND AND WALES

National Registry of Childhood Tumours, 1971–1980

G.J. Draper, C.A. Stiller, H. Fearnley, E.L. Lennox, E.M. Roberts & B.M. Sanders

Cancer registration in England and Wales is carried out by population-based regional cancer registries, with national coverage since 1962. Cancer registration nationally is co-ordinated by the Office of Population Censuses and Surveys (OPCS).

Registration is voluntary and methods of ascertainment vary between regions. Notifications are obtained direct from hospital case notes, computerized in-patient records (hospital activity analysis) and death certificates.

Copies of all records relating to children are sent to the Childhood Cancer Research Group by OPCS and the cancer registries. There, records are linked with notifications from the United Kingdom Children's Cancer Study Group, the Medical Research Council's clinical trials and death certificates. These records, together with those from general practitioners and hospitals, are used to verify and amend the data, particularly the diagnoses, on the original cancer registrations. Comparison with other sources of ascertainment suggest that over 90% of childhood cancers are registered.

Free medical treatment is available under the National Health Service. During the decade covered by the present report, there was an increasing tendency for children with cancer to be treated at centres specializing in paediatric oncology; by 1980, approximately 60% were treated at, or in collaboration with, such centres.

England and Wales have together an area of 151 207 square kilometres. England is predominantly a lowland country with upland regions in the north and south-west; Wales is a country of hills and mountains with extensive tracts of high plateau. The annual mean temperature is about 10° C and average yearly rainfall about 90 cm.

The total population in the 1981 census was 49 634 000, of whom 20.3% were children below age 15.

Population

The population data used here are derived from the annual reports of the Registrar General for England and Wales, and are based on the censuses of 1971 and 1981, together with statistics on births, deaths and migration.

AVERAGE ANNUAL POPULATION: 1971–1980

Age	Male	Female
0	330600	312700
1–4	1398400	1323400
5–9	1970100	1867200
10–14	2008700	1904600
0–14	5707800	5407900

Commentary

The general pattern of rates was similar to that for most European registries, though the total rate for 'All cancers' was rather lower than that for most other predominantly white populations. Approximately one-third of the cases were leukaemias, 80% of these being of the acute lymphocytic type. The next most common categories were brain and spinal tumours, rather less than one-quarter of the cases, and lymphomas, about one-ninth. Retinoblastoma accounted for about one in 40 of all the cases; of these, about 35% were bilateral.

Contd. p. 298

We are grateful to Mr R.T. Benn, Dr N.A. Dent, Mrs S.M. Gravestock, Miss C. Hunt, Prof. C.A.F. Joslin, Dr E.M. Kingsley Pillers, Mr D.S. MacLean, Mr R.A. McNay, Dr R.B. Morley-Davies, Mr R.G. Skeet, Mr M. Slattery, Dr J.A.H. Waterhouse and their colleagues at the Regional Cancer Registries in England and Wales, and also to the Office of Population Censuses and Surveys for providing the original cancer registration data on which the tables for England and Wales in this volume are based.

Great Britain, England and Wales   1971 – 1980   MALE

DIAGNOSTIC GROUP	NUMBER OF CASES 0	1-4	5-9	10-14	All	REL. FREQUENCY(%) Crude	Adj.	Group	RATES PER MILLION 0	1-4	5-9	10-14	Crude	Adj.	Cum	HV(%)
TOTAL	448	2303	1937	1823	6511	100.0	100.0	100.0	135.5	164.7	98.3	90.8	114.1	119.6	1740	94.6
I. LEUKAEMIAS	91	1014	652	453	2210	33.9	33.6	100.0	27.5	72.5	33.1	22.6	38.7	41.8	596	100.0
Acute lymphocytic	47	880	529	307	1763	27.1	26.7	79.8	14.2	62.9	26.9	15.3	30.9	33.7	477	99.9
Other lymphocytic	0	1	0	0	1	–	–	–	–	–	–	–	–	–	–	100.0
Acute non-lymphocytic	25	96	101	123	345	5.3	5.3	15.6	7.6	6.9	5.1	6.1	6.0	6.1	91	100.0
Chronic myeloid	11	17	10	13	51	0.8	0.8	2.3	3.3	1.2	0.5	0.6	0.9	1.0	14	100.0
Other and unspecified	8	21	12	9	50	0.8	0.8	2.3	2.4	1.5	0.6	0.4	0.9	1.0	14	100.0
II. LYMPHOMAS	20	149	336	407	912	14.0	14.4	100.0	6.0	10.7	17.1	20.3	16.0	15.2	235	99.0
Hodgkin's disease	0	28	116	215	359	5.5	5.7	39.4	–	2.0	5.9	10.7	6.3	5.6	91	99.2
Non-Hodgkin lymphoma	7	94	193	172	466	7.2	7.3	51.1	2.1	6.7	9.8	8.6	8.2	7.9	121	99.1
Burkitt's lymphoma	0	6	8	3	17	0.3	0.3	1.9	–	0.4	0.4	0.1	0.3	0.3	4	100.0
Unspecified lymphoma	0	7	5	5	17	0.3	0.3	1.9	–	0.5	0.3	0.2	0.3	0.3	5	94.1
Histiocytosis X	11	12	7	5	35	0.5	0.5	3.8	3.3	0.9	0.4	0.2	0.6	0.7	10	97.1
Other reticuloendothelial	2	2	7	7	18	0.3	0.3	2.0	0.6	0.1	0.4	0.3	0.3	0.3	5	100.0
III. BRAIN AND SPINAL	68	415	553	453	1489	22.9	23.0	100.0	20.6	29.7	28.1	22.6	26.1	26.4	392	79.7
Ependymoma	11	79	54	39	183	2.8	2.8	12.3	3.3	5.6	2.7	1.9	3.2	3.5	49	95.1
Astrocytoma	20	133	192	168	513	7.9	8.0	34.5	6.0	9.5	9.7	8.4	9.0	9.0	135	93.1
Medulloblastoma	14	98	139	90	341	5.2	5.3	22.9	4.2	7.0	7.1	4.5	6.0	6.1	90	97.4
Other glioma	10	55	87	72	224	3.4	3.5	15.0	3.0	3.9	4.4	3.6	3.9	3.9	59	38.4
Other and unspecified *	13	50	81	84	228	3.5	3.6	15.3	3.9	3.6	4.1	4.2	4.0	4.0	60	49.5
IV. SYMPATHETIC N.S.	91	192	65	31	379	5.8	5.6	100.0	27.5	13.7	3.3	1.5	6.6	7.9	107	97.1
Neuroblastoma	89	190	65	30	374	5.7	5.6	98.7	26.9	13.6	3.3	1.5	6.6	7.9	105	97.0
Other	2	2	0	1	5	0.1	0.1	1.3	0.6	0.1	–	0.1	0.1	0.1	1	100.0
V. RETINOBLASTOMA	52	94	5	1	152	2.3	2.2	100.0	15.7	6.7	0.3	–	2.7	3.4	44	94.1
VI. KIDNEY	40	211	73	19	343	5.3	5.1	100.0	12.1	15.1	3.7	0.9	6.0	7.1	96	98.8
Wilms' tumour	40	211	69	13	333	5.1	4.9	97.1	12.1	15.1	3.5	0.6	5.8	6.9	93	98.8
Renal carcinoma	0	0	4	6	10	0.2	0.2	2.9	–	–	0.2	0.3	0.2	0.2	3	100.0
Other and unspecified	0	0	0	0	0	–	–	–	–	–	–	–	–	–	–	–
VII. LIVER	14	19	4	9	46	0.7	0.7	100.0	4.2	1.4	0.2	0.4	0.8	0.9	13	97.8
Hepatoblastoma	12	17	4	2	35	0.5	0.5	76.1	3.6	1.2	0.2	0.1	0.6	0.8	10	100.0
Hepatic carcinoma	2	2	0	7	11	0.2	0.2	23.9	0.6	0.1	–	0.3	0.2	0.2	3	90.0
Other and unspecified	0	0	0	0	0	–	–	–	–	–	–	–	–	–	–	–
VIII.BONE	2	14	77	224	317	4.9	4.9	100.0	0.6	1.0	3.9	11.2	5.6	4.9	80	99.4
Osteosarcoma	0	2	34	136	172	2.6	2.8	54.3	–	0.1	1.7	6.8	3.0	2.6	43	98.8
Chondrosarcoma	0	0	1	6	7	0.1	0.1	2.2	–	–	0.1	0.3	0.1	0.1	2	100.0
Ewing's sarcoma	2	8	37	75	122	1.9	2.0	38.5	0.6	0.6	1.9	3.7	2.1	1.9	31	100.0
Other and unspecified	0	4	5	7	16	0.2	0.3	5.0	–	0.3	0.3	0.3	0.3	0.3	4	100.0
IX. SOFT TISSUE SARCOMAS	42	123	119	114	398	6.1	6.1	100.0	12.7	8.8	6.0	5.7	7.0	7.3	106	99.5
Rhabdomyosarcoma	22	104	93	55	274	4.2	4.2	68.8	6.7	7.4	4.7	2.7	4.8	5.1	74	99.3
Fibrosarcoma	5	4	11	28	48	0.7	0.8	12.1	1.5	0.3	0.6	1.4	0.8	0.8	12	100.0
Other and unspecified	15	15	15	31	76	1.2	1.2	19.1	4.5	1.1	0.8	1.5	1.3	1.4	20	100.0
X. GONADAL & GERM CELL	24	59	16	25	124	1.9	1.9	100.0	7.3	4.2	0.8	1.2	2.2	2.5	34	95.1
Non-gonadal germ cell	4	8	9	16	37	0.6	0.6	29.8	1.2	0.6	0.5	0.8	0.6	0.8	10	83.8
Gonadal germ cell	19	50	7	8	84	1.3	1.2	67.7	5.7	3.6	0.4	0.4	1.5	1.8	24	100.0
Gonadal carcinoma	0	1	0	1	2	–	–	1.6	–	0.1	–	–	–	–	–	100.0
Other and unspecified	1	0	0	0	1	–	–	0.8	0.3	–	–	–	–	–	–	100.0
XI. EPITHELIAL NEOPLASMS	3	8	33	83	127	2.0	2.0	100.0	0.9	0.6	1.7	4.1	2.2	2.0	32	99.1
Adrenocortical carcinoma	1	2	2	1	6	0.1	0.1	4.7	0.3	0.1	0.1	–	0.1	0.1	2	100.0
Thyroid carcinoma	0	0	5	7	12	0.2	0.1	9.4	–	–	0.3	0.3	0.2	0.2	5	100.0
Nasopharyngeal carcinoma	0	1	4	15	20	0.3	0.3	15.7	–	0.1	0.2	0.7	0.3	0.3	9	100.0
Melanoma	1	2	8	25	36	0.6	0.6	28.3	0.3	0.1	0.4	1.2	0.6	0.6	9	95.8
Other carcinoma	1	3	14	35	53	0.8	0.9	41.7	0.3	0.2	0.7	1.7	0.9	0.8	13	100.0
XII. OTHER	1	5	4	4	14	0.2	0.2	100.0	0.3	0.4	0.2	0.2	0.2	0.3	4	76.9
* Specified as malignant	1	8	10	5	24	0.4	0.4	100.0	0.3	0.6	0.5	0.2	0.4	0.4	6	62.5

Great Britain, England and Wales   1971 – 1980   FEMALE

DIAGNOSTIC GROUP	\[NUMBER OF CASES\] 0	1-4	5-9	10-14	All	\[REL. FREQUENCY(%)\] Crude	Adj.	Group	\[RATES PER MILLION\] 0	1-4	5-9	10-14	Crude	Adj.	Cum	HV(%)
TOTAL	396	1779	1377	1416	4968	100.0	100.0	100.0	126.6	134.4	73.7	74.3	91.9	96.8	1405	93.5
I. LEUKAEMIAS	86	737	490	334	1647	33.2	32.9	100.0	27.5	55.7	26.2	17.5	30.5	32.9	469	100.0
Acute lymphocytic	37	627	391	209	1264	25.4	25.2	76.7	11.8	47.4	20.9	11.0	23.4	25.5	361	100.0
Other lymphocytic	0	2	0	0	2	-	-	0.1	-	0.2	-	-	-	-	-	100.0
Acute non-lymphocytic	35	84	85	94	298	6.0	6.0	18.1	11.2	6.3	4.6	4.9	5.5	5.7	84	100.0
Chronic myeloid	5	7	6	15	33	0.7	0.7	2.0	1.6	0.5	0.3	0.8	0.6	0.6	9	100.0
Other and unspecified	9	17	8	16	50	1.0	1.0	3.0	2.9	1.3	0.4	0.8	0.9	1.0	14	100.0
II. LYMPHOMAS	21	65	111	205	402	8.1	8.3	100.0	6.7	4.9	5.9	10.8	7.4	7.1	110	98.0
Hodgkin's disease	0	11	32	105	148	3.0	3.1	36.8	-	0.8	1.7	5.5	2.7	2.4	39	100.0
Non-Hodgkin lymphoma	10	35	72	74	191	3.8	4.0	47.5	3.2	2.6	3.9	3.9	3.5	3.4	52	97.9
Burkitt's lymphoma	0	0	4	5	9	0.2	0.2	2.2	-	-	0.2	0.3	0.2	0.2	3	100.0
Unspecified lymphoma	0	0	1	8	9	0.2	0.2	2.2	-	-	0.1	0.4	0.2	0.1	4	88.9
Histiocytosis X	5	10	3	8	26	0.5	0.5	6.5	1.6	0.8	0.2	0.4	0.5	0.4	6	88.5
Other reticuloendothelial	6	6	2	5	19	0.4	0.4	4.7	1.9	0.5	0.1	0.3	0.4	0.4	6	100.0
III. BRAIN AND SPINAL	54	339	431	372	1196	24.1	24.5	100.0	17.3	25.6	23.1	19.5	22.1	22.4	333	76.9
Ependymoma	14	56	41	34	145	2.9	2.9	12.1	4.5	4.2	2.2	1.8	2.7	2.9	41	95.8
Astrocytoma	16	121	172	169	478	9.6	9.8	40.0	5.1	9.1	9.2	8.9	8.8	8.8	132	93.5
Medulloblastoma	10	67	69	42	188	3.8	3.8	15.7	3.2	5.1	3.7	2.2	3.5	3.6	53	93.0
Other glioma	6	54	98	64	222	4.5	4.6	18.6	1.9	4.1	5.2	3.4	4.1	4.1	61	35.0
Other and unspecified *	8	41	51	63	163	3.3	3.3	13.6	2.6	3.1	2.7	3.3	3.0	3.0	45	47.8
IV. SYMPATHETIC N.S.	69	149	40	27	285	5.7	5.5	100.0	22.1	11.3	2.1	1.4	5.3	6.3	85	96.8
Neuroblastoma	69	145	39	24	277	5.6	5.3	97.2	22.1	11.0	2.1	1.3	5.1	6.1	83	96.7
Other	0	4	1	3	8	0.2	0.2	2.8	-	0.3	0.1	0.2	0.1	0.2	2	100.0
V. RETINOBLASTOMA	55	89	7	1	152	3.1	2.8	100.0	17.6	6.7	0.4	0.1	2.8	3.6	47	90.1
VI. KIDNEY	48	218	63	19	348	7.0	6.7	100.0	15.4	16.5	3.4	1.0	6.4	7.7	103	98.9
Wilms' tumour	47	217	62	14	340	6.8	6.5	97.7	15.0	16.4	3.3	0.7	6.3	7.5	101	98.8
Renal carcinoma	0	0	1	4	5	0.1	0.1	1.4	-	-	0.1	0.3	0.1	0.1	1	100.0
Other and unspecified	1	1	0	1	3	0.1	0.1	0.9	0.3	0.1	-	0.1	0.1	0.1	1	100.0
VII. LIVER	12	24	7	6	49	1.0	0.9	100.0	3.8	1.8	0.4	0.3	0.9	1.1	15	98.0
Hepatoblastoma	12	22	3	2	39	0.8	0.7	79.6	3.8	1.7	0.2	0.1	0.7	0.9	12	97.4
Hepatic carcinoma	0	2	4	4	10	0.2	0.2	20.4	-	0.2	0.2	0.2	0.2	0.2	3	100.0
Other and unspecified	0	0	0	0	0	-	-	-	-	-	-	-	-	-	-	-
VIII. BONE	0	13	73	170	256	5.2	5.4	100.0	-	1.0	3.9	8.9	4.7	4.2	68	98.0
Osteosarcoma	0	4	29	116	149	3.0	3.2	58.2	-	0.3	1.6	6.1	2.8	2.4	39	98.0
Chondrosarcoma	0	0	2	3	5	0.1	0.1	2.0	-	-	0.1	0.2	0.1	0.1	1	100.0
Ewing's sarcoma	0	6	38	48	92	1.9	2.0	35.9	-	0.5	2.0	2.5	1.7	1.5	25	97.8
Other and unspecified	0	3	4	3	10	0.2	0.2	3.9	-	0.2	0.2	0.2	0.2	0.2	3	100.0
IX. SOFT TISSUE SARCOMAS	29	90	80	87	286	5.8	5.8	100.0	9.3	6.8	4.3	4.6	5.3	5.5	81	98.9
Rhabdomyosarcoma	20	66	55	33	174	3.5	3.5	60.8	6.4	5.0	2.9	1.7	3.2	3.0	50	98.8
Fibrosarcoma	6	5	13	24	48	1.0	1.0	16.8	1.9	0.4	0.7	1.2	0.9	0.8	13	97.9
Other and unspecified	3	19	12	30	64	1.3	1.3	22.4	1.0	1.4	0.6	1.5	1.2	1.2	18	100.0
X. GONADAL & GERM CELL	11	32	23	78	144	2.9	2.9	100.0	3.5	2.4	1.2	4.1	2.7	2.6	40	99.3
Non-gonadal germ cell	11	26	8	11	56	1.1	1.1	38.9	3.5	2.0	0.4	0.6	1.0	1.2	16	98.2
Gonadal germ cell	0	5	13	58	76	1.5	1.6	52.8	-	0.4	0.7	3.0	1.4	1.2	20	100.0
Gonadal carcinoma	0	0	0	7	7	0.1	0.1	4.9	-	-	-	0.3	0.1	0.1	3	100.0
Other and unspecified	0	1	2	2	5	0.1	0.1	3.5	-	0.1	0.1	0.1	0.1	0.1	1	100.0
XI. EPITHELIAL NEOPLASMS	9	23	49	110	191	3.8	4.0	100.0	2.9	1.7	2.6	5.8	3.5	3.3	52	98.8
Adrenocortical carcinoma	3	10	3	1	17	0.3	0.3	8.9	1.0	0.8	0.2	0.1	0.3	0.4	5	100.0
Thyroid carcinoma	0	2	6	23	31	0.6	0.7	16.2	-	0.2	0.3	1.2	0.6	0.5	8	100.0
Nasopharyngeal carcinoma	0	1	3	11	15	0.3	0.3	7.9	-	0.1	0.2	0.6	0.3	0.2	4	100.0
Melanoma	2	7	17	24	50	1.0	1.0	26.2	0.6	0.5	0.9	1.3	0.9	0.9	14	97.2
Other carcinoma	4	3	20	51	78	1.6	1.6	40.8	1.3	0.2	1.1	2.7	1.4	1.3	21	98.6
XII. OTHER	2	0	3	7	12	0.2	0.3	100.0	0.6	-	0.2	0.4	0.2	0.2	3	91.7
* Specified as malignant	2	6	1	7	16	0.3	0.3	-	0.6	0.5	0.1	0.4	0.3	0.3	5	62.5

These findings are similar to those for Scotland and for the more recent of the two periods for which data from the Manchester Children's Tumour Registry are presented here.

References

Draper, G.J., Birch, J.M., Bithell, J.F., Kinnier Wilson, L.M., Leck, I., Marsden, H.B., Morris Jones, P.H., Stiller, C.A. & Swindell, R. (1982) *Childhood cancer in Britain: incidence, mortality and survival*, London, HMSO (*Studies in Medical and Population Subjects*, No. 37)

Stiller, C.A. (1985) Descriptive epidemiology of childhood leukaemia and lymphoma in Great Britain. *Leukaemia Res.*, 9, 671-674

Stiller, C.A. & Draper, G.J. (1982) Trends in childhood leukaemia incidence in Britain 1968-78. *Br. J. Cancer*, 45, 543-551

Manchester Children's Tumour Registry 1954–1970 and 1971–1983

J.M. Birch

The Manchester Children's Tumour Registry (MCTR) was founded in September 1953. At that time, little was known about the incidence, morphology and natural history of tumours in children. The initial purpose of the Registry was to study these aspects and to use this information as the basis for organizing a service for the care and treatment of children with cancer. The MCTR is located within the Christie Hospital and Holt Radium Institute, which is the regional centre for radiotherapy and oncology, and is supported by the Cancer Research Campaign.

From the outset, the Registry was population-based and all cases of malignant and certain benign neoplasms in children less than 15 years of age were included. During the early years of the Registry's operation, cases were ascertained by direct and frequent contact with pathologists, paediatricians, surgeons, radiotherapists, haematologists and other medical personnel who might have seen a relevant case. Since 1962, when the Manchester region joined the National Cancer Registration scheme, the Children's Tumour Registry has routinely received copies of cancer registrations for children. Death certificates for children which record a neoplasm as a cause of death (not necessarily the principal cause) have also been obtained since the outset.

Each notification is checked for eligibility. For inclusion, a case must have proven neoplastic disease diagnosed before the 15th birthday and be resident at the time of diagnosis within the defined geographical region covered by the Registry. For each case, either a copy of the hospital notes or a detailed summary containing information on presenting symptoms, diagnostic procedures, treatment and outcome is obtained. For solid tumours, histopathological material is circulated to a panel of expert pathologists to ensure diagnostic accuracy. This material is retained by the Registry so that diagnoses may be reviewed from time to time. For leukaemias, diagnosis is based on bone-marrow examinations. A small number of cases for whom there was no histological confirmation of diagnosis have been included. However, the clinical evidence must leave little doubt about the diagnosis for such cases to be considered eligible. The majority of cases for which histology is unavailable are brain stem tumours. Each case is followed up annually until death, by writing to the clinician in charge. Material from subsequent biopsies, post mortems, etc., is obtained and circulated to the pathologists' panel. Ascertainment has been estimated to be at least 95% complete in the early years, rising to 98% by the early 1970s.

From 1953 to 1973 the MCTR registered all cases from the Manchester Regional Hospital Board area, which included the Greater Manchester conurbation, the county of Lancashire and parts of the counties of Cheshire, Cumbria and Derbyshire. The child population was approximately 1 million. With the reorganization of the National Health Service in 1974, the North Western Regional Health Authority (NWRHA) was created and since that time the MCTR has included all NWRHA cases. This present region consists of Greater Manchester and Lancashire. The effect of the boundary changes was to reduce the population by about 10%. Approximately two-thirds of the total regional population live in Greater Manchester, which is mainly urban. Lancashire has both urban and rural areas, including a coastal strip. The main industries in the region are engineering, textiles and chemicals, with coal mining in some areas. Agricultural areas are found in Lancashire. Along the eastern boundary, the Pennine moorlands rise to about 600 m. The main industrialized and populated areas, however, are below 200 m.

The population of the region is fairly stable and there has been little migration during the period covered by the Registry. The majority of the population are of white European extraction, but there are ethnic minority groups, emanating mainly from the West Indies and the Indian subcontinent.

It was as a direct result of the Registry findings that the paediatric oncology service in the Manchester region was set up. The data have also been used in many epidemiological studies (see references). The Registry data are regularly used by members of the paediatric oncology team for clinical purposes.

The tables presented here relate to two time periods, 1954–1970 and 1971–1983, this uneven division of the 30-year series being the result of

Contd p. 304

Great Britain, Manchester (period 1)   1954 – 1970   MALE

DIAGNOSTIC GROUP	NUMBER OF CASES 0	1-4	5-9	10-14	All	REL. FREQ. Crude	Adj.	Group	RATE 0	1-4	5-9	10-14	Crude	Adj.	Cum	HV(%)
TOTAL	87	377	272	196	932	100.0	100.0	100.0	135.8	141.1	93.6	73.4	104.8	105.7	1535	95.7
I. LEUKAEMIAS	14	142	85	58	299	32.1	31.7	100.0	21.9	53.1	29.2	21.7	33.6	33.9	489	100.0
Acute lymphocytic	10	124	76	39	249	26.7	25.9	83.3	15.6	46.4	26.1	14.6	28.0	28.3	405	100.0
Other lymphocytic	0	2	0	0	2	0.2	0.2	0.7	-	0.7	-	-	0.2	0.2	3	100.0
Acute non-lymphocytic	4	14	8	18	44	4.7	5.2	14.7	6.2	5.2	2.8	6.7	4.9	5.0	75	100.0
Chronic myeloid	0	2	0	1	3	0.3	0.3	1.0	-	0.7	-	0.4	0.3	0.3	5	100.0
Other and unspecified	0	0	1	0	1	0.1	0.1	0.3	-	-	0.3	-	0.1	0.1	2	100.0
II. LYMPHOMAS	10	36	36	34	116	12.4	13.1	100.0	15.6	13.5	12.4	12.7	13.0	13.1	195	97.4
Hodgkin's disease	0	7	10	26	43	4.6	5.7	37.1	-	2.6	3.4	9.7	4.8	4.7	76	100.0
Non-Hodgkin lymphoma	1	17	23	7	48	5.2	5.2	41.4	1.6	6.4	7.9	2.6	5.4	5.4	80	100.0
Burkitt's lymphoma	0	0	0	0	0	-	-	-	-	-	-	-	-	-	-	-
Unspecified lymphoma	0	0	0	0	0	-	-	-	-	-	-	-	-	-	-	-
Histiocytosis X	9	12	3	0	24	2.6	2.1	20.7	14.0	4.5	1.0	-	2.7	2.8	37	87.5
Other reticuloendothelial	0	0	0	1	1	0.1	0.2	0.9	-	-	-	0.4	0.1	0.1	2	100.0
III. BRAIN AND SPINAL	15	61	85	43	204	21.9	22.5	100.0	23.4	22.8	29.2	16.1	22.9	23.0	341	87.3
Ependymoma	1	12	5	3	21	2.3	2.1	10.3	1.6	4.5	1.7	1.1	2.4	2.4	34	100.0
Astrocytoma	4	21	26	24	75	8.0	8.7	36.8	6.2	7.9	8.9	9.0	8.4	8.4	127	100.0
Medulloblastoma	5	20	26	6	57	6.1	5.9	27.9	7.8	7.5	8.9	2.2	6.4	6.5	94	100.0
Other glioma	1	2	3	1	7	0.8	0.7	3.4	1.6	0.7	1.0	0.4	0.8	0.8	12	100.0
Other and unspecified *	4	6	25	9	44	4.7	5.0	21.6	6.2	2.2	8.6	3.4	4.9	4.9	75	40.9
IV. SYMPATHETIC N.S.	19	38	12	2	71	7.6	6.5	100.0	29.7	14.2	4.1	0.7	8.0	8.2	111	100.0
Neuroblastoma	19	38	12	2	71	7.6	6.5	100.0	29.7	14.2	4.1	0.7	8.0	8.2	111	100.0
Other	0	0	0	0	0	-	-	-	-	-	-	-	-	-	-	-
V. RETINOBLASTOMA	8	20	1	0	29	3.1	2.5	100.0	12.5	7.5	0.3	-	3.3	3.4	44	93.1
VI. KIDNEY	7	34	7	5	53	5.7	5.1	100.0	10.9	12.7	2.4	1.9	6.0	6.1	83	96.2
Wilms' tumour	7	31	6	4	48	5.2	4.5	90.6	10.9	11.6	2.1	1.5	5.4	5.5	75	100.0
Renal carcinoma	0	1	1	1	3	0.3	0.3	5.7	-	0.4	0.3	0.4	0.3	0.3	5	100.0
Other and unspecified	0	2	0	0	2	0.2	0.2	3.8	-	0.7	-	-	0.2	0.2	3	-
VII. LIVER	1	3	2	0	6	0.6	0.6	100.0	1.6	1.1	0.7	-	0.7	0.7	9	100.0
Hepatoblastoma	1	3	2	0	6	0.6	0.6	100.0	1.6	1.1	0.7	-	0.7	0.7	9	100.0
Hepatic carcinoma	0	0	0	0	0	-	-	-	-	-	-	-	-	-	-	-
Other and unspecified	0	0	0	0	0	-	-	-	-	-	-	-	-	-	-	-
VIII.BONE	0	2	14	24	40	4.3	5.4	100.0	-	0.7	4.8	9.0	4.5	4.4	72	97.5
Osteosarcoma	0	0	4	13	17	1.8	2.4	42.5	-	-	1.4	4.9	1.9	1.9	31	100.0
Chondrosarcoma	0	0	0	3	3	0.3	0.3	7.5	-	-	-	1.1	0.3	0.3	6	100.0
Ewing's sarcoma	0	2	9	7	18	1.9	2.2	45.0	-	0.7	3.1	2.6	2.0	2.0	32	100.0
Other and unspecified	0	0	1	1	2	0.2	0.3	5.0	-	-	0.3	0.4	0.2	0.2	4	50.0
IX. SOFT TISSUE SARCOMAS	8	22	21	12	63	6.8	6.7	100.0	12.5	8.2	7.2	4.5	7.1	7.2	104	100.0
Rhabdomyosarcoma	4	20	14	6	44	4.7	4.5	69.8	6.2	7.5	4.8	2.2	4.9	5.0	71	100.0
Fibrosarcoma	3	2	1	0	6	0.6	0.5	9.5	4.7	0.7	0.3	-	0.7	0.7	9	100.0
Other and unspecified	1	0	6	6	13	1.4	1.7	20.6	1.6	-	2.1	2.2	1.5	1.4	23	100.0
X. GONADAL & GERM CELL	2	4	2	1	9	1.0	0.9	100.0	3.1	1.5	0.7	0.4	1.0	1.0	14	100.0
Non-gonadal germ cell	1	0	2	1	4	0.4	0.5	44.4	1.6	-	0.7	0.4	0.4	0.5	7	100.0
Gonadal germ cell	1	4	0	0	5	0.5	0.4	55.6	1.6	1.5	-	-	0.6	0.6	8	100.0
Gonadal carcinoma	0	0	0	0	0	-	-	-	-	-	-	-	-	-	-	-
Other and unspecified	0	0	0	0	0	-	-	-	-	-	-	-	-	-	-	-
XI. EPITHELIAL NEOPLASMS	0	4	3	11	18	1.9	2.4	100.0	-	1.5	1.0	4.1	2.0	2.0	32	100.0
Adrenocortical carcinoma	0	0	1	0	1	0.1	0.2	5.6	-	-	-	0.4	0.1	0.1	2	100.0
Thyroid carcinoma	0	0	1	0	1	0.1	0.1	5.6	-	-	0.3	-	0.1	0.1	2	100.0
Nasopharyngeal carcinoma	0	0	0	7	7	0.8	1.1	38.9	-	-	-	2.6	0.8	0.8	13	100.0
Melanoma	0	2	0	1	3	0.3	0.3	16.7	-	0.7	-	0.4	0.3	0.3	5	100.0
Other carcinoma	0	2	2	2	6	0.6	0.7	33.3	-	0.7	0.7	0.7	0.7	0.7	10	100.0
XII. OTHER	3	11	4	6	24	2.6	2.6	100.0	4.7	4.1	1.4	2.2	2.7	2.7	39	75.0
* Specified as malignant	1	3	3	0	7	0.8	0.7	100.0	1.6	1.1	1.0	-	0.8	0.8	11	71.4

Great Britain, Manchester (period 1) 1954 - 1970 FEMALE

DIAGNOSTIC GROUP	NUMBER OF CASES					REL. FREQUENCY(%)			RATES PER MILLION							HV(%)
	0	1-4	5-9	10-14	All	Crude	Adj.	Group	0	1-4	5-9	10-14	Crude	Adj.	Cum	
TOTAL	60	307	196	171	734	100.0	100.0	100.0	99.1	122.0	71.2	67.0	87.1	87.9	1278	95.5
I. LEUKAEMIAS	11	113	68	48	240	32.7	32.3	100.0	18.2	44.9	24.7	18.8	28.5	28.7	415	99.6
Acute lymphocytic	6	95	46	28	175	23.8	23.0	72.9	9.9	37.7	16.7	11.0	20.8	21.0	299	99.4
Other lymphocytic	0	1	1	0	2	0.3	0.3	0.8			0.4		0.2	0.2	3	100.0
Acute non-lymphocytic	5	17	20	18	60	8.2	8.6	25.0	8.3	6.8	7.3	7.1	7.1	7.1	107	100.0
Chronic myeloid	0	0	0	2	2	0.3	0.4	0.8				0.8	0.2	0.2	4	100.0
Other and unspecified	0	0	1	0	1	0.1	0.2	0.4			0.4		0.1	0.1	2	100.0
II. LYMPHOMAS	5	19	16	20	60	8.2	8.6	100.0	8.3	7.5	5.8	7.8	7.1	7.1	107	96.7
Hodgkin's disease	0	0	4	13	17	2.3	2.9	28.3			1.5	5.1	2.0	1.9	33	100.0
Non-Hodgkin lymphoma	0	5	9	6	20	2.7	3.0	33.3		2.0	3.3	2.4	2.4	2.4	36	100.0
Burkitt's lymphoma	0	0	0	0	0											
Unspecified lymphoma	0	0	1	0	1	0.1	0.2	1.7			0.4		0.1	0.1	2	100.0
Histiocytosis X	4	14	2	1	21	2.9	2.4	35.0	6.6	5.6	0.7	0.4	2.5	2.6	34	90.5
Other reticuloendothelial	1	0	0	0	1	0.1	0.1	1.7	1.7				0.1	0.1	2	100.0
III. BRAIN AND SPINAL	7	59	64	46	176	24.0	25.1	100.0	11.6	23.4	23.2	18.0	20.9	20.9	312	88.1
Ependymoma	3	17	4	2	26	3.5	3.1	14.8	5.0	6.8	1.5	0.8	3.1	3.2	43	100.0
Astrocytoma	2	19	33	27	81	11.0	12.1	46.0	3.3	7.5	12.0	10.6	9.6	9.5	146	100.0
Medulloblastoma	1	11	8	4	24	3.3	3.2	13.6	1.7	4.4	2.9	1.6	2.8	2.9	41	100.0
Other glioma	0	3	0	3	6	0.8	0.9	3.4		1.2		1.2	0.7	0.7	11	100.0
Other and unspecified *	1	9	19	10	39	5.3	5.8	22.2	1.7	3.6	6.9	3.9	4.6	4.6	70	46.2
IV. SYMPATHETIC N.S.	13	25	3	2	43	5.9	5.0	100.0	21.5	9.9	1.1	0.8	5.1	5.3	71	100.0
Neuroblastoma	13	25	3	2	43	5.9	5.0	100.0	21.5	9.9	1.1	0.8	5.1	5.3	71	100.0
Other	0	0	0	0	0											
V. RETINOBLASTOMA	12	15	3	0	30	4.1	3.4	100.0	19.8	6.0	1.1		3.6	3.7	49	96.7
VI. KIDNEY	2	38	7	0	47	6.4	5.4	100.0	3.3	15.1	2.5		5.6	5.8	76	93.6
Wilms' tumour	2	35	7	0	44	6.0	5.1	93.6	3.3	13.9	2.5		5.2	5.4	72	100.0
Renal carcinoma	0	0	0	0	0											
Other and unspecified	0	3	0	0	3	0.4	0.3	6.4		1.2			0.4	0.4	5	
VII. LIVER	1	0	0	0	1	0.1	0.1	100.0	1.7				0.1	0.1	2	100.0
Hepatoblastoma	1	0	0	0	1	0.1	0.1	100.0	1.7				0.1	0.1	2	100.0
Hepatic carcinoma	0	0	0	0	0											
Other and unspecified	0	0	0	0	0											
VIII. BONE	0	3	14	32	49	6.7	8.1	100.0		1.2	5.1	12.5	5.8	5.6	93	95.9
Osteosarcoma	0	0	5	17	22	3.0	3.7	44.9			1.8	6.7	2.6	2.5	42	95.5
Chondrosarcoma	0	0	2	1	3	0.4	0.5	6.1			0.7	0.4	0.4	0.3	6	100.0
Ewing's sarcoma	0	3	5	10	18	2.5	2.8	36.7		1.2	1.8	3.9	2.1	2.1	33	100.0
Other and unspecified	0	0	2	4	6	0.8	1.0	12.2			0.7	1.6	0.7	0.7	11	83.3
IX. SOFT TISSUE SARCOMAS	4	21	9	7	41	5.6	5.3	100.0	6.6	8.3	3.3	2.7	4.9	4.9	70	100.0
Rhabdomyosarcoma	3	18	7	4	32	4.4	4.1	78.0	5.0	7.2	2.5	1.6	3.8	3.9	54	100.0
Fibrosarcoma	0	0	0	0	0											
Other and unspecified	1	3	2	3	9	1.2	1.3	22.0	1.7	1.2	0.7	1.2	1.1	1.1	16	100.0
X. GONADAL & GERM CELL	1	9	4	7	21	2.9	2.9	100.0	1.7	3.6	1.5	2.7	2.5	2.5	37	100.0
Non-gonadal germ cell	1	8	2	1	12	1.6	1.5	57.1	1.7	3.2	0.7	0.4	1.4	1.4	20	100.0
Gonadal germ cell	0	0	2	5	7	1.0	1.2	33.3			0.7	2.0	0.8	0.8	13	100.0
Gonadal carcinoma	0	0	0	0	0											
Other and unspecified	0	1	0	1	2	0.3	0.3	9.5		0.4		0.4	0.2	0.2	4	100.0
XI. EPITHELIAL NEOPLASMS	2	0	4	6	12	1.6	1.9	100.0	3.3		1.5	2.4	1.4	1.4	22	100.0
Adrenocortical carcinoma	1	0	1	1	3	0.4	0.4	25.0	1.7		0.4	0.4	0.4	0.4	5	100.0
Thyroid carcinoma	0	0	0	0	0											
Nasopharyngeal carcinoma	0	0	0	2	2	0.3	0.4	16.7				0.8	0.2	0.2	4	100.0
Melanoma	0	0	0	1	1	0.1	0.2	8.3				0.4	0.1	0.1	2	100.0
Other carcinoma	1	0	2	3	6	0.8	0.9	50.0	1.7		0.7	1.2	0.7	0.7	11	100.0
XII. OTHER	2	5	4	3	14	1.9	1.9	100.0	3.3	2.0	1.5	1.2	1.7	1.7	24	78.6
* Specified as malignant	0	3	1	0	4	0.5	0.5	100.0		1.2	0.4		0.5	0.5	7	50.0

Great Britain, Manchester (period 2) 1971 - 1983 MALE

DIAGNOSTIC GROUP	NUMBER OF CASES					REL. FREQUENCY(%)			RATES PER MILLION						Cum	HV(%)
	0	1-4	5-9	10-14	All	Crude	Adj.	Group	0	1-4	5-9	10-14	Crude	Adj.		
TOTAL	48	277	189	193	707	100.0	100.0	100.0	129.3	179.2	88.5	86.1	112.3	119.1	1719	96.5
I. LEUKAEMIAS	4	116	75	57	252	35.6	35.5	100.0	10.8	75.1	35.1	25.4	40.0	42.8	614	100.0
Acute lymphocytic	4	104	59	40	207	29.3	28.9	82.1	10.8	67.3	27.6	17.8	32.9	35.8	507	100.0
Other lymphocytic	0	1	1	0	2	0.3	0.3	0.8	-	0.6	0.5	-	0.3	0.4	5	100.0
Acute non-lymphocytic	0	9	11	13	33	4.7	4.9	13.1	-	5.8	5.2	5.8	5.2	5.1	78	100.0
Chronic myeloid	0	2	0	1	3	1.3	1.3	3.6	-	1.3	-	1.3	1.4	1.4	21	100.0
Other and unspecified	0	0	0	1	1	0.1	0.2	0.4	-	-	-	0.4	0.2	0.1	2	100.0
II. LYMPHOMAS	6	28	28	38	100	14.1	14.5	100.0	16.2	18.1	13.1	16.9	15.9	16.0	239	99.0
Hodgkin's disease	0	3	10	24	37	5.2	5.7	37.0	-	1.9	4.7	10.7	5.9	5.2	85	100.0
Non-Hodgkin lymphoma	0	14	17	14	45	6.4	6.6	45.0	-	9.1	8.0	6.2	7.1	7.2	107	100.0
Burkitt's lymphoma	0	1	0	0	1	0.1	0.1	1.0	-	0.6	-	-	0.2	0.2	3	100.0
Unspecified lymphoma	0	0	0	0	0	-	-	-	-	-	-	-	-	-	-	-
Histiocytosis X	5	9	0	0	14	2.0	1.7	14.0	13.5	5.8	-	-	2.2	2.8	37	92.9
Other reticuloendothelial	1	0	3	0	3	0.4	0.4	3.0	2.7	0.6	0.5	-	0.5	0.6	8	100.0
III. BRAIN AND SPINAL	7	47	59	54	167	23.6	24.4	100.0	18.9	30.4	27.6	24.1	26.5	26.8	399	88.0
Ependymoma	1	12	5	5	23	3.3	3.2	13.8	2.7	7.8	2.3	2.2	3.7	4.0	57	100.0
Astrocytoma	2	14	19	27	62	8.8	9.2	37.1	5.4	9.1	8.9	12.0	9.9	9.6	146	100.0
Medulloblastoma	1	11	17	11	40	5.7	5.9	24.0	2.7	7.1	8.0	4.9	6.4	6.4	95	100.0
Other glioma	0	1	3	1	5	0.7	0.8	3.0	-	0.6	1.4	0.4	0.8	0.8	12	100.0
Other and unspecified *	3	9	15	10	37	5.2	5.4	22.2	8.1	5.8	7.0	4.5	5.9	6.0	89	45.9
IV. SYMPATHETIC N.S.	11	21	5	0	37	5.2	4.7	100.0	29.6	13.6	2.3	-	5.9	7.3	96	97.3
Neuroblastoma	11	21	5	0	37	5.2	4.7	100.0	29.6	13.6	2.3	-	5.9	7.3	96	97.3
Other	0	0	0	0	0	-	-	-	-	-	-	-	-	-	-	-
V. RETINOBLASTOMA	3	8	0	0	11	1.6	1.4	100.0	8.1	5.2	-	-	1.7	2.2	29	90.9
VI. KIDNEY	7	22	5	2	36	5.1	4.7	100.0	18.9	14.2	2.3	0.9	5.7	6.9	92	100.0
Wilms' tumour	7	22	5	0	34	4.8	4.4	94.4	18.9	14.2	2.3	-	5.4	6.6	87	100.0
Renal carcinoma	0	0	0	2	2	0.3	0.3	5.6	-	-	-	0.9	0.3	0.3	4	100.0
Other and unspecified	0	0	0	0	0	-	-	-	-	-	-	-	-	-	-	-
VII. LIVER	3	3	0	0	6	0.8	0.7	100.0	8.1	1.9	-	-	1.0	1.2	16	100.0
Hepatoblastoma	3	3	0	0	6	0.8	0.7	100.0	8.1	1.9	-	-	1.0	1.2	16	100.0
Hepatic carcinoma	0	0	0	0	0	-	-	-	-	-	-	-	-	-	-	-
Other and unspecified	0	0	0	0	0	-	-	-	-	-	-	-	-	-	-	-
VIII. BONE	1	2	6	18	27	3.8	4.1	100.0	2.7	1.3	2.8	8.0	4.3	3.8	62	100.0
Osteosarcoma	0	1	3	11	15	2.1	2.3	55.6	-	0.6	1.4	4.9	2.4	2.1	34	100.0
Chondrosarcoma	0	1	0	1	2	0.3	0.3	7.4	-	0.6	-	0.4	0.3	0.3	5	100.0
Ewing's sarcoma	0	0	2	6	8	1.1	1.3	29.6	-	-	0.9	2.7	1.3	1.1	18	100.0
Other and unspecified	1	0	1	0	2	0.3	0.3	7.4	2.7	-	0.5	-	0.3	0.4	5	100.0
IX. SOFT TISSUE SARCOMAS	4	16	6	8	34	4.8	4.7	100.0	10.8	10.4	2.8	3.6	5.4	6.0	84	100.0
Rhabdomyosarcoma	2	14	6	7	29	4.1	4.0	85.3	5.4	9.1	2.8	3.1	4.6	5.4	71	100.0
Fibrosarcoma	2	2	0	0	4	0.6	0.5	11.8	5.4	1.3	-	-	0.6	0.8	11	100.0
Other and unspecified	0	0	0	1	1	0.1	0.2	2.9	-	-	-	0.4	0.2	0.1	3	100.0
X. GONADAL & GERM CELL	2	12	4	5	23	3.3	3.1	100.0	5.4	7.8	1.9	2.2	3.7	4.1	57	95.7
Non-gonadal germ cell	1	3	2	5	11	1.6	1.6	47.8	2.7	1.9	0.9	2.2	1.7	1.8	26	90.9
Gonadal germ cell	1	9	2	0	12	1.7	1.5	52.2	2.7	5.8	0.9	-	1.9	2.3	31	100.0
Gonadal carcinoma	0	0	0	0	0	-	-	-	-	-	-	-	-	-	-	-
Other and unspecified	0	0	0	0	0	-	-	-	-	-	-	-	-	-	-	-
XI. EPITHELIAL NEOPLASMS	0	1	1	10	12	1.7	1.8	100.0	-	0.6	0.5	4.5	1.9	1.6	27	100.0
Adrenocortical carcinoma	0	0	0	0	0	-	-	-	-	-	-	-	-	-	-	-
Thyroid carcinoma	0	0	0	2	2	0.3	0.3	16.7	-	-	-	0.9	0.3	0.3	4	100.0
Nasopharyngeal carcinoma	0	0	0	3	3	0.4	0.5	25.0	-	-	-	1.3	0.5	0.4	7	100.0
Melanoma	0	0	0	0	0	-	-	-	-	-	-	-	-	-	-	-
Other carcinoma	0	1	1	5	7	1.0	1.1	58.3	-	0.6	0.5	2.2	1.1	1.0	16	100.0
XII. OTHER	0	1	1	0	2	0.3	0.3	100.0	-	0.6	0.5	-	0.3	0.3	5	50.0
* Specified as malignant	2	3	2	0	7	1.0	0.9	100.0	5.4	1.9	0.9	-	1.1	1.3	18	85.7

Great Britain, Manchester (period 2)   1971 - 1983   FEMALE

DIAGNOSTIC GROUP	NUMBER OF CASES					REL. FREQUENCY(%)			RATES PER MILLION							HV(%)
	0	1-4	5-9	10-14	All	Crude	Adj	Group	0	1-4	5-9	10-14	Crude	Adj	Cum	
TOTAL	45	204	166	173	588	100.0	100.0	100.0	128.5	139.1	82.1	81.0	98.4	103.0	1501	95.6
I. LEUKAEMIAS	9	84	56	38	187	31.8	31.6	100.0	25.7	57.3	27.7	17.8	31.3	33.8	482	100.0
Acute lymphocytic	7	73	41	25	146	24.8	24.6	78.1	20.0	49.8	20.3	11.7	24.4	26.9	379	100.0
Other lymphocytic	0	0	1	0	1	0.2	0.2	0.5	-	-	0.5	-	0.2	0.2	2	100.0
Acute non-lymphocytic	1	10	13	11	35	6.0	6.0	18.7	2.9	6.8	6.4	5.2	5.9	5.9	88	100.0
Chronic myeloid	0	1	0	2	3	0.5	0.5	1.6	-	0.7	-	0.9	0.5	0.5	7	100.0
Other and unspecified	1	0	1	0	2	0.3	0.3	1.1	2.9	-	0.5	-	0.3	0.4	7	100.0
II. LYMPHOMAS	2	11	18	22	53	9.0	9.2	100.0	5.7	7.5	8.9	10.3	8.9	8.6	132	98.1
Hodgkin's disease	0	0	3	9	12	2.0	2.1	22.6	-	-	1.5	4.2	2.0	1.7	28	100.0
Non-Hodgkin lymphoma	0	6	11	8	25	4.3	4.3	47.2	-	4.1	5.4	3.7	4.2	4.1	62	100.0
Burkitt's lymphoma	0	0	1	0	1	0.2	0.2	1.9	-	-	-	0.5	0.2	0.1	2	100.0
Unspecified lymphoma	0	0	0	0	0	-	-	-	-	-	-	-	-	-	-	-
Histiocytosis X	1	3	4	2	10	1.7	1.7	18.9	2.9	2.0	2.0	0.9	1.7	1.8	26	90.0
Other reticuloendothelial	1	2	0	2	5	0.9	0.8	9.4	2.9	1.4	-	0.9	0.8	0.9	13	100.0
III. BRAIN AND SPINAL	7	34	60	48	149	25.3	25.8	100.0	20.0	23.2	29.7	22.5	24.9	24.8	373	85.9
Ependymoma	2	8	4	6	20	3.4	3.4	13.4	5.7	5.5	2.0	2.8	3.3	3.6	51	100.0
Astrocytoma	1	11	23	19	54	9.2	9.4	36.2	2.9	7.5	11.4	8.9	9.0	8.8	134	100.0
Medulloblastoma	1	7	14	7	29	4.9	4.9	19.5	2.9	4.8	6.9	3.3	4.9	4.9	73	100.0
Other glioma	0	1	2	3	6	1.0	1.0	4.0	-	0.7	1.0	1.4	1.0	0.9	15	47.5
Other and unspecified *	3	7	17	13	40	6.8	6.9	26.8	8.6	4.8	8.4	6.1	6.7	6.6	106	100.0
IV. SYMPATHETIC N.S.	8	26	3	2	39	6.6	6.4	100.0	22.8	17.7	1.5	0.9	6.5	8.0	106	100.0
Neuroblastoma	8	25	3	2	38	6.5	6.2	97.4	22.8	17.1	1.5	0.9	6.4	7.8	103	100.0
Other	0	1	0	0	1	0.2	0.2	2.6	-	0.7	-	-	0.2	0.2	3	100.0
V. RETINOBLASTOMA	3	6	1	0	10	1.7	1.6	100.0	8.6	4.1	0.5	-	1.7	2.1	27	90.0
VI. KIDNEY	8	21	4	2	35	6.0	5.7	100.0	22.8	14.3	2.0	0.9	5.9	7.1	95	97.1
Wilms' tumour	8	20	4	2	34	5.8	5.6	97.1	22.8	13.6	2.0	0.9	5.7	6.9	92	100.0
Renal carcinoma	0	0	0	0	0	-	-	-	-	-	-	-	-	-	-	-
Other and unspecified	0	1	0	0	1	0.2	0.2	2.9	-	0.7	-	-	0.2	0.2	3	-
VII. LIVER	3	0	0	1	4	0.7	0.7	100.0	8.6	-	-	0.5	0.7	0.8	11	75.0
Hepatoblastoma	3	0	0	0	3	0.5	0.5	75.0	8.6	-	-	-	0.5	0.7	9	66.7
Hepatic carcinoma	0	0	0	1	1	0.2	0.2	25.0	-	-	-	0.5	0.2	0.1	2	100.0
Other and unspecified	0	0	0	0	0	-	-	-	-	-	-	-	-	-	-	-
VIII. BONE	0	0	11	24	35	6.0	6.1	100.0	-	-	5.4	11.2	5.9	5.0	83	100.0
Osteosarcoma	0	0	4	16	20	3.4	3.5	57.1	-	-	2.0	7.5	3.3	2.8	47	100.0
Chondrosarcoma	0	0	1	1	2	0.3	0.4	5.7	-	-	0.5	0.5	0.3	0.3	5	100.0
Ewing's sarcoma	0	0	6	7	13	2.2	2.3	37.1	-	-	3.0	3.3	2.2	1.9	31	100.0
Other and unspecified	0	0	0	0	0	-	-	-	-	-	-	-	-	-	-	-
IX. SOFT TISSUE SARCOMAS	4	7	6	5	22	3.7	3.7	100.0	11.4	4.8	3.0	2.3	3.7	4.0	57	100.0
Rhabdomyosarcoma	1	5	3	4	13	2.2	2.2	59.1	2.9	3.4	1.5	1.9	2.2	2.3	33	100.0
Fibrosarcoma	2	2	2	1	7	1.2	1.2	31.8	5.7	1.4	1.0	0.5	1.2	1.3	19	100.0
Other and unspecified	1	0	1	0	2	0.3	0.3	9.1	2.9	-	0.5	-	0.3	0.4	5	100.0
X. GONADAL & GERM CELL	0	9	3	17	29	4.9	4.9	100.0	-	6.1	1.5	8.0	4.9	4.7	72	100.0
Non-gonadal germ cell	0	9	2	2	13	2.2	2.2	44.8	-	6.1	0.5	0.9	2.2	2.5	34	100.0
Gonadal germ cell	0	0	1	14	15	2.6	2.6	51.7	-	-	0.5	6.6	2.5	2.1	35	100.0
Gonadal carcinoma	0	0	0	0	0	-	-	-	-	-	-	-	-	-	-	-
Other and unspecified	0	0	0	1	1	0.2	0.2	3.4	-	-	-	0.5	0.2	0.1	2	-
XI. EPITHELIAL NEOPLASMS	1	5	2	12	20	3.4	3.4	100.0	2.9	3.4	1.0	5.6	3.3	3.2	50	100.0
Adrenocortical carcinoma	1	4	0	1	6	1.0	1.0	30.0	2.9	2.7	-	0.5	1.0	1.2	16	100.0
Thyroid carcinoma	0	0	0	2	2	0.3	0.3	10.0	-	-	-	0.9	0.3	0.3	5	100.0
Nasopharyngeal carcinoma	0	1	1	3	5	0.9	0.9	25.0	-	0.7	0.5	1.4	0.8	0.8	12	100.0
Melanoma	0	0	1	6	7	1.2	1.2	35.0	-	-	0.5	2.8	1.2	1.0	17	80.0
Other carcinoma	0	0	0	0	0	-	-	-	-	-	-	-	-	-	-	-
XII. OTHER	0	1	2	2	5	0.9	0.9	100.0	-	0.7	1.0	0.9	0.8	0.8	12	80.0
* Specified as malignant	2	3	4	0	9	1.5	1.5	100.0	5.7	2.0	2.0	-	1.5	1.7	24	55.6

changes in the format of the population data available.

Population

Population data for the 30-year period 1954–1983 have been based on figures from the 1951, 1961, 1971 and 1981 censuses, including official published mid-year population estimates, and take into account births, deaths and migration (General

AVERAGE ANNUAL POPULATION

Age	Male	Female
Period 1: 1954-1970		
0	37688	35600
1–4	157182	148064
5–9	170970	161947
10–14	157117	150115
0–14	522957	495726
Period 2: 1971-1983		
0	28561	26946
1–4	118890	112774
5–9	164259	155588
10–14	172451	164226
0–14	484161	459534

Register Office, Office of Population Censuses and Surveys).

Up to 1970, annual estimates were available only for broad age-categories, and subdivision into the four age-groups used in the corresponding tables required some interpolation from census data. Since 1970, annual estimates of population by single year of age have been available.

Commentary

Data for two periods, 1954–1970 and 1971–1983, are presented here. For the latter period, the rates are very similar to the other rates for the United Kingdom presented here, namely, those for England and Wales and those for Scotland. The most notable difference is for histiocytosis X, where the Manchester rates are much higher than those for the rest of the United Kingdom, presumably as a result of better ascertainment. Rates for germ-cell tumours are also high. The rates for retinoblastoma are rather low, possibly because of under-ascertainment as a result of referral of the cases to a centre outside the region.

Comparison with data for the period 1953–1970 shows a slightly increased incidence in the rates for several diagnostic groups, but particularly for acute lymphocytic leukaemia at ages 1–4 reported in Birch *et al.*, 1981) and for germ-cell tumours, also reported previously.

References

Birch, J.M. (1983) Epidemiology of paediatric cancer. In: Duncan, W., ed., *Paediatric Oncology*, Recent Results in Cancer Research, Vol. 88, Berlin, Heidelberg, New York, Springer, pp. 1-10

Birch, J.M., Marsden, H.B. & Swindell, R. (1980) Incidence of malignant disease in childhood: 24 year review of the Manchester Children's Tumour Registry data. *Br. J. Cancer*, 42, 215-223

Birch, J.M., Swindell, R., Marsden, H.B. & Morris Jones, P.H. (1981) Childhood leukaemia in north west England 1954-1977: epidemiology, incidence and survival. *Br. J. Cancer*, 43, 324-329

Marsden, H.B. & Steward, J.K., eds (1968) *Tumours in Children*. Recent Results in Cancer Research, Vol. 13, Berlin, Heidelberg, New York, Springer

UNITED KINGDOM — SCOTLAND

National Registry of Childhood Tumours, 1971–1980

C.A. Stiller, I. Kemp, G.J. Draper, H. Fearnley, E.L. Lennox,
E.M. Roberts & B.M. Sanders

Cancer registration in Scotland was established on a national basis in 1959. There are five regional population-based registries, which together cover the entire country. Registration is voluntary and methods of ascertainment vary from one region to another, but all regions make use of in-patient and day patient discharge summaries and information from pathology departments. Registries also receive quarterly lists of deaths certified with a diagnosis of cancer; there are regional variations regarding the use of these lists for ascertainment of cases and the extent to which further information is sought. Cancer registration is co-ordinated nationally by the Information Services Division (ISD) of the Common Services Agency of the Scottish Health Service, which receives copies of the standard record form for all cases in the regional registries. The ISD in turn sends copies of these registrations for all patients aged under 15 years to the Childhood Cancer Research Group (CCRG) in Oxford, where they form the basis of ascertainment for Scottish cases in the National Registry of Childhood Tumours. Details of the methods used by the CCRG to confirm the diagnoses and other information on registered cases are given in the report for England and Wales (page 297). Comparison with other sources of ascertainment suggests that over 90% of childhood cancer patients in Scotland are notified to the cancer registries.

Free medical treatment is available under the National Health Service throughout Scotland. Cancer patients are treated at major teaching hospitals, radiotherapy centres and district general hospitals. The majority of children with cancer are treated at the paediatric oncology centres in Glasgow, Edinburgh and Aberdeen.

Scotland consists of the northern part of the island of Great Britain, together with nearly 800 islands. The total area is 78 772 square kilometres, about one-third of the total area of Great Britain.

The three main geographical regions are the Highlands (in the north), the Central Lowlands and the Southern Uplands. The Highlands account for more than half the total area. Most of the industry and three-quarters of the population are in the Central Lowlands. The Southern Uplands are less mountainous than the Highlands, and contain much fertile farmland. The climate of Scotland is temperate, but the west has more rainfall than the east, and less variation in temperature between summer and winter.

The total population in the 1981 census was 5 180 000 (of whom 21.2% were aged under 15, which is under 10% of the total for Great Britain. More than 97% of the population were born in the United Kingdom. In the early 1970s, 32% of the employed population worked in manufacturing, 54% in service industries and the remaining 14% in construction, mining, agriculture and energy supply. Since then, the proportion accounted for by manufacturing industry will have decreased.

Population

The population data used here are derived from annual reports of the Registrar General for Scotland, and are based on the censuses of 1971 and 1981 and annual statistics on births, deaths and migration.

AVERAGE ANNUAL POPULATION: 1971–1980

Age	Male	Female
0	36300	34300
1–4	154800	146600
5–9	221300	210200
10–14	232400	220800
0–14	644800	611900

Contd p. 308

We are grateful to Dr M.H. Elia, Dr C.R. Gillis, Dr G. Innes, Dr S. Scott, Dr G. Venters and their colleagues at the Regional Cancer Registries in Scotland, and also to the Information Service Division of the Common Services Agency of the Scottish Health Service for providing the original cancer registration data on which the tables for Scotland in this volume are based.

Great Britain, Scotland   1971 - 1980   MALE

DIAGNOSTIC GROUP	NUMBER OF CASES					REL. FREQUENCY(%)			RATES PER MILLION						Cum	HV(%)
	0	1-4	5-9	10-14	All	Crude	Adj.	Group	0	1-4	5-9	10-14	Crude	Adj.		
TOTAL	49	251	218	175	693	100.0	100.0	100.0	135.0	162.1	98.5	75.3	107.5	114.3	1653	97.7
I. LEUKAEMIAS	10	119	71	42	242	34.9	34.2	100.0	27.5	76.9	32.1	18.1	37.5	41.5	586	100.0
Acute lymphocytic	8	102	55	23	188	27.1	26.2	77.7	22.0	65.9	24.9	9.9	29.2	33.0	459	100.0
Other lymphocytic	0	0	0	0	0	-	-	-	-	-	-	-	-	-	-	-
Acute non-lymphocytic	1	14	15	17	47	6.8	7.0	19.4	2.8	9.0	6.8	7.3	7.3	7.3	109	100.0
Chronic myeloid	1	2	1	1	5	0.7	0.7	2.1	2.8	1.3	0.5	0.4	0.8	0.9	12	100.0
Other and unspecified	0	1	0	1	2	0.3	0.3	0.8	-	0.6	-	0.4	0.3	0.3	5	100.0
II. LYMPHOMAS	0	14	43	42	99	14.3	15.0	100.0	-	9.0	19.4	18.1	15.4	14.3	224	100.0
Hodgkin's disease	0	0	20	28	48	6.9	7.6	48.5	-	-	9.0	12.0	7.4	6.4	105	100.0
Non-Hodgkin lymphoma	0	8	23	13	44	6.3	6.5	44.4	-	5.2	10.4	5.6	6.8	6.6	101	100.0
Burkitt's lymphoma	0	0	0	1	1	0.1	0.2	1.0	-	-	-	0.4	0.2	0.1	2	100.0
Unspecified lymphoma	0	2	0	0	2	0.3	0.3	2.0	-	1.3	-	-	0.3	0.3	5	100.0
Histiocytosis X	0	3	0	0	3	0.4	0.4	3.0	-	1.9	-	-	0.5	0.6	8	100.0
Other reticuloendothelial	0	1	0	0	1	0.1	0.1	1.0	-	0.6	-	-	0.2	0.2	3	100.0
III. BRAIN AND SPINAL	8	38	55	42	143	20.6	20.9	100.0	22.0	24.5	24.9	18.1	22.2	22.6	335	90.2
Ependymoma	2	7	2	5	16	2.3	2.3	11.2	5.5	4.5	0.9	2.2	2.5	2.7	39	93.8
Astrocytoma	2	14	21	19	56	8.1	8.3	39.2	5.5	9.0	9.5	8.2	8.7	8.7	130	100.0
Medulloblastoma	4	11	15	8	38	5.5	5.4	26.6	11.0	7.1	6.8	3.4	5.9	6.2	91	100.0
Other glioma	0	5	12	7	24	3.5	3.5	16.8	-	3.2	5.4	3.0	3.7	3.6	55	62.5
Other and unspecified *	0	1	5	3	9	1.3	1.3	6.3	-	0.6	2.3	1.3	1.4	1.3	20	55.6
IV. SYMPATHETIC N.S.	11	24	11	4	50	7.2	6.9	100.0	30.3	15.5	5.0	1.7	7.8	9.3	126	98.0
Neuroblastoma	10	23	10	4	47	6.8	6.5	94.0	27.5	14.9	4.5	1.7	7.3	8.7	118	97.9
Other	1	1	1	0	3	0.4	0.4	6.0	2.8	0.6	0.5	-	0.5	0.6	8	100.0
V. RETINOBLASTOMA	8	12	1	0	21	3.0	2.8	100.0	22.0	7.8	0.5	-	3.3	4.3	55	100.0
VI. KIDNEY	6	24	14	0	44	6.3	5.9	100.0	16.5	15.5	6.3	-	6.8	8.1	110	100.0
Wilms' tumour	6	24	14	0	44	6.3	5.9	100.0	16.5	15.5	6.3	-	6.8	8.1	110	100.0
Renal carcinoma	0	0	0	0	0	-	-	-	-	-	-	-	-	-	-	-
Other and unspecified	0	0	0	0	0	-	-	-	-	-	-	-	-	-	-	-
VII. LIVER	2	1	1	0	4	0.6	0.5	100.0	5.5	0.6	0.5	-	0.6	0.8	10	100.0
Hepatoblastoma	1	0	0	0	1	0.1	0.1	25.0	2.8	-	-	-	0.2	0.2	-	100.0
Hepatic carcinoma	1	1	1	0	3	0.4	0.4	75.0	2.8	0.6	0.5	-	0.5	0.6	8	100.0
Other and unspecified	0	0	0	0	0	-	-	-	-	-	-	-	-	-	-	-
VIII. BONE	0	1	4	19	24	3.5	3.9	100.0	-	0.6	1.8	8.2	3.7	3.2	52	100.0
Osteosarcoma	0	1	4	10	15	2.2	2.4	62.5	-	0.6	1.8	4.3	2.3	2.0	33	100.0
Chondrosarcoma	0	0	0	0	0	-	-	-	-	-	-	-	-	-	-	-
Ewing's sarcoma	0	0	0	8	8	1.2	1.4	33.3	-	-	-	3.4	1.2	1.0	17	100.0
Other and unspecified	0	0	0	1	1	0.1	0.2	4.2	-	-	-	0.4	0.2	0.1	2	100.0
IX. SOFT TISSUE SARCOMAS	3	11	12	12	38	5.5	5.6	100.0	8.3	7.1	5.4	5.2	5.9	6.1	90	100.0
Rhabdomyosarcoma	1	9	7	5	22	3.2	3.2	57.9	2.8	5.8	3.2	2.2	3.4	3.7	53	100.0
Fibrosarcoma	2	0	0	2	4	0.6	0.5	10.5	5.5	-	-	0.9	0.6	0.7	10	100.0
Other and unspecified	0	2	3	7	12	1.7	1.9	31.6	-	1.3	1.4	3.0	1.9	1.7	27	100.0
X. GONADAL & GERM CELL	0	5	1	2	8	1.2	1.1	100.0	-	3.2	0.5	0.9	1.2	1.4	19	100.0
Non-gonadal germ cell	0	1	1	1	3	0.4	0.4	37.5	-	0.6	0.5	0.4	0.5	0.5	7	100.0
Gonadal germ cell	0	4	0	1	5	0.7	0.7	62.5	-	2.6	-	0.4	0.8	0.9	12	100.0
Gonadal carcinoma	0	0	0	0	0	-	-	-	-	-	-	-	-	-	-	-
Other and unspecified	0	0	0	0	0	-	-	-	-	-	-	-	-	-	-	-
XI. EPITHELIAL NEOPLASMS	1	2	4	12	19	2.7	3.0	100.0	2.8	1.3	1.8	5.2	2.9	2.7	43	100.0
Adrenocortical carcinoma	0	1	0	1	2	0.3	0.3	10.5	-	0.6	-	0.4	0.3	0.3	5	100.0
Thyroid carcinoma	0	0	0	2	2	0.3	0.3	10.5	-	-	-	0.9	0.3	0.2	4	100.0
Nasopharyngeal carcinoma	0	0	0	2	2	0.3	0.3	10.5	-	-	-	0.9	0.3	0.2	4	100.0
Melanoma	0	1	4	4	9	1.3	1.4	47.4	-	0.6	1.8	1.7	1.4	1.3	20	100.0
Other carcinoma	1	0	0	3	4	0.6	0.6	21.1	2.8	-	-	1.3	0.6	0.6	9	100.0
XII. OTHER	0	0	0	1	1	0.1	0.1	100.0	-	-	-	0.4	0.2	0.1	2	-
* Specified as malignant	0	0	0	1	1	0.1	0.2	100.0	-	-	-	0.4	0.2	0.1	2	-

* Specified as malignant

Great Britain, Scotland

1971 – 1980

FEMALE

DIAGNOSTIC GROUP	NUMBER OF CASES 0	1-4	5-9	10-14	All	REL. FREQUENCY(%) Crude	Adj.	Group	RATES PER MILLION 0	1-4	5-9	10-14	Crude	Adj.	Cum	HV(%)
TOTAL	36	188	159	167	550	100.0	100.0	100.0	105.0	128.2	75.6	75.6	89.9	94.2	1374	96.1
I. LEUKAEMIAS	5	82	60	49	196	35.6	35.7	100.0	14.6	55.9	28.5	22.2	32.0	34.1	492	100.0
Acute lymphocytic	2	65	50	30	147	26.7	26.8	75.0	5.8	44.3	23.8	13.6	24.0	25.8	370	100.0
Other lymphocytic	0	0	0	0	0	-	-	-	-	-	-	-	-	-	-	-
Acute non-lymphocytic	1	12	6	13	32	5.8	5.8	16.3	2.9	8.2	2.9	5.9	5.2	5.4	79	100.0
Chronic myeloid	0	1	3	4	8	1.5	1.5	4.1	-	0.7	1.4	1.8	1.3	1.2	19	100.0
Other and unspecified	2	4	1	2	9	1.6	1.8	4.6	5.8	2.7	0.5	0.9	1.5	1.7	24	100.0
II. LYMPHOMAS	3	7	12	21	43	7.8	7.8	100.0	8.7	4.8	5.7	9.5	7.0	6.8	104	100.0
Hodgkin's disease	0	1	5	10	16	2.9	2.9	37.2	-	0.7	2.4	4.5	2.6	2.3	37	100.0
Non-Hodgkin lymphoma	1	4	7	9	21	3.8	3.8	48.8	2.9	2.7	3.3	4.1	3.4	3.3	51	100.0
Burkitt's lymphoma	0	0	0	1	1	0.2	0.2	2.3	-	-	-	0.5	0.2	0.1	2	100.0
Unspecified lymphoma	0	0	0	1	1	0.2	0.2	2.3	-	-	-	0.5	0.2	0.1	2	100.0
Histiocytosis X	1	1	0	0	2	0.4	0.4	4.7	2.9	0.7	-	-	0.4	0.4	6	100.0
Other reticuloendothelial	1	1	0	0	2	0.4	0.4	4.7	2.9	0.7	-	-	0.3	0.4	6	100.0
III. BRAIN AND SPINAL	4	34	44	38	120	21.8	21.9	100.0	11.7	23.2	20.9	17.2	19.6	19.8	295	84.9
Ependymoma	1	4	2	1	8	1.5	1.4	6.7	2.9	2.7	1.0	0.5	1.3	1.5	21	100.0
Astrocytoma	0	20	18	18	56	10.2	10.2	46.7	-	13.6	8.6	8.2	9.2	9.4	138	98.2
Medulloblastoma	2	7	15	5	29	5.3	5.3	24.2	5.8	4.8	7.1	2.3	4.7	4.9	72	100.0
Other glioma	0	2	7	6	15	2.7	2.8	12.5	-	1.4	3.3	2.7	2.5	2.3	36	20.0
Other and unspecified *	1	1	2	8	12	2.2	2.2	10.0	2.9	0.7	1.0	3.6	2.0	1.8	29	58.3
IV. SYMPATHETIC N.S.	6	19	4	3	32	5.8	5.8	100.0	17.5	13.0	1.9	1.4	5.2	6.4	86	100.0
Neuroblastoma	6	19	4	3	32	5.8	5.8	100.0	17.5	13.0	1.9	1.4	5.2	6.4	86	100.0
Other	0	0	0	0	0	-	-	-	-	-	-	-	-	-	-	-
V. RETINOBLASTOMA	4	12	0	0	16	2.9	2.9	100.0	11.7	8.2	-	-	2.6	3.4	44	93.8
VI. KIDNEY	6	20	6	2	34	6.2	6.1	100.0	17.5	13.6	2.9	0.9	5.6	6.8	91	94.1
Wilms' tumour	6	19	6	1	32	5.8	5.8	94.1	17.5	13.0	2.9	0.5	5.2	6.4	86	96.9
Renal carcinoma	0	0	0	1	1	0.2	0.2	2.9	-	-	-	0.5	0.2	0.1	2	100.0
Other and unspecified	0	1	0	0	1	0.2	0.2	2.9	-	0.7	-	-	0.2	0.2	3	-
VII. LIVER	2	2	0	0	4	0.7	0.7	100.0	5.8	1.4	-	-	0.7	0.9	11	100.0
Hepatoblastoma	2	2	0	0	4	0.7	0.7	100.0	5.8	1.4	-	-	0.7	0.9	11	100.0
Hepatic carcinoma	0	0	0	0	0	-	-	-	-	-	-	-	-	-	-	-
Other and unspecified	0	0	0	0	0	-	-	-	-	-	-	-	-	-	-	-
VIII. BONE	0	2	11	21	34	6.2	6.2	100.0	-	1.4	5.2	9.5	5.6	4.9	79	100.0
Osteosarcoma	0	0	4	14	18	3.3	3.3	52.9	-	-	1.9	6.3	2.9	2.5	41	100.0
Chondrosarcoma	0	0	0	1	1	0.2	0.2	2.9	-	-	-	0.5	0.2	0.1	2	100.0
Ewing's sarcoma	0	2	7	6	15	2.7	2.8	44.1	-	1.4	3.3	2.7	2.5	2.3	36	100.0
Other and unspecified	0	0	0	0	0	-	-	-	-	-	-	-	-	-	-	-
IX. SOFT TISSUE SARCOMAS	5	6	11	9	31	5.6	5.7	100.0	14.6	4.1	5.2	4.1	5.1	5.3	77	100.0
Rhabdomyosarcoma	4	4	5	1	14	2.5	2.6	45.2	11.7	2.7	2.4	0.5	2.3	2.8	37	100.0
Fibrosarcoma	0	1	0	5	6	1.1	1.1	19.4	-	0.7	-	2.3	1.0	0.8	14	100.0
Other and unspecified	1	1	6	3	11	2.0	2.0	35.5	2.9	0.7	2.8	1.4	1.8	1.8	27	100.0
X. GONADAL & GERM CELL	0	2	9	6	17	3.1	3.1	100.0	-	1.4	4.3	2.7	2.8	2.6	40	100.0
Non-gonadal germ cell	0	1	2	0	3	0.5	0.6	17.6	-	0.7	1.0	-	0.5	0.5	7	100.0
Gonadal germ cell	0	1	6	6	13	2.4	2.4	76.5	-	0.7	2.9	2.7	2.1	1.9	31	100.0
Gonadal carcinoma	0	0	0	0	0	-	-	-	-	-	-	-	-	-	-	-
Other and unspecified	0	0	1	0	1	0.2	0.2	5.9	-	-	0.5	-	0.2	0.2	2	-
XI. EPITHELIAL NEOPLASMS	1	2	1	17	21	3.8	3.8	100.0	2.9	1.4	0.5	7.7	3.4	3.0	49	100.0
Adrenocortical carcinoma	0	1	0	0	1	0.2	0.2	4.8	-	0.7	-	-	0.2	0.2	3	100.0
Thyroid carcinoma	0	0	0	3	3	0.5	0.5	14.3	-	-	-	1.4	0.5	0.4	7	100.0
Nasopharyngeal carcinoma	0	0	0	1	1	0.2	0.2	4.8	-	-	-	0.5	0.2	0.1	2	100.0
Melanoma	0	1	0	6	7	1.3	1.3	33.3	-	0.7	-	2.7	1.1	1.0	16	100.0
Other carcinoma	1	0	1	7	9	1.6	1.6	42.9	2.9	-	0.5	3.2	1.5	1.3	21	100.0
XII. OTHER	0	0	1	1	2	0.4	0.4	100.0	-	-	0.5	0.5	0.3	0.3	5	100.0
* Specified as malignant	1	0	0	0	1	0.2	0.2	100.0	2.9	-	-	-	0.2	0.2	3	100.0

Commentary

The general pattern of rates was similar to that in most European registries. There were no major differences between the incidence rates in Scotland and in England and Wales.

References

Draper, G.J., Birch, J.M., Bithell, J.F., Kinnier Wilson, L.M., Leck, I., Marsden, H.B., Morris Jones, P.H., Stiller, C.A. & Swindell, R. (1982) *Childhood cancer in Britain: incidence, mortality and survival*, London, HMSO (*Studies in Medical and Population Subjects*, No. 37)

Stiller C.A. (1985) Descriptive epidemiology of childhood leukaemia and lymphoma in Great Britain. *Leukaemia Res.*, 9, 671-674

Stiller, C.A. & Draper, G.J. (1982) Trends in childhood leukaemia incidence in Britain 1968-78. *Br. J. Cancer*, 45, 543-551

YUGOSLAVIA

Cancer Registry of Slovenia, 1971–1980

Vera Pompe-Kirn

The Cancer Registry of Slovenia was founded in 1950 to provide continuing information on cancer incidence and on survival of cancer patients, to serve as a basis for planning and evaluating cancer control services and for epidemiological and clinical studies.

The main sources of data are hospital in-patient and out-patient departments. Additional sources are autopsy reports and death certificates. For those cases brought to the attention of the Registry by death certificate only, additional information is required from the certifying physician. Reporting of cancer cases from all these sources and their registration in the central Registry is compulsory.

Cases are classified by site according to the 8th Revision of the ICD. The coded data are stored on magnetic discs. Each primary cancer in the same person is recorded separately, except for multiple carcinomas of skin, bladder and colon and multiple primary cancers of the same histology in paired organs. For the present study, the histological type of all childhood cancers was coded according to the ICD-O.

A precise assessment of the completeness of registration is not possible, but it is thought to be reasonably complete. There are several reasons for this: compulsory registration and follow-up of cancer patients; the legal requirement that each patient dying in hospital be autopsied, and that every death be certified by a physician; the fact that the costs of cancer patient care are covered by the national health insurance system; the inclusion of the activities and role of the Registry within the framework of formal undergraduate and post-graduate teaching in the medical school; the location of the Registry in the Institute of Oncology; and the regular publication of feedback information (annual reports and special analyses).

Basic health services are provided in Slovenia by 22 out-patient establishments, staffed principally by general practitioners; private practice is virtually non-existent. There is at least one general hospital in each of the nine health regions, and in some there is a specialized hospital as well. In Ljubljana, the capital, there is a Clinical Centre consisting of specialized hospitals providing teaching facilities for the Medical Faculty of the University of Ljubljana, to which the Institute of Oncology is affiliated. This Institute is a comprehensive cancer centre where radiotherapy, chemotherapy and hormone treatment are almost completely centralized for the whole of Slovenia, and it has housed the Cancer Registry since its foundation. This is a great advantage, since sooner or later about 50% of all cancer patients in Slovenia are admitted to the Institute, thus permitting more precise data collection and permanent contact with clinical oncologists. There is a special department for paediatric oncology within the University Paediatric Hospital.

Health care services are provided in Slovenia by the Regional Institutes of Social Medicine and Hygiene, and by the Republic Institute of Health Care. The Registry co-operates closely with the latter, especially for cancer mortality data processing. The Regional Institutes are also users of the Registry's data.

The Registry covers the population of the entire territory of the Socialist Republic of Slovenia, which occupies the north-westernmost part of Yugoslavia; it borders on Italy in the west, Austria in the north, Hungary in the north-east, and the Yugoslav Socialist Republic of Croatia in the east and south.

The population, according to the 1981 census, was 1 891 864, of whom 91% were known to be native Slovenes, 6% other Slavic nationalities and 2% non-Slavic nationalities. The proportion of immigrants from the other Yugoslav Republics in Slovenia is steadily increasing. Of the total population, 49% live in urban areas, but only 18% in conurbations of more than 100 000 inhabitants.

Contd p. 312

Yugoslavia, Slovenia   MALE

1971 - 1980

DIAGNOSTIC GROUP	NUMBER OF CASES					REL. FREQUENCY(%)			RATES PER MILLION						Cum	HV(%)
	0	1-4	5-9	10-14	All	Crude	Adj.	Group	0	1-4	5-9	10-14	Crude	Adj.	Cum	HV(%)
TOTAL	24	88	82	76	270	100.0	100.0	100.0	168.5	147.4	112.1	107.3	123.9	126.0	1855	97.8
I. LEUKAEMIAS	6	31	24	15	76	28.1	27.9	100.0	42.1	51.9	32.8	21.2	34.9	36.1	520	100.0
Acute lymphocytic	0	21	13	2	36	13.3	13.0	47.4	-	35.2	17.8	2.8	16.5	17.4	244	100.0
Other lymphocytic	0	0	0	0	0	-	-	-	-	-	-	-	-	-	-	-
Acute non-lymphocytic	1	7	6	8	22	8.1	8.2	28.9	7.0	11.7	8.2	11.3	10.1	10.1	151	100.0
Chronic myeloid	1	2	1	1	5	1.9	1.8	6.6	7.0	3.4	1.4	1.4	2.3	2.4	34	100.0
Other and unspecified	4	1	4	4	13	4.8	4.8	17.1	28.1	1.7	5.5	5.6	6.0	6.1	90	100.0
II. LYMPHOMAS	0	12	15	22	49	18.1	18.5	100.0	-	20.1	20.5	31.1	22.5	21.9	338	100.0
Hodgkin's disease	0	3	7	11	21	7.8	8.0	42.9	-	5.0	9.6	15.5	9.6	9.2	146	100.0
Non-Hodgkin lymphoma	0	7	6	11	24	8.9	9.0	49.0	-	11.7	8.2	15.5	11.0	10.8	166	100.0
Burkitt's lymphoma	0	0	0	0	0	-	-	-	-	-	-	-	-	-	-	-
Unspecified lymphoma	0	1	2	0	3	1.1	1.1	6.1	-	1.7	2.7	-	1.4	1.4	20	100.0
Histiocytosis X	0	1	0	0	1	0.4	0.4	2.0	-	1.7	-	-	0.5	0.5	7	100.0
Other reticuloendothelial	0	0	0	0	0	-	-	-	-	-	-	-	-	-	-	-
III. BRAIN AND SPINAL	5	20	19	14	58	21.5	21.4	100.0	35.1	33.5	26.0	19.8	26.6	27.2	398	91.4
Ependymoma	1	2	2	1	6	2.2	2.2	10.3	7.0	3.4	2.7	1.4	2.8	2.9	41	100.0
Astrocytoma	0	7	7	5	19	7.0	7.0	32.8	-	11.7	9.6	7.0	8.7	8.8	130	100.0
Medulloblastoma	3	5	4	3	15	5.6	5.5	25.9	21.1	8.4	5.5	4.2	6.9	7.2	103	100.0
Other glioma	0	4	2	3	9	3.3	3.3	15.5	-	6.7	2.7	4.2	4.1	4.2	62	100.0
Other and unspecified *	1	2	4	2	9	3.3	3.3	15.5	7.0	3.4	5.5	2.8	4.1	4.2	62	44.4
IV. SYMPATHETIC N.S.	3	5	4	0	12	4.4	4.3	100.0	21.1	8.4	5.5	-	5.5	6.0	82	100.0
Neuroblastoma	3	5	4	0	12	4.4	4.3	100.0	21.1	8.4	5.5	-	5.5	6.0	82	100.0
Other	0	0	0	0	0	-	-	-	-	-	-	-	-	-	-	-
V. RETINOBLASTOMA	2	0	0	0	2	0.7	0.7	100.0	14.0	-	-	-	0.9	1.1	14	100.0
VI. KIDNEY	2	10	4	1	17	6.3	6.1	100.0	14.0	16.8	5.5	1.4	7.8	8.4	115	100.0
Wilms' tumour	2	10	4	1	17	6.3	6.1	100.0	14.0	16.8	5.5	1.4	7.8	8.4	115	100.0
Renal carcinoma	0	0	0	0	0	-	-	-	-	-	-	-	-	-	-	-
Other and unspecified	0	0	0	0	0	-	-	-	-	-	-	-	-	-	-	-
VII. LIVER	1	4	0	0	5	1.9	1.8	100.0	7.0	6.7	-	-	2.3	2.6	34	100.0
Hepatoblastoma	1	4	0	0	5	1.9	1.8	100.0	7.0	6.7	-	-	2.3	2.6	34	100.0
Hepatic carcinoma	0	0	0	0	0	-	-	-	-	-	-	-	-	-	-	-
Other and unspecified	0	0	0	0	0	-	-	-	-	-	-	-	-	-	-	-
VIII.BONE	0	1	0	9	10	3.7	3.9	100.0	-	1.7	-	12.7	4.6	4.2	70	100.0
Osteosarcoma	0	1	0	5	6	2.2	2.3	60.0	-	1.7	-	7.1	2.8	2.6	42	100.0
Chondrosarcoma	0	0	0	0	0	-	-	-	-	-	-	-	-	-	-	-
Ewing's sarcoma	0	0	0	4	4	1.5	1.6	40.0	-	-	-	5.6	1.8	1.6	28	100.0
Other and unspecified	0	0	0	0	0	-	-	-	-	-	-	-	-	-	-	-
IX. SOFT TISSUE SARCOMAS	3	2	10	6	21	7.8	7.8	100.0	21.1	3.4	13.7	8.5	9.6	9.5	145	100.0
Rhabdomyosarcoma	1	1	5	4	11	4.1	4.1	52.4	7.0	1.7	6.8	5.6	5.0	4.9	76	100.0
Fibrosarcoma	0	0	1	1	2	0.7	0.8	9.5	-	-	1.4	1.4	0.9	0.9	14	100.0
Other and unspecified	2	1	4	1	8	3.0	2.9	38.1	14.0	1.7	5.5	1.4	3.7	3.8	55	100.0
X. GONADAL & GERM CELL	0	3	0	1	4	1.5	1.5	100.0	-	5.0	-	1.4	1.8	2.0	27	100.0
Non-gonadal germ cell	0	0	0	1	1	0.4	0.4	25.0	-	-	-	1.4	0.5	0.4	7	100.0
Gonadal germ cell	0	3	0	0	3	1.1	1.1	75.0	-	5.0	-	-	1.4	1.6	20	100.0
Gonadal carcinoma	0	0	0	0	0	-	-	-	-	-	-	-	-	-	-	-
Other and unspecified	0	0	0	0	0	-	-	-	-	-	-	-	-	-	-	-
XI. EPITHELIAL NEOPLASMS	1	0	6	8	15	5.6	5.7	100.0	7.0	-	8.2	11.3	6.9	6.5	105	93.3
Adrenocortical carcinoma	0	0	0	0	0	-	-	-	-	-	-	-	-	-	-	-
Thyroid carcinoma	0	0	0	3	3	1.1	1.2	20.0	-	-	-	4.2	1.4	1.2	21	100.0
Nasopharyngeal carcinoma	0	0	0	1	1	0.4	0.4	6.7	-	-	-	1.4	0.5	0.4	7	100.0
Melanoma	1	0	4	2	7	2.6	2.6	46.7	7.0	-	5.5	2.8	3.2	3.1	48	85.7
Other carcinoma	0	0	2	2	4	1.5	1.5	26.7	-	-	2.7	2.8	1.8	1.7	28	100.0
XII. OTHER	1	0	0	0	1	0.4	0.4	100.0	7.0	-	-	-	0.5	0.5	7	100.0
* Specified as malignant	1	2	4	2	9	3.3	3.3	100.0	7.0	3.4	5.5	2.8	4.1	4.2	62	44.4

Yugoslavia, Slovenia

FEMALE

1971 – 1980

DIAGNOSTIC GROUP	NUMBER OF CASES 0	1-4	5-9	10-14	All	REL. FREQUENCY(%) Crude	Adj.	Group	RATES PER MILLION 0	1-4	5-9	10-14	Crude	Adj.	Cum	HV(%)
TOTAL	10	71	46	47	174	100.0	100.0	100.0	73.2	127.0	66.2	69.7	84.3	86.6	1260	96.6
I. LEUKAEMIAS	2	34	16	11	63	36.2	35.2	100.0	14.6	60.8	23.0	16.3	30.5	32.1	454	98.4
Acute lymphocytic	0	18	11	7	36	20.7	20.5	57.1	–	32.2	15.8	10.4	17.4	18.1	260	97.2
Other lymphocytic	0	0	0	0	0	–	–	–	–	–	–	–	–	–	–	–
Acute non-lymphocytic	1	6	0	1	8	4.6	4.1	12.7	7.3	10.7	–	1.5	3.9	4.3	58	100.0
Chronic myeloid	0	1	0	1	2	1.1	1.1	3.2	–	1.8	–	1.5	1.0	1.0	15	100.0
Other and unspecified	1	9	5	2	17	9.8	9.5	27.0	7.3	16.1	7.2	3.0	8.2	8.7	122	100.0
II. LYMPHOMAS	1	5	3	10	19	10.9	11.3	100.0	7.3	8.9	4.3	14.8	9.2	9.0	139	100.0
Hodgkin's disease	0	2	1	7	10	5.7	6.1	52.6	–	3.6	1.4	10.4	4.8	4.6	73	100.0
Non-Hodgkin lymphoma	0	3	2	2	7	4.0	4.1	36.8	–	5.4	2.9	3.0	3.4	3.5	51	100.0
Burkitt's lymphoma	0	0	0	0	0	–	–	–	–	–	–	–	–	–	–	–
Unspecified lymphoma	1	0	0	1	2	1.1	1.1	10.5	7.3	–	–	1.5	1.0	1.0	15	100.0
Histiocytosis X	0	0	0	0	0	–	–	–	–	–	–	–	–	–	–	–
Other reticuloendothelial	0	0	0	0	0	–	–	–	–	–	–	–	–	–	–	–
III. BRAIN AND SPINAL	0	9	14	7	30	17.2	18.0	100.0	–	16.1	20.1	10.4	14.5	14.5	217	90.0
Ependymoma	0	4	4	3	11	6.3	6.5	36.7	–	7.2	5.8	4.4	5.3	5.4	80	100.0
Astrocytoma	0	1	6	2	9	5.2	5.7	30.0	–	1.8	8.6	3.0	4.4	4.2	65	100.0
Medulloblastoma	0	2	2	1	5	2.9	2.9	16.7	–	3.6	2.9	1.5	2.4	2.5	36	100.0
Other glioma	0	1	0	0	1	0.6	0.5	3.3	–	1.8	–	–	0.5	0.6	7	100.0
Other and unspecified *	0	1	2	1	4	2.3	2.4	13.3	–	1.8	2.9	1.5	1.9	1.9	29	25.0
IV. SYMPATHETIC N.S.	1	8	0	0	9	5.2	4.4	100.0	7.3	14.3	–	–	4.4	5.0	65	100.0
Neuroblastoma	1	8	0	0	9	5.2	4.4	100.0	7.3	14.3	–	–	4.4	5.0	65	100.0
Other	0	0	0	0	0	–	–	–	–	–	–	–	–	–	–	–
V. RETINOBLASTOMA	1	4	1	0	6	3.4	3.1	100.0	7.3	7.2	1.4	–	2.9	3.2	43	100.0
VI. KIDNEY	1	8	2	1	12	6.9	6.4	100.0	7.3	14.3	2.9	1.5	5.8	6.4	86	100.0
Wilms' tumour	1	8	2	1	12	6.9	6.4	100.0	7.3	14.3	2.9	1.5	5.8	6.4	86	100.0
Renal carcinoma	0	0	0	0	0	–	–	–	–	–	–	–	–	–	–	–
Other and unspecified	0	0	0	0	0	–	–	–	–	–	–	–	–	–	–	–
VII. LIVER	1	0	0	0	1	0.6	0.5	100.0	7.3	–	–	–	0.5	0.6	7	100.0
Hepatoblastoma	1	0	0	0	1	0.6	0.5	100.0	7.3	–	–	–	0.5	0.6	7	100.0
Hepatic carcinoma	0	0	0	0	0	–	–	–	–	–	–	–	–	–	–	–
Other and unspecified	0	0	0	0	0	–	–	–	–	–	–	–	–	–	–	–
VIII. BONE	0	0	0	6	6	3.4	3.8	100.0	–	–	–	8.9	2.9	2.6	44	100.0
Osteosarcoma	0	0	0	2	2	1.1	1.3	33.3	–	–	–	3.0	1.0	0.9	15	100.0
Chondrosarcoma	0	0	0	1	1	0.6	0.6	16.7	–	–	–	1.5	0.5	0.4	7	100.0
Ewing's sarcoma	0	0	0	3	3	1.7	1.9	50.0	–	–	–	4.4	1.5	1.3	22	100.0
Other and unspecified	0	0	0	0	0	–	–	–	–	–	–	–	–	–	–	–
IX. SOFT TISSUE SARCOMAS	2	2	6	1	11	6.3	6.5	100.0	14.6	3.6	8.6	1.5	5.3	5.5	80	100.0
Rhabdomyosarcoma	2	2	2	0	6	3.4	3.9	54.5	14.6	3.6	2.9	–	2.9	3.4	43	100.0
Fibrosarcoma	0	0	2	1	3	1.7	1.9	27.3	–	–	2.9	1.5	1.5	1.4	22	100.0
Other and unspecified	0	0	2	0	2	1.1	1.3	18.2	–	–	2.9	–	1.0	0.9	14	100.0
X. GONADAL & GERM CELL	0	0	2	7	9	5.2	5.8	100.0	–	–	2.9	10.4	4.4	3.9	66	100.0
Non-gonadal germ cell	0	0	2	6	8	4.6	5.1	88.9	–	–	2.9	8.9	3.9	3.5	59	100.0
Gonadal germ cell	0	0	0	0	0	–	–	–	–	–	–	–	–	–	–	–
Gonadal carcinoma	0	0	0	1	1	0.6	0.6	11.1	–	–	–	1.5	0.5	0.4	7	100.0
Other and unspecified	0	0	0	0	0	–	–	–	–	–	–	–	–	–	–	–
XI. EPITHELIAL NEOPLASMS	0	0	1	3	4	2.3	2.6	100.0	–	–	1.4	4.4	1.9	1.8	29	100.0
Adrenocortical carcinoma	0	0	0	0	0	–	–	–	–	–	–	–	–	–	–	–
Thyroid carcinoma	0	0	1	1	2	1.1	1.3	50.0	–	–	1.4	1.5	1.0	0.9	15	100.0
Nasopharyngeal carcinoma	0	0	0	0	0	–	–	–	–	–	–	–	–	–	–	–
Melanoma	0	0	0	1	1	0.6	0.6	25.0	–	–	–	1.5	0.5	0.4	7	100.0
Other carcinoma	0	0	0	1	1	0.6	0.6	25.0	–	–	–	1.5	0.5	0.4	7	100.0
XII. OTHER	1	1	1	1	4	2.3	2.3	100.0	7.3	1.8	1.4	1.5	1.9	2.0	29	50.0
* Specified as malignant	0	1	2	1	4	2.3	2.4	100.0	–	1.8	2.9	1.5	1.9	1.9	29	25.0

Of the male and female population, 53% and 47% respectively, are economically active, with 37% employed in industry and mining, 11% in commerce, hotel-keeping and tourism, 15% in agriculture, fishing and forestry, 5% in education, science and culture, 6% in construction, 5% in transport, 7% in arts and public utility, 5% in health and social care and 9% in other occupations.

Population

The average annual population at risk has been calculated from data from the censuses of 1971 and 1981, published by the Statistical Institute of the Socialist Republic of Slovenia, Ljubljana (1974 and 1983).

AVERAGE ANNUAL POPULATION: 1971–1980

Age	Male	Female
0	14241	13656
1–4	59684	55926
5–9	73158	69497
10–14	70814	67433
0–14	217897	206512

Commentary

Compared with most other European registries, the overall sex ratio was high (M/F = 1.45 for age-standardized incidence rates). However, the excess of males among children with leukaemia was less than usually observed. The ratio of 2.4 for acute lymphocytic to acute non-lymphocytic leukaemia was also fairly low, but 30/139 (22%) of leukaemias were in the 'other and unspecified' category. The incidence of lymphomas, particularly Hodgkin's disease, was relatively high. Retinoblastoma had a low incidence rate.

OCEANIA

AUSTRALIA

New South Wales Cancer Registry, 1972-1982

J. Ford

In 1971, the New South Wales Central Cancer Registry was established to collect cancer statistics for the State from January 1972. The director is a medical administrator, assisted by an advisory committee of representatives from organizations involved in educational, clinical and research programmes directed towards cancer control.

The main source of cancer data is the compulsory notification form completed by hospital staff for each cancer case at every in-patient discharge, transfer or death, by every hospital, independently of all other hospitals and whether the admission was for cancer or not. In addition, each radiotherapy department must notify the first attendance each year of each cancer case. Ancillary sources of data are pathology reports relating to cancer received from all major hospitals and pathology laboratories, on a voluntary basis up to 1985 and then by law. Since 1972, the Registrar-General's Department has supplied listings of all deaths certified as having cancer as the primary cause, with supplementary listings of the secondary cause from 1978.

Case registration, classification of non-medical data, and the keeping of manual and some computer systems, are the responsibility of clerical staff. Disease classification — topography and morphology — is done by medical staff, who seek further advice from specialist pathologists and clinicians as necessary.

The basic filing system at the Registry was converted in 1985 from a manual file of the source documents, linked and stored in alphabetical sequence by surname, to an on-line computer system. Contributing hospitals will eventually be able to forward data on tape or disk. There are approximately 620 000 records currently on file (all ages).

The data recorded for each case include identifying information, the institutions attended, and a broad statement of the treatment given at each admission. The latter is used to determine the proportion of cases treated by some type of major surgery aimed at cure, chemotherapy, radiotherapy or combinations of these; these data are also used to assist in assessment of services for cancer patients.

The area covered by the Registry is the State of New South Wales, one of the six federated States of Australia, with a total area of 801 400 square kilometres. Geographically there are four main zones in New South Wales, extending from north to south — the Coastal Zone, the Tablelands, the Western Slopes of the Tablelands and the Western Plains, occupying two-thirds of the area of the State. The population distribution, however, is largely coastal, 76% of the population being in the Sydney-Newcastle-Wollongong complex of the Central Coast. If an urban settlement is defined as one with 1000 or more persons, 89% of the population is urban and 11% rural.

At the 1976 census, the total population of New South Wales was 4 959 588, of whom 26% were children. The countries of birth of the New South Wales population, according to the 1981 census, were Australia 78.4%, New Zealand 1.3%, European (including United Kingdom) 13.8%, other countries 6.5%.

The principal occupations are professional, administrative and clerical 45%, tradesmen 29% and farmers 5%.

There is no established church in New South Wales, and freedom of worship is accorded to all. In 1981, the religions of the population were Church of England 30.6%, Catholic 27.8%, other Christian 21.1%, non-Christian 1.7%, no religion or not stated 18.7%.

Analyses of the records of the Registry are used in undergraduate and postgraduate teaching, with the emphasis on cancer epidemiology, and to respond to *ad hoc* requests from community, educational and industrial sources.

Contd p. 316

Australia, New South Wales 1972 - 1982 MALE

DIAGNOSTIC GROUP	NUMBER OF CASES 0	1-4	5-9	10-14	All	REL. FREQUENCY(%) Crude	Adj.	Group	RATES PER MILLION 0	1-4	5-9	10-14	Crude	Adj.	Cum.	HV(%)
TOTAL	119	394	266	284	1063	100.0	100.0	100.0	257.2	207.8	109.0	115.6	146.5	153.0	2212	98.7
I. LEUKAEMIAS	23	188	88	67	366	34.4	33.5	100.0	49.7	99.2	36.1	27.3	50.5	54.1	763	100.0
Acute lymphocytic	10	156	73	43	282	26.5	25.7	77.0	21.6	82.3	29.9	17.5	38.9	41.9	588	100.0
Other lymphocytic	0	2	0	0	2	0.2	0.2	0.5	-	1.1	-	-	0.3	0.3	-	100.0
Acute non-lymphocytic	9	21	8	15	53	5.0	4.8	14.5	19.5	11.1	3.3	6.1	7.3	7.8	111	100.0
Chronic myeloid	1	2	1	1	5	0.5	0.5	1.4	2.2	1.1	0.4	0.4	0.7	0.7	10	100.0
Other and unspecified	3	7	6	8	24	2.3	2.3	6.6	6.5	3.7	2.5	3.3	3.3	3.4	50	100.0
II. LYMPHOMAS	13	36	47	60	156	14.7	15.5	100.0	28.1	19.0	19.3	24.4	21.5	21.4	323	100.0
Hodgkin's disease	-	5	13	26	44	4.1	4.6	28.2	-	2.6	5.3	10.6	6.1	5.6	90	100.0
Non-Hodgkin lymphoma	2	18	26	31	77	7.2	7.8	49.4	4.3	9.5	10.7	12.6	10.6	10.4	159	100.0
Burkitt's lymphoma	0	1	1	1	3	0.3	0.3	1.9	-	0.5	0.4	0.4	0.4	0.4	6	100.0
Unspecified lymphoma	0	1	3	1	5	0.5	0.5	3.2	-	0.5	1.2	0.4	0.7	0.7	10	100.0
Histiocytosis X	11	11	4	1	27	2.5	2.3	17.3	23.8	5.8	1.6	0.4	3.7	4.3	57	100.0
Other reticuloendothelial	0	0	0	0	0	-	-	-	-	-	-	-	-	-	-	-
III. BRAIN AND SPINAL	12	63	62	46	183	17.2	17.7	100.0	25.9	33.2	25.4	18.7	25.2	25.9	380	92.9
Ependymoma	1	10	7	3	21	2.0	2.0	11.5	2.2	5.3	2.9	1.2	2.9	3.1	44	100.0
Astrocytoma	5	20	22	18	65	6.1	6.3	35.5	10.8	10.5	9.0	7.3	9.0	9.1	135	100.0
Medulloblastoma	4	22	17	8	51	4.8	4.8	27.9	8.6	11.6	7.0	3.3	7.0	7.5	106	100.0
Other glioma	2	6	8	11	27	2.5	2.7	14.8	4.3	3.2	3.3	4.5	3.7	3.7	56	100.0
Other and unspecified *	0	5	8	6	19	1.8	1.9	10.4	-	2.6	3.3	2.4	2.6	2.6	39	31.6
IV. SYMPATHETIC N.S.	30	33	5	2	70	6.6	5.7	100.0	64.8	17.4	2.0	0.8	9.6	11.3	149	100.0
Neuroblastoma	30	33	5	2	70	6.6	5.7	100.0	64.8	17.4	2.0	0.8	9.6	11.3	149	100.0
Other	0	0	0	0	0	-	-	-	-	-	-	-	-	-	-	-
V. RETINOBLASTOMA	10	10	2	2	24	2.3	2.0	100.0	21.6	5.3	0.8	0.8	3.3	3.8	51	100.0
VI. KIDNEY	6	25	12	1	44	4.1	3.9	100.0	13.0	13.2	4.9	0.4	6.1	6.8	92	100.0
Wilms' tumour	6	24	12	1	43	4.0	3.8	97.7	13.0	12.7	4.9	0.4	5.9	6.6	90	100.0
Renal carcinoma	0	1	0	0	1	0.1	0.1	2.3	-	0.5	-	-	0.1	0.2	2	100.0
Other and unspecified	0	0	0	0	0	-	-	-	-	-	-	-	-	-	-	-
VII. LIVER	2	1	2	2	7	0.7	0.7	100.0	4.3	0.5	0.8	0.8	1.0	1.0	15	100.0
Hepatoblastoma	2	1	0	0	3	0.3	0.2	42.9	4.3	0.5	-	-	0.4	0.5	6	100.0
Hepatic carcinoma	0	0	2	2	4	0.4	0.4	57.1	-	-	0.8	0.8	0.6	0.5	8	100.0
Other and unspecified	0	0	0	0	0	-	-	-	-	-	-	-	-	-	-	-
VIII. BONE	0	3	11	35	49	4.6	5.2	100.0	-	1.6	4.5	14.2	6.8	6.1	100	100.0
Osteosarcoma	0	0	4	20	24	2.3	2.6	49.0	-	-	1.6	8.1	3.3	2.9	49	100.0
Chondrosarcoma	0	0	0	1	1	0.1	0.1	2.0	-	-	-	0.4	0.1	0.1	2	100.0
Ewing's sarcoma	0	3	7	11	21	2.0	2.2	42.9	-	1.6	2.9	4.5	2.9	2.7	43	100.0
Other and unspecified	0	0	0	3	3	0.3	0.3	6.1	-	-	-	1.2	0.4	0.4	6	100.0
IX. SOFT TISSUE SARCOMAS	10	21	22	20	73	6.9	7.0	100.0	21.6	11.1	9.0	8.1	10.1	10.4	152	100.0
Rhabdomyosarcoma	8	20	20	11	59	5.6	5.6	80.8	17.3	10.5	8.2	4.5	8.1	8.6	123	100.0
Fibrosarcoma	0	1	2	4	7	0.7	0.7	9.6	-	0.5	0.8	1.6	1.0	0.9	14	100.0
Other and unspecified	2	0	0	5	7	0.7	0.7	9.6	4.3	-	-	2.0	1.0	0.9	14	100.0
X. GONADAL & GERM CELL	11	11	2	6	30	2.8	2.6	100.0	23.8	5.8	0.8	2.4	4.1	4.6	63	100.0
Non-gonadal germ cell	5	2	2	6	15	1.4	1.4	50.0	10.8	1.1	0.8	2.4	2.1	2.1	31	100.0
Gonadal germ cell	6	9	0	0	15	1.4	1.2	50.0	13.0	4.7	-	-	2.1	2.5	32	100.0
Gonadal carcinoma	0	0	0	0	0	-	-	-	-	-	-	-	-	-	-	-
Other and unspecified	0	0	0	0	0	-	-	-	-	-	-	-	-	-	-	-
XI. EPITHELIAL NEOPLASMS	2	2	12	42	58	5.5	6.1	100.0	4.3	1.1	4.9	17.1	8.0	7.2	119	100.0
Adrenocortical carcinoma	0	0	0	0	0	-	-	-	-	-	-	-	-	-	-	-
Thyroid carcinoma	0	0	0	2	2	0.2	0.2	3.4	-	-	-	0.8	0.3	0.3	4	100.0
Nasopharyngeal carcinoma	0	0	1	2	3	0.3	0.3	5.2	-	-	0.4	0.8	0.4	0.4	6	100.0
Melanoma	1	2	9	27	39	3.7	4.1	67.2	2.2	1.1	3.7	11.0	5.4	4.9	80	100.0
Other carcinoma	1	0	2	11	14	1.3	1.5	24.1	2.2	-	0.8	4.5	1.9	1.7	29	100.0
XII. OTHER	0	1	1	1	3	0.3	0.3	100.0	-	0.5	0.4	0.4	0.4	0.3	6	66.7
* Specified as malignant	0	3	8	6	17	1.6	1.8	-	-	1.6	3.3	2.4	2.3	2.3	35	23.5

Australia, New South Wales

1972 – 1982

FEMALE

DIAGNOSTIC GROUP	NUMBER OF CASES					REL. FREQUENCY(%)			RATES PER MILLION						Cum	HV(%)
	0	1-4	5-9	10-14	All	Crude	Adj.	Group	0	1-4	5-9	10-14	Crude	Adj.		
TOTAL	77	317	212	203	809	100.0	100.0	100.0	174.6	174.5	91.1	87.0	116.9	122.2	1763	98.1
I. LEUKAEMIAS	17	138	90	52	297	36.7	36.2	100.0	38.5	76.0	38.7	22.3	42.9	45.5	647	100.0
Acute lymphocytic	9	114	69	26	218	26.9	26.1	73.4	20.4	62.7	29.7	11.1	31.5	33.8	475	100.0
Other lymphocytic	0	0	1	0	1	0.1	0.1	0.3	-	-	0.4	-	0.1	0.1	2	100.0
Acute non-lymphocytic	5	15	12	21	53	6.6	6.8	17.8	11.3	8.3	5.2	9.0	7.7	7.7	115	100.0
Chronic myeloid	1	5	3	5	14	1.7	1.8	4.7	2.3	2.8	1.3	-	2.0	2.1	30	100.0
Other and unspecified	2	4	5	0	11	1.4	1.3	3.7	4.5	2.2	2.1	-	1.6	1.7	24	100.0
II. LYMPHOMAS	9	15	17	19	60	7.4	7.7	100.0	20.4	8.3	7.3	8.1	8.7	8.9	131	100.0
Hodgkin's disease	0	7	4	13	18	2.2	2.6	30.0	-	0.6	1.7	5.6	2.6	2.3	39	100.0
Non-Hodgkin lymphoma	2	7	8	5	22	2.7	2.8	36.7	4.5	3.9	3.4	2.1	3.2	3.3	48	100.0
Burkitt's lymphoma	0	0	0	0	0	-	-	-	-	-	-	-	-	-	-	-
Unspecified lymphoma	0	0	1	1	2	0.2	0.3	3.3	-	-	0.4	0.4	0.3	0.3	4	100.0
Histiocytosis X	7	7	4	0	18	2.2	2.0	30.0	15.9	3.9	1.7	-	2.6	3.0	40	100.0
Other reticuloendothelial	0	0	0	0	0	-	-	-	-	-	-	-	-	-	-	-
III. BRAIN AND SPINAL	7	57	54	37	155	19.2	19.6	100.0	15.9	31.4	23.2	15.9	22.4	23.0	337	91.0
Ependymoma	1	17	1	1	20	2.5	2.9	12.9	2.3	9.4	0.4	0.4	2.9	3.3	44	100.0
Astrocytoma	4	23	32	19	78	9.6	10.1	50.3	9.1	12.7	13.8	8.1	11.3	11.4	169	100.0
Medulloblastoma	0	9	12	3	24	3.0	3.1	15.5	-	5.0	5.2	1.3	3.5	3.6	52	100.0
Other glioma	1	7	5	5	18	2.2	2.3	11.6	2.3	3.9	2.1	1.3	2.6	2.7	39	100.0
Other and unspecified *	1	1	4	9	15	1.9	2.1	9.7	2.3	0.6	1.7	3.9	2.2	2.0	32	6.7
IV. SYMPATHETIC N.S.	20	27	6	4	57	7.0	6.2	100.0	45.3	14.9	2.6	1.7	8.2	9.4	126	100.0
Neuroblastoma	20	27	6	3	56	6.9	6.1	98.2	45.3	14.9	2.6	1.3	8.1	9.3	124	100.0
Other	0	0	0	1	1	0.1	0.1	1.8	-	-	-	0.4	0.1	0.1	2	100.0
V. RETINOBLASTOMA	6	21	1	0	28	3.5	2.9	100.0	13.6	11.6	0.4	-	4.0	4.8	62	100.0
VI. KIDNEY	8	31	10	3	52	6.4	5.8	100.0	18.1	17.1	4.3	1.3	7.5	8.4	114	100.0
Wilms' tumour	8	31	9	3	51	6.3	5.7	98.1	18.1	17.1	3.9	1.3	7.4	8.3	112	100.0
Renal carcinoma	0	0	1	0	1	0.1	0.1	1.9	-	-	0.4	-	0.1	0.1	2	100.0
Other and unspecified	0	0	0	0	0	-	-	-	-	-	-	-	-	-	-	-
VII. LIVER	2	4	1	0	7	0.9	0.8	100.0	4.5	2.2	0.4	-	1.0	1.2	15	100.0
Hepatoblastoma	2	1	0	0	3	0.4	0.3	42.9	4.5	0.6	-	-	0.4	0.5	7	100.0
Hepatic carcinoma	0	3	1	0	4	0.5	0.4	57.1	-	1.7	0.4	-	0.6	0.6	9	100.0
Other and unspecified	0	0	0	0	0	-	-	-	-	-	-	-	-	-	-	-
VIII. BONE	0	4	7	27	38	4.7	5.4	100.0	-	2.2	3.0	11.6	5.5	5.0	82	100.0
Osteosarcoma	0	2	2	15	19	2.3	2.7	50.0	-	1.1	0.9	6.4	2.7	2.5	41	100.0
Chondrosarcoma	0	0	0	0	0	-	-	-	-	-	-	-	-	-	-	-
Ewing's sarcoma	0	2	5	12	19	2.3	2.7	50.0	-	1.1	2.1	5.1	2.7	2.5	41	100.0
Other and unspecified	0	0	0	0	0	-	-	-	-	-	-	-	-	-	-	-
IX. SOFT TISSUE SARCOMAS	7	10	6	15	38	4.7	4.8	100.0	15.9	5.5	2.6	6.4	5.5	5.6	83	100.0
Rhabdomyosarcoma	2	8	5	9	24	3.0	3.1	63.2	4.5	4.4	2.1	3.9	3.5	3.5	52	100.0
Fibrosarcoma	4	0	1	3	8	1.0	1.0	21.1	9.1	-	0.4	1.3	1.2	1.2	18	100.0
Other and unspecified	1	2	0	3	6	0.7	0.7	15.8	2.3	1.1	-	1.3	0.9	0.9	13	100.0
X. GONADAL & GERM CELL	1	5	5	12	23	2.8	3.1	100.0	2.3	2.8	2.1	5.1	3.3	3.2	50	100.0
Non-gonadal germ cell	1	5	1	1	8	1.0	0.9	34.8	2.3	2.8	0.4	0.4	1.2	1.3	18	100.0
Gonadal germ cell	0	0	4	11	15	1.9	2.2	65.2	-	-	1.7	4.7	2.2	1.9	32	100.0
Gonadal carcinoma	0	0	0	0	0	-	-	-	-	-	-	-	-	-	-	-
Other and unspecified	0	0	0	0	0	-	-	-	-	-	-	-	-	-	-	-
XI. EPITHELIAL NEOPLASMS	0	3	13	31	47	5.8	6.7	100.0	-	1.7	5.6	13.3	6.8	6.2	101	100.0
Adrenocortical carcinoma	0	1	0	0	1	0.1	0.1	2.1	-	0.6	-	-	0.1	0.2	2	100.0
Thyroid carcinoma	0	0	1	5	6	0.7	0.9	12.8	-	-	0.4	2.1	0.9	0.8	13	100.0
Nasopharyngeal carcinoma	0	0	0	0	0	-	-	-	-	-	-	-	-	-	-	-
Melanoma	0	2	10	21	33	4.1	4.7	70.2	-	1.1	4.3	9.0	4.8	4.3	71	100.0
Other carcinoma	0	0	2	5	7	0.9	1.0	14.9	-	-	0.9	2.1	1.0	0.9	15	100.0
XII. OTHER	0	2	2	3	7	0.9	0.9	100.0	-	1.1	0.9	1.3	1.0	1.0	15	85.7
* Specified as malignant	1	1	4	8	14	1.7	2.0	100.0	2.3	0.6	1.7	3.4	2.0	1.9	30	-

Population

Annual estimates of the population are available, and are derived from the censuses of 1971, 1976 and 1981 (Australian Bureau of Statistics).

AVERAGE ANNUAL POPULATION: 1972–1982

Age	Male	Female
0	42055	40095
1–4	172347	165168
5–9	221755	211551
10–14	223338	212092
0–14	659495	628906

Commentary

The rates for 'All cancer' are high, that for leukaemia being among the highest reported in this volume. The most notable finding is the high rate of malignant melanoma. For Australian adults the risk of this disease arising from over-exposure to sun is well-known; it is clear from the data presented here that the risk also exists for children.

Queensland Childhood Malignancy Registry, 1973-1981

W.R. McWhirter

The Queensland Childhood Malignancy Registry (QCMR) was established in 1977. The original purpose was to act as a local collector of data from Queensland which could be supplied to the Australian Paediatric Cancer Registry, at that time based in New South Wales but subsequently transferred to Queensland. The Registry covers the whole of Queensland. Children from areas outside the State who are treated in Queensland are not included. Case ascertainment involves obtaining information from a variety of sources in order to minimize the possibility that cases may be missed. These sources include the clinical departments of the two major children's hospitals in Brisbane, the Pathology Departments of the Royal Brisbane and Mater Hospitals in Brisbane, the Queensland Radium Institute and a number of selected practitioners. No new cases have been found from death certificates. Because cases of retinoblastoma are sometimes not referred to a major centre, a questionnaire is sent out periodically to ophthalmologists requef Statistics, it is estimated that registration is at least 98% complete.

Most paediatric oncology cases are seen at either the Royal Children's Hospital or the Mater Children's Hospital in Brisbane. The public hospital system in Queensland has provided its services free of charge for many years. Cases may be referred to one of the two hospitals mentioned above either from other hospitals within the State or from private medical practitioners. Assistance is available for both travel and accommodation of families from outside Brisbane. Radiotherapy is available only in Brisbane.

The proximity of the Registry to the Oncology Clinic at the Royal Children's Hospital, together with the fact that the Director of the QCMR is also a clinician at the Clinic, results in excellent liaison between clinicians and the Registry.

Queensland is the second largest state in Australia and covers an area of 1 727 200 square kilometres (22% of the area of Australia), of which 54% lies within the tropical zone. The climate varies considerably, most of the rainfall occurring along the coastal regions, particularly in the north, which has distinct wet and dry seasons. The interior of the State is hot and dry and for the most part sparsely populated. The population (1981) was 2.3 million, of whom 26% are children. Much of the population is concentrated along the coastal strip and south-east corner of the State. About 30% of the child population lives in Brisbane city and about 80% of the population live in urban areas.

No accurate data are available on the proportions of the various racial groups and there is considerable intermixing, e.g., between Europeans and aborigines. About 14% of the Queensland population were born overseas (half in the United Kingdom and Ireland). Most of the population belong to one of the Christian denominations. Most of the industry is concentrated in the south-east corner and air pollution is relatively low, particularly in the rural areas. The principal occupations, with the proportion employed in each, are: wholesale/retail trade (18.7%), manufacturing (13.9%), community services (13.1%), agriculture (9.7%) and construction (9.6%).

Data on incidence have been published in annual reports, and by McWhirter and Bacon (1981). Analyses have been done, using the data of the QCMR, to relate social class to both incidence (McWhirter, 1982) and survival (McWhirter et al., 1983) in acute lymphoblastic leukaemia. Some geographical variations in incidence have been studied, e.g., in brain tumours. Information on trends in survival rates over a 25-year period has also been published (McWhirter & Siskind, 1984).

Population

The population at risk is available as a set of annual estimates, obtained from the Australian Bureau of Statistics. Censuses have been held in Australia in 1971, 1976 and 1981. The intercensal estimates take into account net long-term and permanent movements of the population, together with estimates of the natural increase. In addition, adjustment for census under-enumeration has been made.

AVERAGE ANNUAL POPULATION: 1973-1981

Age	Male	Female
0	18568	17654
1-4	78060	74891
5-9	102528	98002
10-14	101933	97351
0-14	301089	287898

Contd p. 320

Australia, Queensland   1973 - 1981   MALE

DIAGNOSTIC GROUP	NUMBER OF CASES					REL. FREQUENCY(%)			RATES PER MILLION						Cum	HV(%)
	0	1-4	5-9	10-14	All	Crude	Adj.	Group	0	1-4	5-9	10-14	Crude	Adj.		
TOTAL	29	146	87	75	337	100.0	100.0	100.0	173.5	207.8	94.3	81.8	124.4	131.9	1885	96.7
I. LEUKAEMIAS	4	51	31	13	99	29.4	28.5	100.0	23.9	72.6	33.6	14.2	36.5	39.3	553	99.0
Acute lymphocytic	3	46	28	11	88	26.1	25.3	88.9	18.0	65.5	30.3	12.0	32.5	34.9	492	98.9
Other lymphocytic	0	0	0	0	0	-	-	-	-	-	-	-	-	-	-	-
Acute non-lymphocytic	1	5	3	2	11	3.3	3.2	11.1	6.0	7.1	3.3	2.2	4.1	4.3	62	100.0
Chronic myeloid	0	0	0	0	0	-	-	-	-	-	-	-	-	-	-	-
Other and unspecified	0	0	0	0	0	-	-	-	-	-	-	-	-	-	-	-
II. LYMPHOMAS	2	14	20	25	61	18.1	20.6	100.0	12.0	19.9	21.7	27.3	22.5	22.0	336	100.0
Hodgkin's disease	0	1	8	16	25	7.4	9.4	41.0	-	1.4	8.7	17.4	9.2	8.3	136	100.0
Non-Hodgkin lymphoma	0	7	11	8	26	7.7	8.6	42.6	-	10.0	11.9	8.7	9.6	9.5	143	100.0
Burkitt's lymphoma	0	0	0	0	0	-	-	-	-	-	-	-	-	-	-	-
Unspecified lymphoma	0	1	0	0	1	0.3	0.2	1.6	-	1.4	-	-	0.4	0.4	6	100.0
Histiocytosis X	0	4	1	1	6	1.8	1.7	9.8	-	5.7	1.1	1.1	2.2	2.4	34	100.0
Other reticuloendothelial	2	1	0	0	3	0.9	0.7	4.9	12.0	1.4	-	-	1.1	1.4	18	100.0
III. BRAIN AND SPINAL	6	24	16	20	66	19.6	20.4	100.0	35.9	34.2	17.3	21.8	24.4	25.3	368	86.2
Ependymoma	1	3	0	2	6	1.8	1.7	9.1	6.0	4.3	-	2.2	2.2	2.4	34	100.0
Astrocytoma	4	10	7	13	34	10.1	10.8	51.5	23.9	14.2	7.6	14.2	12.5	12.8	190	93.9
Medulloblastoma	1	7	4	2	14	4.2	4.0	21.2	6.0	10.0	4.3	2.2	5.2	5.6	78	100.0
Other glioma	0	3	1	2	6	1.8	1.8	9.1	-	4.3	1.1	2.2	2.2	2.3	33	16.7
Other and unspecified *	0	1	4	1	6	1.8	2.0	9.1	-	1.4	4.3	1.1	2.2	2.2	33	66.7
IV. SYMPATHETIC N.S.	9	12	4	2	27	8.0	7.0	100.0	53.9	17.1	4.3	2.2	10.0	11.5	155	100.0
Neuroblastoma	9	12	4	2	27	8.0	7.0	100.0	53.9	17.1	4.3	2.2	10.0	11.5	155	100.0
Other	0	0	0	0	0	-	-	-	-	-	-	-	-	-	-	-
V. RETINOBLASTOMA	3	12	0	0	15	4.5	3.4	100.0	18.0	17.1	-	-	5.5	6.7	86	93.3
VI. KIDNEY	1	16	4	0	21	6.2	5.3	100.0	6.0	22.8	4.3	-	7.7	8.9	119	100.0
Wilms' tumour	1	16	4	0	21	6.2	5.3	100.0	6.0	22.8	4.3	-	7.7	8.9	119	100.0
Renal carcinoma	0	0	0	0	0	-	-	-	-	-	-	-	-	-	-	-
Other and unspecified	0	0	0	0	0	-	-	-	-	-	-	-	-	-	-	-
VII. LIVER	1	1	0	1	3	0.9	0.9	100.0	6.0	1.4	-	1.1	1.1	1.2	17	100.0
Hepatoblastoma	1	0	0	0	1	0.3	0.2	33.3	6.0	-	-	-	0.4	0.5	6	100.0
Hepatic carcinoma	0	1	0	1	2	0.6	0.6	66.7	-	1.4	-	1.1	0.7	0.8	11	100.0
Other and unspecified	0	0	0	0	0	-	-	-	-	-	-	-	-	-	-	-
VIII. BONE	0	3	3	7	13	3.9	4.5	100.0	-	4.3	3.3	7.6	4.8	4.6	71	100.0
Osteosarcoma	0	0	1	0	1	0.3	0.4	7.7	-	-	1.1	-	0.4	0.3	5	100.0
Chondrosarcoma	0	0	1	0	1	0.3	0.3	7.7	-	-	1.1	-	0.4	0.3	5	100.0
Ewing's sarcoma	0	2	1	6	9	2.7	3.2	69.2	-	2.8	1.1	6.5	3.3	3.1	50	100.0
Other and unspecified	0	1	0	1	2	0.6	0.6	15.4	-	1.4	-	1.1	0.7	0.8	11	100.0
IX. SOFT TISSUE SARCOMAS	2	7	7	4	20	5.9	6.1	100.0	12.0	10.0	7.6	4.4	7.4	7.7	112	100.0
Rhabdomyosarcoma	2	7	5	0	14	4.2	4.1	70.0	12.0	10.0	5.4	-	5.2	5.5	78	100.0
Fibrosarcoma	0	0	2	1	3	0.9	0.9	15.0	-	-	2.2	1.1	1.1	1.2	17	100.0
Other and unspecified	0	0	0	3	3	0.9	1.1	15.0	-	-	-	3.3	1.1	1.0	16	100.0
X. GONADAL & GERM CELL	1	2	0	0	3	0.9	0.7	100.0	6.0	2.8	-	-	1.1	1.3	17	100.0
Non-gonadal germ cell	1	0	0	0	1	0.3	0.2	33.3	6.0	-	-	-	0.4	0.5	6	100.0
Gonadal germ cell	0	2	0	0	2	0.6	0.5	66.7	-	2.8	-	-	0.7	0.9	11	100.0
Gonadal carcinoma	0	0	0	0	0	-	-	-	-	-	-	-	-	-	-	-
Other and unspecified	0	0	0	0	0	-	-	-	-	-	-	-	-	-	-	-
XI. EPITHELIAL NEOPLASMS	0	3	2	3	8	2.4	2.6	100.0	-	4.3	2.2	3.3	3.0	3.0	44	100.0
Adrenocortical carcinoma	0	2	0	0	2	0.6	0.5	25.0	-	2.8	-	-	0.7	0.7	11	100.0
Thyroid carcinoma	0	0	1	0	1	0.3	0.3	12.5	-	-	1.1	-	0.4	0.4	5	100.0
Nasopharyngeal carcinoma	0	0	1	0	1	0.3	0.3	12.5	-	-	1.1	-	0.4	0.3	5	100.0
Melanoma	0	0	0	0	0	-	-	-	-	-	-	-	-	-	-	-
Other carcinoma	0	1	0	3	4	1.2	1.4	50.0	-	1.4	-	3.3	1.5	1.4	22	100.0
XII. OTHER	0	1	0	0	1	0.3	0.2	100.0	-	1.4	-	-	0.4	0.4	6	100.0
* Specified as malignant	0	1	2	0	3	0.9	0.9	100.0	-	1.4	2.2	-	1.1	1.1	17	66.7

Australia, Queensland 1973 - 1981 FEMALE

In the table below the column groups are: **NUMBER OF CASES** (0, 1-4, 5-9, 10-14, All); **REL. FREQUENCY(%)** (Crude, Adj., Group); **RATES PER MILLION** (0, 1-4, 5-9, 10-14, Crude, Adj.); **Cum**; **HV(%)**.

DIAGNOSTIC GROUP	0	1-4	5-9	10-14	All	Crude	Adj.	Group	0	1-4	5-9	10-14	Crude	Adj.	Cum	HV(%)
TOTAL	25	98	68	56	247	100.0	100.0	100.0	157.3	145.4	77.1	63.9	95.3	100.6	1444	95.5
I. LEUKAEMIAS	4	39	29	19	91	36.8	37.0	100.0	25.2	57.9	32.9	21.7	35.1	36.8	529	100.0
Acute lymphocytic	4	36	23	13	76	30.8	30.1	83.5	25.2	53.4	26.1	14.8	29.3	31.2	443	100.0
Other lymphocytic	0	1	0	0	1	0.4	0.3	1.1	-	1.5	-	-	0.4	0.5	6	100.0
Acute non-lymphocytic	0	2	6	4	12	4.9	5.4	13.2	-	3.0	6.8	4.6	4.6	4.4	69	100.0
Chronic myeloid	0	0	0	1	1	0.4	0.5	1.1	-	-	-	1.1	0.4	0.3	6	100.0
Other and unspecified	0	0	0	1	1	0.4	0.5	1.1	-	-	-	1.1	0.4	0.3	6	100.0
II. LYMPHOMAS	3	7	10	6	26	10.5	10.9	100.0	18.9	10.4	11.3	6.8	10.0	10.3	151	100.0
Hodgkin's disease	0	1	1	3	5	2.0	2.4	19.2	-	1.5	1.1	3.4	1.9	1.8	29	100.0
Non-Hodgkin lymphoma	0	2	4	1	7	2.8	3.0	26.9	-	3.0	4.5	1.1	2.7	2.7	40	100.0
Burkitt's lymphoma	0	0	1	0	1	0.4	0.4	3.8	-	-	1.1	-	0.4	0.3	6	100.0
Unspecified lymphoma	0	0	1	0	1	0.4	0.4	3.8	-	-	1.1	-	0.4	0.4	6	100.0
Histiocytosis X	2	4	3	0	9	3.6	3.3	34.6	12.6	5.9	3.4	-	3.5	3.9	53	100.0
Other reticuloendothelial	1	0	0	2	3	1.2	1.1	11.5	6.3	-	-	2.3	1.2	1.2	18	100.0
III. BRAIN AND SPINAL	7	15	17	9	48	19.4	19.5	100.0	44.1	22.3	19.3	10.3	18.5	19.5	281	85.4
Ependymoma	2	4	1	0	7	2.8	2.4	14.6	12.6	5.9	1.1	-	2.7	3.2	42	85.7
Astrocytoma	4	2	7	2	15	6.1	6.1	31.3	25.2	3.0	7.9	2.3	5.8	4.7	88	100.0
Medulloblastoma	0	4	6	2	12	4.9	5.0	25.0	-	5.9	6.8	2.3	4.6	3.6	69	100.0
Other glioma	1	3	3	2	9	3.6	3.7	18.8	6.3	4.5	3.4	2.3	3.5	3.6	53	33.3
Other and unspecified *	0	2	0	3	5	2.0	2.3	10.4	-	3.0	-	3.4	1.9	1.9	29	100.0
IV. SYMPATHETIC N.S.	3	13	4	0	20	8.1	7.0	100.0	18.9	19.3	4.5	-	7.7	8.9	119	80.0
Neuroblastoma	3	13	4	0	20	8.1	7.0	100.0	18.9	19.3	4.5	-	7.7	8.9	119	80.0
Other	0	0	0	0	0	-	-	-	-	-	-	-	-	-	-	-
V. RETINOBLASTOMA	3	7	0	0	10	4.0	3.3	100.0	18.9	10.4	-	-	3.9	4.7	60	100.0
VI. KIDNEY	1	12	2	0	15	6.1	5.1	100.0	6.3	17.8	2.3	-	5.8	6.7	89	100.0
Wilms' tumour	1	12	2	0	15	6.1	5.1	100.0	6.3	17.8	2.3	-	5.8	6.7	89	100.0
Renal carcinoma	0	0	0	0	0	-	-	-	-	-	-	-	-	-	-	-
Other and unspecified	0	0	0	0	0	-	-	-	-	-	-	-	-	-	-	-
VII. LIVER	0	0	1	2	3	1.2	1.5	100.0	-	-	1.1	2.3	1.2	1.0	17	100.0
Hepatoblastoma	0	0	0	2	2	0.8	1.1	66.7	-	-	-	2.3	0.8	0.7	11	100.0
Hepatic carcinoma	0	0	1	0	1	0.4	0.4	33.3	-	-	1.1	-	0.4	0.4	6	100.0
Other and unspecified	0	0	0	0	0	-	-	-	-	-	-	-	-	-	-	-
VIII. BONE	0	3	1	7	11	4.5	5.2	100.0	-	4.5	1.1	8.0	4.2	4.1	63	100.0
Osteosarcoma	0	0	0	4	4	1.6	2.1	36.4	-	-	-	4.6	1.5	1.3	23	100.0
Chondrosarcoma	0	0	0	0	0	-	-	-	-	-	-	-	-	-	-	-
Ewing's sarcoma	0	3	1	3	7	2.8	3.0	63.6	-	4.5	1.1	3.4	2.7	2.7	41	100.0
Other and unspecified	0	0	0	0	0	-	-	-	-	-	-	-	-	-	-	-
IX. SOFT TISSUE SARCOMAS	3	0	0	5	8	3.2	3.7	100.0	18.9	-	-	5.7	3.1	3.1	47	100.0
Rhabdomyosarcoma	2	0	0	4	6	2.4	2.8	75.0	12.6	-	-	4.6	2.3	2.3	35	100.0
Fibrosarcoma	1	0	0	0	1	0.4	0.3	12.5	6.3	-	-	-	0.4	0.5	6	100.0
Other and unspecified	0	0	0	1	1	0.4	0.5	12.5	-	-	-	1.1	0.4	0.3	6	100.0
X. GONADAL & GERM CELL	1	1	2	5	9	3.6	4.2	100.0	6.3	1.5	2.3	5.7	3.5	3.3	52	100.0
Non-gonadal germ cell	1	1	1	2	5	2.0	2.2	55.6	6.3	1.5	1.1	2.3	1.9	2.0	29	100.0
Gonadal germ cell	0	0	1	1	2	0.8	1.1	22.2	-	-	1.1	1.1	0.8	0.7	11	100.0
Gonadal carcinoma	0	0	0	1	1	0.4	0.4	11.1	-	-	-	1.1	0.4	0.3	6	100.0
Other and unspecified	0	0	0	1	1	0.4	0.5	11.1	-	-	-	1.1	0.4	0.3	6	100.0
XI. EPITHELIAL NEOPLASMS	0	1	2	3	6	2.4	2.8	100.0	-	1.5	2.3	3.4	2.3	2.2	34	100.0
Adrenocortical carcinoma	0	0	0	0	0	-	-	-	-	-	-	-	-	-	-	-
Thyroid carcinoma	0	0	1	1	2	0.8	1.0	33.3	-	-	1.1	1.1	0.8	0.7	11	100.0
Nasopharyngeal carcinoma	0	0	0	0	0	-	-	-	-	-	-	-	-	-	-	-
Melanoma	0	1	1	1	3	1.2	1.5	50.0	-	1.5	1.1	1.1	1.2	1.0	17	100.0
Other carcinoma	0	0	0	1	1	0.4	0.3	16.7	-	-	-	1.1	0.4	0.5	6	100.0
XII. OTHER	0	0	0	0	0	-	-	-	-	-	-	-	-	-	-	-
* Specified as malignant	0	2	0	3	5	2.0	2.3	100.0	-	3.0	-	3.4	1.9	1.9	29	-

* Specified as malignant

Commentary

The total incidence of childhood cancer is comparable with that in most registries in Europe, North America and Oceania. An unusually high proportion of leukaemias, 86%, were acute lymphocytic. The incidence rates of non-Hodgkin lymphoma and retinoblastoma were rather high. There was a very high ratio of Ewing's sarcoma to osteosarcoma (3.2:1), but this was based on a total of only 16 cases of Ewing's sarcoma and five of osteosarcoma; however, the total incidence of bone tumours is not unusual. Educational programmes in Queensland have resulted in a high level of public awareness of the risks of exposure to sunlight; this may account for the unexpectedly low incidence of melanoma (in comparison with New South Wales and New Zealand non-Maoris) in an area with many hours of sunshine of high intensity.

References

McWhirter, W.R. (1982) The relationship of incidence of childhood lymphoblastic leukaemia to social class. *Br. J. Cancer*, *46*, 640-645

McWhirter, W.R. & Bacon, J.E. (1981) Incidence of childhood tumours in Queensland. *Br. J. Cancer*, *44*, 637-642

McWhirter, W.R. & Siskind, V. (1984) Childhood cancer survival trends in Queensland 1956-80. *Br. J. Cancer*, *49*, 513-519

McWhirter, W.R., Smith, H. & McWhirter, K.M. (1983) Social class as a prognostic variable in childhood acute lymphoblastic leukaemia. *Med. J. Aust.*, *2*, 319-321

FIJI

Cancer Registry of Fiji, 1969–1985

L.M. Seruvatu, K.P. Singh & E. Rausuvanua

The Registry was founded in 1965, and is part of the medical statistics section of the Ministry of Health. The sources of notification are forms completed by medical staff in the divisional hospitals, and copies of histopathology reports mentioning cancer. Death certificates are not used as a source of information.

The population covered by Fiji's health services is divided into four divisions, the Central and Western Divisions accounting for 75% of the population. The Colonial War Memorial (CWM) Hospital in Suva (380 beds) and the Lautoka Hospital (305 beds) are the Central and Western divisional hospitals respectively. They are general hospitals providing medical and nursing care for all specialties and collectively account for 80% of admissions and out-patient attendances at divisional hospital level. They are permanently staffed by full-time specialists and provide a wide range of clinical services and the major medical laboratory services for all divisions. They are the teaching hospitals of the Fiji School of Medicine, and act as major cancer referral centres, although no specialized oncological services, including radiotherapy, are available. Despite this, referral of patients overseas is quite rare. The other divisional hospitals at Labasa (125 beds) and Levuka (50 beds) have a minor role in cancer management, and refer cases requiring investigation and treatment to CWM Hospital. CWM and Lautoka Hospitals provide medical laboratory services, including histopathology, for the whole of Fiji.

Since notification to the Registry is entirely passive, it is probable that under-registration of cancer cases occurs. Furthermore, this has probably varied with time: in the early years of the Registry (up to 1972), about 210 cases were notified annually; this fell to 140 between 1973 and 1979, but since 1980 has averaged 370 cases per year.

The Fiji Islands are situated in the south-west Pacific. There are over 300 islands in the archipelago, with a total area of some 18 000 square kilometres but two large islands, Viti Levu (10 268 square kilometres) and Vanua Levu (5471 square kilometres), account for most of this. The interiors of both main islands are mountainous, rising to a maximum of 1300 m. The climate is tropical oceanic, with temperatures at the coast ranging from 16° C in winter to 35° C in summer. In the windward south-eastern areas, rainfall is about 50 cm per year and the vegetation is tropical forest, whereas leeward areas of the main islands are predominantly grasslands, with a rainfall of 30 cm per year.

The population estimates for 1979 show a total of 627 000, of whom 50% are Indians (the descendants of Indian labourers who arrived in Fiji between 1879 and 1916), 44.5% Melanesian Fijians and 5.5% of other origins (Europeans, Polynesians).

Fiji is an agricultural country, sugar being the main export. In recent years, tourism has also become an important source of foreign exchange.

Population

The population at risk has been derived from annual estimates of the population by ethnic origin,

AVERAGE ANNUAL POPULATION: 1969–1985

Age	Male	Female
Fijian		
0	3959	3664
1–4	14633	13606
5–9	17773	16799
10–14	17052	16269
0–14	53417	50338
Indian		
0	4658	4486
1–4	17210	16554
5–9	19928	19398
10–14	20018	19765
0–14	61814	60203

Contd p. 328

Fiji, Fijian   MALE

1969 – 1985

DIAGNOSTIC GROUP	NUMBER OF CASES						REL. FREQUENCY(%)			HV(%)
	0	1-4	5-9	10-14	15	All	Crude	Adj.	Group	
TOTAL	4	23	11	6	6	**55¤**	**100.0**	**100.0**	**100.0**	98.2
I. LEUKAEMIAS	0	6	6	6	0	**18**	**32.7**	**37.3**	**100.0**	94.4
Acute lymphocytic	0	2	2	3	0	7	12.7	14.4	38.9	100.0
Other lymphocytic	0	1	0	0	0	1	1.8	1.5	5.6	100.0
Acute non-lymphocytic	0	3	2	0	0	5	9.1	12.2	27.8	100.0
Chronic myeloid	0	0	1	0	0	1	1.8	2.0	5.6	80.0
Other and unspecified	0	0	1	3	0	4	7.3	7.2	22.2	100.0
II. LYMPHOMAS	0	5	0	1	4	**10**	**18.2**	**18.1**	**100.0**	**100.0**
Hodgkin's disease	0	0	0	0	1	1	1.8	2.0	10.0	100.0
Non-Hodgkin lymphoma	0	3	0	1	1	5	9.1	9.2	50.0	100.0
Burkitt's lymphoma	0	1	0	0	0	1	1.8	1.5	10.0	100.0
Unspecified lymphoma	0	1	0	0	2	3	5.5	5.5	30.0	100.0
Histiocytosis X	0	0	0	0	0	0	–	–	–	–
Other reticuloendothelial	0	0	0	0	0	0	–	–	–	–
III. BRAIN AND SPINAL	1	1	0	0	0	**2**	**3.6**	**3.0**	**100.0**	**100.0**
Ependymoma	1	0	0	0	0	1	1.8	1.5	50.0	100.0
Astrocytoma	0	1	0	0	0	1	1.8	1.5	50.0	100.0
Medulloblastoma	0	0	0	0	0	0	–	–	–	–
Other glioma	0	0	0	0	0	0	–	–	–	–
Other and unspecified *	0	1	0	0	0	1	1.8	1.5	50.0	100.0
IV. SYMPATHETIC N.S.	0	1	1	0	0	**2**	**3.6**	**3.5**	**100.0**	**100.0**
Neuroblastoma	0	1	1	0	0	2	3.6	3.5	100.0	100.0
Other	0	0	0	0	0	0	–	–	–	–
V. RETINOBLASTOMA	0	3	1	0	0	**4**	**7.3**	**7.2**		**100.0**
VI. KIDNEY	1	3	1	0	0	**6¤**	**10.9**	**8.7**	**100.0**	**100.0**
Wilms' tumour	1	3	1	0	0	6¤	10.9	8.7	100.0	100.0
Renal carcinoma	0	0	0	0	0	0	–	–	–	–
Other and unspecified	0	0	0	0	0	0	–	–	–	–
VII. LIVER	1	2	0	0	0	**4¤**	**7.3**	**4.4**	**100.0**	**100.0**
Hepatoblastoma	1	1	0	0	0	3¤	5.5	3.0	75.0	100.0
Hepatic carcinoma	0	1	0	0	0	1	1.8	1.5	25.0	100.0
Other and unspecified	0	0	0	0	0	0	–	–	–	–
VIII. BONE	0	0	0	2	0	**2**	**3.6**	**4.0**	**100.0**	**100.0**
Osteosarcoma	0	0	0	2	0	2	3.6	4.0	100.0	100.0
Chondrosarcoma	0	0	0	0	0	0	–	–	–	–
Ewing's sarcoma	0	0	0	0	0	0	–	–	–	–
Other and unspecified	0	0	0	0	0	0	–	–	–	–
IX. SOFT TISSUE SARCOMAS	1	1	0	0	2	**4**	**7.3**	**7.7**	**100.0**	**100.0**
Rhabdomyosarcoma	0	1	0	0	0	1	1.8	2.0	25.0	100.0
Fibrosarcoma	0	0	0	0	0	0	–	–	–	–
Other and unspecified	1	0	0	0	2	3	5.5	5.7	75.0	100.0
X. GONADAL & GERM CELL	0	1	0	0	0	**1**	**1.8**	**1.5**	**100.0**	**100.0**
Non-gonadal germ cell	0	1	0	0	0	1	1.8	1.5	100.0	100.0
Gonadal germ cell	0	0	0	0	0	0	–	–	–	–
Gonadal carcinoma	0	0	0	0	0	0	–	–	–	–
Other and unspecified	0	1	0	0	0	1	1.8	1.5	100.0	100.0
XI. EPITHELIAL NEOPLASMS	0	0	0	0	1	**1**	**1.8**	**2.0**	**100.0**	**100.0**
Adrenocortical carcinoma	0	0	0	0	0	0	–	–	–	–
Thyroid carcinoma	0	0	0	0	1	1	1.8	2.0	100.0	100.0
Nasopharyngeal carcinoma	0	0	0	0	0	0	–	–	–	–
Melanoma	0	0	0	0	0	0	–	–	–	–
Other carcinoma	0	0	0	1	1	1	1.8	2.0	100.0	100.0
XII. OTHER	0	0	1	0	1	**1**	**1.8**	**2.7**	**100.0**	**100.0**
Specified as malignant	0	1	0	0	1	1	1.8	1.5	100.0	100.0

* Specified as malignant
¤ Includes age unknown

Fiji, Fijian 1969 - 1985 FEMALE

DIAGNOSTIC GROUP	NUMBER OF CASES					REL. FREQUENCY(%)			HV(%)
	0	1-4	5-9	10-14	All	Crude	Adj.	Group	
TOTAL	7	18	12	14	51	100.0	100.0	100.0	98.0
I. LEUKAEMIAS	2	5	4	1	12	23.5	23.3	100.0	100.0
Acute lymphocytic	1	4	4	1	10	19.6	20.1	83.3	100.0
Other lymphocytic	0	0	0	0	0	–	–	–	–
Acute non-lymphocytic	1	0	0	0	1	2.0	1.6	8.3	100.0
Chronic myeloid	0	0	0	0	0	–	–	–	–
Other and unspecified	0	1	0	0	1	2.0	1.6	8.3	100.0
II. LYMPHOMAS	0	4	3	1	8	15.7	16.0	100.0	100.0
Hodgkin's disease	0	0	0	1	1	2.0	2.1	12.5	100.0
Non-Hodgkin lymphoma	0	4	2	0	6	11.8	11.4	75.0	100.0
Burkitt's lymphoma	0	0	0	0	0	–	–	–	–
Unspecified lymphoma	0	0	1	0	1	2.0	2.5	12.5	100.0
Histiocytosis X	0	0	0	0	0	–	–	–	–
Other reticuloendothelial	0	0	0	0	0	–	–	–	–
III. BRAIN AND SPINAL	0	3	1	0	4	7.8	7.3	100.0	75.0
Ependymoma	0	0	0	0	0	–	–	–	–
Astrocytoma	0	1	0	0	1	2.0	1.6	25.0	100.0
Medulloblastoma	0	1	0	0	1	2.0	1.6	25.0	100.0
Other glioma	0	0	0	0	0	–	–	–	–
Other and unspecified *	0	1	1	0	2	3.9	4.1	50.0	50.0
IV. SYMPATHETIC N.S.	0	1	0	2	3	5.9	5.9	100.0	100.0
Neuroblastoma	0	1	0	2	3	5.9	5.9	100.0	100.0
Other	0	0	0	0	0	–	–	–	–
V. RETINOBLASTOMA	0	2	0	0	2	3.9	3.2	100.0	100.0
VI. KIDNEY	0	3	2	0	5	9.8	9.8	100.0	100.0
Wilms' tumour	0	3	2	0	5	9.8	9.8	100.0	100.0
Renal carcinoma	0	0	0	0	0	–	–	–	–
Other and unspecified	0	0	0	0	0	–	–	–	–
VII. LIVER	2	0	0	2	4	7.8	7.5	100.0	100.0
Hepatoblastoma	1	0	0	0	1	2.0	1.6	25.0	100.0
Hepatic carcinoma	1	0	0	2	3	5.9	5.9	75.0	100.0
Other and unspecified	0	0	0	0	0	–	–	–	–
VIII. BONE	0	0	0	3	3	5.9	6.4	100.0	100.0
Osteosarcoma	0	0	0	1	1	2.0	2.1	33.3	100.0
Chondrosarcoma	0	0	0	0	0	–	–	–	–
Ewing's sarcoma	0	0	0	1	1	2.0	2.1	33.3	100.0
Other and unspecified	0	0	0	1	1	2.0	2.1	33.3	100.0
IX. SOFT TISSUE SARCOMAS	0	0	2	1	3	5.9	7.1	100.0	100.0
Rhabdomyosarcoma	0	0	1	0	1	2.0	2.5	33.3	100.0
Fibrosarcoma	0	0	0	1	1	2.0	2.5	33.3	100.0
Other and unspecified	0	0	1	0	1	2.0	2.5	33.3	100.0
X. GONADAL & GERM CELL	0	0	0	3	3	5.9	6.4	100.0	100.0
Non-gonadal germ cell	0	0	0	1	1	2.0	2.1	33.3	100.0
Gonadal germ cell	0	0	0	1	1	2.0	2.1	33.3	100.0
Gonadal carcinoma	0	0	0	0	0	–	–	–	–
Other and unspecified	0	0	0	1	1	2.0	2.1	33.3	100.0
XI. EPITHELIAL NEOPLASMS	2	0	0	1	3	5.9	5.3	100.0	100.0
Adrenocortical carcinoma	0	0	0	0	0	–	–	–	–
Thyroid carcinoma	0	0	0	0	0	–	–	–	–
Nasopharyngeal carcinoma	0	0	0	0	0	–	–	–	–
Melanoma	0	0	0	0	0	–	–	–	–
Other carcinoma	2	0	0	1	3	5.9	5.3	100.0	100.0
XII. OTHER	1	0	0	0	1	2.0	1.6	100.0	100.0

* Specified as malignant
□ Includes age unknown

FIJI

Fiji, Fijian

1969 – 1985 MALE

DIAGNOSTIC GROUP	NUMBER OF CASES					REL. FREQUENCY(%)			RATES PER MILLION							HV(%)
	0	1-4	5-9	10-14	All	Crude	Adj.	Group	0	1-4	5-9	10-14	Crude	Adj.	Cum	
TOTAL	4	23	11	15	55¤	100.0	100.0	100.0	59.4	92.5	36.4	51.7	60.6	60.0	870	98.2
I. LEUKAEMIAS	0	6	6	6	18	32.7	37.3	100.0	–	24.1	19.9	20.7	19.8	19.9	299	94.4
II. LYMPHOMAS	0	5	1	4	10	18.2	18.1	100.0	–	20.1	3.3	13.8	11.0	11.3	166	100.0
III. BRAIN AND SPINAL	1	1	0	0	2	3.6	3.0	100.0	14.9	4.0	–	–	2.2	2.4	31	100.0
IV. SYMPATHETIC N.S.	0	1	0	1	2	3.6	3.5	100.0	–	4.0	–	3.4	2.2	2.2	33	100.0
V. RETINOBLASTOMA	0	3	1	0	4	7.3	7.2	100.0	–	12.1	3.3	–	4.4	4.8	65	100.0
VI. KIDNEY	1	3	1	0	6¤	10.9	8.7	100.0	14.9	12.1	3.3	–	6.6	6.0	80	100.0
VII. LIVER	1	2	0	0	4¤	7.3	4.4	100.0	14.9	8.0	–	–	4.4	3.6	47	100.0
VIII. BONE	0	0	0	2	2	3.6	4.0	100.0	–	–	–	6.9	2.2	2.0	34	100.0
IX. SOFT TISSUE SARCOMAS	1	1	1	1	4	7.3	7.7	100.0	14.9	4.0	3.3	3.4	4.4	4.5	65	100.0
X. GONADAL & GERM CELL	0	1	0	0	1	1.8	1.5	100.0	–	4.0	–	–	1.1	1.2	16	100.0
XI. EPITHELIAL NEOPLASMS	0	0	0	1	1	1.8	2.0	100.0	–	–	–	3.4	1.1	1.0	17	100.0
XII. OTHER	0	0	1	0	1	1.8	2.7	100.0	–	–	3.3	–	1.1	1.1	17	100.0

¤ Includes age unknown

Fiji, Fijian

1969 – 1985 FEMALE

DIAGNOSTIC GROUP	NUMBER OF CASES					REL. FREQUENCY(%)			RATES PER MILLION							HV(%)
	0	1-4	5-9	10-14	All	Crude	Adj.	Group	0	1-4	5-9	10-14	Crude	Adj.	Cum	
TOTAL	7	18	12	14	51	100.0	100.0	100.0	112.4	77.8	42.0	50.6	59.6	61.0	887	98.0
I. LEUKAEMIAS	2	5	4	1	12	23.5	23.3	100.0	32.1	21.6	14.0	3.6	14.0	14.7	207	100.0
II. LYMPHOMAS	0	4	3	1	8	15.7	16.0	100.0	–	17.3	10.5	3.6	9.3	9.8	140	100.0
III. BRAIN AND SPINAL	0	3	1	0	4	7.8	7.3	100.0	–	13.0	3.5	–	4.7	5.1	69	75.0
IV. SYMPATHETIC N.S.	0	1	0	2	3	5.9	5.9	100.0	–	4.3	–	7.2	3.5	3.4	53	100.0
V. RETINOBLASTOMA	0	2	0	0	2	3.9	3.2	100.0	–	8.6	–	–	2.3	2.7	35	100.0
VI. KIDNEY	0	3	2	0	5	9.8	9.8	100.0	–	13.0	7.0	–	5.8	6.3	87	100.0
VII. LIVER	2	0	0	2	4	7.8	7.5	100.0	32.1	–	–	7.2	4.7	4.6	68	100.0
VIII. BONE	0	0	0	3	3	5.9	6.4	100.0	–	–	–	10.8	3.5	3.1	54	100.0
IX. SOFT TISSUE SARCOMAS	0	0	2	1	3	5.9	7.1	100.0	–	–	7.0	3.6	3.5	3.3	53	100.0
X. GONADAL & GERM CELL	0	0	0	3	3	5.9	6.4	100.0	–	–	–	10.8	3.5	3.1	54	100.0
XI. EPITHELIAL NEOPLASMS	2	0	0	1	3	5.9	5.3	100.0	32.1	–	–	3.6	3.5	3.5	50	100.0
XII. OTHER	1	0	0	0	1	2.0	1.6	100.0	16.1	–	–	–	1.2	1.2	16	100.0

¤ Includes age unknown

Fiji, Indian

MALE

1969 - 1985

DIAGNOSTIC GROUP	NUMBER OF CASES					REL. FREQUENCY(%)			HV(%)
	0	1-4	5-9	10-14	All	Crude	Adj.	Group	
TOTAL	4	18	12	19	54¤	100.0	100.0	100.0	98.1
I. LEUKAEMIAS	1	6	9	8	24¤	44.4	47.9	100.0	95.8
Acute lymphocytic	0	4	9	5	18	33.3	37.7	75.0	100.0
Other lymphocytic	0	0	0	0	0	-	-	-	-
Acute non-lymphocytic	0	0	0	1	1	1.9	1.6	4.2	100.0
Chronic myeloid	1	0	0	0	1	1.9	1.8	4.2	100.0
Other and unspecified	0	2	0	2	4	7.4	6.8	16.7	75.0
II. LYMPHOMAS	0	5	1	4	10	18.5	17.9	100.0	100.0
Hodgkin's disease	0	0	1	1	2	3.7	4.1	20.0	100.0
Non-Hodgkin lymphoma	0	2	0	1	3	5.6	5.2	30.0	100.0
Burkitt's lymphoma	0	0	0	0	0	-	-	-	-
Unspecified lymphoma	0	3	0	2	5	9.3	8.6	50.0	100.0
Histiocytosis X	0	0	0	0	0	-	-	-	-
Other reticuloendothelial	0	0	0	0	0	-	-	-	-
III. BRAIN AND SPINAL	0	0	1	0	1	1.9	2.5	100.0	100.0
Ependymoma	0	0	0	0	0	-	-	-	-
Astrocytoma	0	0	0	0	0	-	-	-	-
Medulloblastoma	0	0	0	0	0	-	-	-	-
Other glioma	0	0	0	0	0	-	-	-	-
Other and unspecified *	0	0	1	0	1	1.9	2.5	100.0	100.0
IV. SYMPATHETIC N.S.	1	1	0	0	2	3.7	3.6	100.0	100.0
Neuroblastoma	1	1	0	0	2	3.7	3.6	100.0	100.0
Other	0	0	0	0	0	-	-	-	-
V. RETINOBLASTOMA	0	4	0	0	4	7.4	7.3	100.0	100.0
VI. KIDNEY	0	0	0	0	1¤	1.9	-	100.0	100.0
Wilms' tumour	0	0	0	0	1¤	1.9	-	100.0	100.0
Renal carcinoma	0	0	0	0	0	-	-	-	-
Other and unspecified	0	0	0	0	0	-	-	-	-
VII. LIVER	0	1	0	0	1	1.9	1.8	100.0	100.0
Hepatoblastoma	0	0	0	0	0	-	-	-	-
Hepatic carcinoma	0	1	0	0	1	1.9	1.8	100.0	100.0
Other and unspecified	0	0	0	0	0	-	-	-	-
VIII. BONE	0	0	0	4	4	7.4	6.3	100.0	100.0
Osteosarcoma	0	0	0	4	4	7.4	6.3	100.0	100.0
Chondrosarcoma	0	0	0	0	0	-	-	-	-
Ewing's sarcoma	0	0	0	0	0	-	-	-	-
Other and unspecified	0	0	0	0	0	-	-	-	-
IX. SOFT TISSUE SARCOMAS	1	0	0	2	3	5.6	5.0	100.0	100.0
Rhabdomyosarcoma	1	0	0	0	1	1.9	1.8	33.3	100.0
Fibrosarcoma	0	0	0	1	1	1.9	1.6	33.3	100.0
Other and unspecified	0	0	0	1	1	1.9	1.6	33.3	100.0
X. GONADAL & GERM CELL	1	1	0	0	2	3.7	3.6	100.0	100.0
Non-gonadal germ cell	0	0	0	0	0	-	-	-	-
Gonadal germ cell	1	1	0	0	2	3.7	3.6	100.0	100.0
Gonadal carcinoma	0	0	0	0	0	-	-	-	-
Other and unspecified	0	0	0	0	0	-	-	-	-
XI. EPITHELIAL NEOPLASMS	0	0	1	1	2	3.7	4.1	100.0	100.0
Adrenocortical carcinoma	0	0	0	0	0	-	-	-	-
Thyroid carcinoma	0	0	0	0	0	-	-	-	-
Nasopharyngeal carcinoma	0	0	0	0	0	-	-	-	-
Melanoma	0	0	0	0	0	-	-	-	-
Other carcinoma	0	0	1	1	2	3.7	4.1	100.0	100.0
XII. OTHER	0	0	0	0	0	-	-	-	-

* Specified as malignant
¤ Includes age unknown

Fiji, Indian   FEMALE

1969 – 1985

DIAGNOSTIC GROUP	NUMBER OF CASES					REL. FREQUENCY(%)			HV(%)
	0	1-4	5-9	10-14	All	Crude	Adj.	Group	
TOTAL	**3**	**13**	**8**	**4**	**28**	**100.0**	**100.0**	**100.0**	**96.4**
I. LEUKAEMIAS	**1**	**6**	**4**	**1**	**12**	**42.9**	**40.0**	**100.0**	**100.0**
Acute lymphocytic	0	5	1	1	7	25.0	18.8	58.3	100.0
Other lymphocytic	1	1	0	0	2	7.1	6.3	16.7	100.0
Acute non-lymphocytic	0	0	1	0	1	3.6	3.8	8.3	100.0
Chronic myeloid	0	0	1	0	1	3.6	3.8	8.3	100.0
Other and unspecified	0	0	1	0	1	3.6	3.8	8.3	100.0
II. LYMPHOMAS	**0**	**0**	**2**	**0**	**2**	**7.1**	**7.5**	**100.0**	**100.0**
Hodgkin's disease	0	0	0	0	0	–	–	–	–
Non-Hodgkin lymphoma	0	0	1	0	1	3.6	3.8	50.0	100.0
Burkitt's lymphoma	0	0	0	0	0	–	–	–	–
Unspecified lymphoma	0	0	1	0	1	3.6	3.8	50.0	100.0
Histiocytosis X	0	0	0	0	0	–	–	–	–
Other reticuloendothelial	0	0	0	0	0	–	–	–	–
III. BRAIN AND SPINAL	**0**	**1**	**0**	**0**	**1**	**3.6**	**2.5**	**100.0**	**100.0**
Ependymoma	0	0	0	0	0	–	–	–	–
Astrocytoma	0	0	0	0	0	–	–	–	–
Medulloblastoma	0	0	0	0	0	–	–	–	–
Other glioma	0	1	0	0	1	3.6	2.5	100.0	100.0
Other and unspecified *	0	0	0	0	0	–	–	–	–
IV. SYMPATHETIC N.S.	**0**	**0**	**0**	**0**	**0**	**–**	**–**	**–**	**–**
Neuroblastoma	0	0	0	0	0	–	–	–	–
Other	0	0	0	0	0	–	–	–	–
V. RETINOBLASTOMA	**0**	**0**	**0**	**0**	**0**	**–**	**–**	**–**	**–**
VI. KIDNEY	**0**	**3**	**1**	**0**	**4**	**14.3**	**11.3**	**100.0**	**100.0**
Wilms' tumour	0	3	0	0	3	10.7	7.5	75.0	100.0
Renal carcinoma	0	0	1	0	1	3.6	3.8	25.0	100.0
Other and unspecified	0	0	0	0	0	–	–	–	–
VII. LIVER	**1**	**0**	**0**	**0**	**1**	**3.6**	**2.5**	**100.0**	**100.0**
Hepatoblastoma	0	0	0	0	0	–	–	–	–
Hepatic carcinoma	1	0	0	0	1	3.6	2.5	100.0	100.0
Other and unspecified	0	0	0	0	0	–	–	–	–
VIII. BONE	**0**	**0**	**1**	**1**	**1**	**3.6**	**7.5**	**100.0**	**100.0**
Osteosarcoma	0	0	1	1	1	3.6	7.5	100.0	100.0
Chondrosarcoma	0	0	0	0	0	–	–	–	–
Ewing's sarcoma	0	0	0	0	0	–	–	–	–
Other and unspecified	0	0	0	0	0	–	–	–	–
IX. SOFT TISSUE SARCOMAS	**1**	**1**	**1**	**0**	**2**	**7.1**	**10.0**	**100.0**	**100.0**
Rhabdomyosarcoma	1	1	0	0	2	7.1	10.0	100.0	100.0
Fibrosarcoma	0	0	0	0	0	–	–	–	–
Other and unspecified	0	0	0	0	0	–	–	–	–
X. GONADAL & GERM CELL	**0**	**0**	**1**	**1**	**1**	**3.6**	**7.5**	**100.0**	**100.0**
Non-gonadal germ cell	0	0	0	0	0	–	–	–	–
Gonadal germ cell	0	0	0	0	0	–	–	–	–
Gonadal carcinoma	0	0	1	1	1	3.6	7.5	100.0	100.0
Other and unspecified	0	0	0	0	0	–	–	–	–
XI. EPITHELIAL NEOPLASMS	**0**	**2**	**1**	**0**	**3**	**10.7**	**8.8**	**100.0**	**100.0**
Adrenocortical carcinoma	0	1	0	0	1	3.6	2.5	33.3	100.0
Thyroid carcinoma	0	0	0	0	0	–	–	–	–
Nasopharyngeal carcinoma	0	0	0	0	0	–	–	–	–
Melanoma	0	0	0	0	0	–	–	–	–
Other carcinoma	0	1	1	0	2	7.1	6.3	66.7	100.0
XII. OTHER	**0**	**1**	**0**	**0**	**1**	**3.6**	**2.5**	**100.0**	**100.0**

* Specified as malignant
¤ Includes age unknown

Fiji, Indian

MALE

1969 - 1985

DIAGNOSTIC GROUP	NUMBER OF CASES					REL. FREQUENCY(%)			RATES PER MILLION						Cum	HV(%)
	0	1-4	5-9	10-14	All	Crude	Adj.	Group	0	1-4	5-9	10-14	Crude	Adj.		
TOTAL	4	18	12	19	54¤	100.0	100.0	100.0	50.5	61.5	35.4	55.8	51.4	50.6	753	98.1
I. LEUKAEMIAS	1	6	9	8	24	44.4	47.9	100.0	12.6	20.5	26.6	23.5	22.8	22.7	345	95.8
II. LYMPHOMAS	0	5	1	4	10	18.5	17.9	100.0	-	17.1	3.0	11.8	9.5	9.7	142	100.0
III. BRAIN AND SPINAL	0	0	1	0	1	1.9	2.5	100.0	-	-	3.0	-	1.0	1.0	15	100.0
IV. SYMPATHETIC N.S.	1	1	0	0	2	3.7	3.6	100.0	12.6	3.4	-	-	1.9	2.0	26	100.0
V. RETINOBLASTOMA	0	4	0	0	4	7.4	7.3	100.0	-	13.7	-	-	3.8	4.2	55	100.0
VI. KIDNEY	0	0	0	0	1¤	1.9	-	100.0	-	-	-	-	1.0	-	-	100.0
VII. LIVER	0	1	0	0	1	1.9	1.8	100.0	-	3.4	-	-	1.0	1.1	14	100.0
VIII. BONE	0	0	0	4	4	7.4	6.3	100.0	-	-	-	11.8	3.8	3.4	59	100.0
IX. SOFT TISSUE SARCOMAS	1	0	0	2	3	5.6	5.0	100.0	12.6	-	-	5.9	2.9	2.7	42	100.0
X. GONADAL & GERM CELL	1	1	0	0	2	3.7	3.6	100.0	12.6	3.4	-	-	1.9	2.0	26	100.0
XI. EPITHELIAL NEOPLASMS	0	0	1	1	2	3.7	4.1	100.0	-	-	3.0	2.9	1.9	1.8	29	100.0
XIII. OTHER	0	0	0	0	0	-	-	-	-	-	-	-	-	-	-	-

¤ Includes age unknown

Fiji, Indian

FEMALE

1969 - 1985

DIAGNOSTIC GROUP	NUMBER OF CASES					REL. FREQUENCY(%)			RATES PER MILLION						Cum	HV(%)
	0	1-4	5-9	10-14	All	Crude	Adj.	Group	0	1-4	5-9	10-14	Crude	Adj.		
TOTAL	3	13	8	4	28	100.0	100.0	100.0	39.3	46.2	24.3	11.9	27.4	28.6	405	96.4
I. LEUKAEMIAS	1	6	4	1	12	42.9	40.0	100.0	13.1	21.3	12.1	3.0	11.7	12.4	174	100.0
II. LYMPHOMAS	0	0	2	0	2	7.1	7.5	100.0	-	-	6.1	-	2.0	2.0	30	100.0
III. BRAIN AND SPINAL	0	1	0	0	1	3.6	2.5	100.0	-	3.6	-	-	1.0	1.1	14	100.0
IV. SYMPATHETIC N.S.	0	0	0	0	0	-	-	-	-	-	-	-	-	-	-	-
V. RETINOBLASTOMA	0	0	0	0	0	-	-	-	-	-	-	-	-	-	-	-
VI. KIDNEY	0	3	1	0	4	14.3	11.3	100.0	-	10.7	3.0	-	3.9	4.3	58	100.0
VII. LIVER	1	0	0	0	1	3.6	2.5	100.0	13.1	-	-	-	1.0	1.0	13	100.0
VIII. BONE	0	0	0	1	1	3.6	7.5	100.0	-	-	-	3.0	1.0	0.9	15	100.0
IX. SOFT TISSUE SARCOMAS	1	0	0	1	2	7.1	10.0	100.0	13.1	-	-	3.0	2.0	1.9	28	100.0
X. GONADAL & GERM CELL	0	0	0	1	1	3.6	7.5	100.0	-	-	-	3.0	1.0	0.9	15	-
XI. EPITHELIAL NEOPLASMS	0	2	1	0	3	10.7	8.8	100.0	-	7.1	3.0	-	2.9	3.2	44	100.0
XIII. OTHER	0	1	0	0	1	3.6	2.5	100.0	-	3.6	-	-	1.0	1.1	14	100.0

¤ Includes age unknown

sex and age taken from the Ministry of Health Annual Reports. The estimates are based on census data for 1966 and 1976.

Commentary

Four sets of tables are included. For each of the two main ethnic groups (Fijians and Indians), numbers and relative frequencies are presented, and incidence rates have been calculated for the 12 major diagnostic groups. Because of the under-enumeration of cases, calculated incidence rates represent minimum estimates of incidence.

The total registration rate was the lowest for any population-based registry and it seems likely that registration is very incomplete.

NEW ZEALAND

New Zealand Cancer Registry, 1970–1979

J. Fraser, F.J. Findlay & J.J. Auld

The New Zealand Cancer Registry was established in 1948. It is located in the National Health Statistics Centre, Wellington. The Registry was initially clinically orientated, only patients admitted to hospital for treatment being registered. In 1972 the Registry became population-based.

Cancer registration in New Zealand is compulsory and involves a network of regional hospital-based registries, all of which report to the central registry. The regional registries receive notifications of in-patients treated for cancer in public and private hospitals within their regions. Notifications are sent to the New Zealand Registry, where linkage is effected with records received by the National Health Statistics Centre. The Centre receives all death certificates as well as case abstracts which include full name, address and diagnosis, for every person discharged from or dying in all public and private hospitals. Reports on every autopsy performed in public hospitals — such autopsies are carried out on approximately one-third of all those dying in New Zealand — are also received by the Centre. Thanks to all these records, only 'silent' tumours, i.e, those existing in persons on whom no autopsy was performed, would be missed. Quarterly lists of deaths are sent to regional registries to complete their records.

When cancer registration began in New Zealand, cancer of all sites was registered. However, after 1968 it was decided no longer to register basal-cell or squamous-cell carcinomas of the skin, partly because an increasing number of cases were being treated as out-patients and partly because it was felt that continued registration each year of a large number of cases for whom prognosis was so favourable would soon increase the size of the Register to the stage where the work needed to maintain it would be beyond the resources available. In general, tumours of benign and unspecified nature (including brain tumours) are not registered.

Selected samples of notifications received from regional registries are compared with notifications re-reported from the case-notes during field visits by a New Zealand Registry staff member to such registries. It is a particularly useful method of reducing the effect of differences in interpretation.

Information is held on computer files and most editing functions are computerized but duplication is prevented by manual means. Multiple primary tumours in one individual are registered and cross-referenced.

The New Zealand Cancer Registry covers the whole of New Zealand, which is situated in the South Pacific, 1600 kilometres south-east of Australia. The area is 267 847 square kilometres.

The 1981 census population was 3 175 737; 8.8% of the population were Maori, 2.8% Pacific Island Polynesian and 88.4% other races, mainly European. The main occupational groups in the full-time labour force were production, transport, equipment operators and labourers (34%); clerical (16%); professional and technical (14%); sales (10%); agricultural, animal husbandry and forest workers, fishermen and hunters (11%); service workers (8%); administrative and managerial (3%); and other workers (4%). Of the total population, 47% lived in conurbations of more than 100 000.

AVERAGE ANNUAL POPULATION: 1970-1979

Age	Male	Female
Maori		
0	3773	3578
1–4	15625	15130
5–9	20359	19787
10–14	19370	18754
0–14	59127	57249
Non-Maori		
0	24645	23671
1–4	103692	99503
5–9	137705	131676
10–14	138684	132172
0–14	404726	387022

Contd p. 334

New Zealand, Maori

1970 – 1979

MALE

DIAGNOSTIC GROUP	NUMBER OF CASES 0	1-4	5-9	10-14	All	REL. FREQUENCY(%) Crude	Adj.	Group	RATES PER MILLION 0	1-4	5-9	10-14	Crude	Adj.	Cum	HV(%)
TOTAL	12	30	34	24	100	100.0	100.0	100.0	318.0	192.0	167.0	123.9	169.1	173.9	2540	93.7
I. LEUKAEMIAS	4	8	7	5	24	24.0	23.9	100.0	106.0	51.2	34.4	25.8	40.6	42.6	612	100.0
Acute lymphocytic	0	5	3	3	11	11.0	11.2	45.8	-	32.0	14.7	15.5	18.6	19.2	279	100.0
Other lymphocytic	0	0	0	0	0	-	-	-	-	-	-	-	-	-	-	-
Acute non-lymphocytic	1	1	4	2	8	8.0	7.9	33.3	26.5	6.4	19.6	10.3	13.5	13.4	202	100.0
Chronic myeloid	1	0	0	0	1	1.0	1.0	4.2	26.5	-	-	-	1.7	2.1	26	100.0
Other and unspecified	2	2	0	0	4	4.0	3.8	16.7	53.0	12.8	-	-	6.8	8.1	104	100.0
II. LYMPHOMAS	0	4	8	4	16	16.0	15.9	100.0	-	25.6	39.3	20.6	27.1	26.6	402	100.0
Hodgkin's disease	0	1	5	0	6	6.0	5.4	37.5	-	6.4	24.6	-	10.1	9.9	148	100.0
Non-Hodgkin lymphoma	0	3	2	3	8	8.0	8.4	50.0	-	19.2	9.8	15.5	13.5	13.6	203	100.0
Burkitt's lymphoma	0	0	0	0	0	-	-	-	-	-	-	-	-	-	-	-
Unspecified lymphoma	0	0	1	1	2	2.0	2.1	12.5	-	-	4.9	5.2	3.4	3.1	50	100.0
Histiocytosis X	0	0	0	0	0	-	-	-	-	-	-	-	-	-	-	-
Other reticuloendothelial	0	0	0	0	0	-	-	-	-	-	-	-	-	-	-	-
III. BRAIN AND SPINAL	1	4	6	4	15	15.0	15.1	100.0	26.5	25.6	29.5	20.6	25.4	25.5	379	100.0
Ependymoma	0	0	0	0	0	-	-	-	-	-	-	-	-	-	-	-
Astrocytoma	1	0	1	2	4	4.0	4.3	26.7	26.5	-	4.9	10.3	6.8	6.6	103	100.0
Medulloblastoma	0	2	4	2	8	8.0	7.9	53.3	-	12.8	19.6	10.3	13.5	13.3	201	100.0
Other glioma	0	0	1	0	1	1.0	0.9	6.7	-	-	4.9	-	1.7	1.6	25	100.0
Other and unspecified *	0	2	0	0	2	2.0	1.9	13.3	-	12.8	-	-	3.4	4.0	51	-
IV. SYMPATHETIC N.S.	3	4	2	0	9	9.0	8.4	100.0	79.5	25.6	9.8	-	15.2	17.3	231	100.0
Neuroblastoma	3	4	2	0	9	9.0	8.4	100.0	79.5	25.6	9.8	-	15.2	17.3	231	100.0
Other	0	0	0	0	0	-	-	-	-	-	-	-	-	-	-	-
V. RETINOBLASTOMA	0	2	0	0	2	2.0	1.9	100.0	-	12.8	-	-	3.4	4.0	51	100.0
VI. KIDNEY	0	4	1	0	5	5.0	4.7	100.0	-	25.6	4.9	-	8.5	9.5	127	80.0
Wilms' tumour	0	4	1	0	5	5.0	4.7	100.0	-	25.6	4.9	-	8.5	9.5	127	80.0
Renal carcinoma	0	0	0	0	0	-	-	-	-	-	-	-	-	-	-	-
Other and unspecified	0	0	0	0	0	-	-	-	-	-	-	-	-	-	-	-
VII. LIVER	0	0	0	2	2	2.0	2.5	100.0	-	-	-	10.3	3.4	3.0	52	-
Hepatoblastoma	0	0	0	0	0	-	-	-	-	-	-	-	-	-	-	-
Hepatic carcinoma	0	0	0	2	2	2.0	2.5	100.0	-	-	-	10.3	3.4	3.0	52	-
Other and unspecified	0	0	0	0	0	-	-	-	-	-	-	-	-	-	-	-
VIII. BONE	0	0	2	5	7	7.0	8.0	100.0	-	-	9.8	25.8	11.8	10.7	178	100.0
Osteosarcoma	0	0	0	1	1	1.0	1.3	14.3	-	-	-	5.2	1.7	1.5	26	100.0
Chondrosarcoma	0	0	1	1	2	2.0	2.1	28.6	-	-	4.9	5.2	3.4	3.1	50	100.0
Ewing's sarcoma	0	0	1	3	4	4.0	4.6	57.1	-	-	4.9	15.5	6.8	6.1	102	100.0
Other and unspecified	0	0	0	0	0	-	-	-	-	-	-	-	-	-	-	-
IX. SOFT TISSUE SARCOMAS	0	1	3	0	4	4.0	3.6	100.0	-	6.4	14.7	-	6.8	6.7	99	100.0
Rhabdomyosarcoma	0	1	3	0	4	4.0	3.6	100.0	-	6.4	14.7	-	6.8	6.7	99	100.0
Fibrosarcoma	0	0	0	0	0	-	-	-	-	-	-	-	-	-	-	-
Other and unspecified	0	0	0	0	0	-	-	-	-	-	-	-	-	-	-	-
X. GONADAL & GERM CELL	2	2	1	0	5	5.0	4.7	100.0	53.0	12.8	4.9	-	8.5	9.7	129	100.0
Non-gonadal germ cell	1	1	1	0	3	3.0	2.8	60.0	26.5	6.4	4.9	-	5.1	5.6	77	100.0
Gonadal germ cell	1	1	0	0	2	2.0	1.9	40.0	26.5	6.4	-	-	3.4	4.0	52	100.0
Gonadal carcinoma	0	0	0	0	0	-	-	-	-	-	-	-	-	-	-	-
Other and unspecified	0	0	0	0	0	-	-	-	-	-	-	-	-	-	-	-
XI. EPITHELIAL NEOPLASMS	1	0	2	4	7	7.0	7.7	100.0	26.5	-	9.8	20.6	11.8	11.2	179	100.0
Adrenocortical carcinoma	1	0	1	0	2	2.0	1.8	28.6	26.5	-	4.9	-	3.4	3.6	51	100.0
Thyroid carcinoma	0	0	0	0	0	-	-	-	-	-	-	-	-	-	-	-
Nasopharyngeal carcinoma	0	0	0	0	0	-	-	-	-	-	-	-	-	-	-	-
Melanoma	0	0	0	0	0	-	-	-	-	-	-	-	-	-	-	-
Other carcinoma	0	0	1	4	5	5.0	5.9	71.4	-	-	4.9	20.6	8.5	7.6	128	100.0
XII. OTHER	1	1	2	0	4	4.0	3.7	100.0	26.5	6.4	9.8	-	6.8	7.2	101	-
* Specified as malignant	0	2	0	0	2	2.0	1.9	100.0	-	12.8	-	-	3.4	4.0	51	-

New Zealand, Maori

FEMALE

1970 – 1979

DIAGNOSTIC GROUP	Cases 0	Cases 1–4	Cases 5–9	Cases 10–14	Cases All	Rel.Freq Crude	Rel.Freq Adj.	Rel.Freq Group	Rate 0	Rate 1–4	Rate 5–9	Rate 10–14	Rate Crude	Rate Adj.	Cum	HV(%)
TOTAL	5	23	12	22	62	100.0	100.0	100.0	139.7	152.0	60.6	117.3	108.3	111.5	1637	97.6
I. LEUKAEMIAS	2	6	2	1	11	17.7	17.8	100.0	55.9	39.7	10.1	5.3	19.2	21.4	292	100.0
Acute lymphocytic	0	2	1	0	3	4.8	5.4	27.3	–	13.2	5.1	–	5.2	5.7	78	100.0
Other lymphocytic	0	0	0	0	0	–	–	–	–	–	–	–	–	–	–	–
Acute non-lymphocytic	2	3	0	1	6	9.7	8.5	54.5	55.9	19.8	–	5.3	10.5	12.0	162	100.0
Chronic myeloid	0	0	0	0	0	–	–	–	–	–	–	–	–	–	–	–
Other and unspecified	0	1	1	0	2	3.2	3.9	18.2	–	6.6	5.1	–	3.5	3.7	52	100.0
II. LYMPHOMAS	0	4	1	3	8	12.9	12.3	100.0	–	26.4	5.1	16.0	14.0	14.5	211	100.0
Hodgkin's disease	0	1	0	1	2	3.2	2.8	25.0	–	6.6	–	5.3	3.5	3.6	53	100.0
Non-Hodgkin lymphoma	0	2	0	1	3	4.8	5.4	37.5	–	13.2	–	5.3	5.2	5.7	78	100.0
Burkitt's lymphoma	0	0	1	0	1	1.6	1.4	12.5	–	–	5.1	–	1.7	1.5	27	100.0
Unspecified lymphoma	0	1	0	0	1	1.6	1.4	12.5	–	6.6	–	–	1.7	2.0	26	100.0
Histiocytosis X	0	0	0	0	0	–	–	–	–	–	–	–	–	–	–	–
Other reticuloendothelial	0	0	0	1	1	1.6	1.4	12.5	–	–	–	5.3	1.7	1.5	27	100.0
III. BRAIN AND SPINAL	0	3	5	6	14	22.6	25.0	100.0	–	19.8	25.3	32.0	24.5	23.6	366	100.0
Ependymoma	0	1	1	1	3	4.8	5.3	21.4	–	6.6	5.1	5.3	5.2	5.2	78	100.0
Astrocytoma	0	0	1	0	1	1.6	1.4	7.1	–	–	5.1	–	1.7	1.5	27	100.0
Medulloblastoma	0	2	1	1	4	6.5	6.7	28.6	–	13.2	5.1	5.3	7.0	7.3	105	100.0
Other glioma	0	0	2	3	5	8.1	9.1	35.7	–	–	10.1	16.0	8.7	7.9	131	100.0
Other and unspecified *	0	0	0	1	1	1.6	2.5	7.1	–	–	–	5.3	1.7	1.6	25	100.0
IV. SYMPATHETIC N.S.	2	2	0	1	5	8.1	7.1	100.0	55.9	13.2	–	5.3	8.7	10.0	135	100.0
Neuroblastoma	2	2	0	1	5	8.1	7.1	100.0	55.9	13.2	–	5.3	8.7	10.0	135	100.0
Other	0	0	0	0	0	–	–	–	–	–	–	–	–	–	–	–
V. RETINOBLASTOMA	1	3	0	0	4	6.5	5.7	100.0	27.9	19.8	–	–	7.0	8.3	107	100.0
VI. KIDNEY	0	3	1	0	4	6.5	6.8	100.0	–	19.8	5.1	–	7.0	7.8	105	100.0
Wilms' tumour	0	3	1	0	4	6.5	6.8	100.0	–	19.8	5.1	–	7.0	7.8	105	100.0
Renal carcinoma	0	0	0	0	0	–	–	–	–	–	–	–	–	–	–	–
Other and unspecified	0	0	0	0	0	–	–	–	–	–	–	–	–	–	–	–
VII. LIVER	0	0	0	0	0	–	–	–	–	–	–	–	–	–	–	–
Hepatoblastoma	0	0	0	0	0	–	–	–	–	–	–	–	–	–	–	–
Hepatic carcinoma	0	0	0	0	0	–	–	–	–	–	–	–	–	–	–	–
Other and unspecified	0	0	0	0	0	–	–	–	–	–	–	–	–	–	–	–
VIII. BONE	0	0	0	3	3	4.8	4.1	100.0	–	–	–	16.0	5.2	4.6	80	100.0
Osteosarcoma	0	0	0	1	1	1.6	1.4	33.3	–	–	–	5.3	1.7	1.5	27	100.0
Chondrosarcoma	0	0	0	0	0	–	–	–	–	–	–	–	–	–	–	–
Ewing's sarcoma	0	0	0	1	1	1.6	1.4	33.3	–	–	–	5.3	1.7	1.5	27	100.0
Other and unspecified	0	0	0	1	1	1.6	1.4	33.3	–	–	–	5.3	1.7	1.5	27	100.0
IX. SOFT TISSUE SARCOMAS	0	0	0	2	2	3.2	2.7	100.0	–	–	–	10.7	3.5	3.1	53	100.0
Rhabdomyosarcoma	0	0	0	0	0	–	–	–	–	–	–	–	–	–	–	–
Fibrosarcoma	0	0	0	0	0	–	–	–	–	–	–	–	–	–	–	–
Other and unspecified	0	0	0	2	2	3.2	2.7	100.0	–	–	–	10.7	3.5	3.1	53	100.0
X. GONADAL & GERM CELL	0	0	2	3	5	8.1	9.1	100.0	–	–	10.1	16.0	8.7	7.9	131	100.0
Non-gonadal germ cell	0	0	1	0	1	1.6	2.5	20.0	–	–	5.1	–	1.7	1.6	25	100.0
Gonadal germ cell	0	0	1	3	4	6.5	6.6	80.0	–	–	5.1	16.0	7.0	6.3	105	100.0
Gonadal carcinoma	0	0	0	0	0	–	–	–	–	–	–	–	–	–	–	–
Other and unspecified	0	0	0	0	0	–	–	–	–	–	–	–	–	–	–	–
XI. EPITHELIAL NEOPLASMS	0	1	1	3	5	8.1	8.0	100.0	–	6.6	5.1	16.0	8.7	8.3	132	100.0
Adrenocortical carcinoma	0	0	0	0	0	–	–	–	–	–	–	–	–	–	–	–
Thyroid carcinoma	0	0	0	0	0	–	–	–	–	–	–	–	–	–	–	–
Nasopharyngeal carcinoma	0	0	0	0	0	–	–	–	–	–	–	–	–	–	–	–
Melanoma	0	0	0	0	0	–	–	–	–	–	–	–	–	–	–	–
Other carcinoma	0	1	1	3	5	8.1	8.0	100.0	–	6.6	5.1	16.0	8.7	8.3	132	100.0
XII. OTHER	0	1	0	0	1	1.6	1.4	100.0	–	6.6	–	–	1.7	2.0	26	100.0

* Specified as malignant | 0 | 0 | 1 | 0 | 1 | 1.6 | 2.5 | 100.0 | – | – | 5.1 | – | 1.7 | 1.6 | 25 | – |

New Zealand, non Maori   1970 - 1979   MALE

DIAGNOSTIC GROUP	NUMBER OF CASES					REL. FREQUENCY (%)			RATES PER MILLION						Cum	HV (%)
	0	1-4	5-9	10-14	All	Crude	Adj.	Group	0	1-4	5-9	10-14	Crude	Adj.		
TOTAL	31	194	168	161	554	100.0	100.0	100.0	125.8	187.1	122.0	116.1	136.9	140.7	2065	97.0
I. LEUKAEMIAS	8	82	63	48	201	36.3	36.2	100.0	32.5	79.1	45.7	34.6	49.7	51.8	751	100.0
Acute lymphocytic	2	65	49	27	143	25.8	25.7	71.1	8.1	62.7	35.6	19.5	35.3	37.2	534	100.0
Other lymphocytic	0	2	1	2	5	0.9	0.9	2.5	-	1.9	0.7	1.4	1.2	1.3	19	100.0
Acute non-lymphocytic	4	9	9	16	38	6.9	6.5	18.9	16.2	8.7	6.5	11.5	9.4	9.4	141	100.0
Chronic myeloid	0	2	1	0	3	0.5	0.5	1.5	-	1.9	0.7	-	0.7	0.8	11	100.0
Other and unspecified	2	4	3	3	12	2.2	2.2	6.0	8.1	3.9	2.2	2.2	3.0	3.2	45	100.0
II. LYMPHOMAS	2	19	24	27	72	13.0	13.1	100.0	8.1	18.3	17.4	19.5	17.8	17.6	266	98.0
Hodgkin's disease	0	3	6	14	23	4.2	4.2	31.9	-	2.9	4.4	10.1	5.7	5.2	84	100.0
Non-Hodgkin lymphoma	2	12	17	11	42	7.6	7.6	58.3	8.1	11.6	12.3	7.9	10.4	10.5	156	96.4
Burkitt's lymphoma	0	2	0	0	2	0.4	0.4	2.8	-	1.9	-	-	0.5	0.6	8	100.0
Unspecified lymphoma	0	0	0	0	0				-	-	-	-	-	-		
Histiocytosis X	0	0	0	0	0				-	-	-	-	-	-		
Other reticuloendothelial	0	2	1	2	5	0.9	0.9	6.9	-	1.9	0.7	1.4	1.2	1.3	19	100.0
III. BRAIN AND SPINAL	7	29	39	29	104	18.8	18.8	100.0	28.4	28.0	28.3	20.9	25.7	26.1	386	95.5
Ependymoma	1	2	0	1	4	0.7	0.7	3.8	4.1	1.9	-	0.7	1.0	1.1	15	100.0
Astrocytoma	3	10	15	8	36	6.5	6.5	34.6	12.2	9.6	10.9	5.8	8.9	9.1	134	100.0
Medulloblastoma	1	11	14	8	34	6.1	6.1	32.7	4.1	10.6	10.2	5.8	8.4	8.6	126	100.0
Other glioma	2	4	8	8	22	4.0	4.0	21.2	8.1	3.9	5.8	5.8	5.4	5.4	81	93.3
Other and unspecified *	0	2	2	4	8	1.4	1.5	7.7	-	1.9	1.5	2.9	2.0	1.9	29	50.0
IV. SYMPATHETIC N.S.	4	12	8	4	28	5.1	5.0	100.0	16.2	11.6	5.8	2.9	6.9	7.6	106	100.0
Neuroblastoma	4	12	7	4	27	4.9	4.8	96.4	16.2	11.6	5.1	2.9	6.7	7.3	102	100.0
Other	0	0	1	0	1	0.2	0.2	3.6	-	-	0.7	-	0.2	0.2	4	100.0
V. RETINOBLASTOMA	2	13	0	0	15	2.7	2.7	100.0	8.1	12.5	-	-	3.7	4.5	58	100.0
VI. KIDNEY	2	19	4	2	27	4.9	4.8	100.0	8.1	18.3	2.9	1.4	6.7	7.7	103	100.0
Wilms' tumour	2	17	4	1	24	4.3	4.3	88.9	8.1	16.4	2.9	0.7	5.9	6.9	92	100.0
Renal carcinoma	0	0	0	0	0				-	-	-	-	-	-		
Other and unspecified	0	2	0	1	3	0.5	0.5	11.1	-	1.9	-	0.7	0.7	0.8	11	100.0
VII. LIVER	1	1	2	1	5	0.9	0.9	100.0	4.1	1.0	1.5	0.7	1.2	1.3	19	100.0
Hepatoblastoma	1	1	0	0	2	0.4	0.4	40.0	4.1	1.0	-	-	0.5	0.6	8	100.0
Hepatic carcinoma	0	0	2	1	3	0.5	0.5	60.0	-	-	1.5	0.7	0.7	0.7	11	100.0
Other and unspecified	0	0	0	0	0				-	-	-	-	-	-		
VIII. BONE	0	2	5	12	19	3.4	3.5	100.0	-	1.9	3.6	8.7	4.7	4.3	69	94.1
Osteosarcoma	0	0	2	8	10	1.8	1.8	52.6	-	-	1.5	5.8	2.5	2.1	36	100.0
Chondrosarcoma	0	0	0	1	1	0.2	0.2	5.3	-	-	-	0.7	0.2	0.2	4	100.0
Ewing's sarcoma	0	1	3	2	6	1.1	1.1	31.6	-	1.0	2.2	1.4	1.5	1.4	22	100.0
Other and unspecified	0	1	0	1	2	0.4	0.4	10.5	-	1.0	-	0.7	0.5	0.5	7	50.0
IX. SOFT TISSUE SARCOMAS	0	5	10	11	26	4.7	4.7	100.0	-	4.8	7.3	7.9	6.4	6.1	95	94.4
Rhabdomyosarcoma	0	3	8	6	17	3.1	3.1	65.4	-	2.9	5.8	4.3	4.2	4.0	62	100.0
Fibrosarcoma	0	1	0	0	1	0.2	0.2	3.8	-	1.0	-	-	0.2	0.3	4	100.0
Other and unspecified	0	1	2	5	8	1.4	1.5	30.8	-	1.0	1.5	3.6	1.4	1.8	29	
X. GONADAL & GERM CELL	4	5	1	3	13	2.3	2.3	100.0	16.2	4.8	0.7	2.2	3.2	3.6	50	100.0
Non-gonadal germ cell	2	2	1	3	8	1.4	1.4	61.5	8.1	1.9	0.7	2.2	2.0	2.1	30	100.0
Gonadal germ cell	2	3	0	0	5	0.9	0.9	38.5	8.1	2.9	-	-	1.2	1.5	20	100.0
Gonadal carcinoma	0	0	0	0	0				-	-	-	-	-	-		
Other and unspecified	0	0	0	0	0				-	-	-	-	-	-		
XI. EPITHELIAL NEOPLASMS	0	2	11	22	35	6.3	6.4	100.0	-	1.9	8.0	15.9	8.6	7.8	127	100.0
Adrenocortical carcinoma	0	0	1	0	1	0.2	0.2	2.9	-	-	0.7	-	0.2	0.2	4	100.0
Thyroid carcinoma	0	0	1	3	4	0.7	0.7	11.4	-	-	0.7	2.2	1.0	0.9	14	100.0
Nasopharyngeal carcinoma	0	0	0	0	0				-	-	-	-	-	-		
Melanoma	0	1	2	14	17	3.1	3.1	48.6	-	1.0	1.5	10.1	4.2	3.7	62	100.0
Other carcinoma	0	1	7	5	13	2.3	2.4	37.1	-	1.0	5.1	3.6	3.2	3.0	47	100.0
XII. OTHER	1	5	1	2	9	1.6	1.6	100.0	4.1	4.8	0.7	1.4	2.2	2.5	34	16.7
* Specified as malignant	0	2	2	4	8	1.4	1.5	100.0	-	1.9	1.5	2.9	2.0	1.9	29	50.0

New Zealand, non Maori

1970 – 1979

FEMALE

DIAGNOSTIC GROUP	NUMBER OF CASES 0	1-4	5-9	10-14	All	REL. FREQUENCY(%) Crude	Adj.	Group	RATES PER MILLION 0	1-4	5-9	10-14	Crude	Adj.	Cum	HV(%)
TOTAL	32	166	118	139	455	100.0	100.0	100.0	135.2	166.8	89.6	105.2	117.6	121.6	1776	97.3
I. LEUKAEMIAS	8	65	33	35	141	31.0	30.7	100.0	33.8	65.3	25.1	26.5	36.4	38.6	553	100.0
Acute lymphocytic	1	48	24	23	96	21.1	21.0	68.1	4.2	48.2	18.2	17.4	24.8	26.2	375	100.0
Other lymphocytic	0	2	0	0	2	0.4	0.4	1.4	-	2.0	-	-	0.5	0.6	8	100.0
Acute non-lymphocytic	5	12	8	9	34	7.5	7.4	24.1	21.1	12.1	6.1	6.8	8.8	9.3	134	100.0
Chronic myeloid	0	2	1	3	6	1.3	1.3	4.3	-	2.0	0.8	2.3	1.6	1.5	23	100.0
Other and unspecified	2	1	0	0	3	0.7	0.6	2.1	8.4	1.0	-	-	0.8	1.0	12	-
II. LYMPHOMAS	0	5	8	13	26	5.7	5.8	100.0	-	5.0	6.1	9.8	6.7	6.4	100	100.0
Hodgkin's disease	0	1	2	7	10	2.2	2.2	38.5	-	1.0	1.5	5.3	2.6	2.3	38	100.0
Non-Hodgkin lymphoma	0	3	2	5	10	2.2	2.2	38.5	-	3.0	1.5	3.8	2.6	2.5	39	100.0
Burkitt's lymphoma	0	0	1	1	2	0.4	0.5	7.7	-	-	0.8	0.8	0.5	0.5	8	100.0
Unspecified lymphoma	0	1	2	0	3	0.7	0.7	11.5	-	1.0	1.5	-	0.8	0.8	12	100.0
Histiocytosis X	0	0	0	0	0	-	-	-	-	-	-	-	-	-	-	-
Other reticuloendothelial	0	0	1	0	1	0.2	0.3	3.8	-	-	0.8	-	0.3	0.2	4	100.0
III. BRAIN AND SPINAL	4	29	29	27	89	19.6	19.9	100.0	16.9	29.1	22.0	20.4	23.0	23.4	346	96.7
Ependymoma	1	1	1	2	5	1.1	1.1	5.6	4.2	1.0	0.8	1.5	1.3	1.3	20	100.0
Astrocytoma	1	12	13	13	39	8.6	8.7	43.8	4.2	12.1	9.9	9.8	10.1	10.1	151	100.0
Medulloblastoma	1	5	8	2	16	3.5	3.7	18.0	4.2	5.0	6.1	1.5	4.1	4.3	62	90.0
Other glioma	0	8	6	4	18	4.0	4.0	20.2	-	8.0	4.6	3.0	4.7	4.9	71	90.0
Other and unspecified *	1	3	1	6	11	2.4	2.4	12.4	4.2	3.0	0.8	4.5	2.8	2.7	42	83.3
IV. SYMPATHETIC N.S.	6	17	3	2	28	6.2	5.8	100.0	25.3	17.1	2.3	1.5	7.2	8.4	113	94.4
Neuroblastoma	6	17	3	1	27	5.9	5.6	96.4	25.3	17.1	2.3	0.8	7.0	8.2	109	94.1
Other	0	0	0	1	1	0.2	0.2	3.6	-	-	-	0.8	0.3	0.2	4	100.0
V. RETINOBLASTOMA	5	13	4	0	22	4.8	4.7	100.0	21.1	13.1	3.0	-	5.7	6.7	89	100.0
VI. KIDNEY	3	10	11	3	27	5.9	6.1	100.0	12.7	10.0	8.4	2.3	7.0	7.4	106	92.6
Wilms' tumour	2	10	11	2	25	5.5	5.7	92.6	8.4	10.0	8.4	1.5	6.5	6.9	98	92.0
Renal carcinoma	1	0	0	1	2	0.4	0.4	7.4	4.2	-	-	0.8	0.5	0.5	8	100.0
Other and unspecified	0	0	0	0	0	-	-	-	-	-	-	-	-	-	-	-
VII. LIVER	1	3	0	1	5	1.1	1.0	100.0	4.2	3.0	-	0.8	1.3	1.5	20	100.0
Hepatoblastoma	0	1	0	1	2	0.4	0.4	40.0	-	1.0	-	0.8	0.5	0.6	8	100.0
Hepatic carcinoma	1	2	0	0	3	0.7	0.6	60.0	4.2	2.0	-	-	0.8	0.8	12	100.0
Other and unspecified	0	0	0	0	0	-	-	-	-	-	-	-	-	-	-	-
VIII. BONE	0	3	12	19	34	7.5	7.8	100.0	-	3.0	9.1	14.4	8.8	8.0	130	100.0
Osteosarcoma	0	1	5	11	17	3.7	3.8	50.0	-	1.0	3.8	8.3	4.4	4.0	65	100.0
Chondrosarcoma	0	0	0	0	0	-	-	-	-	-	-	-	-	-	-	-
Ewing's sarcoma	0	1	5	6	12	2.6	2.8	35.3	-	1.0	3.8	4.5	3.1	2.9	46	100.0
Other and unspecified	0	1	2	2	5	1.1	1.1	14.7	-	1.0	1.5	1.5	1.3	1.2	19	100.0
IX. SOFT TISSUE SARCOMAS	2	10	7	3	22	4.8	4.9	100.0	8.4	10.0	5.3	2.3	5.7	6.1	87	100.0
Rhabdomyosarcoma	1	10	3	2	16	3.5	3.4	72.7	4.2	10.0	2.3	1.5	4.1	4.6	63	100.0
Fibrosarcoma	0	0	1	0	1	0.2	0.3	4.5	-	-	0.8	-	0.3	0.2	4	100.0
Other and unspecified	1	0	3	1	5	1.1	1.2	22.7	4.2	-	2.3	0.8	1.3	1.3	19	100.0
X. GONADAL & GERM CELL	2	3	6	10	21	4.6	4.7	100.0	8.4	3.0	4.6	7.6	5.4	5.3	81	100.0
Non-gonadal germ cell	2	3	1	0	6	1.3	1.3	28.6	8.4	3.0	0.8	-	1.6	1.8	24	100.0
Gonadal germ cell	0	0	4	7	11	2.4	2.5	52.4	-	-	3.0	5.3	2.8	2.5	42	100.0
Gonadal carcinoma	0	0	1	2	3	0.7	0.7	14.3	-	-	0.8	1.5	0.8	0.7	11	100.0
Other and unspecified	0	0	0	1	1	0.2	0.2	4.8	-	-	-	0.8	0.3	0.2	4	100.0
XI. EPITHELIAL NEOPLASMS	0	6	4	25	35	7.7	7.6	100.0	-	6.0	3.0	18.9	9.0	8.3	134	100.0
Adrenocortical carcinoma	0	0	0	0	0	-	-	-	-	-	-	-	-	-	-	-
Thyroid carcinoma	0	0	0	4	4	0.9	0.9	11.4	-	-	-	3.0	1.0	0.9	15	100.0
Nasopharyngeal carcinoma	0	0	0	0	0	-	-	-	-	-	-	-	-	-	-	-
Melanoma	0	3	3	9	15	3.3	3.3	42.9	-	3.0	2.3	6.8	3.9	3.6	57	100.0
Other carcinoma	0	3	1	12	16	3.5	3.5	45.7	-	3.0	0.8	9.1	4.1	3.8	61	100.0
XII. OTHER	1	2	1	1	5	1.1	1.1	100.0	4.2	2.0	0.8	0.8	1.3	1.4	20	-
* Specified as malignant	0	3	1	7	11	2.4	2.4	100.0	-	3.0	0.8	5.3	2.8	2.7	42	83.3

Population

The population at risk was calculated from data from the censuses of 1971, 1976 and 1981, giving the total and Maori population by sex and single year of age.

Commentary

A total of 1171 cases are included in the tables presented here, 162 occurring in the Maori population and the remaining 1009 in the non-Maoris (mainly European). The rates for both groups are among the highest recorded in this volume, though the distribution of tumour types is different. There were 16 colorectal carcinomas, four of which were in the Maori population.

Maoris. The rates for Maoris are based on very small numbers but show a relatively low rate of acute lymphocytic leukaemia and a relatively high rate of the acute non-lymphocytic form. High rates were also recorded for lymphomas and neuroblastoma.

Non-Maoris. Most of the rates are similar to those for European and North American populations, with a slight suggestion that the rate for acute non-lymphocytic leukaemia is higher. The rate for brain and spinal tumours is similar to the European and North American figures even though benign and unspecified tumours are not registered. The rates for melanoma are the second highest recorded here (New South Wales being the highest).

Reference

West, R.C., Skegg, D.C.G. & Fraser, J. (1983) Childhood cancer in New Zealand: incidence and survival, 1961-1976. *N.Z. med. J.*, *96*, 923-927

PAPUA NEW GUINEA

Cancer Registry of Papua New Guinea, 1979-1983

K. Jamrozik, R. White & K. Misch

A cancer registry was first established for the whole of Papua New Guinea in 1958. The method of registration relies on medical personnel in any clinic or hospital completing a cancer notification form, which also serves as a request for a histopathology (or haematology) examination. Since there is only one histopathology department in the country, in the Port Moresby General Hospital, all requests are sent there, and the registry is located in the department. Details of the patient (name, sex, age, province of origin) are copied on to registry cards, and the request form and pathology report retained for future reference. Virtually all pathology requests are made by medical and dental practitioners rather than by other health workers, and only 0.7% of the total registrations in the period 1979-1983 were made on the basis of clinical investigation (other than serum alpha-foetoprotein assay) or clinical findings alone.

For the five-year period reported here, a special *ad hoc* study was undertaken. Care was taken to eliminate multiple registration of individual patients for whom several specimens were submitted, and site and morphology were coded according to the *International Classification of Diseases for Oncology* (ICD-O). Cases in residents not of Melanesian origin have been omitted.

The results for earlier periods show that there has been an increase in the rate of registration since the early years of the Registry, and that there is considerable variation in the level of reporting from different provinces (Jamrozik & Parkin, unpublished). It is clear that the level of registration depends on the ease of communication and on access to medical facilities, as well as biopsy or operation rates for different cancers.

Papua New Guinea comprises the eastern half of the island of New Guinea together with several island groups, including the large islands of New Britain, New Ireland and Bougainville. It became independent in 1975, having formerly been administered by Australia. The mainland and many of the islands are mountainous, rising to an altitude of 4600 m, with extensive fertile and populated valleys 1500 m above sea level, whilst the Papuan gulf to the south is a more lowland area. The coast has a tropical climate with a mean temperature of 26° C; temperatures are lower on the islands. The climate is monsoonal, with annual rainfall varying from 200 to 1000 cm, but with a dryer zone in the lowlands (100-150 cm per year). Large areas are still covered with forest or swamp, with smaller areas of grassland or under cultivation. Agriculture is mainly subsistence, but various cash crops are grown (coconuts, coffee, tea, rubber) and mining (gold, copper), forestry and fishing are carried on.

The indigenous people are Melanesians, comprising some 700 separate language groups. The population at the 1980 census was 2.98 million (a density of about 6 per square kilometre); 43% of this total were aged 0-14 years.

Commentary

The tables show numbers and percentages of cases only; incidence rates are not shown since calculation of rates based on these numbers gives marked under-estimation of the true rates (age-standardized rates, per million, for all sites are 47.8 for boys and 23.3 for girls).

The lymphoma/leukaemia ratio was one of the highest seen outside Africa, over 50% of the lymphomas being of Burkitt's type. In the total of 234 tumours there were six cases of Kaposi's sarcoma, all in boys, and 20 cases of hepatic carcinoma. Retinoblastoma accounted for over 8% of the cases. Leukaemia was rare and, though the numbers were small, there was a relatively high proportion of acute non-lymphocytic cases. Only two brain and spinal tumours were recorded, but this is presumably mainly because registration depends on a request for histopathological examination.

References

Campbell, P.E. & Reid, I.S. (1974) Cancer in children in Papua New Guinea. In: Atkinson, L., Clezy, J.K., Reay-Young, P.S., Scott, G.C. & Wigley, S.G., eds, *The Epidemiology of Cancer in Papua New Guinea*, Erskineville, New South Wales, Star Printery Ltd, pp. 139-148

Papua New Guinea, Histopath. Registry   1979 - 1983   MALE

DIAGNOSTIC GROUP	NUMBER OF CASES					REL. FREQUENCY(%)			HV(%)
	0	1-4	5-9	10-14	All	Crude	Adj.	Group	
TOTAL	2	60	46	52	162¤	100.0	100.0	100.0	91.4
I. LEUKAEMIAS	0	8	12	9	29	17.9	18.2	100.0	100.0
Acute lymphocytic	0	5	6	2	13	8.0	8.3	44.8	100.0
Other lymphocytic	0	0	0	0	0	-	-	-	-
Acute non-lymphocytic	0	3	2	2	7	4.3	4.4	24.1	100.0
Chronic myeloid	0	0	1	1	2	1.2	1.2	6.9	100.0
Other and unspecified	0	0	3	4	7	4.3	4.3	24.1	100.0
II. LYMPHOMAS	0	21	18	16	56¤	34.6	34.5	100.0	100.0
Hodgkin's disease	0	0	2	0	2	1.2	1.2	3.6	100.0
Non-Hodgkin lymphoma	0	6	6	6	18	11.1	11.2	32.1	100.0
Burkitt's lymphoma	0	14	11	6	31¤	19.1	19.1	55.4	100.0
Unspecified lymphoma	0	1	1	2	4	2.5	2.5	7.1	100.0
Histiocytosis X	0	0	0	0	0	-	-	-	-
Other reticuloendothelial	0	0	0	1	1	0.6	0.6	1.8	100.0
III. BRAIN AND SPINAL	0	0	0	0	0	-	-	-	-
Ependymoma	0	0	0	0	0	-	-	-	-
Astrocytoma	0	0	0	0	0	-	-	-	-
Medulloblastoma	0	0	0	0	0	-	-	-	-
Other glioma	0	0	0	0	0	-	-	-	-
Other and unspecified *	0	0	0	0	0	-	-	-	-
IV. SYMPATHETIC N.S.	0	1	2	2	5	3.1	3.1	100.0	100.0
Neuroblastoma	0	1	2	2	5	3.1	3.1	100.0	100.0
Other	0	0	0	0	0	-	-	-	-
V. RETINOBLASTOMA	1	10	2	0	13	8.0	8.4	100.0	100.0
VI. KIDNEY	0	5	2	0	7	4.3	4.5	100.0	100.0
Wilms' tumour	0	5	2	0	7	4.3	4.5	100.0	100.0
Renal carcinoma	0	0	0	0	0	-	-	-	-
Other and unspecified	0	0	0	0	0	-	-	-	-
VII. LIVER	0	1	4	10	16¤	9.9	9.0	100.0	18.8
Hepatoblastoma	0	0	0	0	0	-	-	-	-
Hepatic carcinoma	0	1	4	10	16¤	9.9	9.0	100.0	18.8
Other and unspecified	0	0	0	0	0	-	-	-	-
VIII. BONE	0	0	2	9	11	6.8	6.5	100.0	90.9
Osteosarcoma	0	0	0	5	5	3.1	2.9	45.5	100.0
Chondrosarcoma	0	0	0	1	1	0.6	0.6	9.1	100.0
Ewing's sarcoma	0	0	2	3	5	3.1	3.0	45.5	100.0
Other and unspecified	0	0	0	0	0	-	-	-	-
IX. SOFT TISSUE SARCOMAS	1	10	3	3	17	10.5	10.8	100.0	100.0
Rhabdomyosarcoma	1	4	2	2	9	5.6	5.7	52.9	100.0
Fibrosarcoma	0	0	0	0	0	-	-	-	-
Other and unspecified	0	6	1	1	8	4.9	5.1	47.1	100.0
X. GONADAL & GERM CELL	0	1	0	0	1	0.6	0.6	100.0	100.0
Non-gonadal germ cell	0	0	0	0	0	-	-	-	-
Gonadal germ cell	0	1	0	0	1	0.6	0.6	100.0	100.0
Gonadal carcinoma	0	0	0	0	0	-	-	-	-
Other and unspecified	0	0	0	0	0	-	-	-	-
XI. EPITHELIAL NEOPLASMS	0	2	1	3	6	3.7	3.7	100.0	100.0
Adrenocortical carcinoma	0	0	0	0	0	-	-	-	-
Thyroid carcinoma	0	0	0	0	0	-	-	-	-
Nasopharyngeal carcinoma	0	0	0	0	0	-	-	-	-
Melanoma	0	1	0	0	1	0.6	0.6	16.7	100.0
Other carcinoma	0	1	1	3	5	3.1	3.0	83.3	100.0
XII. OTHER	0	1	0	0	1	0.6	0.6	100.0	100.0

* Specified as malignant
¤ Includes age unknown

Papua New Guinea, Histopath. Registry   1979 - 1983   FEMALE

DIAGNOSTIC GROUP	NUMBER OF CASES					REL. FREQUENCY(%)			HV(%)
	0	1-4	5-9	10-14	All	Crude	Adj.	Group	
TOTAL	1	29	23	18	72¤	100.0	100.0	100.0	95.7
I. LEUKAEMIAS	0	3	6	2	11	15.3	15.2	100.0	100.0
Acute lymphocytic	0	1	3	1	5	6.9	6.9	45.5	100.0
Other lymphocytic	0	0	0	1	1	1.4	1.7	9.1	100.0
Acute non-lymphocytic	0	1	2	0	3	4.2	3.9	27.3	100.0
Chronic myeloid	0	0	0	0	0	-	-	-	-
Other and unspecified	0	1	1	0	2	2.8	2.6	18.2	100.0
II. LYMPHOMAS	0	6	9	6	21	29.2	29.7	100.0	100.0
Hodgkin's disease	0	1	0	0	1	1.4	1.3	4.8	100.0
Non-Hodgkin lymphoma	0	1	1	4	6	8.3	9.3	28.6	100.0
Burkitt's lymphoma	0	3	6	2	11	15.3	15.2	52.4	100.0
Unspecified lymphoma	0	1	2	0	3	4.2	3.9	14.3	-
Histiocytosis X	0	0	0	0	0	-	-	-	-
Other reticuloendothelial	0	0	0	0	0	-	-	-	-
III. BRAIN AND SPINAL	0	2	0	0	2	2.8	2.7	100.0	100.0
Ependymoma	0	2	0	0	2	2.8	2.7	100.0	100.0
Astrocytoma	0	0	0	0	0	-	-	-	-
Medulloblastoma	0	0	0	0	0	-	-	-	-
Other glioma	0	0	0	0	0	-	-	-	-
Other and unspecified *	0	0	0	0	0	-	-	-	-
IV. SYMPATHETIC N.S.	1	2	0	0	3	4.2	4.0	100.0	100.0
Neuroblastoma	1	2	0	0	3	4.2	4.0	100.0	100.0
Other	0	0	0	0	0	-	-	-	-
V. RETINOBLASTOMA	0	6	0	0	6	8.3	8.0	100.0	100.0
VI. KIDNEY	0	2	1	0	3	4.2	4.0	100.0	100.0
Wilms' tumour	0	2	1	0	3	4.2	4.0	100.0	100.0
Renal carcinoma	0	0	0	0	0	-	-	-	-
Other and unspecified	0	0	0	0	0	-	-	-	-
VII. LIVER	0	1	2	1	4	5.6	5.6	100.0	25.0
Hepatoblastoma	0	1	2	1	4	5.6	5.6	100.0	25.0
Hepatic carcinoma	0	0	0	0	0	-	-	-	-
Other and unspecified	0	0	0	0	0	-	-	-	-
VIII. BONE	0	2	1	1	4	5.6	5.6	100.0	100.0
Osteosarcoma	0	0	1	1	2	2.8	3.0	50.0	100.0
Chondrosarcoma	0	1	0	0	1	1.4	1.3	25.0	100.0
Ewing's sarcoma	0	1	0	0	1	1.4	1.3	25.0	100.0
Other and unspecified	0	0	0	0	0	-	-	-	-
IX. SOFT TISSUE SARCOMAS	0	4	2	3	10¤	13.9	12.9	100.0	100.0
Rhabdomyosarcoma	0	3	0	0	3	4.2	4.0	30.0	100.0
Fibrosarcoma	0	0	0	1	1	1.4	1.7	10.0	100.0
Other and unspecified	0	1	2	2	6¤	8.3	7.3	60.0	100.0
X. GONADAL & GERM CELL	0	0	1	4	5	6.9	8.0	100.0	100.0
Non-gonadal germ cell	0	0	1	4	5	6.9	8.0	100.0	100.0
Gonadal germ cell	0	0	0	0	0	-	-	-	-
Gonadal carcinoma	0	0	0	0	0	-	-	-	-
Other and unspecified	0	0	0	0	0	-	-	-	-
XI. EPITHELIAL NEOPLASMS	0	1	1	1	3	4.2	4.3	100.0	100.0
Adrenocortical carcinoma	0	0	0	0	0	-	-	-	-
Thyroid carcinoma	0	0	0	0	0	-	-	-	-
Nasopharyngeal carcinoma	0	0	0	0	0	-	-	-	-
Melanoma	0	0	0	0	0	-	-	-	-
Other carcinoma	0	1	1	1	3	4.2	4.3	100.0	100.0
XII. OTHER	0	0	0	0	0	-	-	-	-

* Specified as malignant
¤ Includes age unknown

6. SUMMARY TABLES

6.1

Age-standardized and cumulative rates

AGE STANDARDIZED AND CUMULATIVE (0-14) INCIDENCE RATES PER MILLION

Acute lymphocytic

	Male ASR	Male CUM	Female ASR	Female CUM	Both ASR	Both CUM
AFRICA						
Nigeria, Ibadan						
Uganda, Kampala						
Zimbabwe, Bulawayo, Residents only						
AMERICA : NORTH						
Canada, Atlantic Provinces	20.5	288	17.2	240	18.8	265
Canada, Western Provinces	33.2	466	26.7	374	30.1	421
USA, Greater Delaware Valley, White	38.3	545	28.8	408	33.7	478
USA, Greater Delaware Valley, non White	23.6	344	8.4	123	16.0	234
USA, Los Angeles, Black	23.0	336	15.2	213	19.2	275
USA, Los Angeles, Hispanic	45.6	647	30.4	433	38.2	542
USA, Los Angeles, Other White	43.2	608	35.5	504	39.4	557
USA, New York (City and State), White	35.5	509	30.8	435	33.2	473
USA, New York (City and State), Black	21.2	305	14.0	196	17.6	251
USA, SEER, White	35.9	510	29.7	417	32.9	464
USA, SEER, Black	14.4	207	15.3	220	14.8	214
AMERICA : OTHER						
Brazil, Fortaleza	28.2	443	28.4	431	28.1	434
Brazil, Recife	9.2	134	7.4	110	8.3	122
Brazil, Sao Paulo	15.9	232	12.4	183	14.2	208
Colombia, Cali	40.0	576	23.2	346	31.6	461
Costa Rica	47.5	698	41.9	619	44.7	659
Cuba	15.0	219	12.1	178	13.6	199
Jamaica	13.2	189	16.4	234	14.8	212
Puerto Rico	27.8	398	29.5	418	28.6	408
ASIA						
China, Shanghai	20.4	307	16.2	242	18.4	276
China, Taipei	21.2	304	16.3	231	18.8	268
Hong Kong	21.1	308	18.0	263	19.6	286
India, Bangalore	10.3	149	3.9	58	7.1	103
India, Bombay Cancer Registry	13.2	195	8.6	128	11.0	163
Israel, Jews	21.2	307	20.0	284	20.6	296
Israel, non Jews	17.2	247	11.2	158	14.3	204
Japan, Kanagawa	17.6	252	16.6	232	17.1	243
Japan, Miyagi	17.3	243	15.5	228	16.4	236
Japan, Osaka	22.6	321	19.3	276	21.0	299
Kuwait, Kuwaiti	10.9	163	12.9	190	11.9	176
Kuwait, non Kuwaiti	35.9	514	29.3	421	32.7	468
Philippines, Metro Manila & Rizal	24.7	365	16.1	238	20.5	302
Singapore, Chinese	25.5	365	20.5	291	23.1	329
Singapore, Malay	29.1	425	11.1	178	20.3	304
EUROPE						
Czechoslovakia, Slovakia	24.2	346	22.3	316	23.2	332
Denmark	33.9	489	26.0	368	30.1	430
FRG, Children's Tumour Registry	39.1	554	33.5	471	36.4	514
FRG, Saarland	22.8	325	18.2	253	20.6	290
Finland	30.2	429	22.4	320	26.4	376
France, Bas Rhin	24.7	341	27.5	394	26.1	367
France, Paediatric Registries	32.2	458	35.3	500	33.7	479
German Democratic Republic	25.3	359	22.7	319	24.0	340
Great Britain, England and Wales	33.7	477	25.5	361	29.7	420
Great Britain, Manchester (period 1)	28.3	405	21.0	299	24.7	354
Great Britain, Manchester (period 2)	35.8	507	26.9	379	31.4	445
Great Britain, Scotland	33.0	459	25.8	370	29.5	416
Hungary	30.9	439	24.4	342	27.7	392
Italy, Torino	33.9	480	25.2	353	29.6	418
Netherlands, DCLSG	33.6	473	28.6	402	31.2	438
Netherlands, SOOZ, Eindhoven	34.1	479	28.0	393	31.1	437
Norway	24.4	343	20.3	280	22.4	312
Poland, Warsaw City	–	–	0.7	10	0.4	5
Spain, Zaragoza	24.2	356	30.4	433	27.2	393
Sweden	28.2	398	25.7	364	27.0	381
Switzerland, Three Western Cantons	42.3	608	32.4	456	37.5	534
Yugoslavia, Slovenia	17.4	244	18.1	260	17.8	252
OCEANIA						
Australia, New South Wales	41.9	588	33.8	475	37.9	533
Australia, Queensland	34.9	492	31.2	443	33.1	468
Fiji, Fijian						
Fiji, Indian						
New Zealand, Maori	19.2	279	5.7	78	12.5	180
New Zealand, non Maori	37.2	534	26.2	375	31.8	456

* Light when fewer than 10 cases

AGE STANDARDIZED AND CUMULATIVE (0-14) INCIDENCE RATES PER MILLION

Acute non-lymphocytic

	Male ASR	Male CUM	Female ASR	Female CUM	Both ASR	Both CUM
AFRICA						
Nigeria, Ibadan						
Uganda, Kampala						
Zimbabwe, Bulawayo, Residents only						
AMERICA : NORTH						
Canada, Atlantic Provinces	3.5	56	2.9	40	3.2	49
Canada, Western Provinces	5.0	73	4.1	61	4.6	67
USA, Greater Delaware Valley, White	6.3	95	6.2	91	6.2	93
USA, Greater Delaware Valley, non White	5.1	79	3.9	58	4.5	69
USA, Los Angeles, Black	5.6	84	5.4	81	5.5	82
USA, Los Angeles, Hispanic	8.4	127	9.6	140	9.0	133
USA, Los Angeles, Other White	7.5	112	5.3	80	6.4	96
USA, New York (City and State), White	6.3	92	5.6	84	6.0	88
USA, New York (City and State), Black	6.5	98	4.3	61	5.4	80
USA, SEER, White	5.6	85	6.5	95	6.1	90
USA, SEER, Black	4.3	66	6.2	93	5.2	80
AMERICA : OTHER						
Brazil, Fortaleza	9.4	151	2.7	38	5.9	92
Brazil, Recife	2.8	45	1.8	27	2.2	35
Brazil, Sao Paulo	6.8	103	4.9	73	5.9	88
Colombia, Cali	2.5	41	7.2	110	4.9	75
Costa Rica	8.7	133	8.9	137	8.8	135
Cuba	3.2	49	3.5	53	3.3	51
Jamaica	6.7	105	1.3	21	3.9	62
Puerto Rico	6.9	99	6.2	97	6.6	98
ASIA						
China, Shanghai	13.5	205	10.5	157	12.1	182
China, Taipei	7.1	107	7.4	109	7.2	108
Hong Kong	2.1	31	4.7	68	3.4	49
India, Bangalore	3.8	61	−	−	1.9	31
India, Bombay Cancer Registry	3.6	53	3.1	46	3.3	50
Israel, Jews	9.8	144	3.3	50	6.6	98
Israel, non Jews	8.3	119	1.5	21	5.0	72
Japan, Kanagawa	11.8	172	10.1	150	11.0	162
Japan, Miyagi	11.7	176	10.1	147	10.9	162
Japan, Osaka	10.8	158	8.6	127	9.7	143
Kuwait, Kuwaiti	1.0	18	1.1	18	1.0	18
Kuwait, non Kuwaiti	1.0	15	2.3	37	1.6	26
Philippines, Metro Manila & Rizal	4.8	75	4.1	60	4.5	67
Singapore, Chinese	6.7	98	6.5	94	6.6	97
Singapore, Malay	10.1	147	7.6	117	8.9	133
EUROPE						
Czechoslovakia, Slovakia	5.6	79	7.4	108	6.5	93
Denmark	7.1	102	4.1	59	5.7	81
FRG, Children's Tumour Registry	5.9	86	5.1	75	5.5	81
FRG, Saarland	4.3	59	3.9	53	4.1	56
Finland	5.8	85	4.8	73	5.3	79
France, Bas Rhin	4.6	73	3.9	51	4.3	62
France, Paediatric Registries	5.5	75	6.4	93	5.9	84
German Democratic Republic	7.1	104	7.0	103	7.1	103
Great Britain, England and Wales	6.1	91	5.7	84	5.9	88
Great Britain, Manchester (period 1)	5.0	75	7.1	107	6.0	90
Great Britain, Manchester (period 2)	5.1	78	5.9	88	5.5	83
Great Britain, Scotland	7.3	109	5.4	79	6.4	95
Hungary	6.9	100	4.1	60	5.5	81
Italy, Torino	6.0	90	3.9	61	5.0	76
Netherlands, DCLSG	4.8	71	4.1	60	4.5	65
Netherlands, SOOZ, Eindhoven	9.4	127	4.9	73	7.2	101
Norway	7.7	118	8.4	124	8.0	121
Poland, Warsaw City	2.8	44	2.4	37	2.6	41
Spain, Zaragoza	2.2	31	7.8	118	4.9	73
Sweden	5.0	73	5.3	76	5.1	75
Switzerland, Three Western Cantons	1.8	30	7.2	102	4.4	65
Yugoslavia, Slovenia	10.1	151	4.3	58	7.3	106
OCEANIA						
Australia, New South Wales	7.8	111	7.7	115	7.7	113
Australia, Queensland	4.3	62	4.4	69	4.4	65
Fiji, Fijian						
Fiji, Indian						
New Zealand, Maori	13.4	202	12.0	162	12.7	182
New Zealand, non Maori	9.4	141	9.3	134	9.4	138

* Light when fewer than 10 cases

AGE STANDARDIZED AND CUMULATIVE (0-14) INCIDENCE RATES PER MILLION

All cancer

	Male ASR	CUM	Female ASR	CUM	Both ASR	CUM
AFRICA						
Nigeria, Ibadan	198.5	3055	111.7	1738	155.6	2406
Uganda, Kampala	101.3	1568	79.9	1242	90.3	1401
Zimbabwe, Bulawayo, Residents only	87.2	1207	82.1	1202	85.1	1212
AMERICA : NORTH						
Canada, Atlantic Provinces	102.6	1497	90.4	1305	96.6	1403
Canada, Western Provinces	148.7	2142	119.4	1725	134.4	1938
USA, Greater Delaware Valley, White	139.2	2024	113.7	1656	126.7	1844
USA, Greater Delaware Valley, non White	114.2	1693	96.5	1411	105.4	1552
USA, Los Angeles, Black	118.4	1732	100.5	1488	109.6	1612
USA, Los Angeles, Hispanic	150.4	2174	130.4	1915	140.6	2048
USA, Los Angeles, Other White	156.8	2286	136.2	1992	146.7	2142
USA, New York (City and State), White	145.5	2136	127.4	1855	136.7	1999
USA, New York (City and State), Black	121.0	1794	82.4	1205	101.8	1500
USA, SEER, White	143.9	2096	126.9	1848	135.6	1975
USA, SEER, Black	107.2	1573	107.9	1587	107.6	1580
AMERICA : OTHER						
Brazil, Fortaleza	138.1	2098	136.3	2035	137.0	2063
Brazil, Recife	106.9	1593	105.2	1581	106.2	1589
Brazil, Sao Paulo	164.1	2411	126.4	1859	145.4	2137
Colombia, Cali	130.1	1911	107.9	1567	119.0	1738
Costa Rica	154.7	2286	119.3	1766	137.4	2031
Cuba	103.1	1516	78.7	1164	91.2	1344
Jamaica	87.8	1304	70.1	1031	78.8	1165
Puerto Rico	116.8	1700	99.0	1445	108.1	1574
ASIA						
China, Shanghai	115.2	1709	98.9	1457	107.3	1587
China, Taipei	88.1	1285	67.0	974	77.8	1134
Hong Kong	151.0	2199	107.3	1582	129.8	1899
India, Bangalore	75.2	1137	41.9	626	58.6	882
India, Bombay Cancer Registry	86.3	1287	54.5	810	70.9	1057
Israel, Jews	148.8	2170	118.9	1732	134.2	1957
Israel, non Jews	121.1	1742	78.2	1125	100.5	1446
Japan, Kanagawa	98.2	1420	85.0	1230	91.7	1328
Japan, Miyagi	99.3	1422	85.3	1250	92.5	1338
Japan, Osaka	127.0	1816	100.5	1455	114.1	1640
Kuwait, Kuwaiti	75.4	1141	63.2	937	69.4	1040
Kuwait, non Kuwaiti	143.0	2077	101.6	1468	122.8	1779
Philippines, Metro Manila & Rizal	95.6	1434	80.9	1206	88.4	1322
Singapore, Chinese	105.2	1542	88.8	1289	97.3	1420
Singapore, Malay	89.0	1314	74.7	1104	82.0	1211
EUROPE						
Czechoslovakia, Slovakia	138.2	2008	111.4	1628	125.1	1822
Denmark	143.5	2099	110.6	1606	127.4	1858
FRG, Children's Tumour Registry	120.2	1727	97.2	1379	109.0	1557
FRG, Saarland	122.0	1773	102.6	1491	112.5	1635
Finland	150.4	2163	118.1	1712	134.6	1943
France, Bas Rhin	136.4	1972	123.5	1763	130.1	1870
France, Paediatric Registries	146.6	2104	115.2	1666	131.2	1889
German Democratic Republic	132.9	1932	113.8	1659	123.6	1799
Great Britain, England and Wales	119.6	1740	96.8	1405	108.5	1577
Great Britain, Manchester (period 1)	105.7	1535	87.9	1278	97.0	1410
Great Britain, Manchester (period 2)	119.1	1719	103.0	1501	111.3	1613
Great Britain, Scotland	114.3	1653	94.2	1374	104.5	1517
Hungary	113.5	1637	82.2	1176	98.3	1413
Italy, Torino	157.0	2282	124.9	1814	141.3	2054
Netherlands, DCLSG						
Netherlands, SOOZ, Eindhoven	141.0	2020	101.1	1465	121.5	1749
Norway	138.1	1995	105.9	1529	122.4	1768
Poland, Warsaw City	107.5	1554	86.9	1260	97.5	1411
Spain, Zaragoza	169.9	2505	101.9	1483	137.0	2010
Sweden	149.9	2170	129.9	1881	140.2	2029
Switzerland, Three Western Cantons	136.0	1976	114.4	1617	125.5	1801
Yugoslavia, Slovenia	126.0	1855	86.6	1260	106.8	1565
OCEANIA						
Australia, New South Wales	153.0	2212	122.2	1763	138.0	1993
Australia, Queensland	131.9	1885	100.6	1444	116.6	1669
Fiji, Fijian	60.0	870	61.0	887	60.5	878
Fiji, Indian	50.6	753	28.6	405	39.7	581
New Zealand, Maori	173.9	2540	111.5	1637	143.2	2097
New Zealand, non Maori	140.7	2065	121.6	1776	131.4	1924

* Light when fewer than 10 cases

AGE STANDARDIZED AND CUMULATIVE (0-14) INCIDENCE RATES PER MILLION

Chronic myeloid

	Male ASR	CUM	Female ASR	CUM	Both ASR	CUM
AFRICA						
Nigeria, Ibadan						
Uganda, Kampala						
Zimbabwe, Bulawayo, Residents only						
AMERICA : NORTH						
Canada, Atlantic Provinces	0.3	4	0.3	5	0.3	5
Canada, Western Provinces	1.4	20	0.6	9	1.0	15
USA, Greater Delaware Valley, White	0.9	14	0.9	12	0.9	13
USA, Greater Delaware Valley, non White	1.0	16	–	–	0.5	8
USA, Los Angeles, Black	1.4	20	–	–	0.7	10
USA, Los Angeles, Hispanic	1.0	14	1.3	18	1.1	16
USA, Los Angeles, Other White	0.2	3	1.1	16	0.6	9
USA, New York (City and State), White	1.6	22	1.0	14	1.3	18
USA, New York (City and State), Black	1.9	27	0.4	7	1.2	17
USA, SEER, White	0.7	10	0.4	6	0.5	8
USA, SEER, Black	1.0	15	1.2	20	1.1	18
AMERICA : OTHER						
Brazil, Fortaleza	–	–	1.2	21	0.7	11
Brazil, Recife	0.3	6	–	–	0.2	3
Brazil, Sao Paulo	0.9	14	0.3	5	0.6	9
Colombia, Cali	1.9	28	1.1	15	1.5	21
Costa Rica	1.6	23	–	–	0.8	12
Cuba	0.6	10	0.5	8	0.6	9
Jamaica	0.7	12	0.6	11	0.7	11
Puerto Rico	0.5	6	1.2	18	0.8	12
ASIA						
China, Shanghai	2.0	29	0.7	12	1.4	21
China, Taipei	0.9	16	0.2	3	0.6	9
Hong Kong	–	–	0.5	7	0.2	4
India, Bangalore	0.6	10	0.6	10	0.6	10
India, Bombay Cancer Registry	1.1	16	1.0	16	1.0	16
Israel, Jews	0.7	10	1.2	17	0.9	13
Israel, non Jews	0.8	10	0.8	11	0.8	10
Japan, Kanagawa	2.2	33	1.0	15	1.6	25
Japan, Miyagi	1.4	21	0.4	7	0.9	14
Japan, Osaka	1.8	27	1.0	16	1.4	22
Kuwait, Kuwaiti	–	–	–	–	–	–
Kuwait, non Kuwaiti	–	–	1.0	16	0.5	8
Philippines, Metro Manila & Rizal ·	1.2	20	1.6	25	1.4	23
Singapore, Chinese	3.9	60	1.9	28	3.0	45
Singapore, Malay	3.8	62	–	–	1.9	31
EUROPE						
Czechoslovakia, Slovakia	1.1	17	1.4	19	1.2	18
Denmark	0.9	12	1.2	21	1.1	16
FRG, Children's Tumour Registry	1.4	20	0.5	7	1.0	14
FRG, Saarland	0.7	9	–	–	0.4	5
Finland	2.2	35	0.7	11	1.5	23
France, Bas Rhin	–	–	–	–	–	–
France, Paediatric Registries	0.8	10	–	–	0.4	5
German Democratic Republic	1.7	25	–	–	0.9	13
Great Britain, England and Wales	1.0	14	0.6	9	0.8	12
Great Britain, Manchester (period 1)	0.3	5	0.2	4	0.3	4
Great Britain, Manchester (period 2)	1.4	21	0.5	7	1.0	15
Great Britain, Scotland	0.9	12	1.2	19	1.0	16
Hungary	1.0	14	0.3	4	0.6	9
Italy, Torino	0.9	12	1.3	20	1.1	16
Netherlands, DCLSG	1.7	23	0.9	13	1.3	18
Netherlands, SOOZ, Eindhoven	5.2	68	–	–	2.7	35
Norway	1.2	16	0.7	10	1.0	13
Poland, Warsaw City	0.5	8	–	–	0.2	4
Spain, Zaragoza	–	–	–	–	–	–
Sweden	1.0	16	0.9	14	0.9	15
Switzerland, Three Western Cantons	0.8	14	–	–	0.4	7
Yugoslavia, Slovenia	2.4	34	1.0	15	1.7	25
OCEANIA						
Australia, New South Wales	0.7	10	2.1	30	1.4	20
Australia, Queensland	–	–	0.3	6	0.2	3
Fiji, Fijian						
Fiji, Indian						
New Zealand, Maori	2.1	26	–	–	1.1	14
New Zealand, non Maori	0.8	11	1.5	23	1.2	17

* Light when fewer than 10 cases

AGE STANDARDIZED AND CUMULATIVE (0-14) INCIDENCE RATES PER MILLION

Lymphomas

	Male ASR	Male CUM	Female ASR	Female CUM	Both ASR	Both CUM
AFRICA						
Nigeria, Ibadan	122.7	1941	70.3	1125	96.8	1539
Uganda, Kampala	33.6	538	22.1	347	27.7	440
Zimbabwe, Bulawayo, Residents only	17.1	235	11.9	182	14.6	210
AMERICA : NORTH						
Canada, Atlantic Provinces	10.9	163	6.9	104	8.9	134
Canada, Western Provinces	21.6	325	10.2	160	16.1	244
USA, Greater Delaware Valley, White	16.9	265	8.7	137	12.9	203
USA, Greater Delaware Valley, non White	15.1	232	9.0	138	12.1	185
USA, Los Angeles, Black	12.9	206	9.8	158	11.4	182
USA, Los Angeles, Hispanic	27.0	413	9.8	155	18.6	286
USA, Los Angeles, Other White	20.9	330	10.7	173	15.9	253
USA, New York (City and State), White	20.2	322	10.0	161	15.2	243
USA, New York (City and State), Black	16.8	265	7.5	121	12.2	193
USA, SEER, White	20.3	318	11.5	182	16.0	251
USA, SEER, Black	14.3	222	6.0	92	10.2	158
AMERICA : OTHER						
Brazil, Fortaleza	39.4	601	15.8	231	27.5	413
Brazil, Recife	20.5	313	13.0	202	16.8	258
Brazil, Sao Paulo	38.5	582	19.4	291	29.0	437
Colombia, Cali	26.8	401	13.2	195	20.0	298
Costa Rica	38.8	566	17.3	251	28.3	412
Cuba	30.3	449	14.1	206	22.4	331
Jamaica	15.9	250	6.7	100	11.2	174
Puerto Rico	20.6	316	10.5	163	15.6	241
ASIA						
China, Shanghai	16.0	241	5.7	89	11.0	168
China, Taipei	9.0	135	8.4	123	8.7	129
Hong Kong	24.3	365	14.1	206	19.3	288
India, Bangalore	21.7	342	3.9	60	12.8	201
India, Bombay Cancer Registry	17.5	275	4.8	73	11.4	178
Israel, Jews	36.0	535	18.5	272	27.5	407
Israel, non Jews	42.5	606	13.0	194	28.3	408
Japan, Kanagawa	7.1	109	6.1	91	6.6	100
Japan, Miyagi	4.8	78	2.6	37	3.7	58
Japan, Osaka	12.0	177	6.7	101	9.4	140
Kuwait, Kuwaiti	32.7	510	18.5	279	25.7	396
Kuwait, non Kuwaiti	38.4	564	22.3	336	30.5	452
Philippines, Metro Manila & Rizal	10.3	157	2.5	39	6.5	99
Singapore, Chinese	13.5	206	8.0	117	10.8	163
Singapore, Malay	10.7	163	7.5	105	9.1	134
EUROPE						
Czechoslovakia, Slovakia	24.1	365	9.5	144	17.0	257
Denmark	17.4	271	8.2	128	12.9	201
FRG, Children's Tumour Registry	20.0	305	9.5	143	14.9	226
FRG, Saarland	15.2	234	6.2	95	10.8	166
Finland	17.7	265	8.7	130	13.3	199
France, Bas Rhin	21.2	312	15.0	219	18.2	266
France, Paediatric Registries	18.4	279	12.1	179	15.3	230
German Democratic Republic	21.9	335	12.5	191	17.3	265
Great Britain, England and Wales	15.2	235	7.1	110	11.2	174
Great Britain, Manchester (period 1)	13.1	195	7.1	107	10.2	152
Great Britain, Manchester (period 2)	16.0	239	8.6	132	12.4	187
Great Britain, Scotland	14.3	224	6.8	104	10.6	165
Hungary	18.8	288	6.9	103	13.0	198
Italy, Torino	21.9	337	10.1	157	16.2	249
Netherlands, DCLSG						
Netherlands, SOOZ, Eindhoven	21.7	316	8.9	132	15.5	226
Norway	11.6	181	4.8	72	8.3	128
Poland, Warsaw City	11.8	179	8.0	120	10.0	150
Spain, Zaragoza	30.3	463	12.3	183	21.6	327
Sweden	17.2	267	6.9	104	12.2	187
Switzerland, Three Western Cantons	19.3	293	7.2	111	13.4	204
Yugoslavia, Slovenia	21.9	338	9.0	139	15.6	241
OCEANIA						
Australia, New South Wales	21.4	323	8.9	131	15.3	229
Australia, Queensland	22.0	336	10.3	151	16.3	246
Fiji, Fijian	11.3	166	9.8	140	10.6	153
Fiji, Indian	9.7	142	2.0	30	5.9	87
New Zealand, Maori	26.6	402	14.5	211	20.6	308
New Zealand, non Maori	17.6	266	6.4	100	12.1	185

* Light when fewer than 10 cases

AGE STANDARDIZED AND CUMULATIVE (0-14) INCIDENCE RATES PER MILLION

Leukaemias

	Male ASR	Male CUM	Female ASR	Female CUM	Both ASR	Both CUM
AFRICA						
Nigeria, Ibadan	18.3	301	4.6	75	11.8	194
Uganda, Kampala	16.9	258	11.8	181	14.3	219
Zimbabwe, Bulawayo, Residents only	15.2	215	16.9	251	16.1	234
AMERICA : NORTH						
Canada, Atlantic Provinces	40.4	579	35.3	498	37.9	539
Canada, Western Provinces	47.9	676	39.6	557	43.8	618
USA, Greater Delaware Valley, White	47.6	684	37.7	537	42.8	612
USA, Greater Delaware Valley, non White	31.2	464	13.5	198	22.4	331
USA, Los Angeles, Black	31.6	460	23.9	342	27.8	402
USA, Los Angeles, Hispanic	56.0	801	44.1	631	50.2	717
USA, Los Angeles, Other White	52.7	747	43.6	623	48.2	686
USA, New York (City and State), White	49.2	708	43.9	623	46.6	666
USA, New York (City and State), Black	35.3	517	20.8	293	28.1	405
USA, SEER, White	47.8	681	39.5	559	43.7	622
USA, SEER, Black	24.0	346	26.3	386	25.2	366
AMERICA : OTHER						
Brazil, Fortaleza	44.3	693	40.0	607	41.9	645
Brazil, Recife	28.0	414	22.8	338	25.4	376
Brazil, Sao Paulo	37.6	549	29.4	429	33.5	489
Colombia, Cali	53.0	771	35.1	525	44.1	648
Costa Rica	62.6	927	56.0	830	59.4	880
Cuba	32.5	480	26.9	398	29.8	440
Jamaica	24.2	357	20.4	294	22.2	325
Puerto Rico	39.8	571	40.5	584	40.2	577
ASIA						
China, Shanghai	45.0	676	36.3	534	40.8	607
China, Taipei	29.8	437	24.5	350	27.3	395
Hong Kong	52.7	770	41.4	610	47.2	692
India, Bangalore	18.4	281	6.9	102	12.7	192
India, Bombay Cancer Registry	26.5	392	19.1	285	22.9	340
Israel, Jews	37.6	543	27.5	395	32.7	471
Israel, non Jews	33.7	482	17.4	246	25.8	369
Japan, Kanagawa	39.6	575	37.0	528	38.3	552
Japan, Miyagi	40.3	579	38.6	567	39.5	573
Japan, Osaka	41.6	595	35.1	507	38.4	552
Kuwait, Kuwaiti	11.9	181	14.0	209	12.9	194
Kuwait, non Kuwaiti	36.8	529	32.6	473	34.7	501
Philippines, Metro Manila & Rizal	50.8	757	36.6	544	43.9	653
Singapore, Chinese	42.7	618	32.5	462	37.8	543
Singapore, Malay	49.0	719	27.7	419	38.6	572
EUROPE						
Czechoslovakia, Slovakia	39.6	568	38.1	549	38.9	559
Denmark	43.1	619	34.1	486	38.7	554
FRG, Children's Tumour Registry	47.1	669	39.6	560	43.4	616
FRG, Saarland	44.4	630	34.8	499	39.7	566
Finland	48.0	686	36.4	522	42.3	605
France, Bas Rhin	36.8	520	39.7	558	38.3	539
France, Paediatric Registries	38.9	551	41.8	593	40.3	572
German Democratic Republic	36.2	518	32.1	458	34.2	489
Great Britain, England and Wales	41.8	596	32.9	469	37.5	534
Great Britain, Manchester (period 1)	33.9	489	28.7	415	31.4	453
Great Britain, Manchester (period 2)	42.8	614	33.8	482	38.4	550
Great Britain, Scotland	41.5	586	34.1	492	37.9	540
Hungary	39.1	558	29.3	414	34.3	488
Italy, Torino	54.2	778	43.8	625	49.2	703
Netherlands, DCLSG	40.9	579	34.2	483	37.6	532
Netherlands, SOOZ, Eindhoven	52.0	719	33.7	479	43.1	602
Norway	50.2	712	38.8	543	44.6	630
Poland, Warsaw City	36.9	528	24.7	356	31.0	444
Spain, Zaragoza	49.1	713	43.8	635	46.5	675
Sweden	45.9	654	42.7	605	44.3	630
Switzerland, Three Western Cantons	46.3	670	41.1	578	43.8	625
Yugoslavia, Slovenia	36.1	520	32.1	454	34.1	488
OCEANIA						
Australia, New South Wales	54.1	763	45.5	647	49.9	706
Australia, Queensland	39.3	553	36.8	529	38.0	541
Fiji, Fijian	19.9	299	14.7	207	17.4	254
Fiji, Indian	22.7	345	12.4	174	17.6	260
New Zealand, Maori	42.6	612	21.4	292	32.2	454
New Zealand, non Maori	51.8	751	38.6	553	45.4	654

* Light when fewer than 10 cases

AGE STANDARDIZED AND CUMULATIVE (0–14) INCIDENCE RATES PER MILLION

Hodgkin's disease

	Male ASR	Male CUM	Female ASR	Female CUM	Both ASR	Both CUM
AFRICA						
Nigeria, Ibadan						
Uganda, Kampala						
Zimbabwe, Bulawayo, Residents only						
AMERICA : NORTH						
Canada, Atlantic Provinces	3.9	61	2.2	36	3.1	49
Canada, Western Provinces	4.6	75	3.7	62	4.2	69
USA, Greater Delaware Valley, White	6.7	110	4.1	69	5.4	90
USA, Greater Delaware Valley, non White	7.5	118	3.8	62	5.6	90
USA, Los Angeles, Black	6.2	101	7.1	118	6.7	110
USA, Los Angeles, Hispanic	11.8	186	5.3	89	8.6	138
USA, Los Angeles, Other White	9.0	149	4.9	83	7.0	117
USA, New York (City and State), White	8.1	134	5.0	85	6.6	110
USA, New York (City and State), Black	8.3	134	3.5	58	5.9	96
USA, SEER, White	6.5	106	5.9	100	6.2	103
USA, SEER, Black	7.5	120	1.9	30	4.7	76
AMERICA : OTHER						
Brazil, Fortaleza	9.1	136	3.9	57	6.5	96
Brazil, Recife	7.8	126	4.3	71	6.0	98
Brazil, Sao Paulo	12.3	192	5.0	79	8.6	136
Colombia, Cali	7.8	123	4.3	68	6.1	95
Costa Rica	14.0	219	7.3	111	10.8	166
Cuba	6.5	103	2.9	47	4.8	75
Jamaica	5.2	81	1.4	21	3.3	51
Puerto Rico	8.1	129	4.5	75	6.3	102
ASIA						
China, Shanghai	3.2	48	1.0	15	2.1	32
China, Taipei	0.8	13	0.2	3	0.5	8
Hong Kong	3.2	48	2.1	29	2.7	39
India, Bangalore	8.3	134	1.1	18	4.7	76
India, Bombay Cancer Registry	7.0	112	1.2	19	4.2	67
Israel, Jews	8.7	134	6.0	97	7.4	116
Israel, non Jews	11.2	165	5.8	91	8.6	129
Japan, Kanagawa	0.7	11	0.5	8	0.6	10
Japan, Miyagi	0.4	7	–	–	0.2	4
Japan, Osaka	0.9	14	0.6	9	0.7	12
Kuwait, Kuwaiti	13.7	218	7.0	111	10.3	165
Kuwait, non Kuwaiti	12.1	184	7.3	113	9.8	149
Philippines, Metro Manila & Rizal	1.8	30	–	–	0.9	15
Singapore, Chinese	2.5	39	0.7	11	1.6	25
Singapore, Malay	2.3	34	1.0	16	1.7	25
EUROPE						
Czechoslovakia, Slovakia	8.8	138	4.1	65	6.5	103
Denmark	4.3	71	3.7	63	4.0	67
FRG, Children's Tumour Registry	6.7	107	3.2	53	5.0	81
FRG, Saarland	3.9	64	2.9	46	3.4	55
Finland	3.2	51	1.7	30	2.5	41
France, Bas Rhin	4.0	59	1.6	27	2.8	44
France, Paediatric Registries	4.9	78	3.2	54	4.0	66
German Democratic Republic	7.8	124	5.2	86	6.6	106
Great Britain, England and Wales	5.6	91	2.4	39	4.1	66
Great Britain, Manchester (period 1)	4.7	76	1.9	33	3.4	55
Great Britain, Manchester (period 2)	5.2	85	1.7	28	3.5	57
Great Britain, Scotland	6.4	105	2.3	37	4.4	72
Hungary	6.1	96	1.8	29	4.0	63
Italy, Torino	8.4	132	5.4	87	6.9	110
Netherlands, DCLSG						
Netherlands, SOOZ, Eindhoven	2.9	42	3.1	52	3.0	47
Norway	3.0	49	1.8	29	2.4	39
Poland, Warsaw City	3.6	55	2.8	39	3.2	47
Spain, Zaragoza	8.2	125	2.0	33	5.2	80
Sweden	5.2	83	1.2	21	3.3	53
Switzerland, Three Western Cantons	4.5	73	3.4	59	4.0	66
Yugoslavia, Slovenia	9.2	146	4.6	73	6.9	110
OCEANIA						
Australia, New South Wales	5.6	90	2.3	39	4.0	65
Australia, Queensland	8.3	136	1.8	29	5.1	84
Fiji, Fijian						
Fiji, Indian						
New Zealand, Maori	9.9	148	3.6	53	6.8	101
New Zealand, non Maori	5.2	84	2.3	38	3.8	61

* Light when fewer than 10 cases

AGE STANDARDIZED AND CUMULATIVE (0-14) INCIDENCE RATES PER MILLION

Non-Hodgkin lymphoma

	Male ASR	CUM	Female ASR	CUM	Both ASR	CUM
AFRICA						
Nigeria, Ibadan						
Uganda, Kampala						
Zimbabwe, Bulawayo, Residents only						
AMERICA : NORTH						
Canada, Atlantic Provinces	6.6	97	2.7	39	4.7	69
Canada, Western Provinces	9.4	141	4.0	61	6.8	102
USA, Greater Delaware Valley, White	5.4	85	2.9	43	4.2	65
USA, Greater Delaware Valley, non White	3.0	48	3.9	58	3.5	53
USA, Los Angeles, Black	4.8	77	1.0	18	2.9	47
USA, Los Angeles, Hispanic	9.0	138	1.9	29	5.5	84
USA, Los Angeles, Other White	7.6	119	4.1	64	5.9	92
USA, New York (City and State), White	6.8	106	2.3	36	4.6	72
USA, New York (City and State), Black	5.4	85	1.6	26	3.5	56
USA, SEER, White	6.9	107	2.8	42	4.9	75
USA, SEER, Black	3.9	61	1.5	21	2.7	41
AMERICA : OTHER						
Brazil, Fortaleza	23.9	366	11.9	174	17.8	268
Brazil, Recife	9.8	145	6.3	95	8.1	120
Brazil, Sao Paulo	22.7	336	12.5	183	17.6	260
Colombia, Cali	3.4	54	5.5	82	4.4	68
Costa Rica	10.8	150	5.9	81	8.4	116
Cuba	19.8	287	9.0	127	14.5	209
Jamaica	7.9	128	3.9	60	5.9	94
Puerto Rico	6.0	91	3.2	48	4.6	70
ASIA						
China, Shanghai	7.1	111	2.8	46	5.0	79
China, Taipei	4.4	68	3.4	51	3.9	60
Hong Kong	11.0	166	7.1	106	9.1	137
India, Bangalore	8.5	130	2.8	43	5.7	86
India, Bombay Cancer Registry	7.2	110	1.8	27	4.6	70
Israel, Jews	16.8	248	6.0	85	11.5	169
Israel, non Jews	17.2	252	2.5	39	10.1	150
Japan, Kanagawa	1.4	22	2.0	31	1.7	26
Japan, Miyagi	1.8	29	-	-	0.9	15
Japan, Osaka	5.6	83	3.0	46	4.3	65
Kuwait, Kuwaiti	15.2	236	4.9	73	10.1	155
Kuwait, non Kuwaiti	14.3	213	11.9	178	13.2	196
Philippines, Metro Manila & Rizal	3.7	57	0.9	14	2.3	36
Singapore, Chinese	7.1	109	5.4	79	6.2	94
Singapore, Malay	7.0	111	3.5	51	5.3	81
EUROPE						
Czechoslovakia, Slovakia	8.6	131	2.5	36	5.6	85
Denmark	4.1	64	1.5	22	2.8	44
FRG, Children's Tumour Registry	7.4	114	2.5	37	5.0	77
FRG, Saarland	7.7	116	2.1	32	5.0	75
Finland	7.7	116	4.6	66	6.2	92
France, Bas Rhin	9.2	143	8.2	124	8.7	134
France, Paediatric Registries	4.0	64	2.4	38	3.2	51
German Democratic Republic	9.5	148	4.5	69	7.1	109
Great Britain, England and Wales	7.9	121	3.4	52	5.7	88
Great Britain, Manchester (period 1)	5.4	80	2.4	36	3.9	58
Great Britain, Manchester (period 2)	7.2	107	4.1	62	5.7	85
Great Britain, Scotland	6.6	101	3.3	51	5.0	76
Hungary	0.6	9	0.3	4	0.4	6
Italy, Torino	9.7	146	3.8	57	6.8	103
Netherlands, DCLSG						
Netherlands, SOOZ, Eindhoven	12.8	193	4.4	62	8.7	129
Norway	5.0	80	2.1	30	3.6	55
Poland, Warsaw City	3.4	52	2.1	30	2.8	41
Spain, Zaragoza	19.2	292	6.9	100	13.3	199
Sweden	8.8	133	4.0	59	6.4	97
Switzerland, Three Western Cantons	6.8	106	2.2	33	4.6	70
Yugoslavia, Slovenia	10.8	166	3.5	51	7.2	110
OCEANIA						
Australia, New South Wales	10.4	159	3.3	48	6.9	105
Australia, Queensland	9.5	143	2.7	40	6.2	93
Fiji, Fijian						
Fiji, Indian						
New Zealand, Maori	13.6	203	5.7	78	9.7	142
New Zealand, non Maori	10.5	156	2.5	39	6.6	98

* Light when fewer than 10 cases

AGE STANDARDIZED AND CUMULATIVE (0-14) INCIDENCE RATES PER MILLION

Burkitt's lymphoma

	Male ASR CUM		Female ASR CUM		Both ASR CUM	
AFRICA						
Nigeria, Ibadan						
Uganda, Kampala						
Zimbabwe, Bulawayo, Residents only						
AMERICA : NORTH						
Canada, Atlantic Provinces	–	–	0.7	10	0.3	5
Canada, Western Provinces	0.6	9	–	–	0.3	4
USA, Greater Delaware Valley, White	1.2	18	0.1	2	0.7	10
USA, Greater Delaware Valley, non White	1.1	16	–	–	0.6	8
USA, Los Angeles, Black	0.5	9	–	–	0.3	4
USA, Los Angeles, Hispanic	1.9	27	–	–	1.0	14
USA, Los Angeles, Other White	1.5	24	0.5	7	1.0	16
USA, New York (City and State), White	1.7	26	0.9	14	1.3	20
USA, New York (City and State), Black	0.8	13	–	–	0.4	6
USA, SEER, White	3.5	54	0.4	6	2.0	31
USA, SEER, Black	0.6	10	–	–	0.3	5
AMERICA : OTHER						
Brazil, Fortaleza	1.2	19	–	–	0.6	10
Brazil, Recife	–	–	–	–	–	–
Brazil, Sao Paulo	0.8	12	0.1	2	0.5	7
Colombia, Cali	11.9	169	–	–	6.0	85
Costa Rica	0.6	8	0.6	9	0.6	8
Cuba	0.3	5	0.2	2	0.3	4
Jamaica	–	–	–	–	–	–
Puerto Rico	2.0	29	0.6	9	1.3	19
ASIA						
China, Shanghai	–	–	–	–	–	–
China, Taipei	–	–	–	–	–	–
Hong Kong	0.9	14	1.3	19	1.1	17
India, Bangalore	1.2	16	–	–	0.6	8
India, Bombay Cancer Registry	0.2	3	0.6	8	0.4	5
Israel, Jews	5.6	81	2.6	37	4.2	60
Israel, non Jews	9.0	120	4.0	52	6.6	87
Japan, Kanagawa	0.5	9	–	–	0.3	5
Japan, Miyagi	0.4	7	–	–	0.2	4
Japan, Osaka	0.3	4	0.3	5	0.3	5
Kuwait, Kuwaiti	0.9	12	5.7	81	3.3	46
Kuwait, non Kuwaiti	3.9	55	–	–	2.0	28
Philippines, Metro Manila & Rizal	0.3	4	–	–	0.2	2
Singapore, Chinese	0.7	11	0.2	4	0.5	7
Singapore, Malay	–	–	–	–	–	–
EUROPE						
Czechoslovakia, Slovakia	0.5	7	–	–	0.2	4
Denmark	4.8	71	0.9	12	2.8	42
FRG, Children's Tumour Registry	–	1	–	–	–	–
FRG, Saarland	1.7	24	1.2	17	1.5	21
Finland	–	–	–	–	–	–
France, Bas Rhin	1.0	15	–	–	0.5	8
France, Paediatric Registries	6.5	98	0.8	10	3.7	55
German Democratic Republic	1.4	21	0.6	8	1.0	15
Great Britain, England and Wales	0.3	4	0.2	2	0.2	4
Great Britain, Manchester (period 1)	–	–	–	–	–	–
Great Britain, Manchester (period 2)	0.2	3	0.1	2	0.2	2
Great Britain, Scotland	0.1	2	0.1	2	0.1	2
Hungary	2.1	32	0.5	7	1.3	19
Italy, Torino	–	–	–	–	–	–
Netherlands, DCLSG						
Netherlands, SOOZ, Eindhoven	–	–	–	–	–	–
Norway	0.9	15	0.2	3	0.6	9
Poland, Warsaw City	–	–	0.7	10	0.3	5
Spain, Zaragoza	2.9	46	2.3	33	2.6	40
Sweden	–	–	–	–	–	–
Switzerland, Three Western Cantons	2.2	31	–	–	1.1	16
Yugoslavia, Slovenia	–	–	–	–	–	–
OCEANIA						
Australia, New South Wales	0.4	6	–	–	0.2	3
Australia, Queensland	–	–	0.3	6	0.2	3
Fiji, Fijian						
Fiji, Indian						
New Zealand, Maori	–	–	1.5	27	0.8	13
New Zealand, non Maori	–	–	0.5	8	0.2	4

* Light when fewer than 10 cases

AGE STANDARDIZED AND CUMULATIVE (0-14) INCIDENCE RATES PER MILLION

Brain and spinal

	Male ASR	Male CUM	Female ASR	Female CUM	Both ASR	Both CUM
AFRICA						
Nigeria, Ibadan	5.5	82	4.6	75	4.9	77
Uganda, Kampala	4.3	66	4.0	60	4.2	63
Zimbabwe, Bulawayo, Residents only	12.5	175	16.9	251	14.8	214
AMERICA : NORTH						
Canada, Atlantic Provinces	21.7	329	17.8	258	19.8	294
Canada, Western Provinces	26.9	400	23.0	338	25.0	370
USA, Greater Delaware Valley, White	25.8	387	26.2	392	26.0	389
USA, Greater Delaware Valley, non White	24.8	367	21.9	332	23.4	350
USA, Los Angeles, Black	21.2	307	17.5	266	19.5	287
USA, Los Angeles, Hispanic	26.2	388	22.4	333	24.4	361
USA, Los Angeles, Other White	31.4	467	27.2	404	29.3	436
USA, New York (City and State), White	30.8	463	25.1	372	28.0	419
USA, New York (City and State), Black	23.7	346	19.2	280	21.5	313
USA, SEER, White	26.4	394	23.3	347	24.9	371
USA, SEER, Black	21.0	318	23.0	341	22.0	329
AMERICA : OTHER						
Brazil, Fortaleza	11.8	189	14.0	225	13.0	209
Brazil, Recife	16.0	244	14.6	222	15.3	233
Brazil, Sao Paulo	21.8	330	21.0	318	21.4	324
Colombia, Cali	16.8	260	16.9	250	16.8	254
Costa Rica	17.9	273	10.0	156	14.0	216
Cuba	12.2	186	11.3	172	11.8	179
Jamaica	14.7	231	11.6	177	13.1	203
Puerto Rico	17.8	260	13.5	200	15.7	231
ASIA						
China, Shanghai	19.7	300	20.2	300	19.9	300
China, Taipei	11.0	164	8.8	134	9.9	149
Hong Kong	15.2	223	12.0	179	13.6	202
India, Bangalore	6.7	102	8.9	137	7.8	120
India, Bombay Cancer Registry	8.5	132	6.9	110	7.7	121
Israel, Jews	25.1	370	22.6	337	23.9	354
Israel, non Jews	15.1	238	18.4	273	16.7	255
Japan, Kanagawa	18.3	270	16.1	240	17.2	255
Japan, Miyagi	8.6	126	10.4	146	9.5	136
Japan, Osaka	26.9	400	21.2	313	24.1	358
Kuwait, Kuwaiti	4.7	65	5.1	84	4.9	75
Kuwait, non Kuwaiti	13.1	194	10.4	158	11.8	176
Philippines, Metro Manila & Rizal	9.5	153	6.6	105	8.0	129
Singapore, Chinese	11.0	170	12.4	190	11.7	179
Singapore, Malay	7.3	114	10.5	153	8.8	133
EUROPE						
Czechoslovakia, Slovakia	25.7	384	19.8	298	22.8	342
Denmark	33.9	508	27.7	406	30.9	458
FRG, Children's Tumour Registry	14.2	207	12.5	180	13.4	194
FRG, Saarland	24.1	347	20.1	296	22.2	322
Finland	33.7	493	28.6	420	31.2	457
France, Bas Rhin	25.0	381	28.9	420	26.9	400
France, Paediatric Registries	33.9	499	19.6	301	26.9	402
German Democratic Republic	27.9	413	23.5	350	25.7	382
Great Britain, England and Wales	26.4	392	22.4	333	24.4	363
Great Britain, Manchester (period 1)	23.0	341	20.9	312	22.0	327
Great Britain, Manchester (period 2)	26.8	399	24.8	373	25.8	387
Great Britain, Scotland	22.6	335	19.8	295	21.2	316
Hungary	20.3	298	16.4	244	18.4	272
Italy, Torino	30.4	447	23.6	357	27.1	403
Netherlands, DCLSG						
Netherlands, SOOZ, Eindhoven	20.6	301	10.0	155	15.4	229
Norway	30.2	447	22.6	342	26.5	396
Poland, Warsaw City	17.1	258	20.1	290	18.6	273
Spain, Zaragoza	30.8	452	17.2	264	24.2	361
Sweden	37.0	546	30.3	449	33.7	499
Switzerland, Three Western Cantons	18.0	257	25.1	353	21.5	304
Yugoslavia, Slovenia	27.2	398	14.5	217	21.0	310
OCEANIA						
Australia, New South Wales	25.9	380	23.0	337	24.5	359
Australia, Queensland	25.3	368	19.5	281	22.5	325
Fiji, Fijian	2.4	31	5.1	69	3.7	50
Fiji, Indian	1.0	15	1.1	14	1.0	14
New Zealand, Maori	25.5	379	23.6	366	24.6	373
New Zealand, non Maori	26.1	386	23.4	346	24.7	367

* Light when fewer than 10 cases

AGE STANDARDIZED AND CUMULATIVE (0-14) INCIDENCE RATES PER MILLION

Ependymoma

	Male ASR	Male CUM	Female ASR	Female CUM	Both ASR	Both CUM
AFRICA						
Nigeria, Ibadan						
Uganda, Kampala						
Zimbabwe, Bulawayo, Residents only						
AMERICA : NORTH						
Canada, Atlantic Provinces	3.5	48	2.4	34	3.0	41
Canada, Western Provinces	3.1	42	2.1	30	2.6	36
USA, Greater Delaware Valley, White	3.6	51	2.4	35	3.0	43
USA, Greater Delaware Valley, non White	2.4	33	2.4	34	2.4	34
USA, Los Angeles, Black	3.1	40	-	-	1.6	21
USA, Los Angeles, Hispanic	3.7	52	2.6	37	3.2	45
USA, Los Angeles, Other White	3.6	51	1.8	25	2.7	38
USA, New York (City and State), White	2.6	38	1.5	21	2.1	30
USA, New York (City and State), Black	1.9	26	1.1	14	1.5	20
USA, SEER, White	2.8	39	1.9	28	2.4	34
USA, SEER, Black	1.3	20	3.0	43	2.1	31
AMERICA : OTHER						
Brazil, Fortaleza	-	-	-	-	-	-
Brazil, Recife	1.4	22	1.7	26	1.5	24
Brazil, Sao Paulo	2.0	31	1.1	17	1.6	24
Colombia, Cali	-	-	2.0	28	1.0	14
Costa Rica	1.6	24	-	-	0.8	12
Cuba	1.2	19	0.7	10	1.0	15
Jamaica	2.7	43	-	-	1.3	21
Puerto Rico	2.6	35	0.5	6	1.6	21
ASIA						
China, Shanghai	0.9	11	0.3	5	0.6	8
China, Taipei	0.7	10	0.2	3	0.5	7
Hong Kong	0.8	12	-	-	0.4	6
India, Bangalore	1.2	16	0.5	8	0.8	12
India, Bombay Cancer Registry	0.5	7	0.5	9	0.5	8
Israel, Jews	2.5	35	1.7	23	2.1	29
Israel, non Jews	2.3	36	3.2	45	2.7	41
Japan, Kanagawa	0.7	10	0.7	9	0.7	10
Japan, Miyagi	0.5	7	0.6	7	0.5	7
Japan, Osaka	1.6	22	1.7	25	1.6	23
Kuwait, Kuwaiti	1.9	24	1.1	18	1.5	21
Kuwait, non Kuwaiti	2.0	28	1.3	22	1.6	25
Philippines, Metro Manila & Rizal	-	-	-	-	-	-
Singapore, Chinese	0.5	7	1.2	16	0.8	12
Singapore, Malay	-	-	-	-	-	-
EUROPE						
Czechoslovakia, Slovakia	1.5	22	1.2	17	1.3	19
Denmark	4.9	72	4.8	67	4.9	70
FRG, Children's Tumour Registry	1.5	21	2.1	29	1.8	25
FRG, Saarland	1.7	24	1.5	19	1.6	22
Finland	3.7	51	4.3	63	4.0	57
France, Bas Rhin	4.5	62	4.3	64	4.4	63
France, Paediatric Registries	3.5	48	1.4	19	2.4	34
German Democratic Republic	5.5	78	3.8	54	4.6	66
Great Britain, England and Wales	3.5	49	2.9	41	3.2	45
Great Britain, Manchester (period 1)	2.4	34	3.2	43	2.8	38
Great Britain, Manchester (period 2)	4.0	57	3.6	51	3.8	54
Great Britain, Scotland	2.7	39	1.5	21	2.1	30
Hungary	3.2	46	2.9	41	3.1	43
Italy, Torino	1.7	24	1.8	29	1.8	26
Netherlands, DCLSG						
Netherlands, SOOZ, Eindhoven	1.3	17	1.4	18	1.3	17
Norway	1.5	22	0.9	13	1.2	18
Poland, Warsaw City	1.4	18	1.0	17	1.2	18
Spain, Zaragoza	-	-	-	-	-	-
Sweden	4.8	66	3.9	57	4.3	62
Switzerland, Three Western Cantons	2.7	34	1.4	18	2.0	26
Yugoslavia, Slovenia	2.9	41	5.4	80	4.1	60
OCEANIA						
Australia, New South Wales	3.1	44	3.3	44	3.2	44
Australia, Queensland	2.4	34	3.2	42	2.8	38
Fiji, Fijian						
Fiji, Indian						
New Zealand, Maori	-	-	5.2	78	2.6	39
New Zealand, non Maori	1.1	15	1.3	20	1.2	17

* Light when fewer than 10 cases

AGE STANDARDIZED AND CUMULATIVE (0-14) INCIDENCE RATES PER MILLION

Astrocytoma

	Male ASR	CUM	Female ASR	CUM	Both ASR	CUM
AFRICA						
Nigeria, Ibadan						
Uganda, Kampala						
Zimbabwe, Bulawayo, Residents only						
AMERICA : NORTH						
Canada, Atlantic Provinces	6.7	106	5.4	78	6.1	92
Canada, Western Provinces	13.4	206	12.0	176	12.7	191
USA, Greater Delaware Valley, White	10.5	162	12.4	187	11.4	174
USA, Greater Delaware Valley, non White	9.7	146	6.1	96	7.9	121
USA, Los Angeles, Black	10.1	151	9.3	139	9.7	145
USA, Los Angeles, Hispanic	7.9	122	11.9	176	9.8	148
USA, Los Angeles, Other White	14.0	212	13.4	202	13.7	207
USA, New York (City and State), White	13.1	200	10.8	164	12.0	182
USA, New York (City and State), Black	11.6	172	7.8	113	9.7	143
USA, SEER, White	12.3	186	12.2	187	12.3	186
USA, SEER, Black	9.2	142	9.0	132	9.1	137
AMERICA : OTHER						
Brazil, Fortaleza	1.4	24	–	–	0.7	11
Brazil, Recife	4.2	63	4.4	69	4.3	66
Brazil, Sao Paulo	5.0	77	4.4	67	4.7	72
Colombia, Cali	7.0	109	4.4	68	5.7	89
Costa Rica	4.4	65	3.8	60	4.1	63
Cuba	3.2	48	3.4	52	3.3	50
Jamaica	7.3	117	8.4	128	7.8	122
Puerto Rico	9.9	146	8.4	127	9.2	137
ASIA						
China, Shanghai	2.8	43	2.6	41	2.7	42
China, Taipei	3.9	61	4.3	64	4.1	62
Hong Kong	2.4	34	2.6	40	2.5	37
India, Bangalore	1.6	24	4.0	59	2.8	42
India, Bombay Cancer Registry	2.7	43	3.2	51	2.9	47
Israel, Jews	7.6	113	8.4	128	8.0	121
Israel, non Jews	2.3	38	5.6	84	3.9	60
Japan, Kanagawa	4.3	66	4.7	72	4.5	69
Japan, Miyagi	2.3	35	3.4	52	2.8	43
Japan, Osaka	2.4	38	3.4	51	2.9	44
Kuwait, Kuwaiti	0.9	14	3.1	51	2.0	32
Kuwait, non Kuwaiti	4.1	61	4.1	60	4.1	61
Philippines, Metro Manila & Rizal	2.4	39	2.5	41	2.5	40
Singapore, Chinese	3.0	46	4.6	69	3.8	57
Singapore, Malay	1.8	31	4.0	64	2.9	47
EUROPE						
Czechoslovakia, Slovakia	4.8	74	3.3	53	4.1	64
Denmark	11.3	172	11.5	174	11.4	173
FRG, Children's Tumour Registry	3.3	50	3.9	57	3.6	53
FRG, Saarland	6.6	92	7.5	113	7.0	102
Finland	–	–	–	–	–	–
France, Bas Rhin	10.4	160	12.8	186	11.6	173
France, Paediatric Registries	13.8	201	9.8	150	11.8	176
German Democratic Republic	9.6	145	10.0	150	9.8	148
Great Britain, England and Wales	9.0	135	8.8	132	8.9	133
Great Britain, Manchester (period 1)	8.4	127	9.5	146	9.0	137
Great Britain, Manchester (period 2)	9.6	146	8.8	134	9.2	140
Great Britain, Scotland	8.7	130	9.4	138	9.0	134
Hungary	6.6	98	6.1	91	6.3	95
Italy, Torino	10.2	145	6.0	88	8.1	117
Netherlands, DCLSG						
Netherlands, SOOZ, Eindhoven	7.9	122	4.7	78	6.3	101
Norway	11.2	169	12.6	192	11.9	180
Poland, Warsaw City	2.2	36	4.1	57	3.2	47
Spain, Zaragoza	3.1	48	3.1	49	3.1	48
Sweden	15.2	226	16.2	240	15.7	233
Switzerland, Three Western Cantons	9.9	144	13.2	185	11.5	164
Yugoslavia, Slovenia	8.8	130	4.2	65	6.6	99
OCEANIA						
Australia, New South Wales	9.1	135	11.4	169	10.3	152
Australia, Queensland	12.8	190	6.1	88	9.5	140
Fiji, Fijian						
Fiji, Indian						
New Zealand, Maori	6.6	103	1.5	27	4.1	65
New Zealand, non Maori	9.1	134	10.1	151	9.6	142

* Light when fewer than 10 cases

AGE STANDARDIZED AND CUMULATIVE (0-14) INCIDENCE RATES PER MILLION

Medulloblastoma

	Male ASR	Male CUM	Female ASR	Female CUM	Both ASR	Both CUM
AFRICA						
Nigeria, Ibadan						
Uganda, Kampala						
Zimbabwe, Bulawayo, Residents only						
AMERICA : NORTH						
Canada, Atlantic Provinces	4.3	64	3.0	44	3.7	54
Canada, Western Provinces	6.0	89	4.1	59	5.1	74
USA, Greater Delaware Valley, White	6.3	93	3.8	58	5.1	76
USA, Greater Delaware Valley, non White	6.5	92	4.9	73	5.7	82
USA, Los Angeles, Black	3.4	48	4.8	71	4.1	59
USA, Los Angeles, Hispanic	8.8	127	2.9	43	5.9	85
USA, Los Angeles, Other White	8.4	124	5.3	75	6.9	100
USA, New York (City and State), White	6.3	91	4.3	62	5.3	77
USA, New York (City and State), Black	2.7	34	3.5	48	3.1	41
USA, SEER, White	6.9	102	4.4	64	5.7	84
USA, SEER, Black	5.3	78	4.6	68	5.0	73
AMERICA : OTHER						
Brazil, Fortaleza	-	-	-	-	-	-
Brazil, Recife	4.5	71	2.4	36	3.5	53
Brazil, Sao Paulo	4.9	73	3.8	57	4.4	65
Colombia, Cali	1.7	27	3.8	55	2.7	41
Costa Rica	7.5	119	0.5	9	4.1	65
Cuba	3.2	49	2.1	31	2.7	40
Jamaica	2.7	41	2.0	28	2.3	34
Puerto Rico	3.4	50	2.2	33	2.8	42
ASIA						
China, Shanghai	1.9	28	1.5	24	1.7	26
China, Taipei	3.2	48	2.8	43	3.0	45
Hong Kong	2.3	36	1.8	25	2.0	31
India, Bangalore	2.4	35	4.4	70	3.4	52
India, Bombay Cancer Registry	1.7	27	1.4	22	1.5	25
Israel, Jews	5.8	84	5.5	79	5.7	82
Israel, non Jews	4.5	70	2.4	37	3.5	54
Japan, Kanagawa	3.0	44	3.0	44	3.0	44
Japan, Miyagi	1.9	28	3.1	44	2.5	36
Japan, Osaka	2.9	42	1.6	25	2.3	34
Kuwait, Kuwaiti	-	-	-	-	-	-
Kuwait, non Kuwaiti	2.0	28	3.0	45	2.5	36
Philippines, Metro Manila & Rizal	2.7	43	0.6	9	1.7	27
Singapore, Chinese	3.6	54	1.8	27	2.7	41
Singapore, Malay	-	-	-	-	-	-
EUROPE						
Czechoslovakia, Slovakia	4.7	69	2.7	40	3.7	55
Denmark	6.0	86	2.6	40	4.4	63
FRG, Children's Tumour Registry	5.4	78	3.6	50	4.5	64
FRG, Saarland	5.1	73	5.1	74	5.1	74
Finland	7.4	103	2.8	38	5.1	71
France, Bas Rhin	4.0	59	3.1	46	3.5	53
France, Paediatric Registries	6.3	93	3.6	56	5.0	75
German Democratic Republic	6.9	103	3.9	56	5.4	80
Great Britain, England and Wales	6.1	90	3.6	53	4.9	72
Great Britain, Manchester (period 1)	6.5	94	2.9	41	4.7	68
Great Britain, Manchester (period 2)	6.4	95	4.9	73	5.7	85
Great Britain, Scotland	6.2	91	4.9	72	5.6	81
Hungary	3.4	50	2.4	36	2.9	43
Italy, Torino	7.6	112	4.5	66	6.1	90
Netherlands, DCLSG						
Netherlands, SOOZ, Eindhoven	3.5	47	2.3	32	2.9	40
Norway	5.9	87	2.4	36	4.2	62
Poland, Warsaw City	5.1	76	1.4	20	3.3	49
Spain, Zaragoza	4.3	62	2.3	34	3.3	49
Sweden	8.0	114	4.8	73	6.4	94
Switzerland, Three Western Cantons	3.1	47	2.2	33	2.7	40
Yugoslavia, Slovenia	7.2	103	2.5	36	4.9	70
OCEANIA						
Australia, New South Wales	7.5	106	3.6	52	5.6	80
Australia, Queensland	5.6	78	4.7	69	5.1	74
Fiji, Fijian						
Fiji, Indian						
New Zealand, Maori	13.3	201	7.3	105	10.3	154
New Zealand, non Maori	8.6	126	4.3	62	6.5	95

* Light when fewer than 10 cases

AGE STANDARDIZED AND CUMULATIVE (0-14) INCIDENCE RATES PER MILLION

Sympathetic nervous system tumours

	Male ASR	CUM	Female ASR	CUM	Both ASR	CUM
AFRICA						
Nigeria, Ibadan	9.8	135	2.2	31	6.0	83
Uganda, Kampala	1.1	19	2.2	38	1.7	29
Zimbabwe, Bulawayo, Residents only	11.1	148	4.8	62	8.0	106
AMERICA : NORTH						
Canada, Atlantic Provinces	7.7	106	5.7	77	6.8	92
Canada, Western Provinces	11.3	151	10.1	134	10.7	142
USA, Greater Delaware Valley, White	12.8	170	8.7	117	10.8	144
USA, Greater Delaware Valley, non White	6.1	84	5.5	77	5.8	81
USA, Los Angeles, Black	10.6	145	9.0	122	9.8	133
USA, Los Angeles, Hispanic	4.2	54	7.2	95	5.7	74
USA, Los Angeles, Other White	9.3	124	9.9	130	9.6	127
USA, New York (City and State), White	11.4	153	10.8	144	11.1	149
USA, New York (City and State), Black	8.7	117	6.2	84	7.4	100
USA, SEER, White	12.8	171	12.6	168	12.7	169
USA, SEER, Black	10.0	132	10.8	145	10.4	139
AMERICA : OTHER						
Brazil, Fortaleza	6.8	88	5.2	74	6.0	81
Brazil, Recife	6.9	96	5.4	78	6.2	87
Brazil, Sao Paulo	9.0	126	6.6	90	7.8	108
Colombia, Cali	5.7	73	6.3	86	6.0	80
Costa Rica	5.6	76	4.2	55	4.9	66
Cuba	6.1	84	4.2	58	5.2	72
Jamaica	9.1	124	8.1	115	8.6	120
Puerto Rico	7.3	100	5.8	76	6.6	88
ASIA						
China, Shanghai	5.5	75	3.5	48	4.6	62
China, Taipei	4.5	60	2.7	37	3.6	49
Hong Kong	6.1	83	3.8	53	5.0	68
India, Bangalore	6.7	94	3.0	44	4.8	69
India, Bombay Cancer Registry	3.8	54	2.5	33	3.2	44
Israel, Jews	14.9	203	10.7	144	12.8	174
Israel, non Jews	9.7	125	7.0	96	8.4	111
Japan, Kanagawa	7.8	105	6.3	84	7.0	95
Japan, Miyagi	7.3	96	6.9	94	7.1	95
Japan, Osaka	10.1	135	7.9	106	9.0	121
Kuwait, Kuwaiti	5.8	79	4.9	71	5.4	75
Kuwait, non Kuwaiti	7.1	102	13.4	175	10.2	138
Philippines, Metro Manila & Rizal	0.5	7	1.5	20	1.0	13
Singapore, Chinese	7.0	92	4.1	57	5.6	75
Singapore, Malay	1.0	15	5.3	73	3.1	43
EUROPE						
Czechoslovakia, Slovakia	4.7	62	6.0	82	5.3	72
Denmark	10.0	134	9.9	135	10.0	135
FRG, Children's Tumour Registry	10.4	137	9.9	132	10.1	135
FRG, Saarland	5.6	77	8.4	111	7.0	94
Finland	9.2	124	9.4	125	9.3	124
France, Bas Rhin	16.7	232	6.5	84	11.7	160
France, Paediatric Registries	17.7	231	10.8	141	14.3	187
German Democratic Republic	9.8	131	7.0	95	8.4	114
Great Britain, England and Wales	7.9	107	6.3	85	7.1	96
Great Britain, Manchester (period 1)	8.2	111	5.3	71	6.8	91
Great Britain, Manchester (period 2)	7.3	96	8.0	106	7.6	101
Great Britain, Scotland	9.3	126	6.4	86	7.9	106
Hungary	11.3	151	9.0	121	10.2	137
Italy, Torino	12.3	164	10.1	138	11.2	151
Netherlands, DCLSG	7.4	98	8.2	106	7.8	102
Netherlands, SOOZ, Eindhoven	7.4	102	6.6	88	7.0	95
Norway	9.4	129	4.6	65	7.1	98
Poland, Warsaw City	11.6	156	7.8	101	9.8	129
Spain, Zaragoza	10.3	137	8.5	113	9.5	125
Sweden	15.9	209	9.5	125	12.8	168
Switzerland, Three Western Cantons	6.0	82	5.0	65	5.5	73
Yugoslavia, Slovenia						
OCEANIA						
Australia, New South Wales	11.3	149	9.4	126	10.4	138
Australia, Queensland	11.5	155	8.9	119	10.2	137
Fiji, Fijian	2.2	33	3.4	53	2.8	43
Fiji, Indian	2.0	26	–	–	1.0	13
New Zealand, Maori	17.3	231	10.0	135	13.7	184
New Zealand, non Maori	7.6	106	8.4	113	8.0	109

* Light when fewer than 10 cases

AGE STANDARDIZED AND CUMULATIVE (0-14) INCIDENCE RATES PER MILLION

Neuroblastoma

	Male ASR	CUM	Female ASR	CUM	Both ASR	CUM
AFRICA						
Nigeria, Ibadan						
Uganda, Kampala						
Zimbabwe, Bulawayo, Residents only						
AMERICA : NORTH						
Canada, Atlantic Provinces	7.5	102	5.7	77	6.6	90
Canada, Western Provinces	11.1	147	10.0	132	10.5	140
USA, Greater Delaware Valley, White	12.8	170	8.7	117	10.8	144
USA, Greater Delaware Valley, non White	6.1	84	5.5	77	5.8	81
USA, Los Angeles, Black	10.6	145	9.0	122	9.8	133
USA, Los Angeles, Hispanic	4.2	54	6.9	91	5.5	72
USA, Los Angeles, Other White	9.1	121	9.7	128	9.4	124
USA, New York (City and State), White	11.2	150	10.8	144	11.0	147
USA, New York (City and State), Black	8.7	117	6.2	84	7.4	100
USA, SEER, White	12.6	168	12.3	164	12.5	166
USA, SEER, Black	9.6	127	10.8	145	10.2	136
AMERICA : OTHER						
Brazil, Fortaleza	6.8	88	5.2	74	6.0	81
Brazil, Recife	6.9	96	5.4	78	6.2	87
Brazil, Sao Paulo	9.0	126	6.5	89	7.8	107
Colombia, Cali	5.7	73	5.2	72	5.4	72
Costa Rica	5.1	69	4.2	55	4.6	62
Cuba	6.1	84	4.2	58	5.2	72
Jamaica	8.3	114	8.1	115	8.2	115
Puerto Rico	7.1	97	5.4	70	6.3	83
ASIA						
China, Shanghai	5.4	73	3.5	48	4.5	61
China, Taipei	4.5	60	2.7	37	3.6	49
Hong Kong	6.1	83	3.8	53	5.0	68
India, Bangalore	6.7	94	3.0	44	4.8	69
India, Bombay Cancer Registry	3.8	54	2.4	32	3.1	43
Israel, Jews	14.6	200	10.4	140	12.6	171
Israel, non Jews	9.7	125	7.0	96	8.4	111
Japan, Kanagawa	7.8	105	6.0	81	6.9	93
Japan, Miyagi	7.3	96	6.9	94	7.1	95
Japan, Osaka	10.1	135	7.9	106	9.0	121
Kuwait, Kuwaiti	5.8	79	4.9	71	5.4	75
Kuwait, non Kuwaiti	7.1	102	13.4	175	10.2	138
Philippines, Metro Manila & Rizal	0.5	7	1.5	20	1.0	13
Singapore, Chinese	7.0	92	3.9	54	5.5	74
Singapore, Malay	1.0	15	5.3	73	3.1	43
EUROPE						
Czechoslovakia, Slovakia	4.5	60	5.8	79	5.2	69
Denmark	9.2	123	9.9	135	9.6	129
FRG, Children's Tumour Registry	10.4	137	9.8	131	10.1	134
FRG, Saarland	5.6	77	8.4	111	7.0	94
Finland	9.0	121	9.4	125	9.2	123
France, Bas Rhin	16.7	232	6.5	84	11.7	160
France, Paediatric Registries	16.9	222	10.0	131	13.5	177
German Democratic Republic	9.8	131	6.8	91	8.3	112
Great Britain, England and Wales	7.8	105	6.1	83	7.0	94
Great Britain, Manchester (period 1)	8.2	111	5.3	71	6.8	91
Great Britain, Manchester (period 2)	7.3	96	7.8	103	7.5	99
Great Britain, Scotland	8.7	118	6.4	86	7.6	102
Hungary	11.0	148	8.7	118	9.9	133
Italy, Torino	12.3	164	10.1	138	11.2	151
Netherlands, DCLSG						
Netherlands, SOOZ, Eindhoven	7.4	98	8.2	106	7.8	102
Norway	7.4	102	6.6	88	7.0	95
Poland, Warsaw City	9.4	129	4.6	65	7.1	98
Spain, Zaragoza	11.6	156	7.8	101	9.8	129
Sweden	10.2	136	8.4	112	9.3	124
Switzerland, Three Western Cantons	15.9	209	8.4	109	12.3	160
Yugoslavia, Slovenia	6.0	82	5.0	65	5.5	73
OCEANIA						
Australia, New South Wales	11.3	149	9.3	124	10.3	137
Australia, Queensland	11.5	155	8.9	119	10.2	137
Fiji, Fijian						
Fiji, Indian						
New Zealand, Maori	17.3	231	10.0	135	13.7	184
New Zealand, non Maori	7.3	102	8.2	109	7.8	106

* Light when fewer than 10 cases

AGE STANDARDIZED AND CUMULATIVE (0-14) INCIDENCE RATES PER MILLION

Retinoblastoma

	Male ASR	Male CUM	Female ASR	Female CUM	Both ASR	Both CUM
AFRICA						
Nigeria, Ibadan	6.5	87	8.7	116	7.6	101
Uganda, Kampala	9.3	120	4.9	63	7.1	92
Zimbabwe, Bulawayo, Residents only	4.6	60	7.2	93	5.9	76
AMERICA : NORTH						
Canada, Atlantic Provinces	2.0	25	2.1	27	2.0	26
Canada, Western Provinces	4.7	61	4.3	57	4.5	59
USA, Greater Delaware Valley, White	6.0	78	3.9	51	5.0	65
USA, Greater Delaware Valley, non White	5.4	70	7.3	96	6.4	83
USA, Los Angeles, Black	5.3	68	4.6	61	4.9	65
USA, Los Angeles, Hispanic	5.7	74	6.7	87	6.2	80
USA, Los Angeles, Other White	5.8	76	4.0	53	4.9	65
USA, New York (City and State), White	2.6	34	2.7	35	2.7	35
USA, New York (City and State), Black	3.2	41	2.0	28	2.6	34
USA, SEER, White	3.7	48	4.4	57	4.0	52
USA, SEER, Black	4.8	63	5.5	71	5.1	67
AMERICA : OTHER						
Brazil, Fortaleza	5.6	73	11.0	149	8.3	111
Brazil, Recife	5.5	74	4.6	61	5.1	68
Brazil, Sao Paulo	5.5	72	6.3	83	5.9	78
Colombia, Cali	4.5	58	8.9	117	6.7	88
Costa Rica	3.4	44	4.0	54	3.7	49
Cuba	3.7	49	3.6	47	3.6	48
Jamaica	5.1	66	4.4	57	4.8	61
Puerto Rico	4.0	53	4.2	54	4.1	54
ASIA						
China, Shanghai	3.0	39	2.9	38	2.9	38
China, Taipei	2.3	29	2.0	25	2.1	27
Hong Kong	4.4	57	2.7	34	3.6	46
India, Bangalore	3.1	42	3.3	42	3.2	42
India, Bombay Cancer Registry	6.2	83	4.2	56	5.2	69
Israel, Jews	2.8	36	3.4	44	3.1	40
Israel, non Jews	3.6	49	3.2	41	3.4	45
Japan, Kanagawa	3.1	41	2.3	30	2.7	36
Japan, Miyagi	5.3	68	3.3	43	4.3	56
Japan, Osaka	5.7	74	4.8	63	5.3	68
Kuwait, Kuwaiti	1.9	24	2.9	38	2.4	31
Kuwait, non Kuwaiti	5.9	79	2.1	27	4.0	53
Philippines, Metro Manila & Rizal	4.1	55	6.7	88	5.4	71
Singapore, Chinese	2.4	32	5.8	75	4.1	53
Singapore, Malay	2.8	36	–	–	1.4	19
EUROPE						
Czechoslovakia, Slovakia	5.4	71	4.9	64	5.1	67
Denmark	2.4	31	2.0	26	2.2	28
FRG, Children's Tumour Registry	2.8	37	3.8	50	3.3	43
FRG, Saarland	2.1	27	0.7	10	1.4	19
Finland	6.4	85	3.1	41	4.8	64
France, Bas Rhin	1.3	16	3.9	51	2.6	33
France, Paediatric Registries	4.5	59	3.1	40	3.8	50
German Democratic Republic	3.4	45	3.9	51	3.7	48
Great Britain, England and Wales	3.4	44	3.6	47	3.5	45
Great Britain, Manchester (period 1)	3.4	44	3.7	49	3.6	47
Great Britain, Manchester (period 2)	2.2	29	2.1	27	2.2	28
Great Britain, Scotland	4.3	55	3.4	44	3.9	50
Hungary	1.2	16	2.1	27	1.6	21
Italy, Torino	4.2	55	4.2	56	4.2	55
Netherlands, DCLSG						
Netherlands, SOOZ, Eindhoven	0.9	13	9.6	124	5.1	67
Norway	3.5	45	3.2	41	3.3	43
Poland, Warsaw City	6.8	88	1.4	18	4.2	54
Spain, Zaragoza	–	–	–	–	–	–
Sweden	4.9	64	4.9	63	4.9	64
Switzerland, Three Western Cantons	–	–	5.5	72	2.7	35
Yugoslavia, Slovenia	1.1	14	3.2	43	2.1	28
OCEANIA						
Australia, New South Wales	3.8	51	4.8	62	4.3	56
Australia, Queensland	6.7	86	4.7	60	5.7	74
Fiji, Fijian	4.8	65	2.7	35	3.8	50
Fiji, Indian	4.2	55	–	–	2.2	28
New Zealand, Maori	4.0	51	8.3	107	6.1	79
New Zealand, non Maori	4.5	58	6.7	89	5.6	73

* Light when fewer than 10 cases

AGE STANDARDIZED AND CUMULATIVE (0-14) INCIDENCE RATES PER MILLION

Kidney

	Male		Female		Both	
	ASR	CUM	ASR	CUM	ASR	CUM
AFRICA						
Nigeria, Ibadan	15.1	204	6.5	90	10.9	147
Uganda, Kampala	9.5	135	6.4	85	7.9	109
Zimbabwe, Bulawayo, Residents only	11.6	150	4.8	62	8.3	107
AMERICA : NORTH						
Canada, Atlantic Provinces	6.9	93	6.2	83	6.5	88
Canada, Western Provinces	8.2	110	7.4	100	7.8	105
USA, Greater Delaware Valley, White	8.2	110	7.0	95	7.6	103
USA, Greater Delaware Valley, non White	10.7	145	16.8	225	13.7	185
USA, Los Angeles, Black	10.1	138	13.6	186	11.8	162
USA, Los Angeles, Hispanic	5.9	79	10.4	144	8.1	111
USA, Los Angeles, Other White	9.4	125	10.6	146	10.0	135
USA, New York (City and State), White	7.7	104	8.7	119	8.2	111
USA, New York (City and State), Black	10.7	144	7.1	97	8.9	121
USA, SEER, White	8.0	109	10.0	137	9.0	123
USA, SEER, Black	11.3	157	13.6	191	12.4	174
AMERICA : OTHER						
Brazil, Fortaleza	4.0	55	16.6	228	10.3	142
Brazil, Recife	4.8	65	9.4	128	7.1	96
Brazil, Sao Paulo	9.2	125	9.2	127	9.2	126
Colombia, Cali	4.0	56	8.0	104	6.0	80
Costa Rica	3.9	53	7.0	99	5.4	76
Cuba	5.2	72	4.9	69	5.1	71
Jamaica	7.7	104	4.6	66	6.2	86
Puerto Rico	8.4	114	6.1	85	7.3	100
ASIA						
China, Shanghai	3.3	44	0.3	5	1.8	25
China, Taipei	3.2	45	3.2	43	3.2	44
Hong Kong	7.2	96	1.9	26	4.6	62
India, Bangalore	6.3	87	3.8	50	5.1	69
India, Bombay Cancer Registry	4.6	62	4.3	57	4.4	60
Israel, Jews	6.2	82	8.3	115	7.2	98
Israel, non Jews	4.5	58	4.7	64	4.6	61
Japan, Kanagawa	3.5	47	2.0	26	2.8	37
Japan, Miyagi	5.1	69	3.2	44	4.2	57
Japan, Osaka	5.6	74	3.4	45	4.5	60
Kuwait, Kuwaiti	4.8	69	5.8	76	5.3	72
Kuwait, non Kuwaiti	7.8	109	5.1	69	6.5	89
Philippines, Metro Manila & Rizal	3.0	41	5.7	76	4.3	58
Singapore, Chinese	4.2	56	3.3	43	3.8	50
Singapore, Malay	3.7	52	5.4	73	4.5	62
EUROPE						
Czechoslovakia, Slovakia	10.2	137	8.3	113	9.2	125
Denmark	8.5	120	10.1	140	9.3	130
FRG, Children's Tumour Registry	7.5	101	8.8	118	8.1	109
FRG, Saarland	8.6	119	6.6	90	7.6	104
Finland	11.6	156	9.5	129	10.6	143
France, Bas Rhin	15.4	207	8.6	115	12.1	162
France, Paediatric Registries	6.0	84	6.0	81	6.0	82
German Democratic Republic	6.9	93	8.6	117	7.7	104
Great Britain, England and Wales	7.1	96	7.7	103	7.4	99
Great Britain, Manchester (period 1)	6.1	83	5.8	76	5.9	80
Great Britain, Manchester (period 2)	6.9	92	7.1	95	7.0	93
Great Britain, Scotland	8.1	110	6.8	91	7.5	101
Hungary	7.3	99	6.4	86	6.9	93
Italy, Torino	7.1	95	8.2	106	7.6	101
Netherlands, DCLSG						
Netherlands, SOOZ, Eindhoven	7.4	98	3.6	49	5.6	74
Norway	9.4	127	7.0	96	8.3	112
Poland, Warsaw City	8.8	121	9.0	124	8.9	123
Spain, Zaragoza	9.0	124	4.7	66	6.9	96
Sweden	9.1	122	9.8	135	9.4	128
Switzerland, Three Western Cantons	5.6	80	10.4	140	8.0	110
Yugoslavia, Slovenia	8.4	115	6.4	86	7.4	101
OCEANIA						
Australia, New South Wales	6.8	92	8.4	114	7.6	103
Australia, Queensland	8.9	119	6.7	89	7.8	104
Fiji, Fijian	6.0	80	6.3	87	6.1	83
Fiji, Indian	-	-	4.3	58	2.1	28
New Zealand, Maori	9.5	127	7.8	105	8.7	116
New Zealand, non Maori	7.7	103	7.4	106	7.6	105

* Light when fewer than 10 cases

AGE STANDARDIZED AND CUMULATIVE (0-14) INCIDENCE RATES PER MILLION

Wilms' tumour

	Male ASR	Male CUM	Female ASR	Female CUM	Both ASR	Both CUM
AFRICA						
Nigeria, Ibadan						
Uganda, Kampala						
Zimbabwe, Bulawayo, Residents only						
AMERICA : NORTH						
Canada, Atlantic Provinces	6.6	88	5.9	78	6.3	84
Canada, Western Provinces	7.8	104	7.3	98	7.5	101
USA, Greater Delaware Valley, White	7.9	106	6.9	94	7.4	100
USA, Greater Delaware Valley, non White	10.7	145	16.8	225	13.7	185
USA, Los Angeles, Black	10.1	138	13.6	186	11.8	162
USA, Los Angeles, Hispanic	5.6	74	10.4	144	7.9	109
USA, Los Angeles, Other White	9.4	125	10.2	140	9.8	132
USA, New York (City and State), White	7.1	95	8.5	115	7.8	105
USA, New York (City and State), Black	8.9	118	6.7	90	7.8	104
USA, SEER, White	7.9	107	10.0	136	8.9	121
USA, SEER, Black	9.9	136	12.3	171	11.1	153
AMERICA : OTHER						
Brazil, Fortaleza	4.0	55	16.6	228	10.3	142
Brazil, Recife	4.4	60	8.0	107	6.2	83
Brazil, Sao Paulo	6.9	94	7.4	101	7.2	98
Colombia, Cali	4.0	56	8.0	104	6.0	80
Costa Rica	3.3	46	7.0	99	5.1	72
Cuba	5.0	69	4.8	67	4.9	68
Jamaica	7.7	104	4.6	66	6.2	86
Puerto Rico	8.2	111	6.1	85	7.2	98
ASIA						
China, Shanghai	0.9	12	–	–	0.5	6
China, Taipei	2.0	28	1.6	22	1.8	25
Hong Kong	6.9	92	1.9	26	4.5	60
India, Bangalore	6.3	87	3.8	50	5.1	69
India, Bombay Cancer Registry	3.7	50	3.9	51	3.8	51
Israel, Jews	6.2	82	7.4	100	6.8	91
Israel, non Jews	4.5	58	4.7	64	4.6	61
Japan, Kanagawa	2.1	28	1.2	16	1.7	23
Japan, Miyagi	3.7	48	2.2	29	3.0	38
Japan, Osaka	4.8	63	3.1	41	4.0	52
Kuwait, Kuwaiti	2.8	39	4.9	63	3.8	51
Kuwait, non Kuwaiti	6.9	94	5.1	69	6.0	82
Philippines, Metro Manila & Rizal	1.8	23	3.8	50	2.8	36
Singapore, Chinese	3.7	48	3.1	40	3.4	44
Singapore, Malay	2.8	36	2.9	38	2.9	37
EUROPE						
Czechoslovakia, Slovakia	9.3	125	7.4	101	8.4	113
Denmark	6.8	97	7.8	108	7.3	102
FRG, Children's Tumour Registry	7.4	98	8.7	117	8.0	107
FRG, Saarland	6.3	86	6.2	82	6.3	84
Finland	11.2	150	8.9	120	10.1	135
France, Bas Rhin	15.4	207	7.8	101	11.7	155
France, Paediatric Registries	5.5	75	6.0	81	5.7	78
German Democratic Republic	6.6	89	8.4	113	7.5	101
Great Britain, England and Wales	6.9	93	7.5	101	7.2	97
Great Britain, Manchester (period 1)	5.5	75	5.4	72	5.5	73
Great Britain, Manchester (period 2)	6.6	87	6.9	92	6.8	90
Great Britain, Scotland	8.1	110	6.4	86	7.3	98
Hungary	7.1	95	6.3	83	6.7	89
Italy, Torino	7.1	95	7.8	102	7.5	98
Netherlands, DCLSG						
Netherlands, SOOZ, Eindhoven	7.4	98	3.6	49	5.6	74
Norway	8.5	114	6.1	83	7.4	99
Poland, Warsaw City	8.2	111	9.0	124	8.6	117
Spain, Zaragoza	9.0	124	4.7	66	6.9	96
Sweden	8.8	118	9.7	133	9.2	126
Switzerland, Three Western Cantons	5.6	80	10.4	140	8.0	110
Yugoslavia, Slovenia	8.4	115	6.4	86	7.4	101
OCEANIA						
Australia, New South Wales	6.6	90	8.3	112	7.5	101
Australia, Queensland	8.9	119	6.7	89	7.8	104
Fiji, Fijian						
Fiji, Indian						
New Zealand, Maori	9.5	127	7.8	105	8.7	116
New Zealand, non Maori	6.9	92	6.9	98	6.9	95

* Light when fewer than 10 cases

AGE STANDARDIZED AND CUMULATIVE (0-14) INCIDENCE RATES PER MILLION

Liver

	Male ASR	CUM	Female ASR	CUM	Both ASR	CUM
AFRICA						
Nigeria, Ibadan	4.3	65	–	–	2.2	34
Uganda, Kampala	–	–	1.1	19	0.6	10
Zimbabwe, Bulawayo, Residents only	–	–	–	–	–	–
AMERICA : NORTH						
Canada, Atlantic Provinces	1.1	15	1.2	16	1.2	15
Canada, Western Provinces	2.1	29	0.9	12	1.5	21
USA, Greater Delaware Valley, White	1.5	21	0.8	10	1.1	16
USA, Greater Delaware Valley, non White	0.5	8	0.7	9	0.6	8
USA, Los Angeles, Black	2.0	28	1.3	20	1.6	23
USA, Los Angeles, Hispanic	3.0	43	1.3	19	2.2	31
USA, Los Angeles, Other White	1.3	19	1.4	21	1.4	20
USA, New York (City and State), White	1.1	16	1.3	18	1.2	17
USA, New York (City and State), Black	2.0	31	1.6	26	1.8	28
USA, SEER, White	2.1	29	1.1	16	1.6	23
USA, SEER, Black	1.0	15	1.7	22	1.4	19
AMERICA : OTHER						
Brazil, Fortaleza	1.4	18	–	–	0.7	9
Brazil, Recife	0.8	10	1.1	16	0.9	13
Brazil, Sao Paulo	2.0	28	0.3	5	1.2	16
Colombia, Cali	0.8	14	1.1	15	1.0	14
Costa Rica	2.6	43	1.8	25	2.2	34
Cuba	0.7	10	0.6	8	0.6	9
Jamaica	–	–	0.7	9	0.4	5
Puerto Rico	1.7	23	0.9	12	1.3	18
ASIA						
China, Shanghai	5.1	75	2.7	38	3.9	57
China, Taipei	6.4	98	1.3	19	4.0	60
Hong Kong	5.8	87	1.8	27	3.9	58
India, Bangalore	1.2	16	–	–	0.6	8
India, Bombay Cancer Registry	2.4	33	0.8	11	1.6	22
Israel, Jews	0.7	10	0.7	10	0.7	10
Israel, non Jews	–	–	–	–	–	–
Japan, Kanagawa	3.6	50	1.3	17	2.5	34
Japan, Miyagi	4.9	70	1.5	22	3.3	46
Japan, Osaka	3.3	45	2.9	39	3.1	42
Kuwait, Kuwaiti	–	–	1.0	13	0.5	6
Kuwait, non Kuwaiti	2.0	26	3.1	40	2.5	33
Philippines, Metro Manila & Rizal	1.4	21	0.6	10	1.1	15
Singapore, Chinese	3.4	44	2.0	26	2.7	36
Singapore, Malay	–	–	2.5	35	1.2	17
EUROPE						
Czechoslovakia, Slovakia	1.8	26	0.9	13	1.3	19
Denmark	1.8	24	2.6	37	2.2	30
FRG, Children's Tumour Registry	1.2	16	1.0	13	1.1	15
FRG, Saarland	0.4	7	–	–	0.2	4
Finland	1.4	18	1.0	15	1.2	16
France, Bas Rhin	0.8	13	–	–	0.4	7
France, Paediatric Registries	2.1	29	2.8	39	2.4	34
German Democratic Republic	1.2	16	0.4	6	0.8	11
Great Britain, England and Wales	0.9	13	1.1	15	1.0	14
Great Britain, Manchester (period 1)	0.7	9	0.1	2	0.4	6
Great Britain, Manchester (period 2)	1.2	16	0.8	11	1.0	13
Great Britain, Scotland	0.8	10	0.9	11	0.8	11
Hungary	0.9	13	1.1	14	1.0	14
Italy, Torino	2.4	32	1.7	25	2.1	29
Netherlands, DCLSG						
Netherlands, SOOZ, Eindhoven	1.3	17	–	–	0.7	9
Norway	3.3	45	0.5	7	1.9	26
Poland, Warsaw City	1.3	18	1.5	19	1.4	19
Spain, Zaragoza	7.4	109	–	–	3.8	56
Sweden	1.5	21	1.7	23	1.6	22
Switzerland, Three Western Cantons	1.4	18	–	–	0.7	9
Yugoslavia, Slovenia	2.6	34	0.6	7	1.6	21
OCEANIA						
Australia, New South Wales	1.0	15	1.2	15	1.1	15
Australia, Queensland	1.2	17	1.0	17	1.1	17
Fiji, Fijian	3.6	47	4.6	68	4.1	57
Fiji, Indian	1.1	14	1.0	13	1.0	13
New Zealand, Maori	3.0	52	–	–	1.5	26
New Zealand, non Maori	1.3	19	1.5	20	1.4	19

* Light when fewer than 10 cases

AGE STANDARDIZED AND CUMULATIVE (0–14) INCIDENCE RATES PER MILLION

Hepatoblastoma

	Male ASR	Male CUM	Female ASR	Female CUM	Both ASR	Both CUM
AFRICA						
Nigeria, Ibadan						
Uganda, Kampala						
Zimbabwe, Bulawayo, Residents only						
AMERICA : NORTH						
Canada, Atlantic Provinces	0.4	5	0.4	5	0.4	5
Canada, Western Provinces	1.0	14	0.4	6	**0.7**	**10**
USA, Greater Delaware Valley, White	1.0	14	0.3	4	0.7	9
USA, Greater Delaware Valley, non White	–	–	0.7	9	0.3	4
USA, Los Angeles, Black	1.5	19	0.8	11	1.1	15
USA, Los Angeles, Hispanic	1.8	24	0.7	9	1.3	17
USA, Los Angeles, Other White	1.1	16	0.6	9	0.9	13
USA, New York (City and State), White	0.9	13	1.2	17	1.1	14
USA, New York (City and State), Black	1.0	13	0.4	7	0.7	10
USA, SEER, White	**1.5**	**19**	**0.6**	**8**	**1.1**	**14**
USA, SEER, Black	0.7	10	1.3	16	1.0	13
AMERICA : OTHER						
Brazil, Fortaleza	1.4	18	–	–	0.7	9
Brazil, Recife	0.4	5	0.8	10	0.6	7
Brazil, Sao Paulo	0.9	11	0.1	1	0.5	7
Colombia, Cali	–	–	1.1	15	0.6	7
Costa Rica	0.6	9	1.2	16	0.9	12
Cuba	–	–	–	–	–	–
Jamaica	–	–	0.7	9	0.4	5
Puerto Rico	1.1	15	0.7	9	0.9	12
ASIA						
China, Shanghai	0.9	12	0.7	11	0.8	11
China, Taipei	1.2	16	0.4	6	0.8	11
Hong Kong	0.8	12	0.3	4	0.5	8
India, Bangalore	–	–	–	–	–	–
India, Bombay Cancer Registry	**1.6**	**21**	0.4	6	**1.0**	**13**
Israel, Jews	0.5	6	–	–	0.2	3
Israel, non Jews	–	–	–	–	–	–
Japan, Kanagawa	1.6	21	0.8	10	**1.2**	**16**
Japan, Miyagi	0.5	7	–	–	0.3	3
Japan, Osaka	**2.0**	**27**	1.3	17	1.6	22
Kuwait, Kuwaiti	–	–	1.0	13	0.5	6
Kuwait, non Kuwaiti	2.0	26	2.1	27	2.0	26
Philippines, Metro Manila & Rizal	–	–	–	–	–	–
Singapore, Chinese	1.6	20	1.4	18	1.5	19
Singapore, Malay	–	–	–	–	–	–
EUROPE						
Czechoslovakia, Slovakia	1.1	16	0.9	13	**1.0**	**14**
Denmark	1.5	19	2.3	32	1.9	25
FRG, Children's Tumour Registry	**0.9**	**12**	**1.0**	**13**	**0.9**	**12**
FRG, Saarland	–	–	–	–	–	–
Finland	1.2	16	0.5	6	0.9	11
France, Bas Rhin	0.8	13	–	–	0.4	7
France, Paediatric Registries	2.1	29	1.5	20	1.8	24
German Democratic Republic	–	–	0.2	2	0.1	1
Great Britain, England and Wales	**0.8**	**10**	**0.9**	**12**	**0.8**	**11**
Great Britain, Manchester (period 1)	0.7	9	0.1	2	0.4	6
Great Britain, Manchester (period 2)	1.2	16	0.7	9	1.0	12
Great Britain, Scotland	0.2	3	0.9	11	0.5	7
Hungary	0.4	6	0.5	6	**0.5**	**6**
Italy, Torino	1.8	24	1.0	13	1.4	19
Netherlands, DCLSG						
Netherlands, SOOZ, Eindhoven	–	–	–	–	–	–
Norway	1.2	16	0.3	3	0.7	10
Poland, Warsaw City	0.6	10	1.5	19	1.1	14
Spain, Zaragoza	4.4	62	–	–	2.3	32
Sweden	0.6	7	0.6	8	**0.6**	**7**
Switzerland, Three Western Cantons	1.4	18	–	–	0.7	9
Yugoslavia, Slovenia	2.6	34	0.6	7	1.6	21
OCEANIA						
Australia, New South Wales	0.5	6	0.5	7	0.5	7
Australia, Queensland	0.5	6	0.7	11	0.6	9
Fiji, Fijian						
Fiji, Indian						
New Zealand, Maori	–	–	–	–	–	–
New Zealand, non Maori	0.6	8	0.6	8	0.6	8

* Light when fewer than 10 cases

AGE STANDARDIZED AND CUMULATIVE (0-14) INCIDENCE RATES PER MILLION

Hepatic carcinoma

	Male ASR	CUM	Female ASR	CUM	Both ASR	CUM
AFRICA						
Nigeria, Ibadan						
Uganda, Kampala						
Zimbabwe, Bulawayo, Residents only						
AMERICA : NORTH						
Canada, Atlantic Provinces	0.3	4	0.4	5	0.3	5
Canada, Western Provinces	1.0	13	0.5	6	**0.7**	**10**
USA, Greater Delaware Valley, White	0.3	5	0.4	6	0.4	6
USA, Greater Delaware Valley, non White	0.5	8	–	–	0.3	4
USA, Los Angeles, Black	0.5	9	0.5	9	0.5	9
USA, Los Angeles, Hispanic	1.2	18	0.6	10	0.9	14
USA, Los Angeles, Other White	0.2	3	0.8	12	0.5	8
USA, New York (City and State), White	0.1	2	0.1	1	0.1	2
USA, New York (City and State), Black	1.0	18	0.4	6	0.7	12
USA, SEER, White	**0.6**	**9**	**0.5**	**8**	0.5	8
USA, SEER, Black	0.3	5	0.4	5	0.4	5
AMERICA : OTHER						
Brazil, Fortaleza	–	–	–	–	–	–
Brazil, Recife	0.4	5	–	–	0.2	2
Brazil, Sao Paulo	0.9	13	0.2	3	**0.6**	**8**
Colombia, Cali	0.8	14	–	–	0.4	7
Costa Rica	2.0	35	0.6	9	1.3	22
Cuba	0.4	6	0.4	6	**0.4**	**6**
Jamaica	–	–	–	–	–	–
Puerto Rico	0.2	3	–	–	0.1	1
ASIA						
China, Shanghai	0.3	5	0.1	2	0.2	3
China, Taipei	**1.9**	**31**	0.4	6	**1.2**	**19**
Hong Kong	**3.7**	**57**	0.4	7	**2.1**	**33**
India, Bangalore	1.2	16	–	–	0.6	8
India, Bombay Cancer Registry	0.5	8	0.1	1	0.3	5
Israel, Jews	0.2	4	0.5	7	0.3	5
Israel, non Jews	–	–	–	–	–	–
Japan, Kanagawa	0.2	4	0.2	3	0.2	3
Japan, Miyagi	2.9	42	1.0	15	2.0	29
Japan, Osaka	0.3	5	0.2	3	0.3	4
Kuwait, Kuwaiti	–	–	–	–	–	–
Kuwait, non Kuwaiti	–	–	1.0	13	0.5	7
Philippines, Metro Manila & Rizal	0.6	9	–	–	0.3	4
Singapore, Chinese	0.2	3	0.7	9	0.4	6
Singapore, Malay	–	–	1.5	19	0.7	9
EUROPE						
Czechoslovakia, Slovakia	0.5	7	–	–	0.3	4
Denmark	0.3	5	0.3	5	0.3	5
FRG, Children's Tumour Registry	0.3	4	–	1	0.2	3
FRG, Saarland	0.4	7	–	–	0.2	4
Finland	0.1	3	0.5	8	0.3	5
France, Bas Rhin	–	–	–	–	–	–
France, Paediatric Registries	–	–	1.3	19	0.6	9
German Democratic Republic	1.0	14	0.3	4	**0.6**	**9**
Great Britain, England and Wales	**0.2**	**3**	**0.2**	**3**	**0.2**	**3**
Great Britain, Manchester (period 1)	–	–	–	–	–	–
Great Britain, Manchester (period 2)	–	–	0.1	2	0.1	1
Great Britain, Scotland	0.6	8	–	–	0.3	4
Hungary	0.4	6	0.6	8	**0.5**	**7**
Italy, Torino	0.2	4	0.5	8	0.4	6
Netherlands, DCLSG						
Netherlands, SOOZ, Eindhoven	1.3	17	–	–	0.7	9
Norway	1.8	26	0.3	4	1.1	15
Poland, Warsaw City	–	–	–	–	–	–
Spain, Zaragoza	1.2	16	–	–	0.6	8
Sweden	**0.9**	**14**	**1.1**	**16**	**1.0**	**15**
Switzerland, Three Western Cantons	–	–	–	–	–	–
Yugoslavia, Slovenia	–	–	–	–	–	–
OCEANIA						
Australia, New South Wales	0.5	8	0.6	9	0.6	8
Australia, Queensland	0.8	11	0.4	6	0.6	8
Fiji, Fijian						
Fiji, Indian						
New Zealand, Maori	3.0	52	–	–	1.5	26
New Zealand, non Maori	0.7	11	0.8	12	0.8	11

* Light when fewer than 10 cases

AGE STANDARDIZED AND CUMULATIVE (0-14) INCIDENCE RATES PER MILLION

Bone

	Male ASR	CUM	Female ASR	CUM	Both ASR	CUM
AFRICA						
Nigeria, Ibadan	2.1	37	3.4	52	2.8	45
Uganda, Kampala	5.4	91	9.6	164	7.5	128
Zimbabwe, Bulawayo, Residents only	1.8	28	2.1	36	2.0	33
AMERICA : NORTH						
Canada, Atlantic Provinces	4.1	68	5.3	86	4.7	77
Canada, Western Provinces	5.4	88	4.1	67	4.8	78
USA, Greater Delaware Valley, White	4.8	80	5.3	86	5.1	83
USA, Greater Delaware Valley, non White	5.2	85	4.7	78	4.9	82
USA, Los Angeles, Black	5.4	90	6.0	100	5.7	95
USA, Los Angeles, Hispanic	2.7	44	7.4	124	5.0	84
USA, Los Angeles, Other White	5.8	93	6.2	100	6.0	96
USA, New York (City and State), White	5.6	92	5.6	92	5.6	92
USA, New York (City and State), Black	4.3	70	4.2	70	4.3	70
USA, SEER, White	5.4	88	5.6	91	5.5	90
USA, SEER, Black	4.2	69	4.5	75	4.3	72
AMERICA : OTHER						
Brazil, Fortaleza	5.4	85	8.8	146	7.2	117
Brazil, Recife	3.1	50	6.9	115	5.0	83
Brazil, Sao Paulo	8.6	143	6.7	109	7.7	126
Colombia, Cali	3.1	54	3.0	52	3.1	53
Costa Rica	3.1	52	3.7	63	3.4	57
Cuba	3.0	49	3.1	51	3.1	50
Jamaica	4.0	68	2.6	41	3.3	54
Puerto Rico	4.2	70	3.9	63	4.1	67
ASIA						
China, Shanghai	2.1	36	5.2	86	3.6	60
China, Taipei	2.2	36	1.6	28	1.9	32
Hong Kong	4.2	69	4.6	73	4.4	71
India, Bangalore	3.9	66	-	-	1.9	33
India, Bombay Cancer Registry	4.9	81	4.3	71	4.6	76
Israel, Jews	6.4	102	5.8	92	6.1	97
Israel, non Jews	2.2	36	5.7	86	3.9	60
Japan, Kanagawa	2.6	42	2.0	34	2.3	38
Japan, Miyagi	3.1	50	5.1	82	4.1	66
Japan, Osaka	3.7	59	3.9	64	3.8	61
Kuwait, Kuwaiti	5.0	82	6.1	95	5.5	88
Kuwait, non Kuwaiti	11.3	184	3.0	47	7.2	117
Philippines, Metro Manila & Rizal	3.3	54	6.1	102	4.7	79
Singapore, Chinese	4.2	70	4.9	78	4.5	74
Singapore, Malay	4.1	65	4.7	79	4.4	72
EUROPE						
Czechoslovakia, Slovakia	4.9	77	6.1	98	5.5	87
Denmark	4.3	68	6.1	98	5.2	83
FRG, Children's Tumour Registry	5.6	90	4.5	73	5.1	82
FRG, Saarland	7.8	128	11.0	172	9.4	150
Finland	6.6	105	4.8	76	5.7	91
France, Bas Rhin	4.2	70	6.4	104	5.3	86
France, Paediatric Registries	4.1	69	5.1	83	4.6	76
German Democratic Republic	7.8	123	5.7	93	6.8	108
Great Britain, England and Wales	4.9	80	4.2	68	4.5	74
Great Britain, Manchester (period 1)	4.4	72	5.6	93	5.0	82
Great Britain, Manchester (period 2)	3.8	62	5.0	83	4.4	72
Great Britain, Scotland	3.2	52	4.9	79	4.0	65
Hungary	3.8	61	3.3	54	3.6	58
Italy, Torino	6.4	105	7.9	127	7.1	116
Netherlands, DCLSG						
Netherlands, SOOZ, Eindhoven	5.8	99	7.3	119	6.5	109
Norway	6.0	95	3.7	61	4.9	79
Poland, Warsaw City	3.5	60	3.9	61	3.7	60
Spain, Zaragoza	11.3	191	4.3	67	7.9	130
Sweden	5.8	96	6.2	100	6.0	98
Switzerland, Three Western Cantons	8.1	132	4.0	62	6.1	98
Yugoslavia, Slovenia	4.2	70	2.6	44	3.4	58
OCEANIA						
Australia, New South Wales	6.1	100	5.0	82	5.6	91
Australia, Queensland	4.6	71	4.1	63	4.3	68
Fiji, Fijian	2.0	34	3.1	54	2.6	44
Fiji, Indian	3.4	59	0.9	15	2.1	37
New Zealand, Maori	10.7	178	4.6	80	7.7	130
New Zealand, non Maori	4.3	69	8.0	130	6.1	99

* Light when fewer than 10 cases

AGE STANDARDIZED AND CUMULATIVE (0-14) INCIDENCE RATES PER MILLION

Osteosarcoma

	Male ASR	CUM	Female ASR	CUM	Both ASR	CUM
AFRICA						
Nigeria, Ibadan						
Uganda, Kampala						
Zimbabwe, Bulawayo, Residents only						
AMERICA : NORTH						
Canada, Atlantic Provinces	1.2	21	2.9	49	2.1	35
Canada, Western Provinces	2.5	43	1.5	26	2.0	35
USA, Greater Delaware Valley, White	2.4	41	2.4	38	2.4	40
USA, Greater Delaware Valley, non White	4.7	78	3.7	62	4.2	70
USA, Los Angeles, Black	4.9	81	4.3	72	4.6	77
USA, Los Angeles, Hispanic	1.2	21	5.6	93	3.4	57
USA, Los Angeles, Other White	2.5	40	2.1	33	2.3	37
USA, New York (City and State), White	2.4	39	2.9	48	2.6	43
USA, New York (City and State), Black	2.3	38	3.9	64	3.1	51
USA, SEER, White	2.3	38	2.7	45	2.5	41
USA, SEER, Black	3.0	49	3.8	64	3.4	57
AMERICA : OTHER						
Brazil, Fortaleza	2.8	48	6.3	103	4.6	76
Brazil, Recife	1.0	16	4.3	72	2.7	45
Brazil, Sao Paulo	4.2	70	3.7	62	3.9	66
Colombia, Cali	2.4	41	3.0	52	2.7	47
Costa Rica	1.1	17	2.1	36	1.6	27
Cuba	1.5	25	1.5	25	1.5	25
Jamaica	3.4	59	1.9	32	2.6	45
Puerto Rico	1.9	32	2.0	33	2.0	33
ASIA						
China, Shanghai	1.5	25	2.3	38	1.9	31
China, Taipei	1.9	31	1.3	22	1.6	27
Hong Kong	1.5	25	2.1	35	1.8	30
India, Bangalore	2.2	37	–	–	1.1	19
India, Bombay Cancer Registry	1.7	27	1.6	27	1.6	27
Israel, Jews	3.3	55	2.6	40	2.9	47
Israel, non Jews	1.6	27	2.4	37	2.0	32
Japan, Kanagawa	0.9	15	0.8	13	0.9	14
Japan, Miyagi	1.3	21	2.7	45	2.0	33
Japan, Osaka	2.3	37	1.9	32	2.1	34
Kuwait, Kuwaiti	3.1	54	2.1	37	2.6	45
Kuwait, non Kuwaiti	2.2	35	1.0	16	1.6	26
Philippines, Metro Manila & Rizal	1.2	21	3.0	52	2.1	36
Singapore, Chinese	2.4	40	3.4	57	2.9	48
Singapore, Malay	1.8	31	2.0	32	1.9	31
EUROPE						
Czechoslovakia, Slovakia	1.6	26	2.2	38	1.9	32
Denmark	1.5	25	2.1	36	1.8	31
FRG, Children's Tumour Registry	2.7	43	2.2	37	2.4	40
FRG, Saarland	3.1	50	4.3	69	3.7	59
Finland	3.5	58	2.8	45	3.2	52
France, Bas Rhin	–	–	4.4	72	2.2	35
France, Paediatric Registries	3.6	60	2.8	46	3.2	53
German Democratic Republic	2.6	42	3.2	52	2.9	47
Great Britain, England and Wales	2.6	43	2.4	39	2.5	41
Great Britain, Manchester (period 1)	1.9	31	2.5	42	2.2	37
Great Britain, Manchester (period 2)	2.1	34	2.8	47	2.4	41
Great Britain, Scotland	2.0	33	2.5	41	2.2	37
Hungary	1.2	20	1.7	29	1.5	25
Italy, Torino	2.8	46	4.8	78	3.8	62
Netherlands, DCLSG						
Netherlands, SOOZ, Eindhoven	2.8	49	4.7	78	3.8	63
Norway	3.5	58	2.2	35	2.8	47
Poland, Warsaw City	1.9	33	1.7	27	1.8	30
Spain, Zaragoza	7.4	128	3.3	50	5.4	90
Sweden	2.7	45	2.3	39	2.5	42
Switzerland, Three Western Cantons	4.6	75	0.9	15	2.8	45
Yugoslavia, Slovenia	2.6	42	0.9	15	1.7	29
OCEANIA						
Australia, New South Wales	2.9	49	2.5	41	2.7	45
Australia, Queensland	0.3	5	1.3	23	0.8	14
Fiji, Fijian						
Fiji, Indian						
New Zealand, Maori	1.5	26	1.5	27	1.5	26
New Zealand, non Maori	2.1	36	4.0	65	3.0	50

* Light when fewer than 10 cases

AGE STANDARDIZED AND CUMULATIVE (0-14) INCIDENCE RATES PER MILLION

Ewing's sarcoma

	Male ASR	CUM	Female ASR	CUM	Both ASR	CUM
AFRICA						
Nigeria, Ibadan						
Uganda, Kampala						
Zimbabwe, Bulawayo, Residents only						
AMERICA : NORTH						
Canada, Atlantic Provinces	2.6	43	1.8	28	2.2	35
Canada, Western Provinces	2.4	37	2.2	36	2.3	36
USA, Greater Delaware Valley, White	2.1	35	2.1	34	2.1	35
USA, Greater Delaware Valley, non White	-	-	0.5	8	0.3	4
USA, Los Angeles, Black	-	-	1.3	19	0.6	9
USA, Los Angeles, Hispanic	1.5	23	1.5	25	1.5	24
USA, Los Angeles, Other White	2.5	41	2.5	42	2.5	41
USA, New York (City and State), White	2.7	44	2.1	35	2.4	40
USA, New York (City and State), Black	0.4	7	-	-	0.2	3
USA, SEER, White	2.5	41	2.4	37	2.4	39
USA, SEER, Black	0.3	5	0.4	5	0.4	5
AMERICA : OTHER						
Brazil, Fortaleza	1.2	19	-	-	0.6	10
Brazil, Recife	1.0	17	2.0	33	1.5	25
Brazil, Sao Paulo	3.3	55	1.6	25	2.5	40
Colombia, Cali	0.8	14	-	-	0.4	7
Costa Rica	1.0	17	1.6	27	1.3	22
Cuba	1.1	17	1.1	18	1.1	18
Jamaica	0.6	10	-	-	0.3	5
Puerto Rico	1.6	26	1.3	21	1.5	24
ASIA						
China, Shanghai	0.3	4	0.4	7	0.3	6
China, Taipei	0.3	5	0.3	5	0.3	5
Hong Kong	0.4	6	0.5	8	0.4	7
India, Bangalore	1.1	19	-	-	0.6	10
India, Bombay Cancer Registry	2.3	38	2.0	33	2.1	36
Israel, Jews	2.2	35	1.8	31	2.0	33
Israel, non Jews	-	-	1.7	25	0.8	12
Japan, Kanagawa	0.2	4	0.3	5	0.2	4
Japan, Miyagi	0.4	7	0.9	15	0.7	11
Japan, Osaka	0.5	7	0.7	11	0.6	9
Kuwait, Kuwaiti	0.9	14	3.0	45	1.9	30
Kuwait, non Kuwaiti	7.9	128	-	-	4.1	66
Philippines, Metro Manila & Rizal	0.6	9	0.3	5	0.5	7
Singapore, Chinese	0.6	10	0.3	4	0.5	7
Singapore, Malay	1.4	18	-	-	0.7	9
EUROPE						
Czechoslovakia, Slovakia	2.4	36	2.0	31	2.2	34
Denmark	2.4	37	4.0	62	3.2	49
FRG, Children's Tumour Registry	2.3	37	2.2	34	2.2	35
FRG, Saarland	3.1	50	4.3	69	3.7	59
Finland	1.5	26	1.3	20	1.4	23
France, Bas Rhin	3.5	56	2.0	31	2.8	44
France, Paediatric Registries	0.5	8	1.7	27	1.1	18
German Democratic Republic	3.2	50	1.3	21	2.3	36
Great Britain, England and Wales	1.9	31	1.5	25	1.7	28
Great Britain, Manchester (period 1)	2.0	32	2.1	33	2.0	32
Great Britain, Manchester (period 2)	1.1	18	1.9	31	1.5	24
Great Britain, Scotland	1.0	17	2.3	36	1.6	26
Hungary	2.1	33	1.3	21	1.7	27
Italy, Torino	2.7	43	1.2	20	2.0	32
Netherlands, DCLSG						
Netherlands, SOOZ, Eindhoven	2.3	38	2.5	41	2.4	39
Norway	0.4	6	0.6	10	0.5	8
Poland, Warsaw City	1.1	18	0.5	9	0.8	14
Spain, Zaragoza	3.8	62	1.0	16	2.5	40
Sweden	2.3	37	2.3	38	2.3	38
Switzerland, Three Western Cantons	3.5	58	0.9	15	2.2	37
Yugoslavia, Slovenia	1.6	28	1.3	22	1.5	25
OCEANIA						
Australia, New South Wales	2.7	43	2.5	41	2.6	42
Australia, Queensland	3.1	50	2.7	41	2.9	45
Fiji, Fijian						
Fiji, Indian						
New Zealand, Maori	6.1	102	1.5	27	3.8	65
New Zealand, non Maori	1.4	22	2.9	46	2.1	34

* Light when fewer than 10 cases

AGE STANDARDIZED AND CUMULATIVE (0-14) INCIDENCE RATES PER MILLION

Soft tissue sarcomas

	Male ASR	CUM	Female ASR	CUM	Both ASR	CUM
AFRICA						
Nigeria, Ibadan	13.0	187	4.3	62	8.7	125
Uganda, Kampala	11.3	179	4.8	78	8.0	128
Zimbabwe, Bulawayo, Residents only	11.0	166	6.3	96	8.6	130
AMERICA : NORTH						
Canada, Atlantic Provinces	4.6	68	3.4	52	4.0	60
Canada, Western Provinces	8.3	124	7.3	110	7.8	117
USA, Greater Delaware Valley, White	8.9	130	7.8	116	8.4	123
USA, Greater Delaware Valley, non White	11.8	183	6.7	99	9.3	141
USA, Los Angeles, Black	9.0	134	5.5	85	7.3	110
USA, Los Angeles, Hispanic	10.7	153	9.8	148	10.2	151
USA, Los Angeles, Other White	11.4	176	10.4	153	10.9	165
USA, New York (City and State), White	9.0	131	8.8	129	8.9	130
USA, New York (City and State), Black	7.6	122	4.1	60	5.9	91
USA, SEER, White	9.0	135	8.2	123	8.6	129
USA, SEER, Black	9.4	143	7.2	113	8.3	128
AMERICA : OTHER						
Brazil, Fortaleza	5.4	85	6.2	107	5.9	98
Brazil, Recife	7.8	120	6.8	100	7.2	110
Brazil, Sao Paulo	9.5	136	6.6	98	8.0	117
Colombia, Cali	6.2	85	4.5	69	5.4	77
Costa Rica	6.1	87	6.5	91	6.3	89
Cuba	4.1	61	4.2	63	4.2	62
Jamaica	5.7	80	3.5	51	4.6	65
Puerto Rico	8.1	120	6.1	91	7.1	106
ASIA						
China, Shanghai	3.1	45	6.8	96	4.9	70
China, Taipei	3.8	56	2.3	36	3.1	46
Hong Kong	5.4	76	5.6	83	5.5	80
India, Bangalore	3.5	54	3.6	53	3.6	53
India, Bombay Cancer Registry	4.3	63	2.4	36	3.4	50
Israel, Jews	10.0	151	8.0	117	9.1	135
Israel, non Jews	3.8	56	4.9	69	4.3	62
Japan, Kanagawa	3.6	53	4.1	62	3.8	58
Japan, Miyagi	7.2	105	3.0	44	5.1	75
Japan, Osaka	4.8	68	4.9	70	4.8	69
Kuwait, Kuwaiti	4.8	71	3.0	45	3.9	58
Kuwait, non Kuwaiti	8.1	110	-	-	4.1	56
Philippines, Metro Manila & Rizal	3.3	48	4.4	64	3.8	55
Singapore, Chinese	4.7	69	4.8	70	4.7	70
Singapore, Malay	0.9	16	3.8	54	2.3	34
EUROPE						
Czechoslovakia, Slovakia	6.1	90	4.7	68	5.4	79
Denmark	9.7	134	2.9	44	6.3	90
FRG, Children's Tumour Registry	8.5	122	4.8	70	6.7	97
FRG, Saarland	6.4	94	7.3	103	6.8	98
Finland	7.4	106	6.2	93	6.8	100
France, Bas Rhin	9.0	133	5.5	78	7.3	106
France, Paediatric Registries	13.4	195	5.5	78	9.6	138
German Democratic Republic	9.7	140	9.2	132	9.5	136
Great Britain, England and Wales	7.3	106	5.5	81	6.4	94
Great Britain, Manchester (period 1)	7.2	104	4.9	70	6.1	87
Great Britain, Manchester (period 2)	6.0	84	4.0	57	5.0	71
Great Britain, Scotland	6.1	90	5.3	77	5.7	84
Hungary	6.5	92	4.1	60	5.3	77
Italy, Torino	9.1	133	5.8	82	7.5	108
Netherlands, DCLSG						
Netherlands, SOOZ, Eindhoven	6.6	98	11.0	156	8.8	126
Norway	4.2	62	7.8	112	6.0	87
Poland, Warsaw City	7.0	99	7.4	110	7.2	105
Spain, Zaragoza	13.1	204	9.6	133	11.4	169
Sweden	7.5	107	7.3	104	7.4	106
Switzerland, Three Western Cantons	11.0	160	5.6	83	8.4	122
Yugoslavia, Slovenia	9.5	145	5.5	80	7.5	113
OCEANIA						
Australia, New South Wales	10.4	152	5.6	83	8.1	118
Australia, Queensland	7.7	112	3.1	47	5.5	80
Fiji, Fijian	4.5	65	3.3	53	3.9	59
Fiji, Indian	2.7	42	1.9	28	2.3	35
New Zealand, Maori	6.7	99	3.1	53	4.9	77
New Zealand, non Maori	6.1	95	6.1	87	6.1	91

* Light when fewer than 10 cases

AGE STANDARDIZED AND CUMULATIVE (0-14) INCIDENCE RATES PER MILLION

Rhabdomyosarcoma

	Male ASR	CUM	Female ASR	CUM	Both ASR	CUM
AFRICA						
Nigeria, Ibadan						
Uganda, Kampala						
Zimbabwe, Bulawayo, Residents only						
AMERICA : NORTH						
Canada, Atlantic Provinces	3.4	50	2.4	37	2.9	44
Canada, Western Provinces	4.3	63	3.4	49	3.8	56
USA, Greater Delaware Valley, White	5.4	75	4.2	60	4.8	68
USA, Greater Delaware Valley, non White	5.3	81	3.0	42	4.2	61
USA, Los Angeles, Black	6.1	88	2.1	31	4.2	60
USA, Los Angeles, Hispanic	6.6	96	4.5	65	5.5	81
USA, Los Angeles, Other White	5.8	88	4.4	64	5.1	76
USA, New York (City and State), White	5.8	84	5.6	79	5.7	82
USA, New York (City and State), Black	4.6	71	2.2	33	3.4	52
USA, SEER, White	5.0	74	4.4	65	4.7	69
USA, SEER, Black	5.2	77	1.7	26	3.5	52
AMERICA : OTHER						
Brazil, Fortaleza	1.2	19	–	–	0.6	10
Brazil, Recife	2.5	35	2.9	42	2.7	38
Brazil, Sao Paulo	3.6	50	2.7	38	3.1	44
Colombia, Cali	2.3	29	2.5	40	2.4	35
Costa Rica	3.4	47	4.8	65	4.1	56
Cuba	1.9	27	2.0	30	1.9	29
Jamaica	2.9	38	2.8	40	2.9	39
Puerto Rico	3.8	56	3.7	54	3.8	55
ASIA						
China, Shanghai	1.6	22	4.2	56	2.9	38
China, Taipei	1.6	23	0.9	14	1.3	18
Hong Kong	2.3	32	2.0	28	2.2	30
India, Bangalore	2.9	44	2.3	36	2.6	40
India, Bombay Cancer Registry	1.9	26	1.5	21	1.7	24
Israel, Jews	4.5	66	2.6	37	3.6	52
Israel, non Jews	0.8	13	2.5	32	1.6	22
Japan, Kanagawa	2.1	29	2.1	33	2.1	31
Japan, Miyagi	3.5	48	1.5	22	2.5	36
Japan, Osaka	2.4	34	1.9	27	2.1	31
Kuwait, Kuwaiti	3.9	57	2.0	31	3.0	44
Kuwait, non Kuwaiti	4.0	51	–	–	2.0	26
Philippines, Metro Manila & Rizal	1.8	25	2.8	38	2.3	31
Singapore, Chinese	2.5	37	2.7	37	2.6	37
Singapore, Malay	–	–	0.9	16	0.5	8
EUROPE						
Czechoslovakia, Slovakia	1.5	21	0.6	7	1.1	14
Denmark	7.2	99	0.9	12	4.1	57
FRG, Children's Tumour Registry	6.3	90	2.9	41	4.7	66
FRG, Saarland	3.0	42	1.2	17	2.1	30
Finland	1.8	26	1.1	17	1.4	21
France, Bas Rhin	6.2	91	4.7	64	5.5	78
France, Paediatric Registries	9.9	141	3.6	50	6.8	97
German Democratic Republic	3.7	53	3.2	45	3.5	49
Great Britain, England and Wales	5.1	74	3.5	50	4.3	62
Great Britain, Manchester (period 1)	5.0	71	3.9	54	4.5	63
Great Britain, Manchester (period 2)	5.0	71	2.3	33	3.7	53
Great Britain, Scotland	3.7	53	2.6	37	3.2	45
Hungary	3.2	44	1.9	26	2.5	36
Italy, Torino	3.3	47	2.9	41	3.1	44
Netherlands, DCLSG						
Netherlands, SOOZ, Eindhoven	4.3	60	5.1	75	4.7	67
Norway	1.4	19	3.8	53	2.6	36
Poland, Warsaw City	5.8	82	5.0	73	5.4	78
Spain, Zaragoza	5.4	77	8.6	116	6.9	96
Sweden	2.1	32	2.3	31	2.2	32
Switzerland, Three Western Cantons	8.4	116	2.9	37	5.7	77
Yugoslavia, Slovenia	4.9	76	3.2	43	4.1	60
OCEANIA						
Australia, New South Wales	8.6	123	3.5	52	6.1	88
Australia, Queensland	5.5	78	2.3	35	3.9	57
Fiji, Fijian						
Fiji, Indian						
New Zealand, Maori	6.7	99	–	–	3.4	50
New Zealand, non Maori	4.0	62	4.6	63	4.3	63

* Light when fewer than 10 cases

AGE STANDARDIZED AND CUMULATIVE (0-14) INCIDENCE RATES PER MILLION

Fibrosarcoma

	Male ASR	CUM	Female ASR	CUM	Both ASR	CUM
AFRICA						
Nigeria, Ibadan						
Uganda, Kampala						
Zimbabwe, Bulawayo, Residents only						
AMERICA : NORTH						
Canada, Atlantic Provinces	0.9	14	0.5	9	0.7	11
Canada, Western Provinces	2.2	34	1.7	27	2.0	30
USA, Greater Delaware Valley, White	1.3	20	1.7	26	1.5	23
USA, Greater Delaware Valley, non White	3.0	47	1.1	16	2.0	32
USA, Los Angeles, Black	1.0	17	1.0	18	1.0	18
USA, Los Angeles, Hispanic	0.7	9	2.2	35	1.4	21
USA, Los Angeles, Other White	2.5	41	1.9	28	2.2	35
USA, New York (City and State), White	1.6	24	1.4	20	1.5	22
USA, New York (City and State), Black	1.6	26	1.5	20	1.5	23
USA, SEER, White	1.7	26	1.5	23	1.6	24
USA, SEER, Black	2.5	40	3.3	51	2.9	46
AMERICA : OTHER						
Brazil, Fortaleza	4.2	66	1.2	21	2.7	43
Brazil, Recife	1.0	18	0.7	11	0.8	14
Brazil, Sao Paulo	2.0	28	1.4	22	1.7	25
Colombia, Cali	1.1	15	2.0	28	1.6	21
Costa Rica	0.5	9	–	–	0.3	4
Cuba	0.3	5	0.3	5	0.3	5
Jamaica	0.7	9	–	–	0.4	5
Puerto Rico	1.1	18	0.5	9	0.8	13
ASIA						
China, Shanghai	0.7	11	0.7	12	0.7	12
China, Taipei	0.9	13	0.9	14	0.9	13
Hong Kong	2.7	40	2.2	34	2.5	37
India, Bangalore	–	–	–	–	–	–
India, Bombay Cancer Registry	1.4	22	0.6	9	1.0	15
Israel, Jews	1.1	16	3.5	52	2.3	33
Israel, non Jews	0.8	10	–	–	0.4	5
Japan, Kanagawa	0.5	7	0.2	4	0.4	6
Japan, Miyagi	0.4	7	0.6	7	0.5	7
Japan, Osaka	0.6	9	0.9	14	0.8	11
Kuwait, Kuwaiti	–	–	–	–	–	–
Kuwait, non Kuwaiti	1.0	13	–	–	0.5	7
Philippines, Metro Manila & Rizal	0.3	4	0.9	16	0.6	10
Singapore, Chinese	0.9	14	0.9	15	0.9	14
Singapore, Malay	–	–	1.5	19	0.7	9
EUROPE						
Czechoslovakia, Slovakia	1.1	17	1.2	17	1.1	17
Denmark	1.6	23	2.0	33	1.8	28
FRG, Children's Tumour Registry	0.8	12	0.6	10	0.7	11
FRG, Saarland	0.4	7	2.1	32	1.2	19
Finland	2.5	37	2.2	34	2.4	36
France, Bas Rhin	0.8	13	–	–	0.4	7
France, Paediatric Registries	1.8	27	0.7	10	1.3	19
German Democratic Republic	3.2	47	2.9	41	3.1	44
Great Britain, England and Wales	0.8	12	0.8	13	0.8	13
Great Britain, Manchester (period 1)	0.7	9	–	–	0.4	5
Great Britain, Manchester (period 2)	0.8	11	1.3	19	1.1	14
Great Britain, Scotland	0.7	10	0.8	14	0.8	12
Hungary	0.6	9	1.1	16	0.9	12
Italy, Torino	2.2	31	1.5	21	1.8	26
Netherlands, DCLSG						
Netherlands, SOOZ, Eindhoven	0.9	13	–	–	0.4	7
Norway	1.5	22	1.7	26	1.6	24
Poland, Warsaw City	0.7	9	0.7	10	0.7	10
Spain, Zaragoza	4.7	80	1.0	17	2.9	49
Sweden	2.0	28	1.5	22	1.8	25
Switzerland, Three Western Cantons	0.8	14	–	–	0.4	7
Yugoslavia, Slovenia	0.9	14	1.4	22	1.1	18
OCEANIA						
Australia, New South Wales	0.9	14	1.2	18	1.1	16
Australia, Queensland	1.2	17	0.5	6	0.9	12
Fiji, Fijian						
Fiji, Indian						
New Zealand, Maori	–	–	–	–	–	–
New Zealand, non Maori	0.3	4	0.2	4	0.3	4

* Light when fewer than 10 cases

AGE STANDARDIZED AND CUMULATIVE (0-14) INCIDENCE RATES PER MILLION

Gonadal & germ cell neoplasms

	Male ASR	CUM	Female ASR	CUM	Both ASR	CUM
AFRICA						
Nigeria, Ibadan	–	–	1.2	21	0.6	10
Uganda, Kampala	1.6	23	2.6	41	2.1	32
Zimbabwe, Bulawayo, Residents only	–	–	4.5	67	2.3	34
AMERICA : NORTH						
Canada, Atlantic Provinces	1.6	20	1.6	24	1.6	22
Canada, Western Provinces	3.3	45	4.6	68	3.9	56
USA, Greater Delaware Valley, White	4.1	57	4.5	67	4.3	62
USA, Greater Delaware Valley, non White	1.1	16	6.4	97	3.7	57
USA, Los Angeles, Black	3.6	48	2.2	37	2.9	43
USA, Los Angeles, Hispanic	6.2	83	4.9	79	5.6	81
USA, Los Angeles, Other White	3.5	47	5.0	77	4.2	62
USA, New York (City and State), White	3.6	50	4.5	69	4.0	59
USA, New York (City and State), Black	1.3	19	4.5	70	2.9	45
USA, SEER, White	4.3	60	4.1	65	4.2	62
USA, SEER, Black	3.2	42	5.2	81	4.2	62
AMERICA : OTHER						
Brazil, Fortaleza	–	–	9.4	134	4.7	67
Brazil, Recife	1.1	15	4.1	64	2.7	40
Brazil, Sao Paulo	5.4	72	4.7	70	5.0	71
Colombia, Cali	–	–	3.8	56	1.9	28
Costa Rica	3.4	45	4.3	71	3.9	58
Cuba	0.7	9	1.6	25	1.1	17
Jamaica	–	–	4.1	64	2.1	32
Puerto Rico	2.3	32	3.0	48	2.6	40
ASIA						
China, Shanghai	4.2	55	5.8	84	5.0	69
China, Taipei	5.8	76	3.8	55	4.8	66
Hong Kong	5.9	79	2.3	36	4.2	58
India, Bangalore	1.3	17	2.9	43	2.1	30
India, Bombay Cancer Registry	2.0	28	1.7	26	1.9	27
Israel, Jews	3.4	46	4.0	61	3.7	53
Israel, non Jews	1.5	19	0.8	11	1.1	15
Japan, Kanagawa	4.8	69	4.1	62	4.4	66
Japan, Miyagi	6.6	90	5.9	97	6.3	93
Japan, Osaka	8.2	112	4.6	70	6.4	92
Kuwait, Kuwaiti	0.9	12	–	–	0.5	6
Kuwait, non Kuwaiti	3.9	55	3.3	51	3.6	53
Philippines, Metro Manila & Rizal	2.0	28	4.4	66	3.2	47
Singapore, Chinese	3.8	51	4.0	63	3.9	57
Singapore, Malay	2.8	36	4.3	67	3.6	51
EUROPE						
Czechoslovakia, Slovakia	2.9	39	4.2	64	3.5	51
Denmark	1.7	24	2.5	39	2.1	31
FRG, Children's Tumour Registry	1.7	25	2.1	29	1.9	27
FRG, Saarland	1.8	25	1.7	29	1.7	27
Finland	4.2	55	3.3	48	3.7	51
France, Bas Rhin	2.5	32	2.9	44	2.7	38
France, Paediatric Registries	2.3	29	4.2	59	3.2	44
German Democratic Republic	3.7	50	5.2	78	4.4	64
Great Britain, England and Wales	2.5	34	2.6	40	2.5	37
Great Britain, Manchester (period 1)	1.0	14	2.5	37	1.7	25
Great Britain, Manchester (period 2)	4.1	57	4.7	72	4.4	64
Great Britain, Scotland	1.4	19	2.6	40	2.0	30
Hungary	2.6	36	2.6	38	2.6	37
Italy, Torino	1.9	27	4.5	67	3.2	46
Netherlands, DCLSG						
Netherlands, SOOZ, Eindhoven	6.5	84	1.5	25	4.1	56
Norway	5.2	71	3.1	49	4.2	60
Poland, Warsaw City	–	–	3.6	56	1.8	27
Spain, Zaragoza	–	–	2.3	34	1.1	16
Sweden	4.6	61	3.8	57	4.2	59
Switzerland, Three Western Cantons	4.9	67	2.2	33	3.6	50
Yugoslavia, Slovenia	2.0	27	3.9	66	2.9	46
OCEANIA						
Australia, New South Wales	4.6	63	3.2	50	3.9	57
Australia, Queensland	1.3	17	3.3	52	2.3	34
Fiji, Fijian	1.2	16	3.1	54	2.2	35
Fiji, Indian	2.0	26	0.9	15	1.5	21
New Zealand, Maori	9.7	129	7.9	131	8.8	130
New Zealand, non Maori	3.6	50	5.3	81	4.4	65

* Light when fewer than 10 cases

AGE STANDARDIZED AND CUMULATIVE (0-14) INCIDENCE RATES PER MILLION

Non-gonadal germ cell neoplasms

	Male ASR	Male CUM	Female ASR	Female CUM	Both ASR	Both CUM
AFRICA						
Nigeria, Ibadan						
Uganda, Kampala						
Zimbabwe, Bulawayo, Residents only						
AMERICA : NORTH						
Canada, Atlantic Provinces	–	–	1.1	15	0.5	7
Canada, Western Provinces	1.3	20	2.8	38	2.0	28
USA, Greater Delaware Valley, White	1.7	24	2.7	38	2.2	31
USA, Greater Delaware Valley, non White	0.4	8	2.2	33	1.3	20
USA, Los Angeles, Black	3.1	40	–	–	1.6	20
USA, Los Angeles, Hispanic	0.9	13	1.2	17	1.0	15
USA, Los Angeles, Other White	1.8	25	2.4	33	2.1	29
USA, New York (City and State), White	1.2	19	1.9	26	1.6	22
USA, New York (City and State), Black	0.8	12	1.9	26	1.4	19
USA, SEER, White	1.9	26	1.6	23	1.7	25
USA, SEER, Black	1.2	16	2.5	36	1.9	26
AMERICA : OTHER						
Brazil, Fortaleza	–	–	–	–	–	–
Brazil, Recife			1.2	15	0.6	7
Brazil, Sao Paulo	1.5	20	1.6	21	1.5	21
Colombia, Cali	–	–	2.3	30	1.1	15
Costa Rica	1.1	16	1.1	17	1.1	16
Cuba	0.2	3	0.3	5	0.3	4
Jamaica	–	–	2.8	41	1.4	21
Puerto Rico	0.8	12	0.5	6	0.6	9
ASIA						
China, Shanghai	2.3	30	3.0	39	2.6	35
China, Taipei	1.1	15	2.1	28	1.6	21
Hong Kong	0.2	3	–	–	0.1	2
India, Bangalore	–	–	1.8	25	0.9	12
India, Bombay Cancer Registry	0.5	7	0.4	6	0.5	6
Israel, Jews	0.4	7	1.7	23	1.0	14
Israel, non Jews	0.7	9	0.8	11	0.8	10
Japan, Kanagawa	2.9	44	1.5	24	2.2	34
Japan, Miyagi	1.4	21	1.0	15	1.2	18
Japan, Osaka	2.4	36	1.6	22	2.0	30
Kuwait, Kuwaiti	–	–	–	–	–	–
Kuwait, non Kuwaiti	1.0	13	2.0	29	1.5	21
Philippines, Metro Manila & Rizal	0.8	12	1.9	25	1.4	18
Singapore, Chinese	0.7	11	1.0	13	0.9	12
Singapore, Malay	1.4	18	–	–	0.7	9
EUROPE						
Czechoslovakia, Slovakia	0.7	9	1.6	21	1.1	15
Denmark	0.8	12	0.5	7	0.7	9
FRG, Children's Tumour Registry	1.3	18	1.3	18	1.3	18
FRG, Saarland	–	–	0.4	7	0.2	4
Finland	1.3	18	2.5	34	1.9	26
France, Bas Rhin	1.3	16	2.1	31	1.7	23
France, Paediatric Registries	2.3	29	3.7	50	3.0	39
German Democratic Republic	0.7	10	2.7	38	1.7	23
Great Britain, England and Wales	0.6	10	1.2	16	0.9	13
Great Britain, Manchester (period 1)	0.5	7	1.5	20	0.9	13
Great Britain, Manchester (period 2)	1.8	26	2.5	34	2.1	30
Great Britain, Scotland	0.5	7	0.5	7	0.5	7
Hungary	1.3	17	1.6	22	1.4	20
Italy, Torino	0.6	8	2.2	30	1.4	19
Netherlands, DCLSG						
Netherlands, SOOZ, Eindhoven	1.3	17	–	–	0.7	9
Norway	0.9	13	1.0	13	0.9	13
Poland, Warsaw City	–	–	–	–	–	–
Spain, Zaragoza	–	–	1.3	17	0.6	8
Sweden	1.2	16	1.5	19	1.3	17
Switzerland, Three Western Cantons	–	–	1.4	18	0.7	9
Yugoslavia, Slovenia	0.4	7	–	–	0.2	4
OCEANIA						
Australia, New South Wales	2.1	31	1.3	18	1.7	25
Australia, Queensland	0.5	6	2.0	29	1.2	17
Fiji, Fijian						
Fiji, Indian						
New Zealand, Maori	5.6	77	1.6	25	3.7	52
New Zealand, non Maori	2.1	30	1.8	24	2.0	27

* Light when fewer than 10 cases

AGE STANDARDIZED AND CUMULATIVE (0-14) INCIDENCE RATES PER MILLION

Gonadal germ cell neoplasms

	Male ASR	Male CUM	Female ASR	Female CUM	Both ASR	Both CUM
AFRICA						
Nigeria, Ibadan						
Uganda, Kampala						
Zimbabwe, Bulawayo, Residents only						
AMERICA : NORTH						
Canada, Atlantic Provinces	1.2	15	0.5	9	0.9	12
Canada, Western Provinces	1.3	17	1.2	21	1.3	19
USA, Greater Delaware Valley, White	2.2	31	1.2	21	1.7	26
USA, Greater Delaware Valley, non White	0.7	9	2.7	41	1.7	25
USA, Los Angeles, Black	0.5	9	1.7	28	1.1	18
USA, Los Angeles, Hispanic	5.4	69	3.7	62	4.6	66
USA, Los Angeles, Other White	1.4	19	2.2	38	1.8	28
USA, New York (City and State), White	2.3	30	2.1	35	2.2	33
USA, New York (City and State), Black	0.4	7	1.8	31	1.1	19
USA, SEER, White	2.4	33	2.1	35	2.3	34
USA, SEER, Black	1.6	21	2.3	40	2.0	30
AMERICA : OTHER						
Brazil, Fortaleza	–	–	6.6	97	3.3	49
Brazil, Recife	0.8	10	1.0	16	0.9	13
Brazil, Sao Paulo	2.0	26	1.7	27	1.8	26
Colombia, Cali	–	–	–	–	–	–
Costa Rica	2.3	29	3.2	54	2.7	42
Cuba	0.2	3	0.7	11	0.4	7
Jamaica	–	–	0.6	11	0.3	6
Puerto Rico	1.3	18	2.2	36	1.7	27
ASIA						
China, Shanghai	1.8	23	1.1	19	1.5	21
China, Taipei	4.5	58	0.9	14	2.7	37
Hong Kong	5.1	68	2.3	36	3.8	53
India, Bangalore	1.3	17	0.6	10	0.9	13
India, Bombay Cancer Registry	1.1	16	1.0	16	1.1	16
Israel, Jews	2.7	36	1.8	31	2.3	34
Israel, non Jews	0.8	10	–	–	0.4	5
Japan, Kanagawa	1.9	25	1.2	19	1.6	22
Japan, Miyagi	4.2	55	2.7	45	3.5	50
Japan, Osaka	4.3	56	2.4	38	3.4	47
Kuwait, Kuwaiti	0.9	12	–	–	0.5	6
Kuwait, non Kuwaiti	2.0	28	1.3	22	1.6	25
Philippines, Metro Manila & Rizal	1.2	15	1.2	21	1.2	18
Singapore, Chinese	2.1	28	2.1	36	2.1	32
Singapore, Malay	–	–	3.4	51	1.7	25
EUROPE						
Czechoslovakia, Slovakia	2.2	30	1.6	27	1.9	29
Denmark	0.9	12	2.0	32	1.4	22
FRG, Children's Tumour Registry	0.5	6	0.7	11	0.6	8
FRG, Saarland	1.1	16	1.3	22	1.2	19
Finland	2.9	37	0.3	5	1.6	22
France, Bas Rhin	1.3	16	0.8	14	1.0	15
France, Paediatric Registries	–	–	0.5	9	0.2	4
German Democratic Republic	2.9	38	1.7	28	2.3	33
Great Britain, England and Wales	1.8	24	1.2	20	1.5	22
Great Britain, Manchester (period 1)	0.6	8	0.8	13	0.7	10
Great Britain, Manchester (period 2)	2.3	31	2.1	35	2.2	33
Great Britain, Scotland	0.9	12	1.9	31	1.4	21
Hungary	1.4	18	0.9	14	1.1	16
Italy, Torino	1.3	19	2.3	37	1.8	28
Netherlands, DCLSG						
Netherlands, SOOZ, Eindhoven	5.2	68	1.5	25	3.4	47
Norway	3.6	48	1.9	32	2.7	41
Poland, Warsaw City	–	–	2.8	47	1.4	23
Spain, Zaragoza	–	–	1.0	17	0.5	8
Sweden	3.3	44	1.3	21	2.3	33
Switzerland, Three Western Cantons	4.9	67	0.9	15	2.9	41
Yugoslavia, Slovenia	1.6	20	3.5	59	2.5	39
OCEANIA						
Australia, New South Wales	2.5	32	1.9	32	2.2	32
Australia, Queensland	0.9	11	0.7	11	0.8	11
Fiji, Fijian						
Fiji, Indian						
New Zealand, Maori	4.0	52	6.3	105	5.1	78
New Zealand, non Maori	1.5	20	2.5	42	2.0	30

* Light when fewer than 10 cases

AGE STANDARDIZED AND CUMULATIVE (0-14) INCIDENCE RATES PER MILLION

Epithelial neoplasms

	Male ASR	Male CUM	Female ASR	Female CUM	Both ASR	Both CUM
AFRICA						
Nigeria, Ibadan	–	–	3.7	63	1.7	30
Uganda, Kampala	7.6	129	7.7	125	7.6	127
Zimbabwe, Bulawayo, Residents only	2.3	30	6.5	102	4.5	68
AMERICA : NORTH						
Canada, Atlantic Provinces	1.6	26	4.9	81	3.2	53
Canada, Western Provinces	6.6	100	7.2	111	6.9	106
USA, Greater Delaware Valley, White	2.5	41	2.5	42	2.5	41
USA, Greater Delaware Valley, non White	2.3	38	3.9	63	3.1	51
USA, Los Angeles, Black	4.0	69	6.3	102	5.1	85
USA, Los Angeles, Hispanic	1.5	25	4.3	73	2.9	49
USA, Los Angeles, Other White	3.4	55	6.0	96	4.7	75
USA, New York (City and State), White	1.9	31	4.4	70	3.1	50
USA, New York (City and State), Black	5.1	85	4.0	63	4.5	74
USA, SEER, White	3.2	52	5.8	94	4.5	72
USA, SEER, Black	4.1	65	3.7	60	3.9	63
AMERICA : OTHER						
Brazil, Fortaleza	5.5	95	1.2	21	3.3	56
Brazil, Recife	4.8	75	9.2	144	7.0	110
Brazil, Sao Paulo	8.0	119	9.2	137	8.6	128
Colombia, Cali	6.1	96	4.8	70	5.4	83
Costa Rica	7.3	118	4.4	71	5.8	95
Cuba	2.4	37	2.5	40	2.5	39
Jamaica	1.4	23	1.9	33	1.7	29
Puerto Rico	1.2	20	3.6	60	2.4	40
ASIA						
China, Shanghai	1.6	26	1.9	30	1.7	28
China, Taipei	2.7	42	2.9	46	2.8	44
Hong Kong	6.0	94	4.3	70	5.2	83
India, Bangalore	1.1	19	5.1	86	3.1	53
India, Bombay Cancer Registry	2.2	37	1.1	18	1.7	28
Israel, Jews	4.4	70	7.0	111	5.7	90
Israel, non Jews	3.1	53	0.8	14	2.0	35
Japan, Kanagawa	0.9	15	1.3	20	1.1	18
Japan, Miyagi	2.3	35	2.7	45	2.5	40
Japan, Osaka	1.5	23	1.7	27	1.6	25
Kuwait, Kuwaiti	3.0	48	1.9	29	2.5	39
Kuwait, non Kuwaiti	3.4	54	3.0	45	3.2	49
Philippines, Metro Manila & Rizal	2.1	37	1.5	26	1.8	31
Singapore, Chinese	4.8	81	3.7	61	4.3	71
Singapore, Malay	2.8	46	0.9	16	1.9	31
EUROPE						
Czechoslovakia, Slovakia	6.2	94	4.0	62	5.1	78
Denmark	4.6	73	2.9	48	3.8	61
FRG, Children's Tumour Registry	1.0	16	0.6	10	0.8	13
FRG, Saarland	4.5	68	3.7	56	4.1	62
Finland	4.0	64	6.4	102	5.2	83
France, Bas Rhin	1.5	26	2.8	45	2.2	35
France, Paediatric Registries	4.5	70	4.2	71	4.3	71
German Democratic Republic	3.5	53	4.8	75	4.1	64
Great Britain, England and Wales	2.0	32	3.3	52	2.6	42
Great Britain, Manchester (period 1)	2.0	32	1.4	22	1.7	27
Great Britain, Manchester (period 2)	1.6	27	3.2	50	2.4	38
Great Britain, Scotland	2.7	43	3.0	49	2.9	46
Hungary	0.9	15	0.5	8	0.7	12
Italy, Torino	4.2	70	2.5	41	3.3	56
Netherlands, DCLSG						
Netherlands, SOOZ, Eindhoven	10.7	177	6.5	106	8.6	142
Norway	3.6	58	4.5	71	4.0	65
Poland, Warsaw City	1.6	26	1.3	21	1.5	24
Spain, Zaragoza	–	–	–	–	–	–
Sweden	3.9	63	6.1	101	5.0	82
Switzerland, Three Western Cantons	4.6	75	2.9	47	3.8	61
Yugoslavia, Slovenia	6.5	105	1.8	29	4.2	68
OCEANIA						
Australia, New South Wales	7.2	119	6.2	101	6.7	110
Australia, Queensland	3.0	44	2.2	34	2.6	39
Fiji, Fijian	1.0	17	3.5	50	2.2	33
Fiji, Indian	1.8	29	3.2	44	2.5	36
New Zealand, Maori	11.2	179	8.3	132	9.8	156
New Zealand, non Maori	7.8	127	8.3	134	8.1	130

* Light when fewer than 10 cases

AGE STANDARDIZED AND CUMULATIVE (0-14) INCIDENCE RATES PER MILLION

Adrenocortical carcinoma

	Male ASR	CUM	Female ASR	CUM	Both ASR	CUM
AFRICA						
Nigeria, Ibadan						
Uganda, Kampala						
Zimbabwe, Bulawayo, Residents only						
AMERICA : NORTH						
Canada, Atlantic Provinces	–	–	0.3	4	0.1	2
Canada, Western Provinces	0.1	2	0.2	2	0.1	2
USA, Greater Delaware Valley, White	0.1	2	–	–	0.1	1
USA, Greater Delaware Valley, non White	0.5	8	–	–	0.3	4
USA, Los Angeles, Black	–	–	–	–	–	–
USA, Los Angeles, Hispanic	–	–	–	–	–	–
USA, Los Angeles, Other White	–	–	0.3	3	0.1	2
USA, New York (City and State), White	–	–	0.2	3	0.1	1
USA, New York (City and State), Black	0.5	7	–	–	0.3	4
USA, SEER, White	0.3	4	0.4	6	**0.4**	**5**
USA, SEER, Black	0.3	5	–	–	0.1	2
AMERICA : OTHER						
Brazil, Fortaleza	–	–	–	–	–	–
Brazil, Recife	–	–	0.3	5	0.2	3
Brazil, Sao Paulo	**1.0**	**15**	**2.0**	**26**	**1.5**	**21**
Colombia, Cali	–	–	–	–	–	–
Costa Rica	–	–	0.5	9	0.3	4
Cuba	–	–	0.1	2	0.1	1
Jamaica	–	–	–	–	–	–
Puerto Rico	–	–	–	–	–	–
ASIA						
China, Shanghai	–	–	–	–	–	–
China, Taipei	0.3	5	0.2	3	0.3	4
Hong Kong	–	–	–	–	–	–
India, Bangalore	–	–	–	–	–	–
India, Bombay Cancer Registry	–	–	–	–	–	–
Israel, Jews	–	–	0.2	3	0.1	2
Israel, non Jews	–	–	–	–	–	–
Japan, Kanagawa	–	–	0.2	3	0.1	2
Japan, Miyagi	–	–	–	–	–	–
Japan, Osaka	–	–	–	–	–	–
Kuwait, Kuwaiti	–	–	–	–	–	–
Kuwait, non Kuwaiti	–	–	–	–	–	–
Philippines, Metro Manila & Rizal	–	–	–	–	–	–
Singapore, Chinese	–	–	–	–	–	–
Singapore, Malay	–	–	–	–	–	–
EUROPE						
Czechoslovakia, Slovakia	0.2	2	–	–	0.1	1
Denmark	–	–	–	–	–	–
FRG, Children's Tumour Registry	0.2	2	0.1	1	0.1	2
FRG, Saarland	–	–	0.7	10	0.4	5
Finland	–	–	0.8	12	0.4	6
France, Bas Rhin	–	–	–	–	–	–
France, Paediatric Registries	0.8	10	–	–	0.4	5
German Democratic Republic	0.6	8	0.1	2	0.4	5
Great Britain, England and Wales	0.1	2	**0.4**	**5**	**0.2**	**3**
Great Britain, Manchester (period 1)	0.1	2	0.4	5	0.2	4
Great Britain, Manchester (period 2)	–	–	1.2	16	0.6	8
Great Britain, Scotland	0.3	5	0.2	3	0.3	4
Hungary	0.1	1	–	–	–	1
Italy, Torino	0.5	8	–	–	0.2	4
Netherlands, DCLSG						
Netherlands, SOOZ, Eindhoven	–	–	–	–	–	–
Norway	0.4	6	–	–	0.2	3
Poland, Warsaw City	–	–	–	–	–	–
Spain, Zaragoza	–	–	–	–	–	–
Sweden	0.2	3	0.2	3	0.2	3
Switzerland, Three Western Cantons	–	–	–	–	–	–
Yugoslavia, Slovenia	–	–	–	–	–	–
OCEANIA						
Australia, New South Wales	–	–	0.2	2	0.1	1
Australia, Queensland	0.9	11	–	–	0.4	6
Fiji, Fijian						
Fiji, Indian						
New Zealand, Maori	3.6	51	–	–	1.9	26
New Zealand, non Maori	0.2	4	–	–	0.1	2

* Light when fewer than 10 cases

AGE STANDARDIZED AND CUMULATIVE (0-14) INCIDENCE RATES PER MILLION

Thyroid carcinoma

	Male ASR CUM		Female ASR CUM		Both ASR CUM	
AFRICA						
Nigeria, Ibadan						
Uganda, Kampala						
Zimbabwe, Bulawayo, Residents only						
AMERICA : NORTH						
Canada, Atlantic Provinces	-	-	1.3	22	0.6	11
Canada, Western Provinces	0.6	10	**1.4**	**24**	**1.0**	**17**
USA, Greater Delaware Valley, White	0.8	12	1.3	21	1.0	17
USA, Greater Delaware Valley, non White	-	-	-	-	-	-
USA, Los Angeles, Black	0.5	9	2.8	47	1.7	27
USA, Los Angeles, Hispanic	0.3	5	2.5	42	1.4	23
USA, Los Angeles, Other White	0.5	9	2.5	41	1.5	25
USA, New York (City and State), White	0.4	6	1.9	32	1.1	19
USA, New York (City and State), Black	1.7	30	0.8	13	1.3	22
USA, SEER, White	**0.9**	15	2.2	36	1.5	25
USA, SEER, Black	0.3	5	1.1	20	0.7	12
AMERICA : OTHER						
Brazil, Fortaleza	-	-	-	-	-	-
Brazil, Recife			1.3	22	0.7	11
Brazil, Sao Paulo	0.1	2	0.7	11	0.4	6
Colombia, Cali	-	-	-	-	-	-
Costa Rica	0.6	9	2.7	44	1.6	26
Cuba	**0.4**	**7**	**1.0**	**17**	**0.7**	**12**
Jamaica	-	-	-	-	-	-
Puerto Rico	0.5	9	1.2	21	**0.9**	**15**
ASIA						
China, Shanghai	0.3	4	0.4	7	0.3	6
China, Taipei	0.3	5	1.1	19	0.7	12
Hong Kong	0.5	9	1.2	20	0.9	15
India, Bangalore	0.6	10	1.7	29	1.1	19
India, Bombay Cancer Registry	0.3	5	0.1	2	0.2	4
Israel, Jews	0.7	11	1.8	32	**1.2**	**21**
Israel, non Jews	2.3	40	-	-	1.2	21
Japan, Kanagawa	-	-	-	-	-	-
Japan, Miyagi	-	-	1.8	30	0.9	15
Japan, Osaka	0.2	3	0.1	2	0.1	2
Kuwait, Kuwaiti	-	-	-	-	-	-
Kuwait, non Kuwaiti	1.2	20	1.0	16	1.1	18
Philippines, Metro Manila & Rizal	0.3	5	0.3	5	0.3	5
Singapore, Chinese	0.6	10	1.6	28	1.1	19
Singapore, Malay	-	-	-	-	-	-
EUROPE						
Czechoslovakia, Slovakia	0.1	2	0.4	7	0.3	5
Denmark	0.6	10	1.2	21	0.9	15
FRG, Children's Tumour Registry	0.3	5	-	1	0.2	3
FRG, Saarland	-	-	-	-	-	-
Finland	0.6	10	0.7	11	0.6	11
France, Bas Rhin	-	-	-	-	-	-
France, Paediatric Registries	-	-	1.1	19	0.6	9
German Democratic Republic	0.4	7	1.2	19	0.8	12
Great Britain, England and Wales	**0.2**	**3**	**0.5**	**8**	**0.3**	**6**
Great Britain, Manchester (period 1)	0.1	2	-	-	0.1	1
Great Britain, Manchester (period 2)	0.3	4	-	-	0.1	2
Great Britain, Scotland	0.2	4	0.4	7	0.3	6
Hungary	0.2	3	0.1	1	0.1	2
Italy, Torino	1.4	23	1.2	21	1.3	22
Netherlands, DCLSG						
Netherlands, SOOZ, Eindhoven	-	-	0.7	13	0.4	6
Norway	0.4	6	1.1	19	0.7	13
Poland, Warsaw City	1.1	18	0.7	10	0.9	14
Spain, Zaragoza	-	-	-	-	-	-
Sweden	0.4	7	**1.6**	**27**	**1.0**	**16**
Switzerland, Three Western Cantons	-	-	-	-	-	-
Yugoslavia, Slovenia	1.2	21	0.9	15	1.1	18
OCEANIA						
Australia, New South Wales	0.2	4	0.8	13	0.5	8
Australia, Queensland	0.3	5	0.7	11	0.5	8
Fiji, Fijian						
Fiji, Indian						
New Zealand, Maori	-	-	-	-	-	-
New Zealand, non Maori	0.9	14	0.9	15	0.9	15

* Light when fewer than 10 cases

AGE STANDARDIZED AND CUMULATIVE (0-14) INCIDENCE RATES PER MILLION

Nasopharyngeal carcinoma

	Male ASR	Male CUM	Female ASR	Female CUM	Both ASR	Both CUM
AFRICA						
Nigeria, Ibadan						
Uganda, Kampala						
Zimbabwe, Bulawayo, Residents only						
AMERICA : NORTH						
Canada, Atlantic Provinces	–	–	0.5	9	0.2	4
Canada, Western Provinces	0.2	2	–	–	0.1	1
USA, Greater Delaware Valley, White	0.2	3	0.1	2	0.1	2
USA, Greater Delaware Valley, non White	0.9	15	1.4	23	1.1	19
USA, Los Angeles, Black	1.5	26	1.5	27	1.5	26
USA, Los Angeles, Hispanic	–	–	–	–	–	–
USA, Los Angeles, Other White	0.3	5	0.2	3	0.2	4
USA, New York (City and State), White	–	–	0.1	1	–	1
USA, New York (City and State), Black	1.4	24	0.4	6	0.9	15
USA, SEER, White	0.2	3	0.1	1	0.1	2
USA, SEER, Black	1.3	20	–	–	0.6	10
AMERICA : OTHER						
Brazil, Fortaleza	–	–	–	–	–	–
Brazil, Recife	–	–	–	–	–	–
Brazil, Sao Paulo	0.2	3	0.2	3	0.2	3
Colombia, Cali	–	–	–	–	–	–
Costa Rica	3.5	61	–	–	1.8	31
Cuba	0.3	5	0.3	4	**0.3**	**5**
Jamaica	0.7	12	0.6	11	0.7	11
Puerto Rico	–	–	0.2	3	0.1	1
ASIA						
China, Shanghai	–	–	–	–	–	–
China, Taipei	0.5	8	0.3	6	0.4	7
Hong Kong	1.2	18	0.6	10	0.9	14
India, Bangalore	–	–	1.1	19	ʲ 0.6	10
India, Bombay Cancer Registry	0.5	8	0.1	2	0.3	5
Israel, Jews	0.7	11	0.5	8	0.6	10
Israel, non Jews	0.8	13	–	–	0.4	7
Japan, Kanagawa	–	–	0.3	5	0.1	2
Japan, Miyagi	–	–	–	–	–	–
Japan, Osaka	0.1	2	–	–	–	1
Kuwait, Kuwaiti	1.0	18	–	–	0.5	9
Kuwait, non Kuwaiti	1.2	20	1.0	16	1.1	18
Philippines, Metro Manila & Rizal	0.6	10	0.6	10	0.6	10
Singapore, Chinese	1.4	23	0.4	7	0.9	15
Singapore, Malay	1.9	31	–	–	1.0	16
EUROPE						
Czechoslovakia, Slovakia	–	–	0.1	2	0.1	1
Denmark	–	–	–	–	–	–
FRG, Children's Tumour Registry	0.3	4	0.1	3	0.2	3
FRG, Saarland	–	–	–	–	–	–
Finland	0.7	11	0.2	3	0.4	7
France, Bas Rhin	0.8	13	–	–	0.4	7
France, Paediatric Registries	–	–	1.5	26	0.7	13
German Democratic Republic	0.2	3	0.2	3	0.2	3
Great Britain, England and Wales	**0.3**	**5**	**0.2**	**4**	**0.3**	**5**
Great Britain, Manchester (period 1)	0.8	13	0.2	4	0.5	9
Great Britain, Manchester (period 2)	0.4	7	0.3	5	0.3	6
Great Britain, Scotland	0.2	4	0.1	2	0.2	3
Hungary	0.2	3	–	–	0.1	1
Italy, Torino	0.7	12	–	–	0.4	6
Netherlands, DCLSG						
Netherlands, SOOZ, Eindhoven	–	–	0.7	13	0.4	6
Norway	0.2	3	0.2	3	0.2	3
Poland, Warsaw City	–	–	–	–	–	–
Spain, Zaragoza	–	–	–	–	–	–
Sweden	0.3	5	0.1	1	0.2	3
Switzerland, Three Western Cantons	0.8	14	–	–	0.4	7
Yugoslavia, Slovenia	0.4	7	–	–	0.2	4
OCEANIA						
Australia, New South Wales	0.4	6	–	–	0.2	3
Australia, Queensland	0.3	5	–	–	0.2	3
Fiji, Fijian						
Fiji, Indian						
New Zealand, Maori	–	–	–	–	–	–
New Zealand, non Maori	–	–	–	–	–	–

* Light when fewer than 10 cases

AGE STANDARDIZED AND CUMULATIVE (0-14) INCIDENCE RATES PER MILLION

Melanoma

	Male ASR CUM		Female ASR CUM		Both ASR CUM	
AFRICA						
Nigeria, Ibadan						
Uganda, Kampala						
Zimbabwe, Bulawayo, Residents only						
AMERICA : NORTH						
Canada, Atlantic Provinces	1.1	18	0.9	14	1.0	16
Canada, Western Provinces	1.2	19	0.6	10	0.9	15
USA, Greater Delaware Valley, White	0.6	10	0.3	5	0.5	8
USA, Greater Delaware Valley, non White	-	-	0.7	9	0.3	4
USA, Los Angeles, Black	-	-	0.7	10	0.4	5
USA, Los Angeles, Hispanic	-	-	-	-	-	-
USA, Los Angeles, Other White	1.4	23	1.5	24	1.4	23
USA, New York (City and State), White	0.4	6	1.0	15	0.7	11
USA, New York (City and State), Black	-	-	0.9	13	0.4	7
USA, SEER, White	0.8	14	1.5	24	1.1	18
USA, SEER, Black	0.4	5	-	-	0.2	3
AMERICA : OTHER						
Brazil, Fortaleza	-	-	-	-	-	-
Brazil, Recife	0.3	5	-	-	0.2	3
Brazil, Sao Paulo	0.6	9	0.7	12	0.7	10
Colombia, Cali	1.7	27	3.9	56	2.8	42
Costa Rica	0.6	8	0.6	9	0.6	8
Cuba	0.2	3	0.1	2	0.2	2
Jamaica	-	-	-	-	-	-
Puerto Rico	0.4	6	0.2	3	0.3	4
ASIA						
China, Shanghai	-	-	0.3	5	0.1	2
China, Taipei	-	-	-	-	-	-
Hong Kong	0.8	12	1.4	22	1.1	17
India, Bangalore	0.6	10	0.6	10	0.6	10
India, Bombay Cancer Registry	0.2	3	-	-	0.1	1
Israel, Jews	1.8	27	1.9	28	1.8	27
Israel, non Jews	-	-	-	-	-	-
Japan, Kanagawa	0.2	4	0.2	3	0.2	3
Japan, Miyagi	1.0	14	0.9	15	0.9	14
Japan, Osaka	0.3	4	0.5	8	0.4	6
Kuwait, Kuwaiti	-	-	-	-	-	-
Kuwait, non Kuwaiti	-	-	-	-	-	-
Philippines, Metro Manila & Rizal	-	-	-	-	-	-
Singapore, Chinese	0.2	3	-	-	0.1	2
Singapore, Malay	0.9	16	-	-	0.5	8
EUROPE						
Czechoslovakia, Slovakia	0.6	10	1.1	17	0.9	13
Denmark	1.6	26	0.8	11	1.2	19
FRG, Children's Tumour Registry	-	1	0.2	2	0.1	2
FRG, Saarland	1.6	24	0.7	10	1.2	17
Finland	0.5	8	1.2	20	0.9	14
France, Bas Rhin	-	-	1.0	16	0.5	8
France, Paediatric Registries	1.0	17	1.0	18	1.0	17
German Democratic Republic	0.7	11	0.8	12	0.7	12
Great Britain, England and Wales	0.6	9	0.9	14	0.7	11
Great Britain, Manchester (period 1)	0.3	5	0.1	2	0.2	3
Great Britain, Manchester (period 2)	-	-	0.8	12	0.4	6
Great Britain, Scotland	1.3	20	1.0	16	1.1	18
Hungary	-	-	0.2	3	0.1	1
Italy, Torino	1.0	15	0.5	8	0.7	12
Netherlands, DCLSG						
Netherlands, SOOZ, Eindhoven	1.6	26	1.5	25	1.5	25
Norway	1.4	21	2.2	32	1.7	27
Poland, Warsaw City	0.5	8	-	-	0.2	4
Spain, Zaragoza	-	-	-	-	-	-
Sweden	0.5	8	0.6	10	0.6	9
Switzerland, Three Western Cantons	-	-	1.9	31	0.9	15
Yugoslavia, Slovenia	3.1	48	0.4	7	1.8	28
OCEANIA						
Australia, New South Wales	4.9	80	4.3	71	4.6	75
Australia, Queensland	-	-	1.0	17	0.5	8
Fiji, Fijian						
Fiji, Indian						
New Zealand, Maori	-	-	-	-	-	-
New Zealand, non Maori	3.7	62	3.6	57	3.7	60

* Light when fewer than 10 cases

6.2
Ratio-tables

LYMPHOMA DISTRIBUTION

	Male			Female		
	Hodgkin's	Burkitt's	Other*	Hodgkin's	Burkitt's	Other*
AFRICA						
Madagascar, Institut Pasteur	30.5	7.8	61.7	13.7	11.0	75.3
Malawi, Histopathology Registry	5.3	63.2	31.6	–	60.7	39.3
Morocco, Children's Hospital, Rabat	36.6	15.2	48.2	24.2	39.4	36.4
Nigeria, Ibadan	8.0	78.8	13.2	3.7	90.0	6.3
Sudan, RICK, Arab	44.2	14.7	41.1	29.4	5.9	64.7
Sudan, RICK, Sudanic	44.4	36.1	19.4	30.0	20.0	50.0
Tanzania	34.6	46.2	19.2	16.2	45.9	37.8
Tunisia, Institut Salah-Azaiz	45.0	22.5	32.4	31.3	34.3	34.3
Uganda, Kampala	14.3	34.3	51.4	24.0	20.0	56.0
Uganda, West Nile	1.1	90.3	8.6	–	90.3	9.7
Zimbabwe, Bulawayo	35.2	13.0	51.9	41.4	10.3	48.3
AMERICA : NORTH						
Canada, Atlantic Provinces	38.9	–	61.1	36.4	9.1	54.5
Canada, Western Provinces	24.2	2.7	73.1	40.9	–	59.1
USA, Greater Delaware Valley, White	43.1	6.5	50.3	52.6	1.3	46.1
USA, Greater Delaware Valley, non White	51.7	6.9	41.4	47.1	–	52.9
USA, Los Angeles, Black	50.0	4.5	45.5	76.5	–	23.5
USA, Los Angeles, Hispanic	44.3	6.8	48.9	54.8	–	45.2
USA, Los Angeles, Other White	46.4	7.1	46.4	50.0	3.4	46.6
USA, New York (City and State), White	43.0	8.0	49.0	55.4	8.3	36.4
USA, New York (City and State), Black	51.2	4.9	43.9	47.4	–	52.6
USA, SEER, White	34.6	16.6	48.7	56.7	3.3	40.0
USA, SEER, Black	54.5	4.5	40.9	33.3	–	66.7
AMERICA : OTHER						
Brazil, Fortaleza	23.3	3.3	73.3	25.0	–	75.0
Brazil, Recife	39.0	–	61.0	34.2	–	65.8
Brazil, Sao Paulo	32.5	2.1	65.4	26.6	0.5	72.9
Colombia, Cali	31.0	41.4	27.6	35.7	–	64.3
Costa Rica	37.1	1.4	61.4	43.3	3.3	53.3
Cuba	23.0	1.2	75.8	23.0	1.1	75.9
Jamaica	33.3	–	66.7	20.0	–	80.0
Puerto Rico	40.7	9.3	50.0	46.3	5.6	48.1
ASIA						
Bangladesh, CERP	41.8	–	58.2	26.1	–	73.9
China, Shanghai	19.7	–	80.3	18.5	–	81.5
China, Taipei	9.3	–	90.7	2.2	–	97.8
Hong Kong	13.0	4.0	83.0	13.2	9.4	77.4
India, Bangalore	38.5	5.1	56.4	28.6	–	71.4
India, Bombay Cancer Registry	40.7	1.0	58.3	25.5	11.8	62.7
India, Tata Hospital, Bombay	57.5	0.5	42.0	41.1	2.1	56.8
Indonesia, Yogyakarta Path. Dept.	22.9	–	77.1	4.2	4.2	91.7
Iraq, Baghdad	32.4	29.3	38.4	28.7	35.4	35.9
Israel, Jews	24.2	15.5	60.2	33.3	14.1	52.6
Israel, non Jews	26.3	21.1	52.6	43.8	31.3	25.0
Japan, Kanagawa	10.0	6.7	83.3	8.3	–	91.7
Japan, Miyagi	9.1	9.1	81.8	–	–	100.0
Japan, Osaka	7.3	2.4	90.3	9.0	4.5	86.6
Kuwait, Kuwaiti	41.2	2.9	55.9	36.8	31.6	31.6
Kuwait, non Kuwaiti	31.6	10.5	57.9	33.3	–	66.7
Pakistan, JPMC	67.8	1.7	30.5	69.2	–	30.8
Philippines, Metro Manila & Rizal	17.6	2.9	79.4	–	–	100.0
Singapore, Chinese	19.0	5.2	75.9	10.0	3.3	86.7
Singapore, Malay	20.0	–	80.0	16.7	–	83.3
Thailand	23.0	8.0	69.0	7.3	5.5	87.3
Vietnam, Ho Chi Minh City	23.5	–	76.5	14.3	–	85.7

Note : Figures are % of total Lymphomas
       Light when fewer than 10 cases

* Other includes: Non-Hodgkin lymphoma
              Unspecified lymphoma
              Histiocytosis X
              Other Reticuloendothelial

LYMPHOMA DISTRIBUTION

	Male			Female		
	Hodgkin's	Burkitt's	Other*	Hodgkin's	Burkitt's	Other*
EUROPE						
Czechoslovakia, Slovakia	37.3	2.0	60.8	44.8	–	55.2
Denmark	27.5	25.5	47.1	52.2	8.7	39.1
FRG, Children's Tumour Registry	36.4	0.3	63.3	40.4	–	59.6
FRG, Saarland	29.0	9.7	61.3	50.0	16.7	33.3
Finland	20.2	–	79.8	25.0	–	75.0
France, Bas Rhin	19.0	4.8	76.2	14.3	–	85.7
France, Paediatric Registries	29.0	35.5	35.5	31.6	5.3	63.2
German Democratic Republic	38.2	6.0	55.8	47.7	3.7	48.6
Great Britain, England and Wales	39.4	1.9	58.8	36.8	2.2	60.9
Great Britain, Manchester (period 1)	37.1	–	62.9	28.3	–	71.7
Great Britain, Manchester (period 2)	37.0	1.0	62.0	22.6	1.9	75.5
Great Britain, Scotland	48.5	1.0	50.5	37.2	2.3	60.5
Hungary	33.0	11.2	55.8	26.3	6.6	67.1
Italy, Torino	39.1	–	60.9	55.3	–	44.7
Netherlands, SOOZ, Eindhoven	13.6	–	86.4	44.4	–	55.6
Norway	27.1	8.5	64.4	40.9	4.5	54.5
Poland, Warsaw City	30.0	–	70.0	33.3	8.3	58.3
Spain, Childhood Cancer Registry	19.7	28.3	51.9	23.6	18.0	58.4
Spain, Zaragoza	26.7	10.0	63.3	18.2	18.2	63.6
Sweden	31.2	–	68.8	20.5	–	79.5
Switzerland, Three Western Cantons	26.3	10.5	63.2	57.1	–	42.9
Yugoslavia, Slovenia	42.9	–	57.1	52.6	–	47.4
OCEANIA						
Australia, New South Wales	28.2	1.9	69.9	30.0	–	70.0
Australia, Queensland	41.0	–	59.0	19.2	3.8	76.9
Fiji, Fijian	10.0	10.0	80.0	12.5	–	87.5
Fiji, Indian	20.0	–	80.0	–	–	100.0
New Zealand, Maori	37.5	–	62.5	25.0	12.5	62.5
New Zealand, non Maori	31.9	–	68.1	38.5	7.7	53.8
Papua New Guinea, Histopath. Registry	3.6	55.4	41.1	4.8	52.4	42.9

Note : Figures are % of total Lymphomas
Light when fewer than 10 cases

* Other includes: Non—Hodgkin lymphoma
Unspecified lymphoma
Histiocytosis X
Other Reticuloendothelial

LYMPHOMA : LEUKAEMIA (1) RATIO

	Male	Female
AFRICA		
Madagascar, Institut Pasteur	47.00	–
Malawi, Histopathology Registry	–	28.00
Morocco, Children's Hospital, Rabat	1.60	1.06
Nigeria, Ibadan	5.82	7.31
Sudan, RICK, Arab	2.97	1.10
Sudan, RICK, Sudanic	6.00	5.00
Tanzania	11.14	7.40
Tunisia, Institut Salah-Azaiz	–	–
Uganda, Kampala	1.84	1.79
Uganda, West Nile	23.25	15.50
Zimbabwe, Bulawayo	1.29	0.81
AMERICA : NORTH		
Canada, Atlantic Provinces	0.29	0.22
Canada, Western Provinces	0.50	0.31
USA, Greater Delaware Valley, White	0.41	0.28
USA, Greater Delaware Valley, non White	0.51	0.71
USA, Los Angeles, Black	0.46	0.50
USA, Los Angeles, Hispanic	0.49	0.23
USA, Los Angeles, Other White	0.47	0.30
USA, New York (City and State), White	0.49	0.29
USA, New York (City and State), Black	0.53	0.44
USA, SEER, White	0.49	0.35
USA, SEER, Black	0.66	0.24
AMERICA : OTHER		
Brazil, Fortaleza	0.91	0.39
Brazil, Recife	0.75	0.59
Brazil, Sao Paulo	1.04	0.67
Colombia, Cali	0.53	0.37
Costa Rica	0.61	0.31
Cuba	0.94	0.52
Jamaica	0.69	0.33
Puerto Rico	0.55	0.28
ASIA		
Bangladesh, CERP	2.33	1.21
China, Shanghai	0.39	0.20
China, Taipei	0.31	0.35
Hong Kong	0.48	0.34
India, Bangalore	1.15	0.58
India, Bombay Cancer Registry	0.69	0.26
India, Tata Hospital, Bombay	0.93	0.52
Indonesia, Yogyakarta Path. Dept.	–	–
Iraq, Baghdad	1.00	0.82
Israel, Jews	0.96	0.67
Israel, non Jews	1.27	0.73
Japan, Kanagawa	0.18	0.16
Japan, Miyagi	0.13	0.06
Japan, Osaka	0.29	0.19
Kuwait, Kuwaiti	2.83	1.36
Kuwait, non Kuwaiti	1.03	0.68
Pakistan, JPMC	3.28	1.30
Philippines, Metro Manila & Rizal	0.20	0.07
Singapore, Chinese	0.35	0.26
Singapore, Malay	0.23	0.24
Thailand	0.37	0.35
Vietnam, Ho Chi Minh City	0.40	0.35

LYMPHOMA : LEUKAEMIA (1) RATIO

	Male	Female
EUROPE		
Czechoslovakia, Slovakia	0.64	0.26
Denmark	0.46	0.28
FRG, Children's Tumour Registry	0.48	0.27
FRG, Saarland	0.40	0.20
Finland	0.40	0.26
France, Bas Rhin	0.62	0.40
France, Paediatric Registries	0.53	0.31
German Democratic Republic	0.70	0.45
Great Britain, England and Wales	0.41	0.24
Great Britain, Manchester (period 1)	0.39	0.25
Great Britain, Manchester (period 2)	0.40	0.28
Great Britain, Scotland	0.41	0.22
Hungary	0.50	0.24
Italy, Torino	0.44	0.25
Netherlands, SOOZ, Eindhoven	0.47	0.29
Norway	0.26	0.13
Poland, Warsaw City	0.34	0.32
Spain, Childhood Cancer Registry	0.88	0.42
Spain, Zaragoza	0.65	0.29
Sweden	0.42	0.17
Switzerland, Three Western Cantons	0.45	0.21
Yugoslavia, Slovenia	0.64	0.30
OCEANIA		
Australia, New South Wales	0.43	0.20
Australia, Queensland	0.62	0.29
Fiji, Fijian	0.56	0.67
Fiji, Indian	0.42	0.17
New Zealand, Maori	0.67	0.73
New Zealand, non Maori	0.36	0.18
Papua New Guinea, Histopath. Registry	1.93	1.91

EMBRYONAL AND BONE TUMOUR RATIOS
(Both sexes)

	Neuroblastoma : Wilms' tumour (1)	Retinoblastoma : Wilms' tumour (1)	Ewing's : Osteosarcoma (1)
AFRICA			
Madagascar, Institut Pasteur	0.17	2.26	0.64
Malawi, Histopathology Registry	0.19	0.93	-
Morocco, Children's Hospital, Rabat	0.72	0.39	0.71
Nigeria, Ibadan	0.61	1.00	-
Sudan, RICK, Arab	0.26	1.53	0.12
Sudan, RICK, Sudanic	0.27	3.27	0.14
Tanzania	0.07	1.73	0.40
Tunisia, Institut Salah-Azaiz	0.53	0.87	0.70
Uganda, Kampala	0.10	0.95	0.08
Uganda, West Nile	-	1.33	-
Zimbabwe, Bulawayo	0.28	1.12	0.08
AMERICA : NORTH			
Canada, Atlantic Provinces	1.09	0.30	1.00
Canada, Western Provinces	1.37	0.57	1.00
USA, Greater Delaware Valley, White	1.43	0.63	0.87
USA, Greater Delaware Valley, non White	0.44	0.44	0.06
USA, Los Angeles, Black	0.84	0.41	0.12
USA, Los Angeles, Hispanic	0.70	0.76	0.45
USA, Los Angeles, Other White	0.96	0.49	1.12
USA, New York (City and State), White	1.42	0.33	0.90
USA, New York (City and State), Black	0.97	0.33	0.06
USA, SEER, White	1.36	0.43	0.93
USA, SEER, Black	0.88	0.43	0.09
AMERICA : OTHER			
Brazil, Fortaleza	0.60	0.80	0.14
Brazil, Recife	1.03	0.82	0.56
Brazil, Sao Paulo	1.10	0.81	0.62
Colombia, Cali	0.91	1.09	0.14
Costa Rica	0.89	0.72	0.83
Cuba	1.05	0.69	0.70
Jamaica	1.33	0.72	0.13
Puerto Rico	0.85	0.55	0.73
ASIA			
Bangladesh, CERP	0.06	5.95	0.19
China, Shanghai	12.00	6.50	0.22
China, Taipei	2.00	1.16	0.20
Hong Kong	1.17	0.76	0.22
India, Bangalore	1.00	0.63	0.50
India, Bombay Cancer Registry	0.85	1.37	1.32
India, Tata Hospital, Bombay	1.02	2.12	1.20
Indonesia, Yogyakarta Path. Dept.	1.00	4.56	-
Iraq, Baghdad	1.15	1.11	0.81
Israel, Jews	1.88	0.45	0.69
Israel, non Jews	1.83	0.75	0.40
Japan, Kanagawa	4.07	1.57	0.29
Japan, Miyagi	2.45	1.45	0.33
Japan, Osaka	2.32	1.33	0.28
Kuwait, Kuwaiti	1.38	0.63	0.80
Kuwait, non Kuwaiti	1.67	0.67	2.33
Pakistan, JPMC	-	2.83	1.50
Philippines, Metro Manila & Rizal	0.39	1.94	0.21
Singapore, Chinese	1.71	1.19	0.14
Singapore, Malay	1.25	0.50	0.25
Thailand	2.03	3.73	0.37
Vietnam, Ho Chi Minh City	0.12	1.68	1.67

EMBRYONAL AND BONE TUMOUR RATIOS
(Both sexes)

	Neuroblastoma : Wilms' tumour (1)	Retinoblastoma : Wilms' tumour (1)	Ewing's : Osteosarcoma (1)
EUROPE			
Czechoslovakia, Slovakia	0.62	0.61	1.04
Denmark	1.20	0.26	1.50
FRG, Children's Tumour Registry	1.25	0.40	0.84
FRG, Saarland	1.11	0.21	1.00
Finland	0.91	0.47	0.45
France, Bas Rhin	1.05	0.21	1.20
France, Paediatric Registries	2.25	0.63	0.33
German Democratic Republic	1.13	0.46	0.75
Great Britain, England and Wales	0.97	0.45	0.67
Great Britain, Manchester (period 1)	1.24	0.64	0.92
Great Britain, Manchester (period 2)	1.10	0.31	0.60
Great Britain, Scotland	1.04	0.49	0.70
Hungary	1.48	0.24	1.14
Italy, Torino	1.54	0.56	0.52
Netherlands, SOOZ, Eindhoven	1.33	0.89	0.60
Norway	0.95	0.43	0.17
Poland, Warsaw City	0.84	0.48	0.43
Spain, Childhood Cancer Registry	1.27	0.31	1.69
Spain, Zaragoza	1.33	–	0.45
Sweden	0.97	0.49	0.89
Switzerland, Three Western Cantons	1.38	0.31	0.83
Yugoslavia, Slovenia	0.72	0.28	0.88
OCEANIA			
Australia, New South Wales	1.34	0.55	0.93
Australia, Queensland	1.31	0.69	3.20
Fiji, Fijian	0.45	0.55	0.33
Fiji, Indian	0.50	1.00	–
New Zealand, Maori	1.56	0.67	2.50
New Zealand, non Maori	1.10	0.76	0.67
Papua New Guinea, Histopath. Registry	0.80	1.90	0.86

7. APPENDIX TABLES

7.1

Miscellaneous intracranial and intraspinal neoplasms

MISCELLANEOUS INTRACRANIAL AND INTRASPINAL NEOPLASMS (Group IIIe)

REGION	ALL CANCER	MISCEL. INTRACRANIAL AND INTRASPINAL NEOPLASMS	Pituitary Adenomas 8270-8281, 8300	Cranio-pharyngioma 9350	Pineal Tumours 9360-9362	Ganglio-glioma 9505	Meningiomas 9530-9539	Benign Teratoma 9060-9102 /0,1	Malignant NOS 8000-8004, 9990/3,6,9	Benign or Uncertain NOS 9990/0,1
AFRICA										
Madagascar, Institut Pasteur	555	1	-	-	-	-	-	-	-	-
Malawi, Histopathology Registry	238	-	-	-	-	-	-	-	-	-
Morocco, Children's Hospital, Rabat	444	-	-	-	-	-	-	-	-	-
Nigeria, Ibadan	957	30	-	6	-	-	2	-	19	1
Sudan, RICK, Arab	558	6	1	1	1	-	1	1	3	-
Sudan, RICK, Sudanic	217	4	1	-	-	-	2	-	1	-
Tanzania	258	-	-	-	-	-	-	-	-	-
Tunisia, Institut Salah-Azaiz	900	-	-	-	-	-	-	-	-	-
Uganda, Kampala	203	2	-	2	-	-	-	-	-	-
Uganda, West Nile	205	-	-	-	-	-	-	-	-	-
Zimbabwe, Bulawayo	543	12	-	3	-	-	1	-	8	-
AMERICA : NORTH										
Canada, Atlantic Provinces	591	25	-	2	2	-	2	-	21	-
Canada, Western Provinces	2072	31	-	6	2	-	2	-	21	-
USA, Greater Delaware Valley, White	1970	56	-	23	11	9	3	-	10	-
USA, Greater Delaware Valley, non White	379	13	-	10	1	1	-	-	2	-
USA, Los Angeles, Black	334	10	-	4	-	-	-	-	4	2
USA, Los Angeles, Hispanic	891	26	-	11	2	4	-	-	9	-
USA, Los Angeles, Other White	1368	38	-	13	4	1	-	-	14	6
USA, New York (City and State), White	2853	112	1	25	9	6	11	-	60	6
USA, New York (City and State), Black	454	14	1	4	2	-	1	-	6	-
USA, SEER, White	5142	35	-	-	1	-	5	-	29	-
USA, SEER, Black	610	5	-	-	2	-	-	-	3	-
AMERICA : OTHER										
Brazil, Fortaleza	207	16	-	-	-	-	-	-	16	-
Brazil, Recife	602	33	-	2	-	-	1	-	30	-
Brazil, Sao Paulo	2806	192	-	8	2	-	2	-	180	-
Colombia, Cali	249	15	-	-	-	-	-	-	15	-
Costa Rica	491	1	-	-	-	-	-	-	1	-
Cuba	3478	96	-	5	4	-	4	-	83	-
Jamaica	232	2	-	-	-	-	-	-	1	1
Puerto Rico	1059	9	-	-	-	-	-	-	9	1
ASIA										
Bangladesh, CERP	1293	8	-	1	-	-	3	-	4	-
China, Shanghai	828	101	-	7	5	-	2	-	87	-
China, Taipei	873	23	-	-	1	-	-	-	22	-
Hong Kong	999	61	-	-	-	-	-	-	61	-
India, Bangalore	204	-	-	-	-	-	-	-	-	-
India, Bombay Cancer Registry	1528	47	1	8	-	-	-	-	38	1
India, Tata Hospital, Bombay	2366	35	-	-	-	-	-	-	35	1
Indonesia, Yogyakarta Path. Dept.	215	-	-	-	-	-	-	-	-	-

MISCELLANEOUS INTRACRANIAL AND INTRASPINAL NEOPLASMS (Group IIe)

REGION	ALL CANCER	MISCEL. INTRACRANIAL AND INTRASPINAL NEOPLASMS	Pituitary Adenomas 8270-8281, 8300	Cranio-pharyngioma 9350	Pineal Tumours 9360-9362	Ganglio-glioma 9505	Meningiomas 9530-9539	Benign Teratoma 9060-9102 /0,1	Malignant NOS 8000-8004, 9990/3,6,9	Benign or Uncertain NOS 9990/0,1
Iraq, Baghdad	2410	18	–	4	–	–	5	–	9	27
Israel, Jews	1167	61	–	1	–	–	5	1	27	12
Israel, non Jews	260	16	–	1	–	–	–	–	3	–
Japan, Kanagawa	751	62	–	2	1	–	1	–	58	–
Japan, Miyagi	374	14	1	1	–	–	–	–	12	–
Japan, Osaka	2288	324	1	24	28	–	5	10	256	–
Kuwait, Kuwaiti	142	2	–	1	–	–	–	–	2	–
Kuwait, non Kuwaiti	238	5	–	1	–	–	–	–	4	–
Pakistan, JPMC	331	15	–	–	–	–	–	–	15	–
Philippines, Metro Manila & Rizal	579	21	–	4	–	–	1	–	13	8
Singapore, Chinese	746	36	–	–	–	–	–	1	30	–
Singapore, Malay	145	9	–	4	1	–	2	–	9	–
Thailand	1098	18	–	4	1	–	–	–	10	–
Vietnam, Ho Chi Minh City	240	–	–	–	–	–	–	–	–	–
EUROPE										
Czechoslovakia, Slovakia	1511	52	1	3	2	2	14	1	32	10
Denmark	653	43	–	7	2	2	5	2	14	3
FRG, Children's Tumour Registry	2992	93	–	22	8	2	2	1	55	2
FRG, Saarland	401	30	–	2	2	–	5	–	24	–
Finland	1318	79	–	16	1	–	–	–	58	–
France, Bas Rhin	243	11	–	3	3	–	–	–	7	–
France, Paediatric Registries	400	20	2	8	2	–	11	6	4	5
German Democratic Republic	1992	83	–	21	2	8	42	–	39	–
Great Britain, England and Wales	11479	391	2	126	47	1	–	2	96	138
Great Britain, Manchester (period 1)	1666	83	1	19	3	4	6	2	30	40
Great Britain, Manchester (period 2)	1295	77	–	13	3	–	2	–	8	36
Great Britain, Scotland	1243	21	–	8	2	3	6	2	12	6
Hungary	2193	135	–	26	1	1	1	–	5	60
Italy, Torino	1023	77	–	14	1	–	–	–	47	–
Netherlands, SOOZ, Eindhoven	235	6	–	1	1	–	–	–	–	–
Norway	1104	48	–	1	1	–	–	–	32	1
Poland, Warsaw City	304	34	–	–	6	1	3	–	–	–
Spain, Childhood Cancer Registry	2111	104	–	25	1	1	–	–	69	–
Spain, Zaragoza	250	30	–	–	13	–	14	–	29	–
Sweden	2898	113	1	29	–	–	1	–	55	–
Switzerland, Three Western Cantons	220	5	–	–	–	–	–	–	3	–
Yugoslavia, Slovenia	444	13	–	–	–	–	–	–	13	–
OCEANIA										
Australia, New South Wales	1872	34	–	2	1	–	3	1	28	–
Australia, Queensland	584	11	–	5	3	–	–	–	2	–
Fiji, Fijian	106	3	–	2	–	–	–	–	1	–
Fiji, Indian	82	1	–	1	–	–	–	–	–	–
New Zealand, Maori	162	3	–	–	–	–	–	–	3	–
New Zealand, non Maori	1009	19	–	3	3	–	3	–	10	–
Papua New Guinea, Histopath. Registry	234	–	–	–	–	–	–	–	–	–

7.2

Soft tissue sarcomas

SOFT TISSUE SARCOMAS (Group IX)

REGION	ALL CANCER	SOFT TISSUE SARCOMAS	RHABDOMYO-SARCOMA IX a)	FIBRO-SARCOMA IX b)	OTHER SARCOMAS (by ICD-0 Histology)									
					Total	Myxo. 8840	Lipo. 8850–8860	Myo. 8890–8895	Malig. Mesen. 8990	Synovial 9040–9044	Angio. 9120–9150[1]	Kaposi 9140	NOS 8800–8804	Other[2]
AFRICA														
Madagascar, Institut Pasteur	555	72	18	21	33	–	1	2	–	3	4	2	20	1
Malawi, Histopathology Registry	238	40	19	5	16	–	1	2	–	–	–	12	–	–
Morocco, Children's Hospital, Rabat	444	20	18	1	1	–	–	1	–	1	–	1	–	–
Nigeria, Ibadan	957	46	27	9	10	–	3	1	1	1	1	1	3	–
Sudan, RICK, Arab	558	46	8	33	5	–	1	–	–	3	–	1	–	–
Sudan, RICK, Sudanic	217	15	2	10	3	–	1	–	–	–	1	1	1	–
Tanzania	258	51	11	7	33	–	2	–	–	1	1	26	4	–
Tunisia, Institut Salah-Azaiz	900	97	53	18	26	–	7	4	2	2	4	–	6	–
Uganda, Kampala	203	17	8	3	6	–	–	–	–	–	1	4	1	–
Uganda, West Nile	205	6	3	–	3	–	–	1	–	–	–	1	1	–
Zimbabwe, Bulawayo	543	75	15	18	42	5	1	7	–	1	2	19	7	–
AMERICA : NORTH														
Canada, Atlantic Provinces	591	26	19	5	2	–	–	–	–	–	–	–	2	–
Canada, Western Provinces	2072	128	61	34	33	2	8	4	2	5	6	–	11	1
USA, Greater Delaware Valley, White	1970	132	71	26	35	2	–	2	2	4	6	–	18	2
USA, Greater Delaware Valley, non White	379	35	15	8	12	–	2	2	2	1	2	1	1	1
USA, Los Angeles, Black	334	23	12	4	7	–	–	1	2	1	1	–	1	1
USA, Los Angeles, Hispanic	891	65	35	9	21	–	2	1	6	1	1	1	8	3
USA, Los Angeles, Other White	1368	108	49	23	36	1	1	2	6	3	5	–	15	1
USA, New York (City and State), White	2853	186	115	32	39	–	1	4	4	11	6	–	13	3
USA, New York (City and State), Black	454	28	16	7	5	–	1	–	1	1	2	–	1	1
USA, SEER, White	5142	340	180	66	94	–	1	4	19	18	11	–	36	5
USA, SEER, Black	610	50	20	18	12	–	1	1	3	1	–	–	6	–
AMERICA : OTHER														
Brazil, Fortaleza	207	9	1	4	4	–	1	–	–	1	1	–	1	1
Brazil, Recife	602	41	15	5	21	1	1	1	1	6	3	–	13	1
Brazil, Sao Paulo	2806	154	59	33	62	2	11	4	–	6	8	–	31	–
Colombia, Cali	249	11	5	3	3	–	–	–	1	1	1	–	1	–
Costa Rica	491	22	14	1	7	–	–	–	1	1	1	–	3	2
Cuba	3478	160	74	13	73	2	5	2	–	1	10	4	48	1
Jamaica	232	13	8	1	4	1	1	1	–	1	2	–	–	–
Puerto Rico	1059	71	37	9	25	–	4	3	2	4	2	–	8	2
ASIA														
Bangladesh, CERP	1293	86	9	16	61	1	4	12	–	2	8	–	34	–
China, Shanghai	828	34	15	8	11	–	2	2	1	3	2	–	1	–
China, Taipei	873	35	14	10	11	–	1	1	1	2	2	–	4	1
Hong Kong	999	41	15	20	6	–	1	1	1	–	1	–	3	–
India, Bangalore	204	12	9	–	3	–	–	1	1	–	1	–	3	–
India, Bombay Cancer Registry	1528	72	35	22	15	–	4	1	1	1	2	–	7	1
India, Tata Hospital, Bombay	2366	177	103	34	40	–	2	1	1	6	4	–	26	1
Indonesia, Yogyakarta Path. Dept.	215	29	22	2	5	–	1	–	1	1	2	–	2	–

[1] Excludes 9140
[2] Includes 9170,9240,9251,9581

SOFT TISSUE SARCOMAS (Group IX)

REGION	ALL CANCER	SOFT TISSUE SARCOMAS	RHABDOMYO-SARCOMA IX a)	FIBRO-SARCOMA IX b)	OTHER SARCOMAS (by ICD-O Histology)								
					Total	Myxo. 8840	Lipo. 8850–8860	Myo. 8890–8895	Malig. Mesen. 8990	Synovial 9040–9044	Angio. 9120–9150[1]	Kaposi 9140	NOS 8800–8804	Other[2]
Iraq, Baghdad	2410	119	50	34	35	–	7	1	2	1	11	1	11	1
Israel, Jews	1167	79	31	20	28	–	2	3	2	3	6	2	9	1
Israel, non Jews	260	11	4	1	6	–	–	3	1	1	1	–	–	–
Japan, Kanagawa	751	31	17	3	11	–	1	3	–	1	3	–	2	1
Japan, Miyagi	374	21	10	2	9	–	2	3	–	1	–	–	3	–
Japan, Osaka	2288	96	43	15	38	–	5	3	–	2	13	–	11	4
Kuwait, Kuwaiti	142	8	6	–	2	–	–	–	–	–	2	–	–	–
Kuwait, non Kuwaiti	238	8	4	1	3	–	1	–	–	1	–	–	1	–
Pakistan, JPMC	331	16	2	4	10	–	–	3	–	2	1	–	4	–
Philippines, Metro Manila & Rizal	579	25	15	4	6	–	2	1	–	–	3	–	–	–
Singapore, Chinese	746	37	19	8	10	–	1	1	–	5	1	–	2	–
Singapore, Malay	145	4	1	1	2	–	1	–	–	1	–	–	–	–
Thailand	1098	68	32	13	23	–	1	4	3	1	3	–	11	–
Vietnam, Ho Chi Minh City	240	7	2	4	1	1	–	–	–	–	–	–	–	–
EUROPE														
Czechoslovakia, Slovakia	1511	66	12	14	40	1	3	1	1	3	5	–	26	–
Denmark	653	31	19	10	2	–	–	–	–	–	–	–	1	1
FRG, Children's Tumour Registry	2992	188	127	23	38	–	1	1	1	17	4	–	13	1
FRG, Saarland	401	24	7	5	12	1	1	–	–	2	–	–	8	–
Finland	1318	69	15	25	29	1	2	–	8	6	1	–	10	1
France, Bas Rhin	243	14	10	1	3	1	–	–	–	1	–	–	1	–
France, Paediatric Registries	400	29	20	4	5	1	–	–	–	–	–	–	4	–
German Democratic Republic	1992	152	53	49	50	6	14	2	2	4	4	–	18	–
Great Britain, England and Wales	11479	684	448	96	140	–	8	15	8	15	17	1	75	1
Great Britain, Manchester (period 1)	1666	104	76	6	22	–	–	4	1	4	6	–	6	1
Great Britain, Manchester (period 2)	1295	56	42	11	3	–	–	–	1	1	–	–	1	–
Great Britain, Scotland	1243	69	36	10	23	–	6	–	1	11	3	–	1	1
Hungary	2193	119	56	19	44	1	7	–	2	1	1	–	32	–
Italy, Torino	1023	54	22	13	19	1	1	1	2	1	1	–	9	1
Netherlands, SOOZ, Eindhoven	235	17	9	1	7	–	1	–	–	1	3	–	2	–
Norway	1104	54	22	15	17	–	1	1	1	3	–	–	8	3
Poland, Warsaw City	304	23	17	2	4	–	–	2	1	–	2	–	–	–
Spain, Childhood Cancer Registry	2111	175	123	22	30	–	2	3	3	3	3	–	16	–
Spain, Zaragoza	250	21	12	6	3	–	2	–	–	–	1	–	–	–
Sweden	2898	150	45	35	70	2	2	3	38	5	5	–	14	1
Switzerland, Three Western Cantons	220	15	9	1	5	–	1	–	–	1	–	–	2	1
Yugoslavia, Slovenia	444	32	17	5	10	–	3	–	1	–	2	–	4	–
OCEANIA														
Australia, New South Wales	1872	111	83	15	13	–	1	2	–	1	1	–	8	–
Australia, Queensland	584	28	20	4	4	–	–	–	–	1	–	–	3	–
Fiji, Fijian	106	7	2	1	4	–	–	–	–	1	1	–	2	–
Fiji, Indian	82	5	3	1	1	–	–	–	–	1	1	–	–	–
New Zealand, Maori	162	6	4	–	2	–	1	1	–	–	–	–	–	–
New Zealand, non Maori	1009	48	33	2	13	–	1	1	–	1	6	–	5	–
Papua New Guinea, Histopath. Registry	234	27	12	1	14	–	–	2	–	2	–	6	6	–

[1] Excludes 9140
[2] Includes 9170, 9240, 9251, 9581

7.3
Melanoma

MELANOMA (Group XId)

REGION	ALL CANCER	MELANOMA	Skin Head & Neck 173.0–173.4	Skin Trunk 173.5	Skin Upper Limb 173.6	Skin Lower Limb 173.7	Other Skin 173.8–173.9	Eye 190.0–190.9	All other
AFRICA									
Madagascar, Institut Pasteur	555	6	3	1	–	–	–	1	1
Malawi, Histopathology Registry	238	3	1	1	–	–	–	–	1
Morocco, Children's Hospital, Rabat	444	1	–	–	–	–	–	–	1
Nigeria, Ibadan	957	1	–	–	–	–	–	1	–
Sudan, RICK, Arab	558	2	–	–	–	–	1	–	1
Sudan, RICK, Sudanic	217	1	–	–	–	–	–	–	1
Tanzania	258	1	1	–	–	–	–	–	–
Tunisia, Institut Salah-Azaiz	900	–	–	–	–	–	–	–	–
Uganda, Kampala	203	2	–	–	–	–	2	–	–
Uganda, West Nile	205	–	–	–	–	–	–	–	–
Zimbabwe, Bulawayo	543	2	–	–	–	–	2	–	–
AMERICA : NORTH									
Canada, Atlantic Provinces	591	7	1	3	2	1	–	–	–
Canada, Western Provinces	2072	17	4	2	3	4	2	1	1
USA, Greater Delaware Valley, White	1970	9	2	1	–	5	–	–	1
USA, Greater Delaware Valley, non White	379	1	–	–	–	1	–	–	–
USA, Los Angeles, Black	334	1	–	–	–	1	–	–	–
USA, Los Angeles, Hispanic	891	–	–	–	–	–	–	–	–
USA, Los Angeles, Other White	1368	16	4	4	3	3	1	1	–
USA, New York (City and State), White	2853	16	5	4	2	–	1	2	2
USA, New York (City and State), Black	454	2	–	1	–	–	1	–	–
USA, SEER, White	5142	51	8	13	11	11	1	6	1
USA, SEER, Black	610	1	–	1	–	–	–	–	–
AMERICA : OTHER									
Brazil, Fortaleza	207	1	–	–	–	–	1	–	–
Brazil, Recife	602	1	–	–	–	–	1	–	–
Brazil, Sao Paulo	2806	13	1	–	2	1	4	4	1
Colombia, Cali	249	6	–	1	3	2	–	–	–
Costa Rica	491	2	–	1	–	–	–	–	1
Cuba	3478	6	–	1	1	1	–	3	–
Jamaica	232	–	–	–	–	–	–	–	–
Puerto Rico	1059	3	–	1	–	2	–	–	–
ASIA									
Bangladesh, CERP	1293	5	1	–	–	–	4	–	–
China, Shanghai	828	2	–	–	–	–	1	–	1
China, Taipei	873	–	–	–	–	–	–	–	–
Hong Kong	999	9	–	–	–	–	8	–	1
India, Bangalore	204	2	–	2	–	–	–	–	–
India, Bombay Cancer Registry	1528	2	1	–	–	–	1	–	–
India, Tata Hospital, Bombay	2366	1	–	–	–	–	1	–	–
Indonesia, Yogyakarta Path. Dept.	215	2	1	–	–	–	–	–	1

MELANOMA (Group XId)

REGION	ALL CANCER	MELANOMA	Skin Head & Neck 173.0-173.4	Skin Trunk 173.5	Skin Upper Limb 173.6	Skin Lower Limb 173.7	Other Skin 173.8-173.9	Eye 190.0-190.9	All Other
Iraq, Baghdad	2410	7	1	-	-	1	4	-	1
Israel, Jews	1167	16	3	4	2	5	2	-	-
Israel, non Jews	260	2	-	-	2	-	-	-	-
Japan, Kanagawa	751	4	2	-	-	-	1	1	-
Japan, Miyagi	374	8	2	1	-	2	2	-	1
Japan, Osaka	2288	-	-	-	-	-	-	-	-
Kuwait, Kuwaiti	142	-	-	-	-	-	-	-	-
Kuwait, non Kuwaiti	238	-	-	-	-	-	-	-	-
Pakistan, JPMC	331	3	3	-	-	-	-	-	-
Philippines, Metro Manila & Rizal	579	1	-	-	-	-	1	-	-
Singapore, Chinese	746	1	-	1	-	-	-	-	-
Singapore, Malay	145	1	-	1	-	-	2	-	-
Thailand	1098	2	-	-	-	-	-	-	-
Vietnam, Ho Chi Minh City	240	-	-	-	-	-	-	-	-
EUROPE									
Czechoslovakia, Slovakia	1511	11	-	1	1	5	2	2	-
Denmark	653	7	3	2	-	2	3	-	-
FRG, Children's Tumour Registry	2992	3	-	1	-	1	2	-	-
FRG, Saarland	401	4	-	4	-	-	-	-	-
Finland	1318	10	-	1	1	5	2	1	-
France, Bas Rhin	243	1	1	-	-	-	-	-	-
France, Paediatric Registries	400	4	2	1	1	-	-	-	-
German Democratic Republic	1992	14	2	3	1	3	5	-	-
Great Britain, England and Wales	11479	86	12	31	11	20	5	5	2
Great Britain, Manchester (period 1)	1666	4	1	-	1	1	-	1	-
Great Britain, Manchester (period 2)	1295	5	2	3	-	-	-	-	-
Great Britain, Scotland	1243	16	2	3	1	5	2	3	-
Hungary	2193	2	-	-	1	1	-	-	-
Italy, Torino	1023	6	-	-	1	3	2	-	-
Netherlands, SOOZ, Eindhoven	235	4	1	-	-	-	1	1	1
Norway	1104	17	16	-	-	-	-	1	-
Poland, Warsaw City	304	1	-	-	-	-	1	-	-
Spain, Childhood Cancer Registry	2111	-	-	-	-	-	-	-	-
Spain, Zaragoza	250	-	-	-	-	-	-	-	-
Sweden	2898	13	3	3	-	3	1	3	-
Switzerland, Three Western Cantons	220	2	-	-	2	-	-	-	-
Yugoslavia, Slovenia	444	8	4	2	2	-	-	-	-
OCEANIA									
Australia, New South Wales	1872	72	12	-	21	12	24	3	-
Australia, Queensland	584	3	1	-	-	-	1	1	-
Fiji, Fijian	106	-	-	-	-	-	-	-	-
Fiji, Indian	82	-	-	-	-	-	-	-	-
New Zealand, Maori	162	-	-	-	-	-	-	-	-
New Zealand, non Maori	1009	32	8	1	9	6	4	4	-
Papua New Guinea, Histopath. Registry	234	1	1	-	-	-	-	-	-

7.4

Miscellaneous carcinomas

MISCELLANEOUS CARCINOMAS (Group XI excluding XId)

REGION	ALL CANCER	MISCEL. CARCIN.	ADRENO. 194.0	THYROID 193.9	NASOPH. 147	OTHER (By ICD-O Site)												
						Total	140–149[1]	153–154	157	162	164	173	174–175	179–184	188–189[2]	190	191–192	Other
AFRICA																		
Madagascar, Institut Pasteur	555	10	–	1	–	9	2	1	–	–	–	4	–	–	–	–	–	2
Malawi, Histopathology Registry	238	27	1	–	2	24	7	1	–	–	–	7	–	1	3	1	–	4
Morocco, Children's Hospital, Rabat	444	19	–	–	12	7	3	2	–	–	–	1	–	–	–	–	–	1
Nigeria, Ibadan	957	9	–	5	1	3	2	–	–	–	–	1	–	1	–	–	1	1
Sudan, RICK, Arab	558	89	–	2	46	41	11	3	–	–	–	5	–	1	–	6	1	14
Sudan, RICK, Sudanic	217	56	–	–	32	24	6	–	–	–	–	8	–	–	–	3	–	7
Tanzania	258	17	–	–	–	17	3	–	–	–	–	5	–	2	–	1	–	6
Tunisia, Institut Salah-Azaiz	900	160	1	5	63	91	2	2	–	–	–	81	–	2	–	–	–	4
Uganda, Kampala	203	13	–	–	3	10	2	–	–	–	–	2	–	1	–	3	–	2
Uganda, West Nile	205	2	–	–	1	1	–	–	–	–	–	1	–	–	–	–	–	–
Zimbabwe, Bulawayo	543	23	1	6	–	16	5	–	–	1	–	6	–	–	–	1	–	3
AMERICA : NORTH																		
Canada, Atlantic Provinces	591	17	1	5	2	9	2	1	–	–	–	1	–	1	–	–	–	4
Canada, Western Provinces	2072	101	2	20	1	78	4	9	1	4	1	32	2	1	3	–	10	11
USA, Greater Delaware Valley, White	1970	39	1	19	3	16	6	1	1	–	2	3	1	1	1	–	1	–
USA, Greater Delaware Valley, non White	379	12	1	–	5	6	3	1	–	–	–	1	–	–	–	1	–	3
USA, Los Angeles, Black	334	18	–	6	6	6	1	–	1	1	1	–	–	–	–	–	–	3
USA, Los Angeles, Hispanic	891	19	1	9	–	10	–	7	1	2	1	–	–	1	–	–	–	–
USA, Los Angeles, Other White	1368	35	1	17	3	14	5	4	–	1	1	–	1	2	–	1	–	3
USA, New York (City and State), White	2853	60	2	30	1	27	3	3	1	2	1	1	1	1	–	–	4	10
USA, New York (City and State), Black	454	22	–	7	5	9	4	–	1	–	–	–	–	3	–	1	2	–
USA, SEER, White	5142	151	13	71	6	61	17	19	1	4	4	–	–	3	7	–	–	6
USA, SEER, Black	610	24	1	5	4	14	7	2	–	3	–	–	–	1	–	–	–	2
AMERICA : OTHER																		
Brazil, Fortaleza	207	5	–	–	–	5	2	–	–	–	–	3	–	–	–	–	–	–
Brazil, Recife	602	40	1	4	–	35	1	4	1	4	1	8	2	1	2	2	3	14
Brazil, Sao Paulo	2806	154	28	8	4	114	17	11	–	4	1	35	–	2	2	2	7	34
Colombia, Cali	249	6	1	–	–	6	–	–	–	3	–	2	–	1	–	–	–	3
Costa Rica	491	20	1	6	7	6	2	1	–	–	1	1	–	–	–	–	–	2
Cuba	3478	94	2	32	12	48	5	2	2	2	2	10	–	1	–	2	1	22
Jamaica	232	5	–	–	2	3	2	–	–	–	–	1	–	1	–	1	–	–
Puerto Rico	1059	24	–	10	1	13	6	–	2	–	1	1	–	–	–	1	–	2
ASIA																		
Bangladesh, CERP	1293	111	–	1	31	79	42	2	–	–	–	10	1	1	–	3	–	20
China, Shanghai	828	18	–	5	–	13	3	3	–	–	5	1	–	–	–	–	–	1
China, Taipei	873	33	3	9	5	16	2	2	–	3	2	1	1	–	1	–	–	4
Hong Kong	999	38	–	9	8	21	3	3	–	3	–	2	1	3	3	1	–	7
India, Bangalore	204	9	–	4	2	3	1	–	–	–	–	–	1	1	–	–	–	1
India, Bombay Cancer Registry	1528	37	–	5	7	25	8	3	–	1	2	2	1	1	–	1	–	9
India, Tata Hospital, Bombay	2366	91	–	16	36	39	12	2	–	1	1	2	2	1	1	1	–	20
Indonesia, Yogyakarta Path. Dept.	215	27	–	–	5	22	3	–	–	–	–	7	–	–	–	1	–	11

[1] Excludes 147
[2] Excludes 189.0

MISCELLANEOUS CARCINOMAS (Group XI excluding XId)

REGION	ALL CANCER	MISCEL. CARCIN.	ADRENO. 194.0	THYROID 193.9	NASOPH. 147	Total	OTHER (By ICD–O Site) 140–149¹	153–154	157	162	164	173	174–175	179–184	188–189²	190	191–192	Other
Iraq, Baghdad	2410	95	–	11	14	70	10	6	–	3	1	15	3	–	5	7	2	18
Israel, Jews	1167	34	1	11	5	17	6	4	1	–	3	1	–	1	1	1	–	1
Israel, non Jews	260	5	–	3	1	1	–	1	–	–	–	1	–	–	–	–	–	2
Japan, Kanagawa	751	7	1	–	1	5	1	1	–	1	–	1	–	–	–	–	–	1
Japan, Miyagi	374	7	–	4	–	3	1	–	–	–	–	1	–	1	–	–	–	1
Japan, Osaka	2288	25	–	3	1	21	2	2	3	–	3	6	–	–	–	–	–	4
Kuwait, Kuwaiti	142	5	–	–	2	4	1	–	–	–	–	2	–	–	–	–	–	1
Kuwait, non Kuwaiti	238	6	–	2	2	2	–	1	–	–	–	2	–	–	1	2	–	4
Pakistan, JPMC	331	14	1	1	2	10	1	–	–	–	–	1	1	–	1	–	–	4
Philippines, Metro Manila & Rizal	579	12	–	2	4	6	2	1	–	2	3	2	1	–	–	2	2	5
Singapore, Chinese	746	40	–	11	9	20	4	3	1	–	1	2	–	–	–	–	–	16
Singapore, Malay	145	3	–	–	2	1	1	–	–	1	–	–	–	–	–	–	–	1
Thailand	1098	57	–	14	11	32	8	2	–	1	1	4	–	–	–	–	–	16
Vietnam, Ho Chi Minh City	240	11	–	–	3	8	4	1	–	–	–	2	–	–	–	–	–	1
EUROPE																		
Czechoslovakia, Slovakia	1511	54	1	4	1	48	8	4	1	2	3	14	1	4	2	–	1	8
Denmark	653	16	–	6	–	10	–	–	1	–	1	4	–	–	1	1	3	1
FRG, Children's Tumour Registry	2992	24	3	6	8	7	2	1	1	–	–	1	–	1	–	–	2	2
FRG, Saarland	401	12	1	–	–	11	1	6	–	–	–	16	2	2	–	–	–	4
Finland	1318	50	4	8	5	33	7	1	1	–	–	–	1	–	1	2	–	1
France, Bas Rhin	243	4	–	–	1	3	1	–	–	–	–	–	–	–	1	–	–	1
France, Paediatric Registries	400	12	1	2	3	6	1	1	–	–	5	4	–	1	1	–	2	2
German Democratic Republic	1992	61	5	15	4	37	5	3	5	8	8	17	1	3	2	3	1	12
Great Britain, England and Wales	11479	232	23	43	35	131	25	9	–	2	8	54	1	1	2	3	1	3
Great Britain, Manchester (period 1)	1666	26	4	1	9	12	4	2	–	1	–	3	–	3	–	–	–	3
Great Britain, Manchester (period 2)	1295	27	6	2	5	14	3	1	–	2	2	4	–	1	1	1	1	1
Great Britain, Scotland	1243	24	3	5	3	13	1	1	–	2	2	2	–	–	–	1	–	4
Hungary	2193	15	1	3	2	9	–	1	–	–	–	1	–	–	1	–	2	1
Italy, Torino	1023	22	2	11	3	6	–	1	2	–	–	1	–	–	1	–	–	2
Netherlands, SOOZ, Eindhoven	235	18	–	1	1	16	1	5	–	–	–	8	–	–	2	–	2	2
Norway	1104	24	2	8	2	12	1	2	–	1	2	6	–	–	–	–	–	4
Poland, Warsaw City	304	4	–	3	–	1	–	–	–	2	–	–	1	–	–	4	4	–
Spain, Childhood Cancer Registry	2111	31	4	8	4	15	2	1	1	–	–	1	1	1	2	–	–	5
Spain, Zaragoza	250	–	–	–	–	–	–	–	–	–	–	–	–	3	–	–	–	1
Sweden	2898	106	4	24	5	73	12	49	–	1	1	–	1	–	2	–	–	1
Switzerland, Three Western Cantons	220	6	–	–	1	5	1	–	–	1	1	–	1	–	–	–	2	1
Yugoslavia, Slovenia	444	11	–	5	1	5	1	2	–	–	1	1	–	–	1	–	–	1
OCEANIA																		
Australia, New South Wales	1872	33	1	8	3	21	10	3	–	–	2	–	–	–	1	–	2	3
Australia, Queensland	584	11	2	3	1	5	1	–	–	1	–	2	–	–	1	1	1	1
Fiji, Fijian	106	4	–	–	–	4	–	1	–	–	–	2	–	–	1	–	–	3
Fiji, Indian	82	5	1	–	–	4	1	1	–	–	–	–	–	–	–	–	1	2
New Zealand, Maori	162	12	2	–	–	10	3	4	–	–	1	–	–	–	2	–	1	7
New Zealand, non Maori	1009	38	1	8	1	29	1	12	–	–	1	4	–	–	2	–	7	7
Papua New Guinea, Histopath. Registry	234	8	–	–	–	8	1	–	–	–	–	–	–	–	1	–	–	3

¹ Excludes 147
² Excludes 189.0

7.5

Other and unspecified tumours

OTHER AND UNSPECIFIED TUMOURS (Group XII)

REGION	ALL CANCER	OTHER AND UNSPECIFIED TUMOURS	140–149	151	153–154	162	163	164	171	173	179–184	188–189[1]	190	191–192	193–194[2]	Other
AFRICA																
Madagascar, Institut Pasteur	555	21	1	-	1	-	-	-	3	1	2	-	-	-	-	13
Malawi, Histopathology Registry	238	7	1	-	-	-	-	-	2	-	-	-	-	-	-	4
Morocco, Children's Hospital, Rabat	444	-	-	-	-	-	-	-	-	-	-	-	-	-	-	-
Nigeria, Ibadan	957	23	4	-	-	1	-	-	1	-	1	-	4	-	-	13
Sudan, RICK, Arab	558	11	-	1	-	1	-	-	2	-	-	2	1	1	1	4
Sudan, RICK, Sudanic	217	3	-	-	-	-	-	-	1	-	-	1	1	-	-	-
Tanzania	258	8	2	-	-	-	-	-	1	1	1	-	1	-	-	4
Tunisia, Institut Salah-Azaiz	900	6	1	-	-	-	1	-	1	-	1	-	1	-	-	2
Uganda, Kampala	203	4	-	-	-	-	-	-	1	-	1	-	-	-	-	3
Uganda, West Nile	205	8	-	-	-	-	-	-	-	-	1	-	6	-	-	2
Zimbabwe, Bulawayo	543	10	-	-	-	-	-	-	-	1	2	-	3	-	-	4
AMERICA : NORTH																
Canada, Atlantic Provinces	591	1	-	-	-	-	-	-	-	-	-	-	-	-	-	1
Canada, Western Provinces	2072	24	-	-	-	-	-	2	2	4	1	-	2	-	1	16
USA, Greater Delaware Valley, White	1970	5	-	-	-	-	-	-	1	1	1	-	-	-	-	3
USA, Greater Delaware Valley, non White	379	-	-	-	-	-	-	-	-	-	-	-	-	-	-	-
USA, Los Angeles, Black	334	5	1	-	-	-	-	-	2	-	-	-	-	-	-	2
USA, Los Angeles, Hispanic	891	10	-	-	-	-	-	1	1	-	-	-	1	-	-	7
USA, Los Angeles, Other White	1368	14	1	1	3	-	-	-	5	1	1	1	1	-	-	7
USA, New York (City and State), White	2853	40	1	-	-	-	-	-	5	1	1	1	6	-	9	17
USA, New York (City and State), Black	454	8	1	-	-	-	-	-	6	-	1	1	1	-	1	3
USA, SEER, White	5142	28	-	-	-	2	-	2	6	-	-	-	-	-	-	18
USA, SEER, Black	610	2	-	-	-	-	-	-	1	-	-	-	-	-	-	1
AMERICA : OTHER																
Brazil, Fortaleza	207	12	-	-	1	1	-	1	2	1	-	2	2	-	-	5
Brazil, Recife	602	43	4	1	1	4	1	1	3	6	2	2	2	-	2	16
Brazil, Sao Paulo	2806	154	11	3	7	6	-	8	18	11	2	2	12	-	10	66
Colombia, Cali	249	5	-	-	-	-	-	-	1	-	-	-	-	-	-	4
Costa Rica	491	-	-	-	-	-	-	-	-	-	-	-	-	-	-	-
Cuba	3478	71	3	6	4	-	2	1	4	2	3	2	8	-	2	34
Jamaica	232	2	-	-	-	-	-	1	1	-	-	-	-	-	-	1
Puerto Rico	1059	10	-	-	-	-	-	1	1	-	-	-	-	-	-	9
ASIA																
Bangladesh, CERP	1293	78	20	-	1	-	1	22	4	1	-	-	6	-	5	24
China, Shanghai	828	55	12	1	7	1	-	4	1	6	-	1	4	-	5	13
China, Taipei	873	71	2	-	-	-	-	-	2	-	-	1	14	-	-	52
Hong Kong	999	101	11	2	2	13	1	-	10	2	11	14	11	-	6	18
India, Bangalore	204	3	-	-	-	-	-	-	-	-	-	-	-	-	-	3
India, Bombay Cancer Registry	1528	60	6	1	1	1	1	1	3	1	1	1	6	-	3	34
India, Tata Hospital, Bombay	2366	44	1	1	1	1	-	1	4	5	2	-	7	-	1	22
Indonesia, Yogyakarta Path. Dept.	215	-	-	-	-	-	-	-	-	-	-	-	-	-	-	-

(By ICD-O Site)

1 Excludes 189.0
2 Excludes 194.3–194.4

OTHER AND UNSPECIFIED TUMOURS (Group XII)

(By ICD-O Site)

REGION	ALL CANCER	OTHER AND UNSPECIFIED TUMOURS	140–149	151	153–154	162	163	164	171	173	179–184	188–189[1]	190	191–192	193–194[2]	other
Iraq, Baghdad	2410	29	–	–	2	3	–	1	5	2	–	–	1	–	–	16
Israel, Jews	1167	17	2	1	–	1	–	1	1	–	2	–	1	–	1	8
Israel, non Jews	260	5	1	–	–	–	–	1	2	–	–	–	2	–	–	1
Japan, Kanagawa	751	23	1	–	1	–	–	1	2	–	2	–	1	–	5	13
Japan, Miyagi	374	12	1	–	1	–	–	1	3	–	1	–	1	–	1	4
Japan, Osaka	2288	72	2	2	1	3	1	6	8	2	1	1	7	–	6	32
Kuwait, Kuwaiti	142	–	–	–	–	–	–	–	–	–	–	–	–	–	–	–
Kuwait, non Kuwaiti	238	8	–	–	–	1	–	1	–	–	–	–	2	–	1	4
Pakistan, JPMC	331	59	4	–	–	1	–	1	1	5	–	2	2	–	1	33
Philippines, Metro Manila & Rizal	579	32	2	2	–	1	–	–	1	1	1	1	12	–	2	19
Singapore, Chinese	746	25	2	1	1	1	–	–	2	–	1	1	3	–	1	10
Singapore, Malay	145	5	1	–	–	–	–	–	2	–	–	–	6	–	–	–
Thailand	1098	21	4	–	3	–	–	–	2	1	1	1	1	–	2	6
Vietnam, Ho Chi Minh City	240	14	2	–	–	–	–	–	1	2	–	–	3	–	–	6
EUROPE																
Czechoslovakia, Slovakia	1511	72	6	3	2	4	1	8	4	3	–	2	2	–	2	35
Denmark	653	20	1	–	–	1	1	1	2	–	–	–	1	–	1	14
FRG, Children's Tumour Registry	2992	5	–	–	–	–	–	2	2	1	1	–	1	–	–	5
FRG, Saarland	401	6	–	–	–	–	–	2	1	–	–	–	2	–	–	2
Finland	1318	6	1	–	–	–	–	1	3	–	1	–	1	–	1	2
France, Bas Rhin	243	5	1	–	–	–	–	–	–	–	–	1	1	–	1	1
France, Paediatric Registries	400	1	–	–	–	–	–	–	–	–	–	–	–	–	–	1
German Democratic Republic	1992	15	2	–	–	1	–	2	2	1	1	–	1	–	–	5
Great Britain, England and Wales	11479	26	4	–	–	1	–	3	2	3	3	1	1	–	2	12
Great Britain, Manchester (period 1)	1666	38	1	–	–	2	–	1	18	–	1	1	2	–	2	11
Great Britain, Manchester (period 2)	1295	7	–	–	–	1	–	–	1	1	1	–	1	–	–	2
Great Britain, Scotland	1243	3	1	–	–	2	–	2	3	–	–	–	3	–	–	2
Hungary	2193	13	1	–	–	2	1	2	3	–	–	1	3	–	–	14
Italy, Torino	1023	18	1	–	–	–	–	1	–	–	–	1	–	–	1	14
Netherlands, SOOZ, Eindhoven	235	1	–	–	–	1	–	1	5	1	–	–	3	–	1	12
Norway	1104	30	3	–	–	–	–	2	2	–	3	–	2	–	–	1
Poland, Warsaw City	304	7	–	–	–	–	–	3	–	–	–	–	1	–	6	8
Spain, Childhood Cancer Registry	2111	19	–	–	1	1	–	–	1	1	1	–	1	–	–	4
Spain, Zaragoza	250	6	–	–	–	2	–	–	2	–	–	–	–	–	–	16
Sweden	2898	42	6	–	–	–	–	–	8	1	1	–	8	3	–	1
Switzerland, Three Western Cantons	220	2	–	–	–	–	–	–	1	–	–	–	–	–	–	5
Yugoslavia, Slovenia	444	5	–	–	–	–	1	–	–	–	–	1	–	–	–	–
OCEANIA																
Australia, New South Wales	1872	10	1	–	–	–	–	2	3	–	3	–	–	–	1	1
Australia, Queensland	584	1	–	–	–	–	–	–	–	–	–	–	–	–	1	1
Fiji, Fijian	106	2	–	–	–	–	–	–	–	–	–	–	–	–	–	2
Fiji, Indian	82	1	–	–	–	–	–	–	1	–	–	–	–	–	–	1
New Zealand, Maori	162	5	–	–	–	–	–	–	3	–	–	–	–	5	–	–
New Zealand, non Maori	1009	14	–	–	–	–	–	–	1	–	–	–	–	8	–	3
Papua New Guinea, Histopath. Registry	234	1	–	–	–	–	–	–	–	–	–	–	1	–	–	–

1 Excludes 189.0
2 Excludes 194.3–194.4

PUBLICATIONS OF THE INTERNATIONAL AGENCY FOR RESEARCH ON CANCER
SCIENTIFIC PUBLICATIONS SERIES

(Available from Oxford University Press)
through local bookshops

No. 1 LIVER CANCER
1971; 176 pages; out of print

No. 2 ONCOGENESIS AND HERPESVIRUSES
Edited by P.M. Biggs, G. de-Thé & L.N. Payne
1972; 515 pages; out of print

No. 3 N-NITROSO COMPOUNDS: ANALYSIS AND FORMATION
Edited by P. Bogovski, R. Preussmann & E. A. Walker
1972; 140 pages; out of print

No. 4 TRANSPLACENTAL CARCINOGENESIS
Edited by L. Tomatis & U. Mohr
1973; 181 pages; out of print

*No. 5 PATHOLOGY OF TUMOURS IN LABORATORY ANIMALS. VOLUME 1. TUMOURS OF THE RAT. PART 1
Editor-in-Chief V.S. Turusov
1973; 214 pages

*No. 6 PATHOLOGY OF TUMOURS IN LABORATORY ANIMALS. VOLUME 1. TUMOURS OF THE RAT. PART 2
Editor-in-Chief V.S. Turusov
1976; 319 pages
*reprinted in one volume, Price £50.00

No. 7 HOST ENVIRONMENT INTERACTIONS IN THE ETIOLOGY OF CANCER IN MAN
Edited by R. Doll & I. Vodopija
1973; 464 pages; £32.50

No. 8 BIOLOGICAL EFFECTS OF ASBESTOS
Edited by P. Bogovski, J.C. Gilson, V. Timbrell & J.C. Wagner
1973; 346 pages; out of print

No. 9 N-NITROSO COMPOUNDS IN THE ENVIRONMENT
Edited by P. Bogovski & E. A. Walker
1974; 243 pages; £16.50

No. 10 CHEMICAL CARCINOGENESIS ESSAYS
Edited by R. Montesano & L. Tomatis
1974; 230 pages; out of print

No. 11 ONCOGENESIS AND HERPESVIRUSES II
Edited by G. de-Thé, M.A. Epstein & H. zur Hausen
1975; Part 1, 511 pages; Part 2, 403 pages; £65.-

No. 12 SCREENING TESTS IN CHEMICAL CARCINOGENESIS
Edited by R. Montesano, H. Bartsch & L. Tomatis
1976; 666 pages; £12.-

No. 13 ENVIRONMENTAL POLLUTION AND CARCINOGENIC RISKS
Edited by C. Rosenfeld & W. Davis
1976; 454 pages; out of print

No. 14 ENVIRONMENTAL N-NITROSO COMPOUNDS: ANALYSIS AND FORMATION
Edited by E.A. Walker, P. Bogovski & L. Griciute
1976; 512 pages; £37.50

No. 15 CANCER INCIDENCE IN FIVE CONTINENTS. VOLUME III
Edited by J. Waterhouse, C. Muir, P. Correa & J. Powell
1976; 584 pages; out of print

No. 16 AIR POLLUTION AND CANCER IN MAN
Edited by U. Mohr, D. Schmähl & L. Tomatis
1977; 311 pages; out of print

Prices, valid for October 1987, are subject to change without notice

SCIENTIFIC PUBLICATIONS SERIES

SCIENTIFIC PUBLICATIONS SERIES

No. 54 LABORATORY DECONTAMINATION
AND DESTRUCTION OF CARCINOGENS IN
LABORATORY WASTES: SOME HYDRAZINES
Edited by M. Castegnaro, G. Ellen, M. Lafontaine,
H.C. van der Plas, E.B. Sansone & S.P. Tucker
1983; 87 pages; £9.-

No. 55 LABORATORY DECONTAMINATION
AND DESTRUCTION OF CARCINOGENS IN
LABORATORY WASTES: SOME N-NITROSAMIDES
Edited by M. Castegnaro, M. Benard,
L.W. van Broekhoven, D. Fine, R. Massey,
E.B. Sansone, P.L.R. Smith, B. Spiegelhalder,
A. Stacchini, G. Telling & J.J. Vallon
1984; 65 pages; £7.50

No. 56 MODELS, MECHANISMS AND ETIOLOGY
OF TUMOUR PROMOTION
Edited by M. Börszönyi, N.E. Day, K. Lapis
& H. Yamasaki
1984; 532 pages; £32.50

No. 57 N-NITROSO COMPOUNDS:
OCCURRENCE, BIOLOGICAL EFFECTS
AND RELEVANCE TO HUMAN CANCER
Edited by I.K. O'Neill, R.C. von Borstel, C.T. Miller,
J. Long & H. Bartsch
1984; 1011 pages; £80.-

No. 58 AGE-RELATED FACTORS IN
CARCINOGENESIS
Edited by A. Likhachev, V. Anisimov & R. Montesano
1985; 288 pages; £20.-

No. 59 MONITORING HUMAN EXPOSURE TO
CARCINOGENIC AND MUTAGENIC AGENTS
Edited by A. Berlin, M. Draper, K. Hemminki
& H. Vainio
1984; 457 pages; £27.50

No. 60 BURKITT'S LYMPHOMA: A HUMAN
CANCER MODEL
Edited by G. Lenoir, G. O'Conor & C.L.M. Olweny
1985; 484 pages; £22.50

No. 61 LABORATORY DECONTAMINATION
AND DESTRUCTION OF CARCINOGENS IN
LABORATORY WASTES: SOME HALOETHERS
Edited by M. Castegnaro, M. Alvarez, M. Iovu,
E.B. Sansone, G.M. Telling & D.T. Williams
1984; 53 pages; £7.50

No. 62 DIRECTORY OF ON-GOING RESEARCH
IN CANCER EPIDEMIOLOGY 1984
Edited by C.S. Muir & G.Wagner
1984; 728 pages; £26.-

No. 63 VIRUS-ASSOCIATED CANCERS IN AFRICA
Edited by A.O. Williams, G.T. O'Conor, G.B. de-Thé
& C.A. Johnson
1984; 774 pages; £22.-

No. 64 LABORATORY DECONTAMINATION
AND DESTRUCTION OF CARCINOGENS IN
LABORATORY WASTES: SOME AROMATIC
AMINES AND 4-NITROBIPHENYL
Edited by M. Castegnaro, J. Barek, J. Dennis,
G. Ellen, M. Klibanov, M. Lafontaine, R. Mitchum,
P. Van Roosmalen, E.B. Sansone, L.A. Sternson
& M. Vahl
1985; 85 pages; £6.95

No. 65 INTERPRETATION OF NEGATIVE
EPIDEMIOLOGICAL EVIDENCE FOR
CARCINOGENICITY
Edited by N.J. Wald & R. Doll
1985; 232 pages; £20.-

No. 66 THE ROLE OF THE REGISTRY IN
CANCER CONTROL
Edited by D.M. Parkin, G. Wagner & C. Muir
1985; 155 pages; £10.-

No. 67 TRANSFORMATION ASSAY OF
ESTABLISHED CELL LINES: MECHANISMS
AND APPLICATION
Edited by T. Kakunaga & H. Yamasaki
1985; 225 pages; £20.-

No. 68 ENVIRONMENTAL CARCINOGENS:
SELECTED METHODS OF ANALYSIS
VOLUME 7. SOME VOLATILE HALOGENATED
HYDROCARBONS
Edited by L. Fishbein & I.K. O'Neill
1985; 479 pages; £20.-

No. 69 DIRECTORY OF ON-GOING RESEARCH
IN CANCER EPIDEMIOLOGY 1985
Edited by C.S. Muir & G. Wagner
1985; 756 pages; £22.

No. 70 THE ROLE OF CYCLIC NUCLEIC ACID
ADDUCTS IN CARCINOGENESIS AND
MUTAGENESIS
Edited by B. Singer & H. Bartsch
1986; 467 pages; £40.-

No. 71 ENVIRONMENTAL CARCINOGENS:
SELECTED METHODS OF ANALYSIS
VOLUME 8. SOME METALS: As, Be, Cd, Cr, Ni,
Pb, Se, Zn
Edited by I.K. O'Neill, P. Schuller & L. Fishbein
1986; 485 pages; £20.

No. 72 ATLAS OF CANCER IN SCOTLAND
1975-1980: INCIDENCE AND EPIDEMIOLOGICAL
PERSPECTIVE
Edited by I. Kemp, P. Boyle, M. Smans & C. Muir
1985; 282 pages; £35.-

SCIENTIFIC PUBLICATIONS SERIES

IARC MONOGRAPHS ON THE EVALUATION OF THE CARCINOGENIC RISK OF CHEMICALS TO HUMANS
(English editions only)

(Available from booksellers through the network of WHO Sales Agents*)

Volume 1
Some inorganic substances, chlorinated hydrocarbons, aromatic amines, N-nitroso compounds, and natural products
1972; 184 pages; out of print

Volume 2
Some inorganic and organometallic compounds
1973; 181 pages; out of print

Volume 3
Certain polycyclic aromatic hydrocarbons and heterocyclic compounds
1973; 271 pages; out of print

Volume 4
Some aromatic amines, hydrazine and related substances, N-nitroso compounds and miscellaneous alkylating agents
1974; 286 pages;
Sw. fr. 18.-

Volume 5
Some organochlorine pesticides
1974; 241 pages; out of print

Volume 6
Sex hormones
1974; 243 pages;
out of print

Volume 7
Some anti-thyroid and related substances, nitrofurans and industrial chemicals
1974; 326 pages; out of print

Volume 8
Some aromatic azo compounds
1975; 357 pages; Sw.fr. 36.-

Volume 9
Some aziridines, N-, S- and O-mustards and selenium
1975; 268 pages; Sw. fr. 27.-

Volume 10
Some naturally occurring substances
1976; 353 pages; out of print

Volume 11
Cadmium, nickel, some epoxides, miscellaneous industrial chemicals and general considerations on volatile anaesthetics
1976; 306 pages; out of print

Volume 12
Some carbamates, thiocarbamates and carbazides
1976; 282 pages; Sw. fr. 34.-

Volume 13
Some miscellaneous pharmaceutical substances
1977; 255 pages; Sw. fr. 30.-

Volume 14
Asbestos
1977; 106 pages; out of print

Volume 15
Some fumigants, the herbicides 2,4-D and 2,4,5-T, chlorinated dibenzodioxins and miscellaneous industrial chemicals
1977; 354 pages; Sw. fr. 50.-

Volume 16
Some aromatic amines and related nitro compounds — hair dyes, colouring agents and miscellaneous industrial chemicals
1978; 400 pages; Sw. fr. 50.-

Volume 17
Some N-nitroso compounds
1978; 365 pages; Sw. fr. 50.

Volume 18
Polychlorinated biphenyls and polybrominated biphenyls
1978; 140 pages; Sw. fr. 20.-

Volume 19
Some monomers, plastics and synthetic elastomers, and acrolein
1979; 513 pages; Sw. fr. 60.-

Volume 20
Some halogenated hydrocarbons
1979; 609 pages; Sw. fr. 60.-

*A list of these Agents may be obtained by writing to the World Health Organization, Distribution and Sales Service, 1211 Geneva 27, Switzerland

IARC MONOGRAPHS SERIES

Volume 21
Sex hormones (II)
1979; 583 pages; Sw. fr. 60.-

Volume 22
Some non-nutritive sweetening agents
1980; 208 pages; Sw. fr. 25.-

Volume 23
Some metals and metallic compounds
1980; 438 pages; Sw. fr. 50.-

Volume 24
Some pharmaceutical drugs
1980; 337 pages; Sw. fr. 40.-

Volume 25
Wood, leather and some associated industries
1981; 412 pages; Sw. fr. 60.-

Volume 26
Some antineoplastic and immunosuppressive agents
1981; 411 pages; Sw. fr. 62.-

Volume 27
Some aromatic amines, anthraquinones and nitroso compounds, and inorganic fluorides used in drinking-water and dental preparations
1982; 341 pages; Sw. fr. 40.-

Volume 28
The rubber industry
1982; 486 pages; Sw. fr. 70.-

Volume 29
Some industrial chemicals and dyestuffs
1982; 416 pages; Sw. fr. 60.-

Volume 30
Miscellaneous pesticides
1983; 424 pages; Sw. fr. 60.-

Volume 31
Some food additives, feed additives and naturally occurring substances
1983; 14 pages; Sw. fr. 60.-

Volume 32
Polynuclear aromatic compounds, Part 1, Chemical, environmental and experimental data
1984; 477 pages; Sw. fr. 60.-

Volume 33
Polynuclear aromatic compounds, Part 2, Carbon blacks, mineral oils and some nitroarenes
1984; 245 pages; Sw. fr. 50.-

Volume 34
Polynuclear aromatic compounds, Part 3, Industrial exposures in aluminium production, coal gasification, coke production, and iron and steel founding
1984; 219 pages; Sw. fr. 48.-

Volume 35
Polynuclear aromatic compounds, Part 4, Bitumens, coal-tars and derived products, shale-oils and soots
1985; 271 pages; Sw. fr.70.-

Volume 36
Allyl compounds, aldehydes, epoxides and peroxides
1985; 369 pages; Sw. fr. 70.-

Volume 37
Tobacco habits other than smoking; betel-quid and areca-nut chewing; and some related nitrosamines
1985; 291 pages; Sw. fr. 70.-

Volume 38
Tobacco smoking
1986; 421 pages; Sw. fr. 75.-

Volume 39
Some chemicals used in plastics and elastomers
1986; 403 pages; Sw. fr. 60.-

Volume 40
Some naturally occurring and synthetic food components, furocoumarins and ultraviolet radiation
1986; 444 pages; Sw. fr. 65.-

Volume 41
Some halogenated hydrocarbons and pesticide exposures
1986; 434 pages; Sw. fr. 65.-

Volume 42
Silica and some silicates
1987; 289 pages; Sw. fr. 65.-

*Volume 43
Man-made mineral fibres and radon
(in press)

Volume 44
Alcohol and alcoholic beverages
(in preparation)

Supplement No. 1
Chemicals and industrial processes associated with cancer in humans (IARC Monographs, Volumes 1 to 20)
1979; 71 pages; out of print

Supplement No. 2
Long-term and short-term screening assays for carcinogens: a critical appraisal
1980; 426 pages; Sw. fr. 40.-

Supplement No. 3
Cross index of synonyms and trade names in Volumes 1 to 26
1982; 199 pages; Sw. fr. 60.-

IARC MONOGRAPHS SERIES

Supplement No. 4
*Chemicals, industrial processes and industries
associated with cancer in humans (IARC Monographs,
Volumes 1 to 29)*
1982; 292 pages; Sw. fr. 60.-

Supplement No. 5
*Cross index of synonyms and trade names in
Volumes 1 to 36*
1985; 259 pages; Sw. fr. 60.-

*Supplement No. 6
*Genetic and related effects: An updating of selected
IARC Monographs from Volumes 1-42*
1987; 729 pages; Sw. fr. 80.

*Supplement No. 7
*Overall evaluations of carcinogenicity: An updating of
IARC Monographs Volumes 1-42*
1987; 440 pages; Sw. fr. 65

*From Volume 43 onwards, the series title has been changed to: IARC MONOGRAPHS ON THE EVALUATION OF
CARCINOGENIC RISKS TO HUMANS

INFORMATION BULLETINS ON THE SURVEY OF CHEMICALS BEING TESTED FOR CARCINOGENICITY

(Available from IARC and WHO Sales Agents)

No. 8 (1979)
Edited by M.-J. Ghess, H. Bartsch
& L. Tomatis
604 pages; Sw. fr. 40.-

No. 9 (1981)
Edited by M.-J. Ghess, J.D. Wilbourn,
H. Bartsch & L. Tomatis
294 pages; Sw. fr. 41.-

No. 10 (1982)
Edited by M.-J. Ghess, J.D. Wilbourn
& H. Bartsch
362 pages; Sw. fr. 42.-

No. 11 (1984)
Edited by M.-J. Ghess, J.D. Wilbourn,
H. Vainio & H. Bartsch
362 pages; Sw. fr. 50.-

No. 12 (1986)
Edited by M.-J. Ghess, J.D. Wilbourn,
A. Tossavainen & H. Vainio
385 pages; Sw. fr. 50.-

NON-SERIAL PUBLICATIONS

(Available from IARC)

ALCOOL ET CANCER
By A. Tuyns (in French only)
1978; 42 pages; Fr. fr. 35.-

CANCER MORBIDITY AND CAUSES OF
DEATH AMONG DANISH BREWERY
WORKERS
By O.M. Jensen
1980; 143 pages; Fr. fr. 75.-

DIRECTORY OF COMPUTER SYSTEMS
USED IN CANCER REGISTRIES
By H.R. Menck & D.M. Parkin
1986; 236 pages; Fr. fr. 50.-